A Clinical Guide to Applied Dental Materials

Representative values of various mechanical and physical properties of generic dental materials

	Compressive strength (MPa)	Tensile strength (MPa)	Modulus (GPa)	Hardness*	Thermal expansion (10⁻⁶/°C)	Thermal conductivity cal/s/cm/°C	Thermal diffusivity (cm²/sec)	Bond strength to enamel (MPa)	Bond strength to dentine (MPa)	Water uptake (mg/cm² at 7 days) ISO standard test	Water solubility (mg/cm²)
Tooth											
Enamel	261–288	10	46–48	272–500K	11.4	0.0022	0.0042			Negligible	Negligible
Dentine	248–305	50	12.5–16	50–70K	8.3	0.0015	0.0026			Negligible	Negligible
Filling materials											
Amalgam											
High copper amalgam	388–400	43	34	100K	23–25	0.057	1.7			Negligible	Negligible
Unicompositional amalgam	455–510	48–56	42	Similar	24–27	0.055	Similar			Negligible	Negligible
Conventional amalgam	302–366	51–58	36	Similar	23–26	0.053	Similar			Negligible	Negligible
Composite											
Microfine	230–290	22–33	3.2–6	22–36K	55–65	0.0012–0.0015	0.0015–0.0024	20	10.5–17	1.2–2.2	0.01–0.06
Hybrid	250–390	70–90	7.5–20	55–80K	25–38	0.0026–0.0030	0.0025–0.0056	24	5–20	0.4–0.8	0.01–0.06
Glass ionomer	170–280	11.5–19	9.5–18	48K	11.5–12.4	0.0018–0.0011	0.0015–0.0021	4.1–6.9	2.2–5.1		0.13–0.7
Resin modified glass ionomer	105–170	19.1–21.6	0.4	40K	20–23	0.0012–0.0008	0.0018–0.0022	5.1–9.2	10–12		
Compomer	270–349	14.8	5.1	68V	46.7	0.0022–0.0025	0.0017–0.0021	11	19.51–19.7	0.37	0.02–0.08
Fissure sealant	130–170	24–31	2.1–5.2	20–25K	71–94	0.0008	0.0015–0.0020	0–unetched	0–unetched	1.3–2.0	0.02
Cements											
Zinc Phosphate	70–160	3.1–8	13.7–22		26	0.0028	0.0029–0.0035	0	0		0.2
Zinc Polycarboxylate	57–99	3.1–17	4		28	0.0031	0.0014–0.0034	4.9–6.7	2.1		<0.05
Zinc oxide/eugenol	38–52	3.8–7.4	2.7		35	0.0011	0.0031–0.0061	0	0		0.08
Calcium hydroxide	12.3–28	1	0.4		32	x		0	0		
EBA cement	40–70	5.5–7.0	5.4		32	0.0021	0.0034–0.0054	0	0		0.065
Resin Adhesive	32–224	37–41	1.2–10.7	15–18K	60–67	x	0.0018–0.0024	15–27	8.5–30		
Metal alloys											
High noble	425–525		77	175–180	13.5	0.9–0.7	8				
Noble	650–1300		185–235	210–410V	14.8	0.17	9				
Base											
Co-Cr	530–820		186–216	210V	9.8–13	0.32	5–9.5				
Titanium	242–900		80–110	125–353V	8.4–8.6	0.052					
Ceramic											
Dental porcelain	172–356	34	69	460K	12	0.003	0.0011				
Methacrylate polymer											
Resins (PMMA)	74–80	50	2.2–3.5	15–18K	81	0.39–0.49	0.0012–0.0018			0.69	0.02

*K, Knoop; V, Vickers; B, Brinell.

A Clinical Guide to Applied Dental Materials

Stephen J. Bonsor BDS(Hons) MSc FHEA

General Dental Practitioner, Aberdeen, Scotland, UK,

Honorary Fellow, University of Edinburgh, Edinburgh, Scotland, UK,

Former Honorary Clinical Teacher, University of Dundee, Dundee, Scotland, UK

Gavin J. Pearson PhD BDS LDS

Former Professor of Biomaterials in Relation to Dentistry

Queen Mary, University of London, London, UK

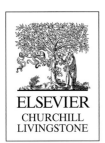

ELSEVIER
CHURCHILL
LIVINGSTONE

Amsterdam • Boston • Heidelberg • London • New York • Oxford
Paris • San Diego • San Francisco • Singapore • Sydney • Tokyo

CHURCHILL
LIVINGSTONE
ELSEVIER

ISBN 978-0-7020-3158-8
eBook ISBN 9780702046964

British Library Cataloguing-in-Publication Data
A catalogue record for this book is available from the British Library

Library of Congress Cataloging-in-Publication Data
A catalog record for this book is available from the Library of Congress

Notices
Knowledge and best practice in this field are constantly changing. As new research and experience broaden our understanding, changes in research methods, professional practices, or medical treatment may become necessary.

Practitioners and researchers must always rely on their own experience and knowledge in evaluating and using any information, methods, compounds, or experiments described herein. In using such information or methods they should be mindful of their own safety and the safety of others, including parties for whom they have a professional responsibility.

With respect to any drug or pharmaceutical products identified, readers are advised to check the most current information provided (i) on procedures featured or (ii) by the manufacturer of each product to be administered, to verify the recommended dose or formula, the method and duration of administration, and contraindications. It is the responsibility of practitioners, relying on their own experience and knowledge of their patients, to make diagnoses, to determine dosages and the best treatment for each individual patient, and to take all appropriate safety precautions.

To the fullest extent of the law, neither the Publisher nor the authors, contributors, or editors, assume any liability for any injury and/or damage to persons or property as a matter of products liability, negligence or otherwise, or from any use or operation of any methods, products, instructions, or ideas contained in the material herein.

ELSEVIER your source for books, journals and multimedia in the health sciences

www.elsevierhealth.com

Working together to grow
libraries in developing countries

www.elsevier.com | www.bookaid.org | www.sabre.org

ELSEVIER BOOK AID International Sabre Foundation

The Publisher's policy is to use paper manufactured from sustainable forests

Printed in China

Senior Content Strategist: Alison Taylor
Content Development Specialist: Lotika Singha/Carole McMurray
Project Manager: Caroline Jones
Design: Russell Purdy
Illustration Manager: Jennifer Rose
Illustrator: Robert Britton

Contents

For additional information, please visit the website www.bonsorandpearson.com

Acknowledgements

The authors wish to acknowledge the help and support given so readily and kindly by the many dental material and instrument manufacturers and companies. In particular Coltène Whaledent, Ivoclar Vivadent and W & H were especially helpful during the research and development of this book. Thanks also to those companies and individuals who gave their permission to use diagrams and photographs.

Some people must get a special and personal acknowledgement for their contribution so willingly given despite their own heavy workload: Herr Silvan Benz at Coltène Whaledent, Ing. Michael Pointner of W & H Dentalwerk Buermoos GmbH, Mr Mark Jones and Mr Michael Powell of the Ceramic Arts Dental Laboratory, Nottingham and Mr Jim Simpson at Albyn Dental Laboratory, Aberdeen. Thank you too to the many representatives of the dental companies for supplying information and products to play with and photograph. There are too many people to mention but you will know who you are!

Thanks also go to Miss Suzy Peters and Miss Sarah Styles, dental nurses, for their help in the production of many of the clinical photographs.

The authors owe a huge debt of gratitude to Dr R Graham Chadwick for proofreading the entire manuscript, to Dr Sarah Manton for reviewing the chapter on Preventive and periodontal materials, implants and biomaterials, Mr Charles Meadows of W & H (UK) for commenting on the handpiece section in the cutting instruments chapter and to Mr John Maloney, Optident for his input on the bleaching chapter. Thank you also to Professor Trevor Burke for contributing the foreword and to the Elsevier team for their help during the genesis of the text.

Lastly, to our wives Lindsay and Margaret for patiently putting up with our absences from home during the research phase and for their support and encouragement during the many evenings, (late) nights and weekends spent writing.

FIGURE CREDITS

The illustrations listed below have been reproduced or adapted with permission from the following publications/organizations/individuals:

3M ESPE: 1.3A, 1.4A, 19.37A, 22.30, 22.31A, 22.32A

Mount GJ, Hume WR. Preservation and Restoration of Tooth Structure, 2nd edition, Knowledge Books and Software, Brisbane, Australia, 2005: 7.26

American Medical Technologies and PrepStart H2O Danville Engineering: 19.33A

Blackwell Supplies: 17.25

BP: 1.1

Colgate: 17.26

Coltène Whaledent: 7.3

DenMed Technologies: 2.17A

Dental Update: 4.1A, 7.21A, 7.22, 7.23, 11.20

Dr D Nisand, Paris (Straumann) 17.28A

Dux Dental 15.13A

Elementist.com esweb 13.3

Frank Mikley 16.2A

Barry TI, Clinton DJ, Wilson AD. The structure of a glass-ionomer cement and its relationship to the setting process. Journal of Dental Research 1979; 58:1072–1079: 9.1

Prosser HJ, Wilson AD. Zinc oxide eugenol cements. VI. Effect of zinc oxide type on the setting reactions. Journal of Biomedical Materials Research 1982; 16:585–598: 12.3A

Wilson AD, Clinton DJ, Miller RP. Zinc oxide–eugenol cements IV. Microstructure and hydrolysis. Journal of Dental Research 1973; 52: 253–260: 12.12

GC 17.22B

Brunner TJ, Grass RN, Stark WJ. Glass and bioactive glass nanopowders by flame synthesis. Chemistry and Applied Biosciences, ETH Zurich, Zurich, 8093, Switzerland, (http://aiche.confex.com/aiche/2006/techprogram/P59557.HTM): 17.30A

http://www.rtmat.com/start_en.htm: 17.32

Ivoclar Vivadent: 2.18B, 17.19A, 17.20, 17.22A, 18.3, 23.13A

KaVo: 19.34A, 19.35, 19.41A

Mineraly a horniny Slovenska (http://www.mineraly.sk/): 15.15

MNF Petroleum: 16.4A

Méndez-Vilas A, Díaz J (eds) Modern Research and Educational Topics in Microscopy: 21.2A

Mr Richard Buckle: 11.27

National Institute of Science and Technology: 4.17C

Panadent: 2.12

Hargreaves KM, Cohen S. Pathways to the Pulp, edition. Mosby: 13.11

Peninsula Business Services: 3.4

Prestige Dental: 14.28

Rob Lavinsky: 22.23

Robert Gougaloff Wikopedia: 17.37

Technicare: 17.29A

The Seaweed Site (http://www.seaweed.ie/): 15.14A

University of Sheffield: 3.3

Valplast: 23.17A

Vita Fabrik: 22.7, 22.8A, 22.11A, Box Figure 22.1A

Voco and Kuraray: 17.21A

W&H: 19.1, 19.4, 19.5, 19.6, 19.8A–C, 19.10, 19.13, 19.16, 19.17, 19.18, 19.19, 19.20, 19.21

Wikimedia: 21.2B

Wilcopedia: 16.1A

Wilkopedia: 22.3A

Zwick: 4.3A

Foreword

It may be considered that Dental Materials Science is the foundation upon which restorative dentistry is built, this tenet being true for the dental student, general dental practitioner and specialist alike. Get the material wrong for a given clinical situation, and there is a lessened chance that the subsequent restoration will perform optimally in terms of, for example, its appearance, its structural adequacy and/or its protection of the vital tooth tissues, dentine and pulp. Forty years ago, the choices available to the clinician were small – amalgam, early composite, silicate cement, gold and elementary ceramics. Today, the choice is vast, with the number of dentine bonding agents currently available worldwide approaching three figures. It is therefore a bonus that this book is written by a practising clinician and by one of the UK's best dentist/scientists, thereby contributing a broad range of expertise from the authors. In this regard, areas of best clinical practice are marked with a good practice tick.

Today's buzz word in dental research is 'translational research', broadly meaning, the translation of laboratory research on a material or technique into research into the performance of that material or technique in the clinical setting. This book, very effectively, does this for dental materials, translating their performance into clinical relevance. As such, it fills a gap in the market and it should be essential reading for students and more experienced clinicians. For example, it translates the relevance of sell-by date into efficient surgery stock control, also stressing the fact that the directions for use should not be discarded when the pack is opened! It explains the significance of the various test methodologies, adding that some of these must not be extrapolated into clinical performance and also pointing out that graphs may provide misleading data by altering the scales on the graphs

The text is incredibly broad in its coverage of dental materials. Amalgam, resin-based materials, glass ionomer, alloys and impression materials might be what the reader might expect, but there are extensive sections on endodontic materials, materials for temporisation, preventive and periodontal materials, implants, bleaching systems, and cutting instruments. The increasing impact of aesthetic dentistry is reflected by sections on bleaching and on the state of the art ceramics available to the contemporary dental profession.

In summary, *A Clinical Guide to Applied Dental Materials* is a comprehensive resource for dental students and practising dentists alike, presenting, as it does, a blend of science and the clinical application of dental materials. In an area complicated by the views of self-appointed opinion-leaders who present their convincing anecdotal views, this book presents a refreshing, scientific, comprehensive, evidence-based approach to dental materials and their clinical applications. It is therefore an important text for those who wish to achieve clinical excellence.

FJT Burke   DDS, MSc, MDS, FDS MGDS (RCS Edin.), FDS RCS (Eng.), FFGDP, FADM

Professor of Primary Dental Care, University of Birmingham, UK.

SCOPE OF THE BOOK AND BACKGROUND

The teaching of dental materials at undergraduate level has traditionally been provided prior to students' first contact with patients or at an early stage thereafter. Unfortunately, these courses have been perceived by students as abstract and irrelevant as their emphasis is often not practically based, with little detail provided on the clinical manipulation and usage of dental materials. The result is that students feel they cannot appreciate the relationship of the (essential) subject matter with its clinical application and their interest in materials quickly wanes.

This book aims to bridge this gap between the knowledge gained in the basic dental materials science course and the clinical restorative disciplines. Written by a practising dentist with academic experience and an academic in biomaterials with extensive clinical experience, the preparation of this text has been uniquely approached from two perspectives, with the emphasis being very much on the practical aspects of dental materials' use. It is not intended to serve as a definitive dental materials or restorative dentistry text, and the reader is referred to appropriate texts throughout the book for more theoretical background information. This text attempts to give the reader a thorough understanding of the dental materials they are using clinically: how to properly select a given material for any given situation, how they can use them to best effect and, how not to use them! It is also important to consider the impact on the performance of dental materials in the mouth, an often hostile environment filled with microorganisms, bacteria, acids and saliva. It has been said that the oral cavity is a far more hostile environment in which materials are expected to survive when compared to those used in North Sea oil exploration. All of these factors are critical for clinical success and good patient care.

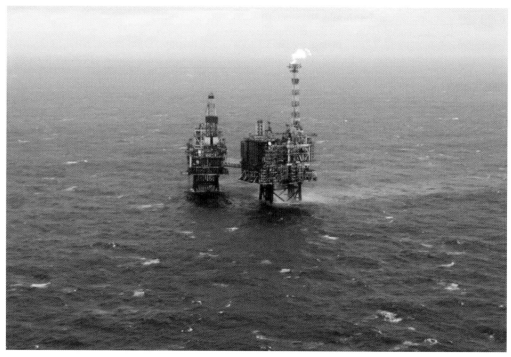

The environment in the mouth can be more corrosive to dental materials than the North Sea is to oil platforms.
Photograph courtesy of BP.

As well as undergraduate students providing care for patients, postgraduate students will also find this book of use when preparing for examinations in subjects allied to clinical dentistry. Practising dentists will find the information containing in the book invaluable and very relevant to their daily work by enhancing their understanding of the materials they are handling and developing their decision-making skills. The dental team (nurses, hygienists, therapists and technicians) will benefit from the many practical tips contained within the text and be able to relate it to their daily work. This book will also be of interest to dental manufacturers and retailers as it provides an overview of many of the dental materials currently commercially available (and from a dentist's perspective,) not to mention the principles and applications which underpin them.

HOW TO USE THIS BOOK

The text systematically deals with the commonly available dental materials and equipment. While the reader could work their way through the chapters, it could also be used to "dip in" to a particular section as each chapter dealing with a family of materials stands alone and appropriate cross-references are provided where relevant. The first section deals with many important points and principles which are common to many materials and underpin their handling and behaviour. It includes a chapter which discusses the usage of materials with special reference to general dental practice. Thereafter the text visits all the material families with the second section dealing with materials which are generally directly placed and includes a chapter on materials and equipment used in endodontics. The third section introduces materials which are used in conjunction with indirect techniques, namely temporization, impression materials, and bite registration materials and waxes. The fourth section is concerned with other materials used in the dental clinic, namely preventive and periodontal materials, biomaterials, dental implants, bleaching systems and cutting instruments. The last section covers those materials more commonly seen in a dental laboratory, but which the practitioner needs to be familiar with to prescribe effectively and when discussing cases with their technical colleagues.

Important practical aspects of each material are presented in boxes to highlight them:

- The boxes with a 'tick' include **good practice** tips.
- The boxes with an 'exclamation mark' provide information about a **potential interaction or problem or precautions** to be taken while using a material.

The text contains more details and knowledge underpinning the highlighted points where relevant. Important words and terms are either given in bold and defined within the text or they are defined in boxes following the text where the term has been used. The concise definitions will be a useful aide memoire during examination preparation. This also includes technical terms, which are introduced as necessary throughout the text. By using this approach these terms are illustrated in context and build the reader's understanding in a gradual and relevant manner.

In an attempt to bridge the knowledge gap between the generic and the proprietary names, trade names used within the European Union have been used throughout the text. However, the same material may be referred to by an alternative name in other parts of the world. It is possible that some products with the same name may in fact differ in composition in different countries because of local legislation. Readers outside the European Union should contact the manufacturer for questions about the availability of a particular product in their country. To facilitate this, the contact details of each manufacturer mentioned in this text is available online at www.bonsorandpearson.com.

Each chapter ends with a series of self-assessment questions. These are designed to evaluate the readers' understanding and application of knowledge gained within the chapter by posing 'real-life' clinical problems. Completion of this section will enhance knowledge and consolidate understanding. Answers to the questions are provided online at www.bonsorandpearson.com.

For the convenience of the reader, 'Basic dental terminology' appears on the inside front cover of this book , a table containing information on 'Representative values of various mechanical and physical properties of generic dental materials ' is available on prelim page ii and 'Regulation of dental materials and the ISO' appears on the inside back cover.

The commercial products featured do not imply any recommendation or endorsement by the authors and are included to either illustrate a point or as an example of a particular material. The commercial products tables are not exhaustive and list only examples of products. It is important to stress that neither the Publisher nor the Authors assume any responsibility for any loss or injury and/or damage to persons or property arising out of or related to any use of the material contained in this book. It is the responsibility of the treating practitioner, relying on independent expertise and knowledge of the patient, to determine the best treatment and method of application for the patient.

While much care has been taken to ensure every fact contained in this text is evidence based, no references are provided. This has been done deliberately so as not to detract from the practical, user-friendly approach of the book. However, a list of standard dental material texts or review research papers is given in each chapter for readers requiring further material to complement their knowledge.

With new materials being constantly introduced to the market, this book may, by definition, become quickly dated. Every effort has been taken to ensure that all information contained in it is correct at the time of going to press. However, the principles and applications described here provide a blueprint by which new materials can be evaluated such that the practitioner can determine whether the manufacturer's claims can be justified. These precepts should remain good for some time to come. It is a requirement of each practising dentist to ensure that their knowledge keeps pace with this change as, medicolegally, they are responsible for the dental materials used in the course of their work including the prostheses made for them by independent contractors. It is hoped that with a better appreciation of applied dental materials, the reader's interest will be stimulated and that they will extrapolate their increased understanding and knowledge to practise with increased satisfaction and more effectively to the betterment of their patients.

SB, Aberdeen
GP, London

Section | I |

General principles

Dental materials in the oral environment

INTRODUCTION

Perhaps surprisingly, when considering their diversity, the materials that are used across the various branches of dentistry have much in common. They are conceived, developed, tested, manufactured and marketed in the same way by only a small group of dental material manufacturing companies. When they arrive in the clinic, they are kept in the same storeroom. When required for use, they are mixed and manipulated by the dental team in similar ways as they are available in only a small number of presentations. Unfortunately, incorrect handling during this phase could compromise their properties on subsequent placement into the mouth and in some cases they may be ruined. Dental materials may set chemically, or the setting may be initiated by light energy, or a combination of both. They are subjected to the hostile environment which is the human mouth, where they are asked to endure similar stresses and strains during function. With all things being equal their lifespan does not vary significantly either. The first section of this book, consisting of five chapters, discusses these general principles and the commonalities between the different material groups.

This chapter describes the oral environment into which a material is placed. Failure of the clinician to understand the conditions in which a material is expected to perform may lead to incorrect material selection – which will surely compromise clinical success. The way in which the material is presented and handled by chairside dental staff will influence its properties. In order to minimize

operator error, manufacturers have developed less technique-sensitive presentations. Chapter 2 examines how the dental team may influence success by considering clinical factors such as the importance of moisture control when using materials which may be damaged by exposure to water prior to their complete setting. The invention and extensive use in modern dentistry of setting dental materials by exposure to light energy extends across material types. However, this useful technique has the potential to be compromised by various factors and the dentist must be aware of the potential pitfalls.

It is an important criterion that it is undesirable for any dental material to interact with the host, i.e. dental patient. Chapters 3 and 4 deal with the biological considerations of dental materials and how potential interactions may be minimized by the manufacturers and dental team. Clearly all materials must be fit for purpose and conform to various safety, legal and quality standards.

Prior to their launch to market, all dental materials are tested extensively. It is desirable that the end user (the dentist) understands which laboratory tests each material has been subjected to and how relevant this may be clinically. Often promotional and technical literature may be difficult to interpret, yet it is vital that the dentist is equipped to understand this information. By understanding why certain chemicals are contained in the materials it may be possible to make an educated assessment as to how the material is likely to behave with respect to handling and function. This will enable the clinician to make informed decisions as to whether a particular material is suitable for a given situation. Lastly, Chapter 5 describes how materials may be stored and managed in a clinic or dental practice prior to use. Storage in the correct manner will ensure that the material reaches the dentist in optimum condition.

THE HOSTILE ORAL ENVIRONMENT

When dental materials are placed in the mouth, they enter a very hostile environment. In fact, they are asked to perform and survive in conditions more extreme than those found on the oil platforms in the North Sea. There are numerous microorganisms in the oral cavity, and many bacteria produce acids as a by-product of their metabolism. This has the effect of lowering the intraoral pH. Ingested foodstuffs and liquids can also rapidly change the pH of the mouth, swinging between mildly alkaline and strongly acid. Saliva plays a role as a protective fluid barrier by acting as a buffer. However, some of the constituents of saliva such as acids and organic fluids can cause degradation of the dental restoration with time by reacting with it chemically.

During function, restorative materials may well be subjected to intermittent loading and unloading. This is **cyclical loading**. The material will have to resist this mechanical loading, the magnitude and direction of which contributes to stresses and strains within the material and the tooth structure supporting it. Furthermore, the material may be subjected to a variety of fluids at varying temperatures during the course of a day ranging from freezing to 60°C. This is called **thermal cycling**.

> **pH:** stands for the **p**ower of the **H**ydrogen ion and is a measure of the acidity or basicity of a solution. It ranges from 0.1 (highly acid) to 14 (highly alkaline), with pH 7 being neutral.
> **Buffer solution:** an aqueous solution in which the change in pH of the solution is limited when a small amount of acid or base is added to it. Buffer solutions are used as a means of maintaining pH at a nearly constant value.
> **(Dental) restoration:** a form composed of a dental material designed to restore both form and function of dental hard tissue.
> **Stress:** measure of the intensity or internal distribution of the total internal forces acting within a deformable body. Stress is measured in N/m^2 (newtons/metre^2).
> **Strain:** the change in the dimension of a material per unit length when an external force is applied to it.

The combination of these chemical, mechanical and thermal challenges is often synergistic. It is therefore obvious that over long periods of clinical use, the effects of these challenges will profoundly influence a material's behaviour and therefore a restoration's performance and longevity.

The influence of the presentation of materials on success

Unfortunately the harsh oral environment is not the only hazard which can influence material performance. In many cases, the material may not be supplied in a controlled and metered form by the manufacturer.

Instead the dental nurse or dentist must mix the components supplied by the manufacturer just prior to the placement of the material in the mouth. This means that the manufacturer may have only a limited influence over the final state of the material being used clinically. This is problematic as failure to correctly manipulate the constituents can have a major influence in the failure of the material to perform as expected. This potential for error by the end user (i.e. dental team) is very high. To minimize these types of error and maximize clinical success, dental material manufacturers have evolved a range of material presentations to minimize the risk of mishandling. An example of this is the reduction in the use of powder and liquid formulations in favour of ready-mixed pastes which only require to be light cured. These presentations optimize both the proportioning of the ingredients and the mixing of the materials.

Powder and liquid presentations

As the name suggests, these materials, usually cements, are provided as components which the user must mix and place at the site of use. This presents a number of problems. Firstly, the proportions of each component should ideally be similar as it is often difficult to mix a much smaller volume of one with a large volume of the second and still ensure even distribution of the two components. Secondly, the components need to be dispensed in a manner that ensures that the correct proportion of each component is metered out. It is also important that the proportions do not require too much precision as the dispensation process in the clinic is fraught with problems.

Dispensation of powder is subject to considerable variability. During storage, undisturbed powder in a bottle or tub for a period of time will settle and compact. It is important that the powder is **fluffed** by shaking the container so that the correct amount of powder is dispensed. Failure to do this will mean that more powder is dispensed thus affecting the powder to liquid ratio.

Always shake the bottle or tub before dispensing the powder (Figure 1.1). This fluffs the powder so that the correct amount is dispensed and mixes the contents thoroughly as these materials frequently contain mixtures of different powder compositions.

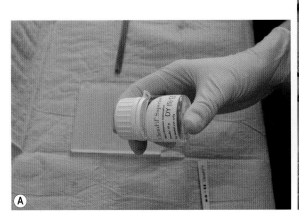
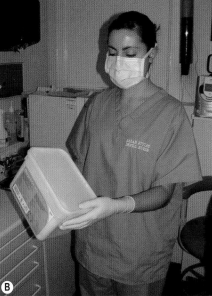

Fig. 1.1A,B A bottle of glass ionomer cement (ChemFil Superior, Dentsply) and a tub of alginate impression material (Blueprint, Dentsply) being shaken by the dental nurse to ensure the correct dispensation of the powder.

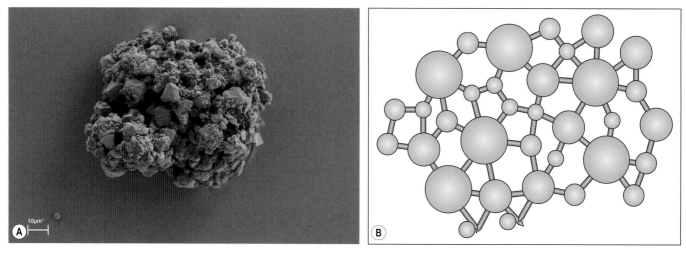

Fig. 1.2A,B A scanning electron micrograph and pictorial representation of a conventional glass ionomer powder. This illustrates the considerable range in particle sizes present in a cement. This can influence the rate of set of the material.

Fig. 1.3 A scanning electron micrograph and pictorial representation of a granular glass ionomer powder.

Powder versus granules

The ease with which the solute dissolves affects the rate of reaction. Generally, speaking dental cements are presented in either powder, or in the case of newer materials, granular form. A **powder** (Figure 1.2) is a fine precipitate produced by grinding or milling small particles. The finer the particle the more rapid the initiation of the chemical reaction as the surface area to volume ratio increases. **Granules** are larger agglomerates of semi-fused particles with a porous structure (Figure 1.3), which facilitates the permeability of a liquid into the agglomerated mass and the surface area available is greater for reaction. This is a similar presentation to the popular coffee granules found in some instant coffees. Figure 1.4 shows the granular and powered presentations of instant coffee. The granular variety was introduced to improve the rapidity with which the coffee may dissolve when hot water is added to it.

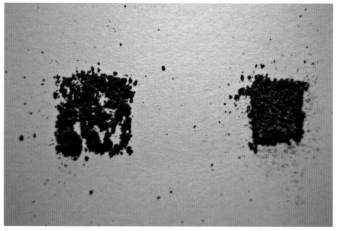

Fig. 1.4 The coffee powder on the left has a granular presentation whilst the other is ground (powdered) coffee. Note the difference in appearance of the two samples.

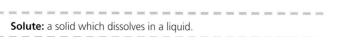

Solute: a solid which dissolves in a liquid.

Rate of reaction

When mixing the ingredients it is important to realize that as soon as the constituents are bought together then the setting reaction commences. Many manufacturers incorporate a **retarder** into the solute to prevent the setting phase commencing immediately so slowing the reaction initially. This has the effect of increasing the working time but there is still a fixed amount of time during which mixing and placement of the material can take place. Once this time has been exceeded, the setting phase will commence (Figure 1.5).

It is desirable to have a long working time and short setting time but this is not possible because once the chemical reaction has been initiated the setting reaction accelerates until the reactive components are exhausted.

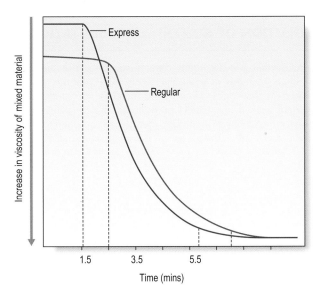

Fig. 1.5 The change in viscosity of two cements. At the beginning of mixing, the viscosity of the paste is low. This viscosity remains the same for 1.5 minutes with the express set material and 2.25 minutes for the regular cement. After this time the cement begins to set and thicken and the viscosity decreases. Once the cement has set the viscosity is the same again.

Working time: the time between the commencement of mix and the first indication of setting.
Setting time: the time from the commencement of mixing to the time at which the material has set clinically.

Effect of temperature and humidity

The temperature and humidity of the clinic or laboratory during the mixing and setting phases will influence the rate of reaction. In general any increase in temperature above ambient will lead to an acceleration of the setting reaction. This can have considerable significance in a clinic which does not have a controlled temperature. On a cold day the material will have a longer working time while on a hot and humid day the material will begin to set prematurely. It is often advisable to store susceptible materials in a refrigerator, the effect of which will be to increase mixing and working time. However, this can create problems. Water-based cements have an optimum level of water to achieve their best performance. If the

slab on which they are mixed is cooled to a temperature which is below the dew point (Figure 1.6), once the slab is back at room temperature, condensation of water from the atmosphere will lead to beads of moisture on the surface which will then be incorporated into the mix, thus reducing the powder to liquid ratio and producing a weakened cement. This can be overcome by using paper mixing pads. However, these pads are unsuitable for mixing of stiff (highly viscous) acid-base cements as the paper curls at the edges as the material is spatulated.

> **!**
>
> It is important to remember that the temperature of the oral cavity is generally between 10 and 14°C above that of the clinic. Once a material is placed in the mouth the setting rate will be increased substantially.

Dew point: the temperature that air must be cooled for water vapour to condense into water.
Viscosity: the resistance of a liquid to flow

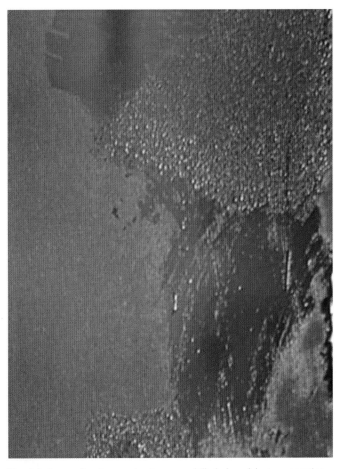

Fig. 1.6 Drops of water condensing on a chilled glass slab. Incorporation of this water into a powder/liquid mix will alter the ratio, so affecting the final properties of the cement.

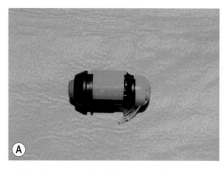
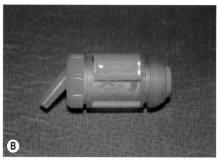

Fig. 1.7A,B Examples of capsules, the one on the left is manufactured by 3M ESPE and contains resin-modified glass ionomer cement (Photacfil) and the other is ChemFil Supreme (Dentsply), a glass ionomer cement. Note the black plastic of the Photacfil capsule protects the constituents from ambient light as this material is light activated.

Clinical implications of the setting phase

To achieve the optimal properties of the material, it should not be disturbed during the setting phase. Manipulation of the material during this phase will have long-term deleterious consequences. Restorative materials must be maintained in a steady state during the period between the end of the working time and the completion of set. Failure to do this will lead to the material being stressed and weakened so impairing its clinical performance and longevity. For example, in the case of elastomeric impression materials (such as silicone rubbers, see Chapter 15), if they are disturbed during the cross-linking phase, they will stress relax on removal from the mouth. This leads to distortion resulting in the cast restoration failing to fit. The impression tray should be evenly supported during the setting phase. The reliance on the patient to support the tray or leaving the tray unsupported is likely to lead to deformation of the impression.

> **Elastomer:** a material which has elastic properties, allowing it to recover to its original shape after distortion.
> **Cross-linking:** covalent or ionic bonds that link one polymer chain to another to form a solid structure.
> **Stress relaxation:** the phenomenon of a material under stress to return to its unstressed original form once any restraint is removed.
> **Impression material:** a material used to record the shape of the structure in the mouth so that a model may be constructed.
> **Impression tray:** A prefabricated U-shaped carrying device which supports the fluid impression material (see Chapter 15).
> **Cast restoration:** restoration produced external to the mouth and cemented into place.

EVOLUTION OF MATERIAL PRESENTATIONS

The traditional powder/liquid cement system is the presentation most likely to result in most significant user variability as already discussed. If the components of the material can be delivered to the dental team in the correct proportions and in such a way that minimal or no mixing is required, then the risk of operator-induced variability can be reduced or even largely eliminated. A number of currently available presentations address these problems, namely:

- Capsules
- Compules
- Automated paste/paste delivery systems.

Encapsulation

A **capsule** is a container that holds the active ingredients of a material in separate compartments until activation. It then becomes the mixing chamber (Figure 1.7). The activated capsule is then placed into a mechanical mixing machine to blend the components of the material together. Manufacturers have designed capsules that allow powders and liquids to be mixed in the correct proportions to achieve the desired mix and consistency. Figure 1.8 shows the design of a capsule and its contents.

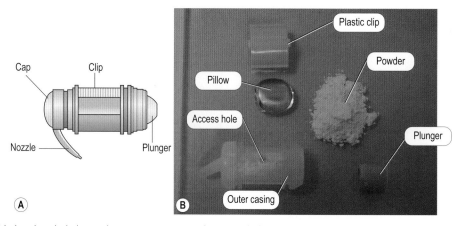

Fig. 1.8A,B The assembled and exploded capsule components. Note the access hole to the main chamber and the pillow which lies over this. The grey cylinder which lies over the end acts a plunger, forcing the cement out through the nozzle after mixing is complete.

Most capsules consist of a chamber with a nozzle at one end through which the mixed material may be extruded. The chamber, internally, is a rounded cylinder with a small hole either on one side or at one end. The powder is stored in this central chamber. Over the small hole lies an aluminium pillow which contains the liquid. This pillow is covered by a plastic clip. When pressure is applied to the plastic clip, this ruptures the pillow and the liquid is expelled into the chamber containing the metered amount of powder. Alternative systems have the liquid in a pillow at the opposite end from the nozzle and are activated by a half turn of the bung.

Some encapsulated glass ionomer cements require the capsule bung to be twisted through 180° prior to syringing. Failure to do this will result in no material being dispensed from the capsule as the nozzle is occluded forcing the outer casing of the capsule apart (Figure 1.9).

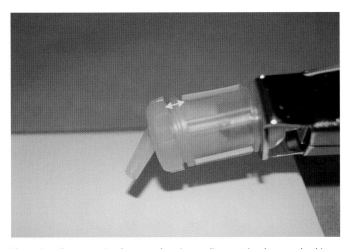

Fig. 1.9 Failure to twist the capsule prior to dispensation has resulted in no material being expressed from the capsule and the capsule rupturing under the pressure being applied to it by the syringe driver.

When using capsules containing ingredients for a cement or restorative which require activation, the dental nurse should ensure that pressure is applied to the clip for a period of time long enough to expel all the liquid into the chamber. The liquid is frequently rather viscous and a minimum time for pressure to be applied is 2 seconds (Figure 1.10). Failure to expel all the liquid will adversely affect the powder to liquid ratio and may lead to difficulties in expelling the mixed material through the syringe nozzle.

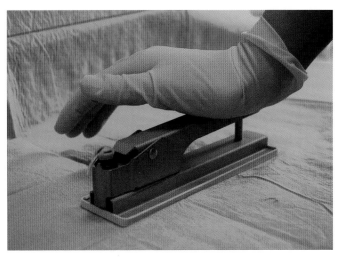

Fig. 1.10 Pressure being applied to the activator device for 2 seconds so that all of the liquid is expressed from the pillow into the mixing chamber.

The powder in capsules will compact on storage with the compacted powder settling at the end of the capsule near the exit nozzle. It is therefore important to always shake the capsule prior to use. Failure to do so will result in a puff of unmixed powder being expressed first, which may interfere with clinical placement.

Once the powder and liquid are in the mixing chamber, the capsule is placed in a mechanical mixer. This machine agitates the capsule for a fixed period of time as recommended by the manufacturer and the mixed material is then extruded into the cavity. Dental amalgam is presented in capsules but in this case the capsule is used solely for mixing the alloy powder and mercury. The mercury is stored in a pillow which is within the body of the capsule. This is ruptures by the movement of the high density mercury once mixing commences. Once mixed, the material is placed in a dispensing dish to be picked up and inserted into the cavity using an amalgam gun.

Amalgam gun: a carrier device used to inject unset amalgam into the cavity.

Mechanical mixers

Mechanical mixers (Figure 1.11) operate either by **rotational** or an **oscillating figure of eight** movement of the capsule. The speed is variable and each machine should be provided with mixing times for each encapsulated material. The reason for this is the **throw** of the mixing arm of each manufacturer varies as does the **speed of oscillation**. This imparts a different amount of energy during the mixing process. The movement of the powder and liquid within the capsule allows the surfaces of the particles to be wetted and the chemical reaction to commence. The movement of the mass within the mixing chamber generates heat, the amount being dependent on the mass of the components involved. At the end of mixing a paste of uniform consistency should be obtained.

Wetting: the ability of a liquid to maintain contact with a solid surface due to intermolecular interactions when they are in close proximity.

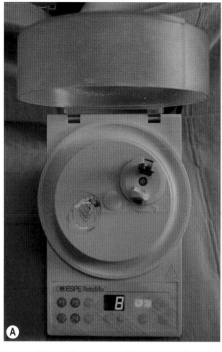
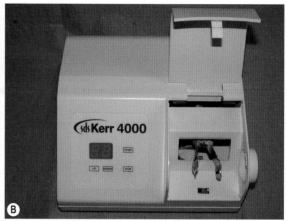

Fig. 1.11 (A) A mixing machine with a rotary mixing motion (3M ESPE Rotomix) and (B) another mixing machine that utilizes a figure-of-eight motion (SDS Kerr 4000).

Limitation of capsules

Even though the proportioning of the components is carried out by the manufacturer under standardized conditions, it is difficult to provide a metered dose precisely. This is because the powders are usually delivered by a hopper and there is some variation in the amount dispensed as the hopper empties. The filling of the pillow has a similar problem as the metering of small volumes of liquid produces some variation. Variations in the portioning of either the powder or liquid will affect the power/liquid ratio and therefore the properties of the mixed material.

The most significant disadvantage of capsule mixes is in those cases where the material is injected via a nozzle to the site. Here the diameter of the orifice of the nozzle will influence the powder to liquid ratio. Too high a powder to liquid ratio will make the material difficult to extrude via a small nozzle which may indeed be the most appropriate for delivery.

It is important that the correct mixing time is adhered to. Too short a time will lead to an incoherent mass with the powder and liquid inadequately mixed. Too long a mixing time will reduce working time and accelerate set.

Compules

A compule is a small cylindrical container with a delivery tip and plunger. They are also sometimes referred to by some manufacturers as **tips** or **Cavifils**™ (Ivoclar Vivadent). An example of a product presented in compule form is shown in Figure 1.12. Compules have been designed to deliver materials where all the active ingredients have already been mixed together by the manufacturer into an injectable paste. This reduces the risk of incorrect mixing and produces a material almost free of air voids. As such those materials suitable for use in compules are limited to polymer systems activated by light.

Polymer: large molecule composed of repeating structural units typically connected by covalent chemical bonds.

During the manufacturing process the material is loaded into the compule chamber in paste form and then a plastic plunger is inserted on top and driven down a fixed distance (Figure 1.13). The process is

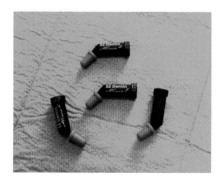

Fig. 1.12 Compules containing a resin-based composite (Miris 2, Coltène Whaledent).

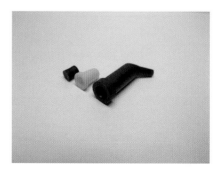

Fig. 1.13 A dismantled compule demonstrating its components.

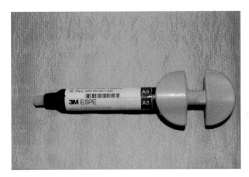

Fig. 1.14 Two compules with different nozzle sizes. The wider one permits the extrusion of a regular viscosity resin composite material (Miris 2, Coltène Whaledent) and the narrower one a flowable resin composite material (X-Flow, Dentsply).

Fig. 1.15 P60 (3M ESPE), a packable resin composite material, is so viscous, it is only supplied in the syringe form. Note the wide bore size.

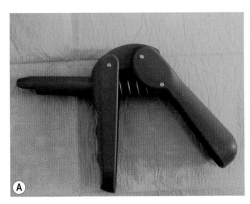

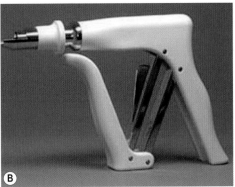

Fig. 1.16A,B Two examples of guns used to express material from compules: (A) single lever delivery gun (B) gun configured to permit plunger to be delivered centally on capsule plunger.

usually carried out in an environment illuminated by amber lights so the material will not be set prematurely. This ensures that the material is packed firmly into the base of the compule and up to the nozzle. The cap covering the nozzle is then placed. The light-resistant material forming the compule walls provides protection from ambient light so preventing premature polymerization. Dispensation is achieved by inserting the compule into a gun which is designed to drive the plunger further into the compule chamber, extruding the material via the nozzle for direct placement into the cavity being restored. The nozzle diameter varies with the viscosity of the material, the thicker the paste the wider the nozzle (Figure 1.14).

Some materials are so viscous that they cannot be delivered from compules but are only supplied in a syringe presentation, e.g. P60 (3M ESPE) (Figure 1.15). The use of a syringe can result in the material being affected by the ambient clinic lighting as the material is not delivered directly to the cavity.

The compule is placed into a gun for ease of delivery and Figure 1.16 illustrates two examples from the range of guns available. Most work on the single lever delivery of the plunger. This can result in the plunger not passing horizontally down the internal surface of the compule so an erratic injection rate occurs. To overcome this shortcoming, another more sophisticated form of gun is available whose plunger is driven down the barrel of the compule centrally and evenly.

After the paste has been injected into the cavity, it is activated by an external energy source such as a light polymerizing unit. The mechanism of light curing is explained in detail in Chapter 2.

Limitations of compules

Compules are considered to be a **unit dose** and should not be reused. This means that inevitably some material is wasted, as not all

of the material will be required to fill the cavity. Similarly there may be a small volume of the material that cannot be expelled out of the compule tip. This is reduced to a minimum by the conical shape of the plunger which will push the bulk of the material into the nozzle. However, the remaining amount is very small in comparison with the amount frequently wasted when materials are dispensed from a syringe and left unused on a mixing pad.

Automated paste/paste delivery systems

Where it is not possible to put all the active ingredients together in one paste, alternative systems have been developed (Figure 1.17). Here, the

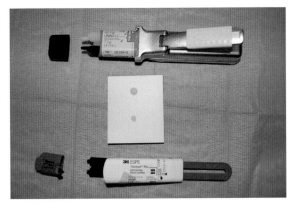

Fig. 1.17 Two automated paste/paste delivery systems. 3M ESPE's Clicker™ system (illustrated by Vitrebond Plus) and GC's Paste Pak Dispenser (illustrated by Fuji Lining LC).

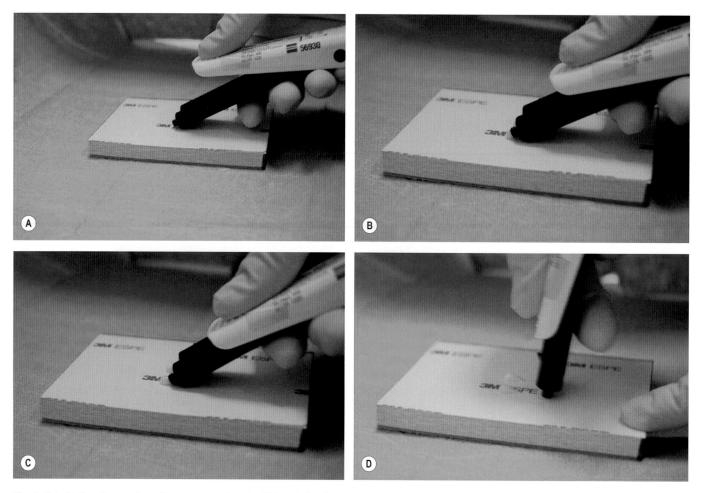

Fig. 1.18A–D The dispensation of two pastes using the Clicker device dispenser (3M ESPE): the pastes are released as the Clicker lever is depressed. Full depression of the lever ends the delivery.

two pastes are presented in **double barrel syringes** and by applying force to a lever, unit doses of the two pastes may be dispensed onto a mixing pad for manual mixing. The advantage of this delivery presentation is that the pastes are delivered in the correct proportions to one another and it obviates the proportion estimation carried out by the dental nurse from two individual tubes. A more accurate mix is therefore achieved (Figure 1.18). Different material types are now available in this presentation (Figure 1.19).

Cartridges

A subgroup of automated paste/paste delivery systems consists of cartridges. Their main indication is for mixing two semi-viscous pastes where a larger volume is required, such as impression materials or materials specifically designed for temporary replacement of tooth structure removed during crown preparation. Cartridges are designed to permit two pastes to be mixed in ratios of 1:1 up to 1:10 (Figure 1.20). A spiral delivery tube is needed to mix the material (Figure 1.21). The number of helical turns depends on the material's viscosity. The more viscous the material, the fewer helical turns are available to thoroughly blend the two pastes together. The two constituent pastes are injected down the spiral and slowly blend together allowing the mixed paste to be extruded at the site of use. A larger-scale variant of this design is the

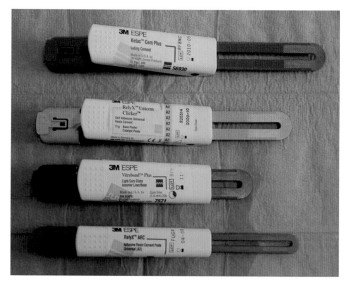

Fig. 1.19 Four different materials presented in 3M ESPE's Clicker™ delivery system. From top to bottom, a resin-modified glass ionomer luting cement, self-etching dual-cured resin composite, a resin-modified glass ionomer lining cement and a dual-cured resin composite adhesive.

mechanical impression material mixer which dispenses the material directly into an impression tray (Figure 1.22).

As has been discussed earlier, the mouth is a hostile environment in which materials are asked to survive. For a material to perform satisfactorily in this environment, its properties must be optimized. In order to achieve this, modern presentations of materials provide a means of standardizing proportions of constituents and quality of mixing. This overcomes the variability associated with hand-mixing and proportioning, which was commonplace previously. However, as will become apparent in the following chapters, there are other variables that impact on a material during use and which may have significantly detrimental effects on the performance of dental materials.

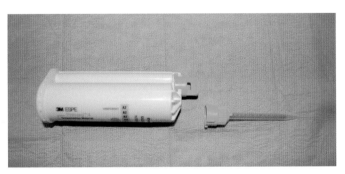

Fig. 1.20 A cartridge mixing system (Protemp 4, 3M ESPE). The difference in the ratio of paste and catalyst is determined by the differing size of the two tubes. In this case the ratio of the two pastes is 4:1.

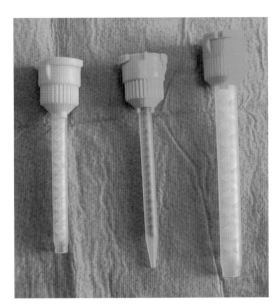

Fig. 1.21 Three mixing and delivery nozzles with different diameters. Note the difference in numbers of turns in the helix. The smaller the number, the more viscous the material.

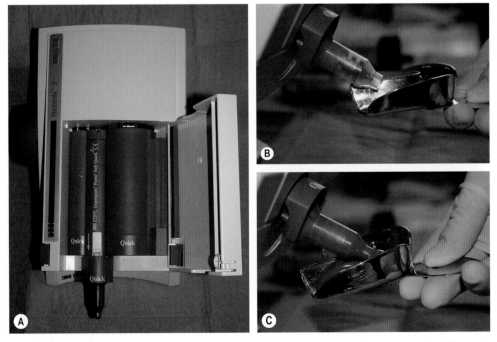

Fig. 1.22A–C Pentamix 3 (3M ESPE) impression material dispensing machine. (A) The two reservoirs of pastes: note the different sizes as the proportions are 4:1. (B) The material is being mixed in the helix of the mixing nozzle. (C) The material is being expressed into the impression tray.

SUMMARY

- The mouth is an extremely hostile environment.
- Materials need to be optimized to achieve the appropriate properties.
- Presentations are now designed to deliver materials as closely matched in performance to that tested in the manufacturers' laboratories to minimize operator mishandling.

SELF-ASSESSMENT QUESTIONS

1. What environmental factors found in the mouth will affect the performance of a dental restorative material?
2. What are the problems with presenting materials in a powder/liquid form for hand mixing?
3. What are the advantages of using pre-dispensed materials in the clinic? Are there any disadvantages?
4. What factors should be considered in establishing the clinic environment?

Chapter | 2 |

Clinical manipulation of materials

LEARNING OBJECTIVES

From this chapter, the reader will:

- Understand the importance of achieving a favourable environment for material manipulation
- Understand the factors which influence shade taking
- Appreciate the benefits and shortcomings of light polymerization as a means of controlled setting
- Understand the need for good preventive maintenance for dental hardware.

INTRODUCTION

There are a number of direct clinical placement factors which the clinician must be mindful of when working intraorally. The manufacturers can only do so much and it is incumbent on the dentist to use dental materials as instructed to ensure maximal success. This chapter will discuss the factors relating to clinical manipulation of dental materials.

MOISTURE CONTROL

A substantial number of dental materials are hydrophobic or are adversely affected by water. They will perform suboptimally if water contamination occurs during their placement and before their final setting. This is a major problem in clinical dentistry as the mouth is full of fluid and has high relative humidity.

> **Hydrophobic:** a material which repels water.

It is well accepted that unless the moisture control is carefully controlled, the clinical behaviour of the restoration and its longevity may be significantly compromised. Poor moisture control is a major cause of adhesive bonding failure and also leads to decreased mechanical properties of the material. There are many methods of moisture control, namely **cotton wool rolls**, **dry guards**, **high volume aspiration**, use of **saliva ejectors** (Figure 2.1) and some clinicians have even advocated the use of **systemic medications** to reduce salivary flow. This latter approach is not recommended because there can be systemic side effects which are undesirable. The most effective and predictable method of moisture control, however, is **rubber dam** (Figure 2.2).

The many advantages of this technique will be readily found in operative dentistry textbooks but from a material's perspective, it can provide the closest conditions to an 'ideal' environment for material placement. Its use will allow the clinician to control the operating field more precisely and with respect to humidity and moisture control. It also greatly improves the dentist's access when placing the material. The different types of rubber dam and other materials used in connection with it are discussed in Chapter 13.

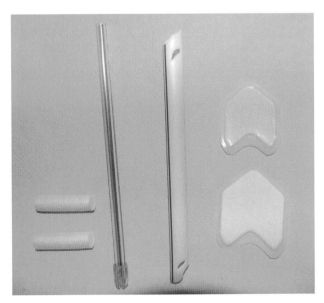

Fig. 2.1 A selection of devices for moisture control. From left to right: cotton wool rolls, saliva ejector, aspiration tip and dry guards (small and large).

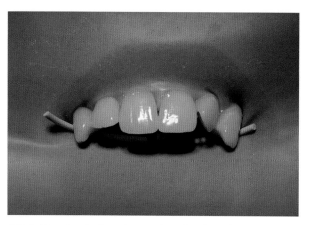

Fig. 2.2 Rubber dam in situ prior to restorative treatment.

SHADE TAKING

Shade taking is an important aspect of restorative dentistry where the dentist attempts to match the colour of the adjacent teeth or tooth with the restorative material, be it a directly placed restorative material such as resin-based composite or one constructed in the dental laboratory such as ceramic. Often the patient will judge the success of the restoration by its appearance, with an imperceptible restoration being considered ideal by them.

> **Resin composites:** hydrophobic materials consisting of an inert glass and a polymerizable resin.
>
> **Ceramic:** an inorganic, non-metallic solid prepared by the action of heat and subsequent cooling.

Some dentists favour a slight mismatch between the shade of the restoration and surrounding natural teeth when providing a posterior restoration. There are two reasons for this:
1. The margins of the restoration are easier to finish.
2. When the restoration needs to be replaced it is easier to identity the tooth-coloured material to be removed and tooth tissue can be preserved.

Shade taking is renowned for being one of the most challenging aspects of restorative dentistry for the dental team. Although the techniques for shade taking are beyond the scope of this book, advice relevant to dental materials is included here.

Matching like with like

It is obvious that to most easily achieve a consistent and predictable result when selecting a shade of restorative material to match the tooth tissue being restored, the material of the shade guide should be the same as the restorative material. Unfortunately this may not be achieved as many manufacturers' shade guides are made from a dissimilar material to the restorative material being used.

One of the most commonly used shade guides is the **Vita Shade Guide** (Figure 2.3), which is used to shade match for ceramics. Unfortunately, the tabs of the shade guide are made of a bulk of material whereas the crown is usually in much thinner sections, altering translucency and shade substantially. It is also possible to get small tabs of the various stains that are available to characterize the ceramic (Figure 2.4).

Some shade guides are designed such that a dentist can select both a shade for ceramic and acrylic when crowns and dentures are being

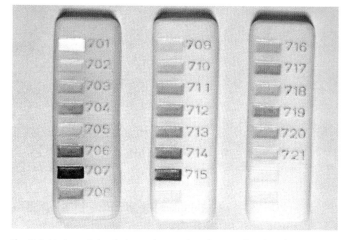

Fig. 2.4 Various stains that may be used to characterize dental ceramic.

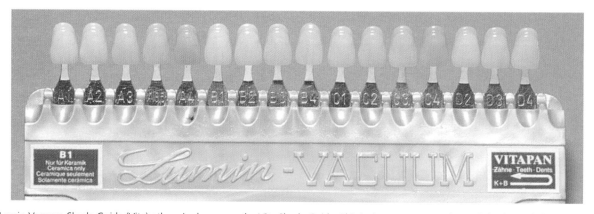

Fig. 2.3 Lumin Vacuum Shade Guide (Vita) otherwise known as the Vita Shade Guide. This is the most commonly used shade guide for matching ceramic restorations.

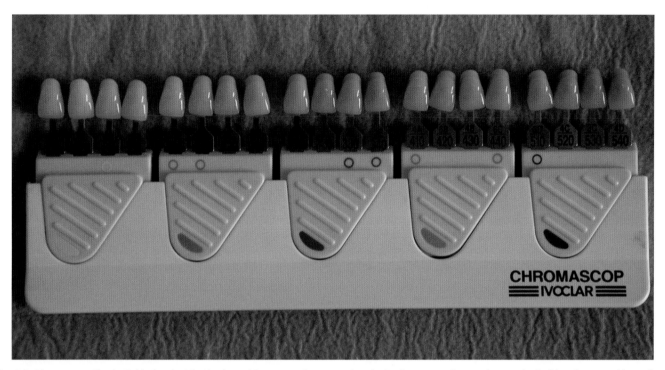

Fig. 2.5 Chromascop Shade Guide (Ivoclar Vivadent) used for cases when ceramic units (such as crowns) are to be matched with a denture with acrylic teeth on it.

provided for the same patient as the shades for the two materials correspond (Figure 2.5). Several manufacturers have recommended using the Vita Shade Guide to shade match for the resin-based composites, and a form of recipe wheel (Figure 2.6) guides the dentist in using the shades in the kit.

To reduce the risk of error, some manufacturers have produced shade guides which are made of the same resin-based composite that is in the kit. This has the benefit that similar types of material are being matched. There is a greater chance that a good shade match will be achieved. Figure 2.7 illustrates two shade guides. One is a simple tab system composed of the resin composite in the kit and the other involves inserting a core of the 'dentine' shade in the shell of 'enamel'. If a small drop of glycerine (or water) is placed to remove the air barrier between the two shade tabs, the dentist can see the final shade result with some certainty.

The other and probably most reliable method of correctly ascertaining shade is applying a small piece of the composite to be used to the tooth without any bond and curing it for 10 seconds. This must be cured as there is a change in shade (**shade shift**) on curing.

 Shade taking (using Miris 2, Coltène Whaledent)

1. Take the dentine shade by matching it with the cervical region of the tooth. This area has the most dentine and less enamel (Figure 2.8).
2. Select the enamel shade by comparing it with the incisal edge. This region has most enamel and less dentine (Figure 2.9).
3. Put the two pieces together with a drop of glycerine between them (Figure 2.10).

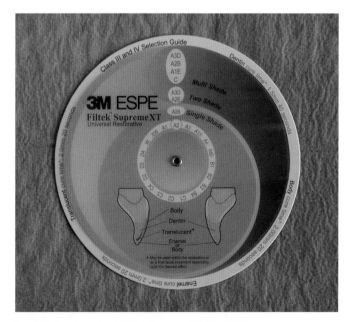

Fig. 2.6 A recipe wheel (Filtek Supreme XT, 3M ESPE).

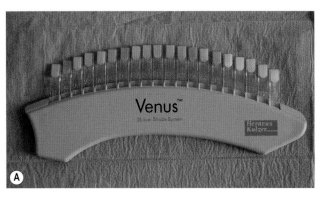

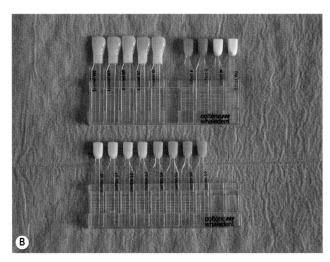

Fig. 2.7 Two shade guides constructed using the material in the kit: (A) Venus (Heraeus) and (B) Miris 2 (Coltène Whaledent).

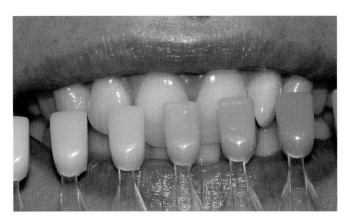

Fig. 2.8 The dentine shade is taken from the cervical region of the tooth. The resin composite 'cores' correspond to dentine.

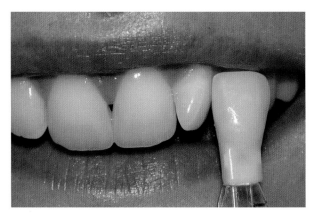

Fig. 2.10 The dentine 'core' is placed inside the enamel 'shell' with a drop of glycerine between them and the product is the matched shade of the tooth.

Similarly when matching ceramic, ceramic should be used. Furthermore different batches of ceramic can differ slightly in their appearance and so ideally the technician should supply the clinician a shade guide manufactured using the same batch of ceramic which will be used to construct the restoration being fitted. For obvious financial reasons this rarely happens.

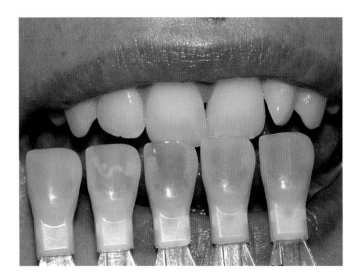

Fig. 2.9 The enamel shade is selected by using the resin composite 'shells' and by matching the tooth colour at the incisal edge where enamel predominates.

- Women have better eyesight for colour perception as they have more cones (colour-sensitive cells) in their retinas. It is therefore advisable for male dentists to ask a female colleague to take the shade or to at least verify it!
- The purest light is the northern light at noon and so if possible take the patient to a (north facing) window to take shade in natural light. A shade should never be taken under the operating light or in non-colour-corrected artificial lighting. It is also advisable to have neutral colours for the surroundings and ensure that a red background is avoided.
- Eyes tire quickly and therefore it is advisable to take a shade at the start of the appointment so that the best result may be obtained.

✓

The shade should always be taken prior to the application of rubber dam. As rubber dam provides such an effective method of isolation so the teeth pushed through the dam will dehydrate quite quickly. Dehydrated teeth appear white and chalky. If the shade assessment was made at this point, then the final composite would be too light after the teeth have rehydrated after rubber dam removal. Figure 2.11 illustrates this phenomenon. This patient has had rubber dam placed to restore 11 and 21 after trauma. The dam was anchored on 13, so the incisal two-thirds was through the dam and the cervical third was in the mouth. Note the obvious demarcation between these parts of the tooth.

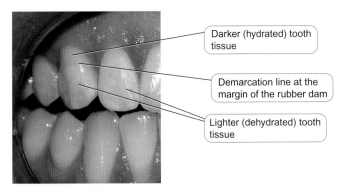

Darker (hydrated) tooth tissue

Demarcation line at the margin of the rubber dam

Lighter (dehydrated) tooth tissue

Fig. 2.11 Tooth 13 illustrating the dehydrating effect of isolating the tooth using rubber dam, so causing a shade change.

New digital technology for shade taking

Digital technology is now available to take the shade to increase the accuracy of the prescription with the intention of decreasing remakes. Bespoke digital shade analysis systems are commercially available which calculate the shade. This information is then corrected to ensure that the true tooth colour is sent to the dental laboratory. This analysed data can then be used by the technician to accurately reproduce the shade of the tooth in ceramic. An example of the type of device available is shown in Figure 2.12. The guide is positioned over a number of points on the tooth surface and the results are mapped.

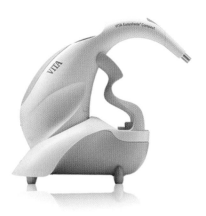

Fig. 2.12 Easy shade compact (Panadent).

LIGHT POLYMERIZATION

Many polymeric materials are prepared in an unset form in the factory and delivered to the dentist in a sealed container. The unset material is then dispensed at the site where it is to be used. The setting reaction is initiated by applying an external energy source – which is usually light. This section explains the mechanics of the light polymerization process.

Modern dental polymers generally **cure** or set into a solid mass, and this process is catalysed either chemically or by the application of external energy such as light. This light polymerization process has been used in dentistry since the early 1970s, the idea originally being developed in the car industry to speed up the set of car paint. The original intention was to save substantial time on the production line by irradiating the painted surface in a light chamber, instead of having to wait for it to dry by a chemical reaction. Although the idea has fallen into disuse in the car industry, its potential for dentistry was realized and as a result there has been a major trend in recent years towards the production of polymeric dental materials which are cured by the application of light.

Advantages and disadvantages of light curing

Light curing offers a number of advantages:

- The material has an extended **working time** so it can be manipulated for a long time without setting. This means that the unset material may be sculpted into a form without time pressure. This is particularly useful if complex aesthetic restorations are being provided. Only when the dentist is happy with the desired shape is the light applied and the material set. This is known as a **command set**.

- It delivers a more **consistent means of polymerization** as a more even distribution of the chemicals within the paste can be obtained because the blending of the paste is optimized by the manufacturer in the factory.

- The **amount and concentration of amine required in the material can be lowered**. A **tertiary amine** is one of the essential components in the (chemical or light) curing process. Unfortunately the presence of any residual amine after curing leads to darkening and yellowing of the set material with time. Restorations in the anterior sextants of the mouth which are subsequently exposed to sunlight are particularly affected, which is clearly not desirable. As the bulk of the amine is used up during the light-curing polymerization process, a decrease in the amount and concentration of amine reduces colour change and enhances colour stability.

- There is a saving in **clinic time** as there is no need to wait for a chemical reaction to go to completion before moving on to the next stage of the operative procedure, such as finishing and polishing.

- The **quality of cure** is improved. The level of conversion of the monomeric component to the polymer varies with the method of initiation of the reaction. The level of conversion is lower for two paste (chemical cured) materials compared to light activated materials. Most light activated materials convert between 50% and 70% monomer to polymer. However, this still leaves some unconverted monomer, which can lead to leaching out of material in the long term and degradation of the restoration with time. Conversion of up to 95–97% of the monomer can be achieved in the laboratory. This increases the mechanical properties but makes the set material more brittle. To achieve this optimum conversion, heat, light and pressure are required and this can only be achieved extraorally.

> **Polymerization reaction:** is a process of reacting monomer molecules together in a chemical reaction to form three-dimensional networks or polymer chains.
> **Monomer:** a small molecule that has the potential of chemically bonding to other monomers of the same species to form a polymer.

Light polymerization also has some disadvantages:

- The **hardware** required to provide the light energy is relatively expensive. A number of light curing units are currently available for the clinician to choose from.
- The systems needs to be **compatible** in that the excitation wavelength of the chemicals in the material and the wavelength of light emitted from the curing lamp must be matched to achieve acceptable cure.
- There is still a **risk of darkening and yellowing** of the restoration as a small amount of residual amine still remains.
- **Failure to deliver adequate energy** to the material will result in a suboptimal restoration.
- **Attenuation of the light** occurs as it passes through the material. This means that the deeper parts of a restoration are not as well polymerized as the surface. This is exacerbated with some materials where the light penetration is limited by the addition of opacifiers and tints.

Mechanism of photo-polymerization

The initiation of the reaction process relies on the use of a **photo-initiator**, a chemical activated by light of a specific wavelength. This activated chemical in turn reacts with an **amine** in the material so producing free radicals. The action of the light on the photo-initiator molecule causing it to break down is called a photolytic reaction. It is these free radicals which initiate the polymerization reaction, and once the initiation phase has been started the reaction propagates until all the chemical has been reacted in the classic chain reaction. The process of activation of a light curing system is illustrated in Table 2.1.

Table 2.1 The mechanism for the setting reaction of light activated resin systems

Photo-initiator (e.g. an α diketone)	+	Light of a specific wavelength	→	activated diketone
(e.g. camphorquinone)		(470 nm)		
Activated diketone	+	amine	→	Free radical [R]
[R] + monomer	+	copolymer	→	Polymer

> **Free radicals:** are atoms, molecules, or ions with unpaired electrons. These unpaired electrons are highly chemically reactive.
> **Photolytic reaction:** is initiated by light energy breaking down a chemical to produce atoms or molecules to initiate a chemical reaction.
> **Chain reaction:** a series of reactions in which the product or by product of the initial stages of the reaction causes further reactions to occur.
> **Copolymer:** a polymer derived from two or more monomeric species. It is also termed a **heteropolymer**.

This is similar to the older (chemically cured) paste systems where one material contained amine and the other **benzoyl peroxide**. When the two pastes were mixed, free radicals were produced. This initiated the polymerization reaction.

Photo-initiator

A widely used photo-initiator used in dentistry is the **α diketone, camphorquinone**. This chemical is yellow in colour (Figure 2.13) and may present manufacturers with a problem when a lighter shade of resin composite is being manufactured as the inclusion of this yellow chemical will have an effect on the final shade. With the increasing use of dental bleaching, lighter resin-based composite materials are required in order to match the lighter shades achieved by the bleaching process. This has meant that camphorquinone cannot be used

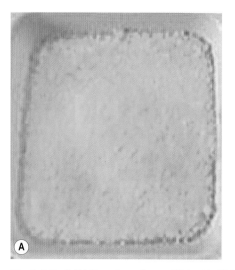 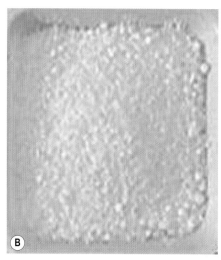 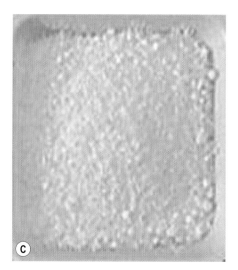

Fig. 2.13A–C (A) Camphorquinone, (B) Lucirin TPO and (C) PPD powders. Note the yellow colour of the camphorquinone; the PPD and Lucirin TPO powders are whiter.

and so other photo-initiators such as **phenylpropanedione (PPD)** or **2,4,6-trimethylbenzoyldiphenylphosphine oxide (Lucirin TPO)** are now becoming more common.

Wavelength of light

Different photo-initiators react with different wavelengths of light. Camphorquinone is most sensitive at wavelengths of between 390 and 510 nm with a **peak absorption** of 470 nm whereas PPD and Lucirin TPO are most effective at between 380 and 430 nm. Most current light cured materials are most sensitive to light at 470 nm. However, there are now some materials available where the peak absorption of the activator is different, whereas other products contain two photo-initiators, increasing the peak excitation waveband. Examples of these materials are:

- Some conventional resin composites, e.g. Solitaire 2 (Hereaus)
- Adhesives, e.g. Touch & Bond (Parkell)
- Luting composites, e.g. Panavia F (Kuraray)
- Light-cured protective varnishes, e.g. Palaseal (Hereaus).

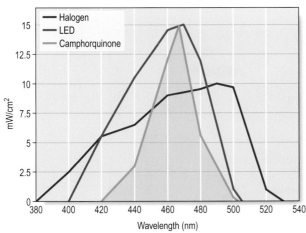

Fig. 2.14 Superimposition of the spectral bands of an LED and halogen curing light with that of camphorquinone. Note that camphorquinone corresponds with both lights but particularly the LED light meaning this is a more efficient curing device.

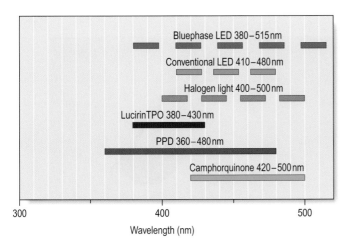

Fig. 2.15 Absorption spectra of three photo-initiators (solid line) and operating wavelength of three light sources (dash line). Bluephase is a light source using a polywave LED (Ivoclar Vivadent).

It is therefore essential to ensure that the wavelength of the light and the peak absorption of the photo-initiator material are compatible, otherwise the materials will not set.

Figure 2.14 illustrates the peak excitation wavelengths for a photo-initiator and two types of light. Different types of curing light emit light at different wavelengths. The excitation wavelength for camphorquinone is shown with those for a halogen and a light emitting diode (LED) light superimposed. The excitation wavelengths of the photo-initiator and the curing light must correspond otherwise the curing lamp is not able to deliver sufficient energy at the photo-initiator's wavelength so ensuring adequate cure. This may be problematic with a narrower, more concentrated **spectral band** seen with the LED's footprint. As halogen lights have a wider spectral output they will tend to cure all material types but it is advisable to verify with the material manufacturer that the light-curing unit used by the clinician will be suitable for purpose. Lucirin TPO, the most common alternative photo-initiator, has a peak excitation which is outside the bulk of spectral spread of both lamps (Figure 2.15).

> **!**
>
> The dentist should use a light-curing source that is compatible with the material to ensure that it will be completely polymerized.

> **Peak absorption:** the wavelength at which the maximum excitation of a photolytic chemical occurs. Also called **peak excitation wavelength**.
> **Spectral band:** the part of the spectrum at which the light polymerizing unit may produce chemical excitation.

Types of lights available

Three types of light are available to initiate light activation:

- Halogen
- Plasma
- LED.

Halogen light

The halogen light (Figure 2.16) has the longest track record and has proved to be very successful. There is considerable variation between lights in terms of the wavelengths over which they deliver light but in general they exhibit a broad spectral range. The intensity of light at the wavelength where peak excitation of the photo-initiator may occur may also vary. The halogen bulb itself emits white light and, in order to produce the required blue light, filters are required. Furthermore, the reflector behind the bulb can become dull and also covered in dust, reducing the efficiency of the system. Much of the energy produced by the light is in the form of heat and cooling fans are therefore required to prevent the bulb overheating.

One of the particular problems associated with a halogen light is that the filament in the bulb ages with time in the same way as a domestic light bulb filament ages. This leads to thinning of the wire filament and also a change in its operating temperature. Changes in the operating temperature will result in an alteration in the wavelength of light delivered from the bulb. As the bulb ages, the amount of energy at 470 nm available (peak absorption for camphorquinone) is reduced. This is difficult to detect as the light will remain blue but

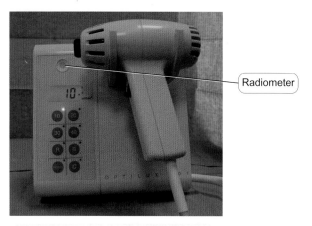

Fig. 2.16 A halogen curing light (Optilux 501, Kerr Hawe). The radiometer is highlighted.

there will be a steady drift in peak intensity. The consequence of this is that the curing efficiency is diminished and the material is less well cured. The only effective way of dealing with this is to change the bulb

on regular basis, such as every 3–6 months, depending on the usage. Many light-curing lamps are now fitted with a light checker. This is called a **radiometer** (Figure 2.16). However many of these are not sophisticated enough to differentiate the variations in wavelength sufficiently well and so should be used with caution.

Plasma light

This light (Figure 2.17) is a **plasma arc** lamp using xenon gas. It provides a very high intensity light but has a narrow spectral band and as discussed earlier, may mean that not all resin composites are cured effectively by this type of lamp. Furthermore, the high energy also leads to the risk of very high shrinking stresses – both within the resin composite and at the tooth–material interface. These stresses will be set up during the short (3 seconds) curing time, which allows no chance of stress relief when compared with the halogen light where this occurs during the initial 7–8 seconds before the material solidifies. This light has been superseded by the LED light and is now primarily used as an adjunct to tooth bleaching as it is possible to fit adaptors to the tip to permit irradiation over a large area (see Chapter 18). The system is also quite bulky when compared with the LED systems, another reason why their use is reducing.

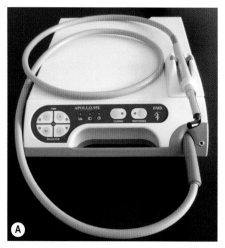
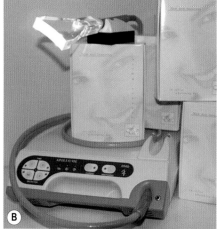

Fig. 2.17A,B Commercially available plasma light (Apollo Elite, DenMed Technologies).

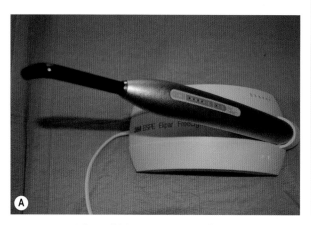
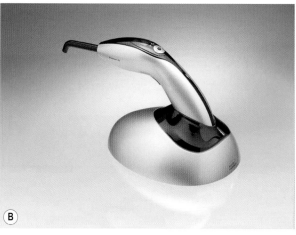

Fig. 2.18 Two commercially available LED curing lights: (A) 3M ESPE's Elipar light and (B) Ivoclar Vivadent's Bluephase light.

Light-emitting diodes (LEDs)

LED lights are the most recent addition to the range of lights available and can produce very effective polymerization of light-sensitive dental materials. Initially they were arrays of LEDs but now generally only one LED is used. They are now very powerful, emitting in excess of 1 W of energy.

The problems of a narrow spectral band is discussed earlier. In order to increase compatibility where the peak excitation wavelength does not correspond to that of the photo-initiator in the composite material, new LED lights are being developed. An example of this is the polywave LED light, which is composed of more than one LED, each operating at a different wavelength. The long-term performance of LEDs is good as the wavelength of light delivered does not change. Even with the high-powered lights, it is unnecessary to have any cooling fans. Two currently available products are shown in Figure 2.18, and Table 2.2 summarizes the key features of the LED and halogen lights.

Effects of incomplete curing

The failure of the clinician to ensure that the correct wavelength is being used with a light cured material will result in an uncured or partially cured material. This will have significant clinical consequences (Figure 2.19):

- **Pulpal inflammation**. Some light cured materials have acidic components. If they are not fully cured, the acid in the unset material may cause chemical trauma. If the pulp is already compromised, tooth sensitivity and pulpal pain may occur.
- **Discolouration**. Oral fluids will diffuse into the partially set material and along the interface between tooth and restoration causing discolouration of the material and **marginal staining**.
- **Decreased wear resistance**. Partially set material will not achieve optimum mechanical properties, resulting in decreased compressive and flexural strengths. Clinically this will manifest as increased wear and abrasion of the material and an inability to withstand forces experienced by the restoration during function.
- **Formation of marginal gaps (microgap)**. These may be generated as the partially set resin will be more elastic and pull away from the tooth surface (**debonding**) during occlusal loading (chewing). This leads to microleakage and subsequently secondary caries.

Table 2.2 Comparison of LED and halogen light sources

Quartz halogen	LED
Relatively cheap	Consistent output
Extended history of use	No filter required
Mains operated	High efficiency
	Limited temperature rise: no fan
Low efficiency	Easily disinfected
High temperature; needs cooling fan	Long life expectancy of LED
Bulb ages	Battery operated
Requires filters	Narrow band width
Reflector must be cleaned	Compatibility of photo-initiator
Difficult to disinfect	Heating with powerful LED

(green = advantage, red = disadvantage, yellow = neither advantage nor disadvantage)

Microgap: the microscopic interface between a restoration and the tooth.
Microleakage: the permeation of fluid, debris and bacteria down the interface between a restoration and the walls of a cavity preparation in the tooth.
Secondary (recurrent) caries: carious lesion developing between an existing dental restoration and the cavity margin.

Factors affecting cure

Several factors will influence the effectiveness of the light-curing process. These can be divided into factors either under the manufacturer's or the clinician's control.

Factors under the manufacturer's control

The variables that the manufacturer can control and which influence the rate of cure are:

- **Refractive index of glass/resin**. The manufacturer tries to match the optical properties of the resin and the glass but this is sometimes difficult. Any mismatch will cause some **refraction** of the light at the interface of each filler particle and some **light attenuation**, leading to a reduction in polymerization efficiency.
- **The shade of material**. A darker shade will require a longer curing time as the light intensity is reduced during passage through the material when compared with a lighter shade of material.
- **The opacity/translucency of the material**. The more opaque a material the longer the curing time must be as the light's intensity through the material is reduced by the increased opacity of the material.

It takes longer for the light to cure darker and/or opaque shades of light-cured, tooth-coloured materials. It is therefore advisable to decrease the depth of each increment of material placed and to increase the curing time of each increment.

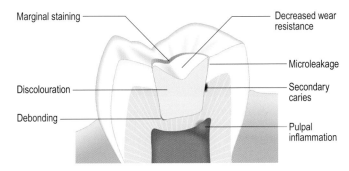

Marginal staining — Decreased wear resistance

Discolouration — Microleakage

— Secondary caries

Debonding — — Pulpal inflammation

Fig. 2.19 A diagrammatic representation of the clinical consequences of incomplete curing of a polymeric material in a cavity.

Clinicians often discuss the **depth of cure** of a light-cured material, which is the maximum depth at which adequate polymerization of a material is achieved on exposure to light energy. Achieving the correct depth of cure is important as insufficient light energy may only adequately cure the material at the surface, leaving a softened mass underneath which will rapidly start to degrade. This has been described by some as the '**soggy bottom**' of a restoration (Figure 2.20). This is a worst case scenario (as opposed to the material not curing at all) because the clinician is lulled into a false sense of security, thinking that the material has been adequately cured through the bulk of the restoration.

- **Variables in diketone/amine chemistry**. A number of manufacturers have altered the diketone/amine concentrations in order to accelerate the polymerization reaction. This means that some materials are more susceptible to ambient light than others and may start to set under the operating light. Additionally, it has been found that the use of excess diketone/amine can lead to the materials forming shorter polymer chains and having poorer mechanical properties. This impairs the performance of the material.
- **Particle size**. A reduction in particle size to improve finish and enhance mechanical properties has been the main goal of manufacturers for a number of years. This creates problems as the light is attenuated more quickly during passage through the bulk of finer particle sizes, due to the larger surface area to volume ratio created, leading to lower light penetration and a reduction in the depth of cure.

The manufacturer assesses the variations described above in the laboratory and provides instructions so that the clinician may achieve the optimum properties for their material. This is set out in the **directions for use** (DFU) or instructions which are supplied with every material.

Factors under the clinician's control

The clinician does not have the manufacturer's advantage of checking the optimum properties and should therefore ensure that the DFU are followed precisely. Failure to do this will inevitably lead to a material that will underperform. The factors over which the clinician has an influence are:

- **Reduction in thickness of each increment** of darker, more opaque and smaller filler particle materials to facilitate light penetration.
- **Distance of light from restoration**. It is essential that the light is as close to the surface of the restoration as possible. The light radiates out and the amount of energy delivered per square millimetre is reduced as the light is moved further away from the surface (Figure 2.21).

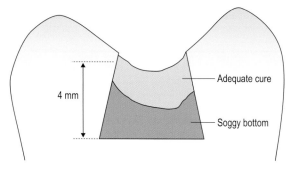

Fig. 2.20 The so called 'soggy bottom' of a resin-based composite where the outer layer is set giving the impression that all the restoration has cured. Unfortunately insufficient polymerization has occurred and in the deeper areas of the cavity unset resin-based composite remains. This is often a result of attempting to cure more than 2 mm thickness of resin composite at once.

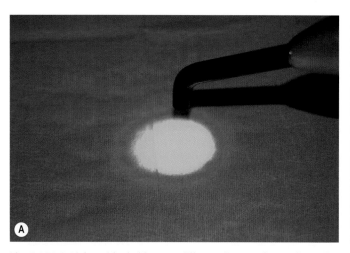

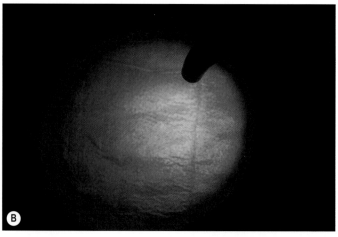

Fig. 2.21A,B Light guides held at two different distances from a flat surface. Note that the area exposed to light increases with the distance from the tip of the light guide. Light intensity is proportion to the area exposed to the beam. The intensity in (B) is less than in (A), this amount being proportional to the ratios of the two surface areas exposed. A flat surface presents ideal conditions, but even here it can be seen that the intensity even at the centre of the illuminated area is reduced and the light distribution is uneven.

- The light guide should not be held away from the material to increase the area illuminated. This will lead to inadequate polymerization.
- Additionally, the clinician should be mindful to increase the curing time when restoring the base of deep cavities as the curing tip to restorative material distance is greater.

- **Choice of curing cycle.** Most lights today have a range of curing programs including a **ramp cure**, **soft start**, **boost** and **slow cure**. This means that the amount of the energy being emitted by the curing light is not the same for every program. These purport to reduce the degree of shrinkage which occurs during the polymerization process. There is little or no scientific evidence that these have effect on shrinkage. It has to be accepted that the degree of shrinkage which occurs is directly related to the degree of conversion of the resin system.
- **Light exposure time.** Any shortening of the exposure time for light curing will decrease the amount of energy transmitted to the material so reducing its cure. It is the amount of energy applied which is the significant factor. Koran and Kürschner postulated the **total energy concept**, which is a useful way of calculating the correct curing time. The energy needed (i.e. rate of cure) is the product of the intensity of the light with the time of application. It can be shown as:

Dose (energy required) = maximum curing time × intensity

The factors which affect the required dose depends on many factors as mentioned earlier (e.g. shade etc.) but it is generally accepted that an energy dose of **16 000 mW/cm²** is required to adequately cure a 2 mm increment of resin composite. For example, how long should a composite be cured for with a curing lamp whose output is 1000 mW/cm²?

Dose (energy required) = maximum curing time × intensity
→ Maximum curing time = dose/intensity
→ Maximum curing time = $16\,000\,\text{mW/cm}^2 / 1000\,\text{mW/cm}^2$
→ Maximum curing time = **16 s**

This also assumes that the light is in direct contact with the surface of the resin to be cured.

> **Ramp cure:** light energy increases linearly with respect to time over period of cure.
> **Soft start:** light energy starts at low level and then reverts to maximum output.
> **Boost/high power:** constant emission of light energy at maximum output.
> **Slow cure/low power:** light energy remains at intermediate level and curing time is increased.

Irradiance

The ideal intensity (**irradiance**) of a curing light has been reported to be 1000 mW/cm². However, many lights do not achieve sufficient intensity with even LEDs outputs varying between 275 and 1050 mW.

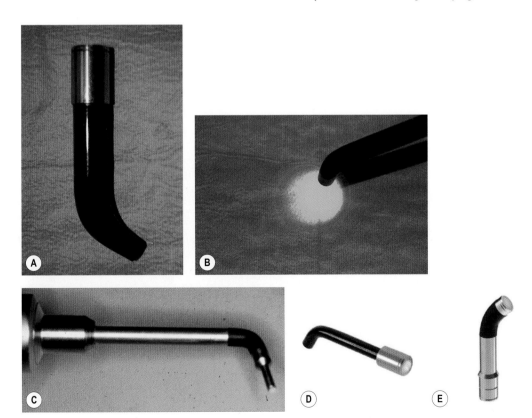

Fig. 2.22A–E An assortment of light guides for use in different situations. Note the difference in size of the light guide's exit portal. The light guide on the top left (picture A) is the turbo tip.

It is therefore important to ask the manufacturer for the minimum light intensity or consult the DFU to ensure the exposure times are appropriate for the curing light to be used. The light may also be checked using a radiometer (Figure 2.16).

The above formula will calculate how long a light-cured material should be exposed to a certain intensity of light. It is important to remember that light-cured materials are only cured by light energy and have no means of self-curing. It is better to increase the curing time slightly to ensure a full cure as the clinical ramifications of under-curing are significant whereas light-cured materials are not affected by over-curing. The only downside of this is that with increasing amount of energy applied, more heat is generated and this may be transmitted to the tooth with the possibility of pulpal thermal trauma. This balance should be considered when working clinically, and it becomes more significant as more higher-powered LED lights become available, as these can generate substantial heat.

- **Tip size.** The exit portal of the light guide can vary and this can be used for various applications. Some tips are very small (2 mm in diameter) and these can be used for tacking restorations, for example, veneers so that they are stabilized on the preparation allowing the dentist to remove the excess cement without disturbing the veneer. Some tips may be wider to irradiate a larger area when working with larger restorations, and others are tapered. These are called **turbo tips** (Figure 2.22). In general, widening the light guide tip from exit portal to end of light guide results in a lower light intensity at the tip. The amount of light delivered remains the same but is distributed over a larger area. The reverse in not necessarily the case as the light is reflected at the surface of the sleeve on the light guide, leading to dissipation of the light within the light guide itself. This may well further lead to the guide becoming warm.

- **Light probe design.** The design of the light guide has an effect on light intensity produced. A fibreglass rod will markedly reduce the amount of light loss due to scattering opposed to the designs of LED lights where the LED is mounted at front of the light emission window. The light guides consist of many individual fibres. The standard parallel-sided light guides are preferred for normal working as they exhibit excellent light distributing characteristics.

Clinical staff should always use the orange eye shield supplied to reduce the amount of light energy reaching the eyes. This decreases the possibility of retinal damage with exposure to high intensity light during light curing (Figure 2.23).

Curing light maintenance and care

As with any dental equipment curing lights should be regularly examined for any defects and maintained according to the manufacturer's recommendations.

The importance of good clinical technique when placing materials has been stressed. Good moisture control will affect shade taking and facilitate the successful placement of hydrophobic materials such as those requiring to be light polymerized. The benefits and pitfalls of light activation have been highlighted and the need for dental

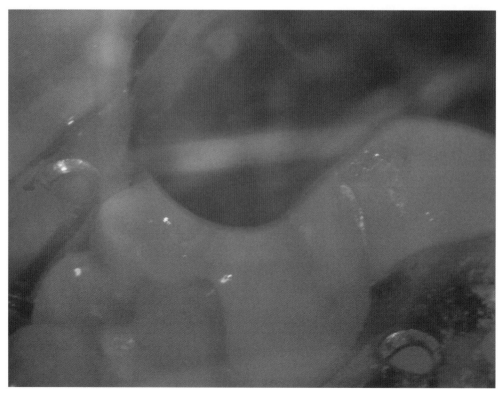

Fig. 2.23 A resin composite material being cured with the use of an orange light shield to decrease the intensity of light transmitted to the eyes.

A suggested protocol for checking curing lights

- Avoid contamination of the light guide with set material (Figure 2.24).
- Ensure that the light guide is decontaminated between patients.
- Protect light and base unit such that it cannot be easily knocked onto the floor.
- Regularly inspect all components for damage.
- Check light output regularly, ideally weekly. This can be done using a radiometer but as previously mentioned care should be exercised and the dentist should not rely on this method of curing light verification. Cure a 3 mm deep cylinder of universal shade composite. If soft material remains on the base (Figure 2.25) the light is not functioning adequately.
- Where a halogen light is used, the bulb should be changed on a regular basis every 3–6 months when used regularly. If the casing of the bulb is becoming darkened, the bulb should be changed immediately.
- Check the reflector behind the bulb or LED is clean and free from dust and debris.
- Clean the light guide immediately after each use.
- Review the conductance of the light guide by viewing daylight through the distal end. Any black spots or speckling indicates damaged fibre in the fibre bundle. Replace the light guide if more than 10% of the fibres are damaged (Figure 2.26).
- Examine the outer casing for cracking and crazing and replace the light guide if damage is observed (Figure 2.27).
- Ensure that any cooling fans and vents are clear of dust and debris.

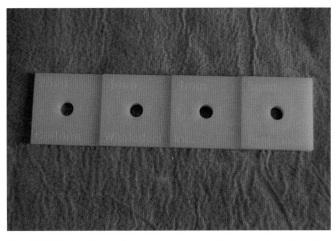

Fig. 2.25 Polytetrafluoroethylene step-wedge with prepared cavities of given thicknesses. Resin-based composite is packed into the cavity and cured. After inverting the step wedge any soft composite may be noted at the base of the cavity.

preventive maintenance outlined. Care should be taken by the dental team when using light-cured materials. Some materials, particularly when uncured have potentially harmful biological effects. It is important that these are handled carefully to minimize any detrimental long-term effects to those exposed to them. The next chapter discusses the biological effects of dental materials and will highlight measures which can be employed to mitigate these problems.

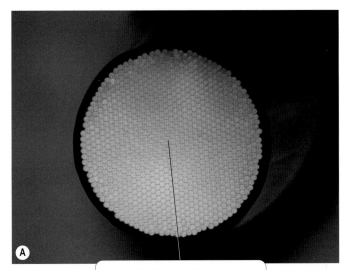

(A) End of light guide showing undamaged end. Nearly all fibre bundles are clearly defined.

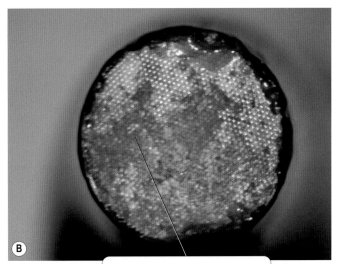

(B) Resin composite covering part of the end of a light guide.

Fig. 2.24 (A) New light guide with no damage and (B) a light guide where set resin composite had been allowed to accumulate on the tip end. This will lead to a reduction in light emission.

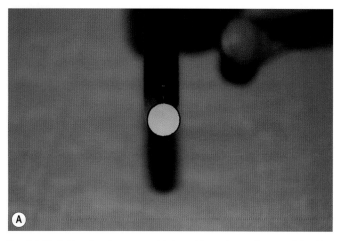 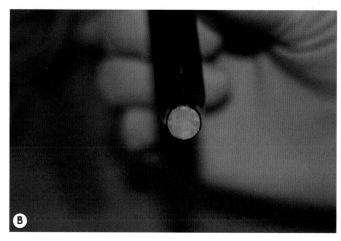

Fig. 2.26A,B The tip of an unused light guide and one after considerable use with daylight shining through. Note the blotching of the surface of the used one where the fibres are damaged.

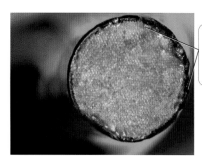

Damaged light guide which has been dropped. The edge has been chipped and the adjacent fibres will not transmit light adequately.

Fig. 2.27 A light guide where the external casing and adjacent fibre optic bundles have been damaged.

SUMMARY

- Good moisture is essential particularly when hydrophobic materials are being placed to achieve a satisfactory outcome.
- Shade taking is a challenging aspect of restorative dentistry. There are many factors which influence the outcome, namely control of the surrounding lighting, the intraoral environment and the material used in the shade matching.
- Light polymerization plays an essential part in the setting reaction of many modern restorative dental materials.
- There are many advantages and disadvantages of this technique (see pp. 17–26).
- It is very important that good care and maintenance is employed with the hardware used to light cure.

FURTHER READING

Malhotra, N., Kundabala, M., Acharya, S., 2010. Strategies to overcome polymerisation shrinkage – materials and techniques – a review. Dent. Update 37, 115–125.

Mitton, B.A., Wilson, N.H., 2001. The use and maintenance of light activation units in general practice. Br. Dent. J. 191, 82–86.

Powers, J.M., Sakaguchi, R.L. (Eds.), 2006. (twelfth ed.). Mosby Elsevier, St Louis (See Chapters 3 and 10).

Santini, A., 2010. Current status of light activation units and the curing of light activated resin based composites. Dent. Update 37, 214–227.

van Noort, R., 2007. Introduction to Dental Materials, third ed. Mosby Elsevier, Edinburgh. (See Chapters 1.7 and 2.2).

SELF-ASSESSMENT QUESTIONS

1. What are the effects of holding a curing light at a distance from the surface of the material being cured?
2. Why is it desirable to maintain a dry field during the placement of a restorative material?
3. How may the manufacturer manipulate the setting properties of the material when it is light activated?
4. What precautions should the dental staff take to ensure that a light-curing unit is operating at an optimum level?
5. What are the advantages and disadvantages of halogen-curing lights?
6. What are the desirable conditions for shade taking?

Chapter | **3** |

Biological effects and safety aspects of dental materials

From this chapter, the reader will:

- Appreciate the interrelation between dental materials and the tissues and environment of the oral cavity
- Appreciate the significance of thermal change during the setting of a material within the mouth and the potential hazards associated with this
- Understand the risks to the dental team as a result of hypersensitivity reactions associated with the materials
- Appreciate the legislation which governs the safe use of materials
- Be aware of the monitoring and reporting systems which are in place and know what to do if a reaction occurs in a patient.

INTRODUCTION

Many long-term biological effects can come to light in the fullness of time. These have significant effects for the patient and the dental team. It is important that the implications of these long-term effects are understood and also notified to the appropriate authorities to ensure that any untoward effect can be investigation for the health and safety of the population.

INTERACTION WITH THE HOST (THE PATIENT)

It is important to compare the properties of the tissue being replaced. An 'ideal' material will match or be very close to the properties of the material to be replaced. One of the most important criteria for any material used within the human body is biocompatibility or more significantly bioactivity. Unlike some implanted materials, the biocompatibility of a dental material can vary with its form and status. An unmixed or unset material may cause a mild adverse reaction whereas the set material may be biologically inert. The assessment of these properties is frequently subjective and ultimately is an informed opinion based on a selection of tests which screen the materials initially. All materials' biological behaviour must be evaluated and this is done by simulating conditions which attempt to match those of the intended use.

>
>
> No dental material is 'ideal' nor as good as the natural dental tissues it is intended to replace. Emphasis should therefore always be placed on prevention by the whole dental team.

> **Biocompatibility:** the ability to support life and having no toxic or injurious effects on the tissues.
> **Bioactivity:** the ability to actively promote activity within the tissue.

THERMAL CHANGES DURING SETTING

All materials will undergo an **exothermic** reaction during setting. In many cases this temperature rise is small and will have no clinical impact. However, there are a number of materials where the temperature rise during the setting reaction is marked. This is particularly the case with any resin systems. Additionally it must not be forgotten that light-curing units including LEDs radiate significant heat, which may be transmitted to the tooth causing thermal trauma to the pulp. Generally speaking, the higher the intensity, the more energy is released as heat. This is illustrated in Figure 3.1. It has been reported that the temperature of the pulp should not be raised by more than 3°C for longer than 1 minute to prevent irreversible pulpal damage occurring.

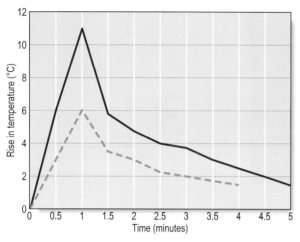

Fig. 3.1 The temperature rise when a curing light is used alone on the surface of a tooth (green line) and the additional temperature rise (red line) which occurs during the setting of a light-cured, resin-based material.

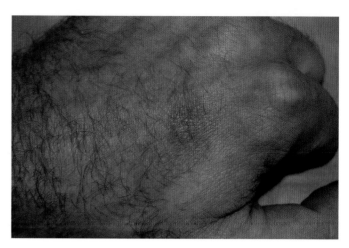

Fig. 3.2 The effects of hypersensitivity to HEMA. Note the area of erythema (redness) and cracking of the skin caused by wiping a HEMA-contaminated instrument on the back of the hand to remove unset resin composite during clinical placement.

ALLERGY AND HYPERSENSITIVITY

In the modern age, with the increasing use of a wide range of chemicals which come into contact with human tissue, it is not uncommon for individuals to become **sensitized** to certain components. The dental clinic is no exception to this. Those members of the dental team involved, in decreasing order of risk, are:

- Dental nurse
- Clinician
- Patient
- Dental technician.

Some of the commonest allergies are associated with polymers and monomers used in dentistry including methylmethacrylate (MMA), hydroxyethylmethacrylate (HEMA) and other methacrylates. Allergies frequently manifest as contact dermatitis (Figure 3.2) and the best ways of reducing the risk of developing an allergy is to avoid, where possible, any direct contact with the material (especially the liquids) employing a **no-touch technique** and practising good **resin hygiene**. The common usage of protective gloves in dental practice has decreased the risk of skin contamination with resins. However, surgical gloves are porous and chemicals such as HEMA may easily penetrate them.

If any contact occurs between gloves (or skin) and chemical, it is advised that the gloves are removed as soon as possible. Hands should be thoroughly washed and dried before donning a fresh pair of gloves and continuing with the procedure.

REPORTING OF HAZARDS/INTERACTIONS

There is an obligation on the clinician to inform any relevant regulatory body of any confirmed or possible adverse reaction to a dental material. This information may be used by manufacturers to improve their products and by government departments to disseminate information to clinicians to safeguard and protect the public. In the UK, adverse reactions are reported an official website run by Medicines and Healthcare products Regulatory Agency (MHRA), but this is primarily concerned with adverse effects related to drugs (www.mhra.gov.uk). An adverse reaction reporting agency for dental materials is run by the University of Sheffield in the UK (www.arrp.group.shef.ac.uk) and has built up a substantial database which is available to enquirers. A sample of the form which should be completed in shown in Figure 3.3. The reporting of adverse reactions to dental materials is particularly important as an adverse reaction is generally associated with an allergic reaction to one or more of the constituents of the product. The mode of use and the history of the application should be reported in detail.

In the UK, there is an ever-increasing burden of health and safety legislation with which the dental team must comply. The **COSHH (Control of Substances Hazardous to Health)** regulations cover any and all chemicals used in the workplace and there is a legal requirement to produce a risk assessment of every chemical and product used. The following pieces of information should be recorded:

- *PPE (personal protective equipment)*: Precautions taken by the individual to protect themselves such as the need for protective clothing, gloves and eye protection. Often this may be obtained from the Materials Safety Data Sheet (MSDS) sheet provided by the manufacturer or from the manufacturer's website.
- *Risk phrases and exposure limits*: At what stage in the placement processes are the team members at risk and what the duration of these risk periods? What is the maximum exposure limit for the particular material used under conditions of use?
- *Material properties which are hazardous*: These include such properties as risk of inflammability, risk of inhalation, risk of swallowing, etc.
- *Precautions to be taken*: These include requirements related to wearing protective clothing, protective glasses, ventilation etc.
- *First aid*: This should describe the action which is to be taken if any member of the team is inadvertently exposed to the hazard.
- *Risk assessment and procedures* to minimize risk.
- *Spillage procedure*: This should indicate how to contain the hazardous material and how to decontaminate the site after the spillage has occurred.
- *Handling and storage*: This should describe the recommended way of handling and storing the hazardous material.

Figure 3.4 shows a typical COSHH assessment form.

Dental Adverse Reactions Reporting Form

ARRP

- This form can be used for patient and occupational adverse reactions.
- Please report all suspected adverse reactions, including minor ones.
- Please order further green forms or photocopy, as required.

Data regarding person affected:

Reporters identification of affected person: _____

Person affected is: Patient   Dentist   Dental nurse
Dental hygienist   Dental technician   Other:_____

Age: under 20   20–29   30–39   40–49   50–59   60+

Gender: ☐ Male ☐ Female

Was the adverse reaction first noticed by?   Affected person   Yourself

What month/year was the reaction first noticed: Month _____ Year _____

If the reaction occurred after dental treatment/handling dental materials, did it occur:

within 1 hour   within 1 day   within 1 week
within 1 month   months to years   unknown

General diseases:

Medications:

Known allergies:

Reactions (objective findings and subjective symptoms):

Local reaction – intraoral:

Reaction – lip/face:

General reaction (other than mouth, lip and face):

PTO

Type of material(s) suspected:

_____

Suspected products: (state brand name and manufacturer if known)

_____

Type of dental treatment(s) suspected:

Fillings
Inlays, veneers
Dentures
Crowns and bridges
Endodontic treatment
Temporary restorations
Periodontal treatment
Oral surgery
Orthodontics
Preventive dentistry
Other (please specify):

Assessment of relationship:

Reporters assessment of relationship between material(s) and reaction(s):

Probable   Possible   Uncertain   Unlikely

Degree of the reaction:

Mild   Moderate   Severe

Referrals:

Has or will the affected person be referred for further investigation?   No   Yes
If yes, to whom?

General practitioner
Dentist
Dermatologist
Allergist
Oral physician
Other (please specify):

Reporters details (Please print clearly)

Title: _____

Name: _____

Address: _____

_____

Post code: _____

Dentist   Physician
Hygenist   Dental technician
Other (please specify):

_____

Telephone: _____

Email: _____

Date: _____

Number of additional form(s) required

_____

Postal address:
Adverse Reaction Reporting Project (ARRP),
The University of Sheffield,
Department of Adult Dental Care,
FREEPOST NEA5451, Sheffield S10 1BQ

E-mail: arrp@sheffield.ac.uk
Tel: 0114 271 7939
Fax: 0114 266 5326
Website: http://www.shef.ac.uk/-arrp

Fig. 3.3 The University of Sheffield adverse reaction to dental materials form, which should be completed by any clinician in the UK suspecting an adverse reaction by a patient to a dental material.

Fortunately, all manufacturers are required to produce a materials safety data sheet with the information on each material, the **MSDS**. It is essential that a risk assessment is done for each material or chemical used in the dental practice or clinic. Failure to do this can lead to prosecution in the UK. It is curious, however, that the failure to carry out an assessment is far more onerous than doing the risk assessment incorrectly, which does not have the same legal gravitas.

HAZARDOUS SUBSTANCES SAFETY INFORMATION SHEET

Form HSSI

Use this form to provide information to employees and others in relation to a particular substance in use for work purposes – it should be made available or displayed in the area where the substance is used.

This information sheet links to Hazardous Substances Risk Assessment No.-	NAME OF PRODUCT/SUBSTANCE: MANUFACTURER'S NAME:
USE/EXPOSURE (DETAILS OF THE WAY IT IS USED):	DATE OF SAFETY DATA SHEET (SDS): LOCATION OF SDS:
IS THE HAZARDOUS SUBSTANCE GENERATED AS A RESULT OF A PROCESS? YES/NO Workspace Exposure Limit (WEL): Stated Risk or Safety Phrases on SDS:	HAZARD WARNING SYMBOL ON CONTAINER LABEL: Identify
POTENTIAL HARM OR ILL EFFECTS: (state what harm may occur) Is health surveillance required?	**ACTION TO BE TAKEN IN CASE OF EMERGENCY:** FIRST AID ARRANGEMENT: SPILLAGE RELEASE ACTION: MANAGEMENT (contact in case of emergency): Name: Telephone No:
DESCRIBE WORK METHOD: (including precautions and control to be implemented) *Continue overleaf if necessary*	
Date of issue:	Date of Review:
Name of Assessor:	Name of Assessor:
Position	Position

(c) PBS 2010/1

PENINSULA

Fig. 3.4 A typical COSHH assessment form.
Courtesy of Peninsula Business Services.

The significance of long-term effects on both the patient and the dental team are of great importance to the manufacturer who has to take account of these in the production of new materials. The sequence of planning and development of a new or modified material is a complex process involving laboratory, clinical and regulatory investigations. The next chapter explains the procedures a manufacturer adopts to produce a new material and the various regulatory mechanisms which they are required to pursue to confirm a material is safe and efficacious for use.

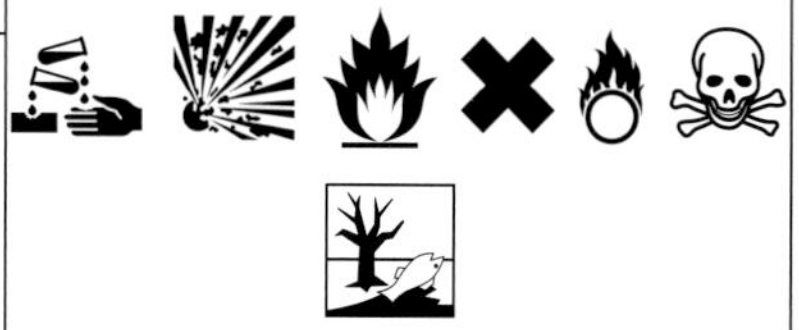

SUMMARY

- Ingredients in many dental materials may by themselves be biologically active and potentially hazardous. This may have an effect on the patient and the dental team depending on their level of contact with the material. The problems may be exacerbated by inadequate manipulation of the material.
- The process of setting generates heat which is potentially hazardous to the dental pulp and the implications of this needs to be considered in the material selection.
- Adverse reactions to materials should be notified both to the manufacturer and to the regulatory authorities.
- There are a number of mechanisms by which reporting of adverse reactions may be achieved. It is essential that the dental team members are cognizant of their legal and ethical obligations to the public while carrying out their duties.

SELF-ASSESSMENT QUESTIONS

1. What the consequences of an excessive exothermic reaction during the setting of a restorative?
2. What should a clinician do if they observe an adverse reaction to a dental material?
3. What requirements should the dental team observe when a new material arrives in the clinic?

Chapter | 4 |

The role of the manufacturer

INTRODUCTION

It is obvious that the manufacturer has a major role in the production of new materials which are suitable for use in the mouth. Over the past 40 years there has been a large increase in both the generic types of material and number of manufacturers producing them. This proliferation of products with their varied applications, particularly in restorative dentistry, has contributed significantly to the way modern dentistry is now practised compared with traditional techniques. The most obvious example is the ability of the dentist to prepare a tooth as conservatively as possible and then select the most appropriate material for the application. This compares with times gone by when the reverse was true as the few materials available determined the clinical preparation, often resulting in the needless loss of tooth tissue (Figure 4.1). This has

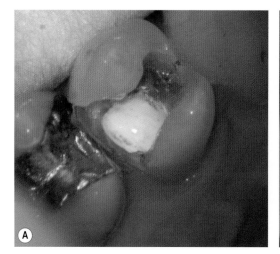 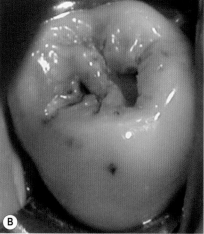

Fig. 4.1 (A) A large cavity relative to the size of the tooth after the removal of an old amalgam restoration showing substantial loss of tooth tissue. Compare this with (B), where the excision of only the small carious lesion is now necessary due to the availability of more modern materials. In this case, there is no need to remove excess tooth tissue to accommodate a traditional restorative material such as dental amalgam where mechanical retention is required to retain the material. This cavity was restored with a flowable resin composite material.
(Photo on the right courtesy of Dental Update.*)*

resulted in a change in philosophy in clinical dentistry. Each advance in dental materials science commonly leads to the production of new products. This increases the treatment options for the clinician, thus theoretically contributing to better care for the patient.

That said in the majority of cases, dental materials manufacturers use previously developed materials as a guide to what may be expected in clinical performance. These performance parameters are used in the development of new materials. New prototype materials which are subsequently produced are then judged against these criteria.

MATERIAL DEVELOPMENT

Problem identification and means of resolution

Most dental materials development is incremental. Only very rarely is an entirely new material developed from scratch. Usually, the manufacturer identifies a problem with an existing material and determines how to improve on or eliminate this shortcoming. Deficiencies are frequently identified in focus meetings with clinicians worldwide and from comments fed back by the sales team from their discussions with the end users, the dental team. New technology usually comes from the larger companies who have their own in-house research and development departments. These research teams examine the alternatives which may enhance material performance. Sometimes the developments come from outside the world of medicine and dentistry such as the astronautic industry (Figure 4.2).

Much of the work in recent years has been aimed to enhance the longer-term performance of the materials and their handling. These are probably the two most significant factors which influence dentists in their search for the 'ideal' material.

Prototype production

Certainly a number of advances in material technology in elastomeric impression materials and resin composites have never been launched for clinical use because their handling properties could not be resolved adequately. Initially, any prototype material is evaluated in the laboratory using a range of mechanical and physical tests to determine what experimental materials might be considered for use.

Dental materials testing

Clearly, the manufacturers of dental materials have no control over the oral environment. Furthermore, they have little control over chairside handling of the materials, but they can influence this by attempting to limit the variables that can contribute to failure. It is obvious that materials require to be extensively tested in the laboratory prior to becoming available to the dental profession.

Laboratory tests and their clinical relevance

It is important to be aware of the tests that manufacturers carry out, the limitations of these tests and the information yielded from them. This will assist in understanding technical information supplied by manufacturers. It will also aid extrapolation of the results to clinical usage. It should be remembered that the tests used are the same as those used in the evaluation of materials for other general applications. This presents a problem, as the size of the sample used in the testing is larger than it would be used in the mouth and therefore is not comparable.

Test specimen size

In order to be able to make a direct comparison between the test result and what happens in the mouth, it is desirable that the test specimen should be sized and shaped approximately to that used clinically. Unfortunately this is rarely possible due to:

- The small volumes of materials used in the mouth. Specimen sizes used in the laboratory are, of necessity, larger than their clinical equivalents. This leads to difficulty manipulating the material during specimen preparation as larger amounts are required to be handled than is used in the mouth.
- The difficulty of mixing these large volumes by hand or mechanically. Air is often incorporated into the mix and this will weaken the test sample. Any defect in the test specimen will result in erroneous results.
- Having to mix several capsules simultaneously. Frequently this will be required to prepare one specimen. This is difficult to achieve as multiple mixing machines are required and dispensation must be rapid otherwise the material will begin to set, which means that part of the test specimen will be prepared with material that has exceeded the working time and is in the setting phase.

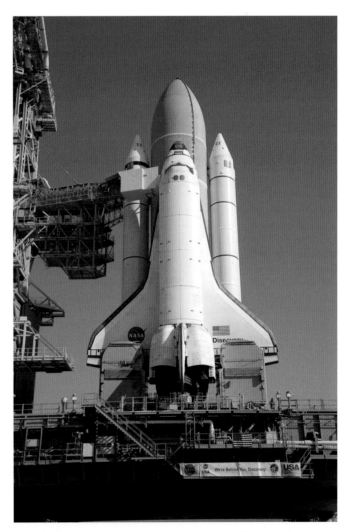

Fig. 4.2 The ceramic tiles used on NASA's space shuttles were the precursor to a cast ceramic restorative material.

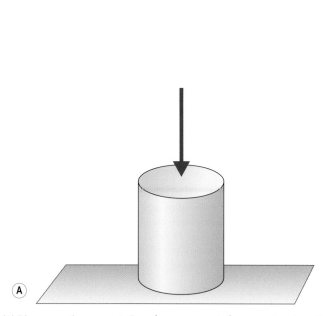
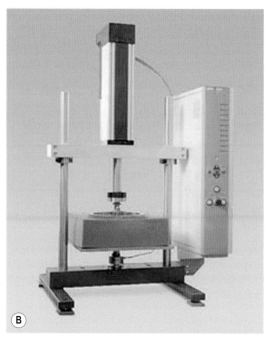

Fig. 4.3 (A) Diagrammatic representation of measurement of compressive strength. A load is applied vertically and the ability of the sample to resist the axial load is measured. (B) A Universal Load Testing Machine being used to measure the compressive strength of foam rubber (ZWICK).

MECHANICAL TESTS

Compressive, **tensile** and **flexural strengths** together with the **modulus of elasticity** of the material can be measured using a series of standard mechanical tests. **Compressive strength** is the ability of a material to withstand *axially* loaded pushing forces (i.e. applied along the long axis of the object, Figure 4.3) and has some relevance in demonstrating reproducibility and reliability of materials from batch to batch during production.

Firstly, a sample of the material to be tested is constructed in the shape of a cylinder of known dimensions, usually 6×4 mm in diameter. It is then conditioned for up to 24 hours at mouth temperature and often in water to simulate intraoral conditions after placement. The cylinder is placed between the platens of a **load testing machine** and the upper platen is driven down at a constant speed until the specimen fractures. The ultimate load applied over the surface area of the end of the cylinder is then calculated. To reduce the variation that may occur during specimen preparation, a number of specimens are produced and tested. The mean of the values at fracture are used to determine the compressive strength of the material.

The test for compressive strength is not a very good discriminator between different material types. The manner in which the test is carried out is obviously not representative of what occurs in the mouth. When a masticatory load is applied to the restoration, the tooth tissue surrounding the restoration will act as a support and help to withstand the occlusal forces encountered.

Platen: heavy duty sheet of metal which supports a test specimen without distortion during loading.

Masticatory load: the load applied to the biting (occlusal) surface of a tooth by the dynamic movement of the jaws and teeth together to shred food.

Tensile strength is the ability of a material to withstand pulling forces in an axial direction. There are two types of tensile test, one for brittle materials which do not deform (Figure 4.4) and the other for elastic materials which will elongate before breaking. The **diametral tensile strength test**, as its name implies, uses a cylinder of material of similar dimensions to the compressive test specimen, but in this case it is loaded along the long axis across its diameter. The compressive forces which are applied at the surface form stress concentrations within the specimen, which is equivalent to pulling the cylinder

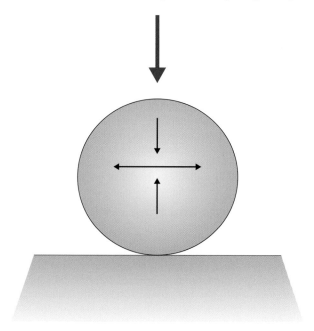

Fig. 4.4 Measurement of tensile strength. A load is applied vertically downward on a cylindrical object. As the cylinder is compressed, its centre is placed under tension. Failure is a result of this tensile stress.

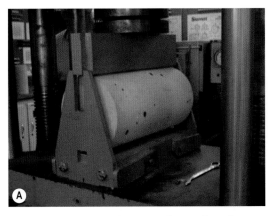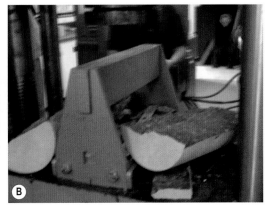

Fig. 4.5 A sample of Portland cement undergoing a diametral tensile strength test: (A) prior to loading and (B) after fracture.

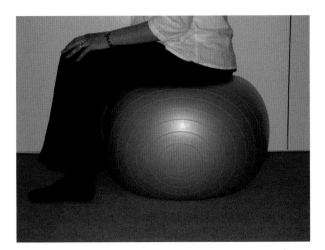

Fig. 4.6 An exercise ball under compression. Note distortion rather than fracture. Diametral tensile testing is unsuitable for materials of this type.

apart along the midline. This test is used for brittle materials, but it is not used very frequently as the reproducibility with dental materials is low (Figure 4.5).

The diametral tensile strength test is unsuitable for materials that are easily compressible as the material distorts before fracture. The calculation of the strength value relies on the measurement of the diameter of the sample prior to commencement of the test remaining the same throughout the test. As can be seen from Figure 4.6, an easily compressible material such as an exercise ball will deform with the horizontal diameter increasing by a substantial amount, while the vertical diameter is reduced, without any fracture occurring.

Tensile strength testing has greater significance with materials such as elastomeric impression materials as they may tear or stretch when withdrawn from between the teeth. If they stretch but do not return to their original shape, then the cast restoration constructed may not fit the prepared tooth. For these materials, a paddle-shaped specimen is prepared and connected to the two crossheads of a loading machine. The upper crosshead is then moved away from the lower and the paddle-shaped strip of material is stretched until it fractures. The elongation of the sample and the ultimate breaking strength are noted (Figure 4.7).

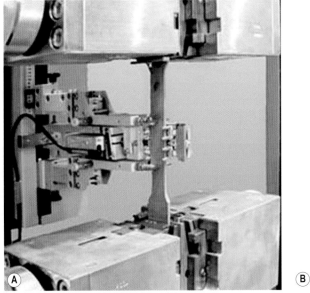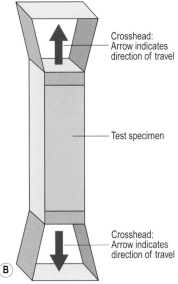

Crosshead: Arrow indicates direction of travel

Test specimen

Crosshead: Arrow indicates direction of travel

Fig. 4.7A,B (A) A laboratory test jig set up for tensile testing with specimen in place. (B) A paddle-shaped sample used in tensile tests for elastomeric materials.

Flexural strength is the ability of a material to resist load when unsupported. It is most closely related to a load being applied to a restorative material as the upper surface of the specimen is placed in compression whereas the underside is bent downward and is in tension. Flexural strength is also called **transverse strength**. Figure 4.8 shows the **three-point bend** test. Load is applied to the unsupported beam. Matchstick-shaped specimens are prepared, 2 × 2 × 25 mm in dimension. The ends of the sample are supported on two knife-edged blades which are positioned on the lower platen of the load testing machine. A knife edged blade is brought down onto the centre of the sample at a constant loading rate and the load is recorded when the sample breaks. This is then used to calculate the flexural strength.

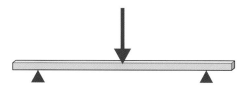

Fig. 4.8 Flexural strength being measured either using an unsupported beam as shown here or a disc supported in a ring, as shown in Figure 4.9.

Figure 4.9 demonstrates a **biaxial** system where the specimen is a disc supported on a ring. As with the three-point bend text, the top of the sample is put under compression while the underneath surface is

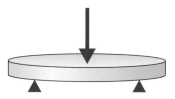

Fig. 4.9 A specimen under biaxial loading.

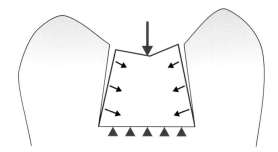

Fig. 4.10 An intracoronal restoration under load, showing support from the cavity floor and the risk of pull away from the walls.

placed in tension on the specimen. Here, however, any edge defects of the sample will not affect the test result since the edge of the sample is outside the area of material being tested, i.e. the supported area. In this case, a sample is prepared 1 mm thick and approximately 1 to 1.2 cm in diameter. The sample is positioned on an annular ring placed on the lower platen of a load testing machine and a load applied at the midpoint of the sample, the centre of the diameter of the ring, using the upper crosshead. The flexural strength is calculated from the ultimate breaking strain recorded. As with the test for compressive strength, it is difficult to extrapolate any results to the clinical situation as the floor of any cavity will provide support to this surface and as such this cannot be easily simulated in the laboratory (Figure 4.10).

There is often a lack of relevance and direct extrapolation between laboratory tests and clinical performance. The results of these tests are frequently used in product promotional literature and therefore should be interpreted with caution.

Modulus of elasticity

Modulus of elasticity describes the relative **stiffness** or **rigidity** of a material. Brittle materials have a high modulus of elasticity while **flexible** materials have a low value (Figure 4.11). Glass is a brittle material that exhibits little distortion before cracking when a load is applied to it (Figure 4.12).

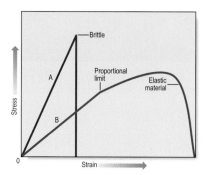

Fig. 4.11 A stress/strain diagram showing the effect of loading a brittle and an elastic material. Curve A illustrates a rapid increase in stress with very much less change in strain (the specimen does not bend). The point at which fracture occurs is where the plot drops to zero. Curve B represents an elastic material such as a rubber band. As a load is applied the rubber band stretches. A rapid increase in the strain occurs but the stress only rises slowly. After a period of time the rubber band passes the proportional limit.

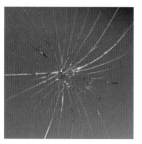

Fig. 4.12 A sheet of glass that has been subjected to a load, causing it to fracture. The force applied therefore rises quickly to a point where the glass breaks. This is explained in Figure 4.11.

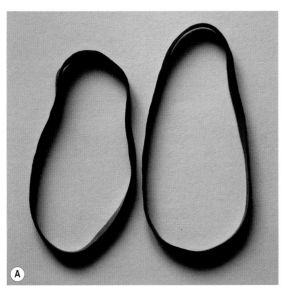 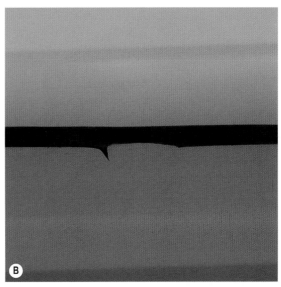

Fig. 4.13 (A) Two elastic bands, one of which has been strained such that it has passed the proportional limit. The increase in length can be seen in the one on the right when the band is allowed to return to unstressed condition. (B) Rubber band just prior to failure. The defect is just about to extend across the rest of the band. This means if the applied load is removed the rubber band will not go back to its original size. It will always be slightly bigger (A). Finally, if extension is continued after passing the proportional limit, the rubber band will break. This is again the point at which the plot in Figure 4.11 returns to zero.

> **Elastic deformation:** the ability of an object to return to its original shape when the applied stress is removed.
>
> **Plastic deformation:** permanent and non-reversible deformation of part or all of the object when stress is applied to it (Figure 4.13A).
>
> **Proportional limit:** The point at which a material begins to deform plastically when a stress is applied to it. Sometimes termed the **yield strength** or **yield point** (Figure 4.13B).

Combination of properties

It is readily apparent that any measurement of a single material property will only give some guide to the behaviour of the material within the mouth. Furthermore the forces applied to any material will be a combination of compression, tension and flexure, which will vary with the type of application and the surrounding tissue. A useful guide to the material's general behaviour is to consider the effect of compressive strength and modulus of elasticity together. As an example, a high compressive strength and high modulus indicates a strong but brittle material such as a ceramic.

The limitations of laboratory testing

Unfortunately testing is not straightforward and there are problems that need to be overcome.

- It is impossible to exactly replicate the oral conditions in the laboratory and this makes it difficult to properly test materials in a similar environment into which they will be placed.
- Many of the tests are limited in that they only address individual properties without necessarily looking at the interactions between the various properties evaluated. In contrast in the mouth a restoration may be subjected to several differing stresses at the same time. The outcome of this is difficult to predict with one test alone.
- The effects of ageing cannot be easily replicated out of the mouth. The ability to understand and predict how the

material will behave as it ages is clearly desirable for both the manufacturer and clinician. The only way of overcoming this is for the manufacturer to use experimental data previously gained, and they use these data to make an informed estimate of the minimum requirements for certain mechanical and physical properties for the material and its intended use.

Other properties to consider

Hardness is also reported for some materials, including both restorative and impression materials. This property can be misleading as there are various scales of hardness measurement. The principle in most cases involves the indentation of the surface and a subsequent measurement of the size and shape of the indentation. The indentations are very small and as such only give an indication of the surface behaviour of the material, which can be misleading particularly if the material has only set at the surface.

While these mechanical properties are often used as an indication of material benefit there are other tests which are of either similar or greater significance. These include properties such as thermal diffusivity, thermal conductivity, thermal expansion, water sorption, solubility, translucency, dimensional stability, fatigue, wear, corrosion and radiodensity.

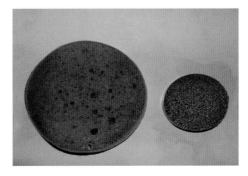

Fig. 4.14 Polymer disc before and after immersion in water for 6 hours, showing hygroscopic expansion due to water uptake and sorption.

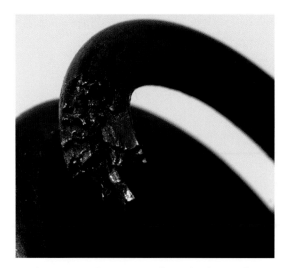

Fig. 4.15 A lorry spring where constant flexing has led to a fatigue fracture.

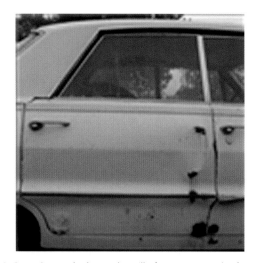

Fig. 4.16 Corrosion to the lower doorsill of a car as a result of water becoming trapped within the door frame and in the presence of oxygen starting a corrosion cell.

Hardness: resistance to permanent deformation by a constant load from a sharp object.

Thermal diffusivity: rate of transfer of heat from one side of a sample to the other.

Thermal conductivity: the ability of a material to conduct heat.

Thermal expansion: the change in a material's volume in response to a change in temperature.

Water sorption: increasing weight and volume of a sample of a material with respect to time on emersion in water due to water uptake. This increase in the bulk of a material due to the uptake of water is termed **hygroscopic expansion** (Figure 4.14).

Solubility: loss of weight of sample (**solute**) with respect to time when immersed in a liquid.

Translucency: ability of a material to permit the transmission of light.

Dimensional stability: ability to maintain shape and size with respect to time.

Fatigue: continual stressing of a material eventually leading to fracture (Figure 4.15).

Wear: loss of material occurring as a result of function.

Fracture toughness: an estimate of the stress required to cause a crack already present to propagation. It is generally associated with brittle materials such as ceramics and glasses.

Corrosion: a chemical reaction between the environment and the material leading to degradation of the material. Corrosion may be the result of interaction of the material with a chemical in the atmosphere. A good example of this is rust on a car body where contamination with salt on the road will lead to breakdown of the car body part (Figure 4.16.) Corrosion may also be initiated within a material after it has been stressed. A defect at a site within the material can then in the presence of chemical cause **stress corrosion**. An example of this is the Silver Bridge in Ohio, USA, where the stressing of an eye-bar led to a corrosive defect, which under load eventually failed, leading to the collapse of the bridge with catastrophic results (Figure 4.17).

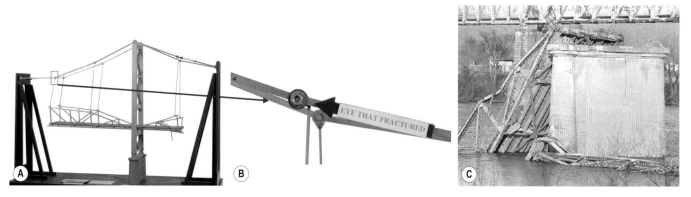

Fig. 4.17 (A) The Silver Bridge showing the eye bar where a defect occurred around the pin (B). This eventually led to a stress corrosion fracture and the collapse of the bridge (C).

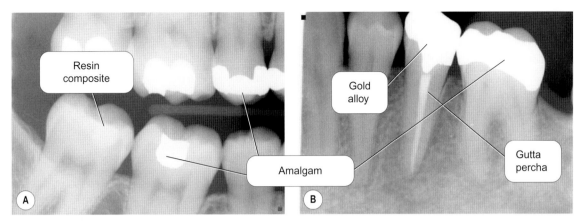

Fig. 4.18A,B Two dental radiographs showing the relative radiodensities of four commonly used restorative materials: gold, amalgam, resin composite and gutta percha.

Radiodensity

Restorative materials meant for either the crown of the tooth or for use within the root canal system should preferably be radiopaque. Modern materials are radiopaque either by virtue of being metallic (e.g. dental amalgam or gold) or because they have elements added to them to confer radiopacity, such as barium or strontium to the glass used in glass ionomer cements and resin composite. The relative radiopacities of various dental restorative materials are illustrated in Figure 4.18. Although the level of radiodensity may be different, their radiopacities contrast with the radiolucent (dark) appearance of dental caries thus facilitating caries diagnosis (Figure 4.19). In the past, some materials (e.g. some linings materials such as the original glass ionomer cements) were radiolucent and this posed a difficult dilemma for the dentist (Figure 4.20): Was caries present or had a radiolucent lining material been used?

In the case of an **endodontic** (root) filling, the whole root canal system needs to be obturated, and this may be seen more easily on a radiograph when a radiopaque material had been used. Any voids, over or under-fills may then be easily examined (Figure 4.21).

> **Radiodensity:** the property of the relative transparency of a material to the passage of X-rays through it.
>
> **Radiopaque:** any material that does not permit X-rays to penetrate it, the beam being absorbed by the material.
>
> **Radiolucent:** any material that permits the passage and penetration of X-rays through it.

Clinical handling properties

While the foregoing properties are important, the material will be judged mainly by its clinical performance, provided that is it being used as intended and directed. This includes ease of **mixing** and **handling**, the length of the **working** and **setting times**, ease of finishing and long-term durability. This is shown in Figure 4.22. While a restoration can be retained in the mouth for a long period of time (**longevity**), it may well have degraded substantially and this is a measure of its durability.

> **Finishing:** contouring and polishing of a material.
>
> **Durability:** the long-term stability of the material in function.

Fig. 4.19 Tooth 24 shows an area of radiolucency under the radiopaque filling material. The radiolucent area is dental caries which had started under a cracked dental amalgam restoration.

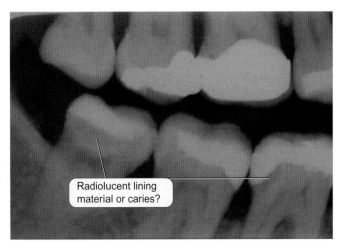

Fig. 4.20 A right bitewing radiograph with radiolucent areas under the radiopaque restorations in 46 and 48. Both of these radiolucent areas represent lining material.

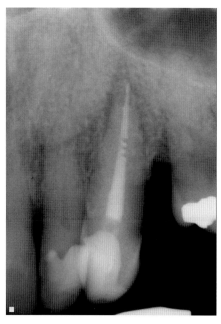

Fig. 4.21 A periapical radiograph of 23, which has been root filled. Note the void in the middle third of the otherwise well-obturated root canal system, which is easily seen due to the radiopacity of the root canal filling materials.

International Standards: these are documents produced by consensus between national specialist groups which lay down a series of minimum requirements for a generic type of material. Manufacturers may claim compliance with a standard. When they do this, any testing facility worldwide may carry out the recommended tests on a sample of the material. The test house results should be similar to those provided by the manufacturer and match those in the standard. The standards are produced by the **ISO**. This organization receives contributions from national standards bodies such as the **British Standards Institute** (**BSI**). In Europe, group standards for generic types of material are produced by the **European Standards Organization** (**ESO**). The contributions to all of the Standards are provided by experts in the specific field. These experts may come from manufacturers, retailers or academia. The principal purposes of standards are to:

♦ To provide protection to the consumer, in this case the dentist and the patient, from inadequate products
♦ To facilitate international trade, since the ISO standard is accepted worldwide. This has the advantage that each country does not have to produce its own requirements and standards.

Laboratory versus 'ideal' intraoral conditions

The closest environment to the ideal which can be created intraorally is when a rubber dam is placed. This means that any material placed under rubber dam may perform more as predicted in laboratory tests. That said, even here the humidity, temperature and the conditions in which the restoration is constructed can vary. This emphasizes the caution with which clinicians should treat the results of laboratory tests and is further emphasized and reinforced as normal intraoral conditions are even more different from those in a laboratory.

Minimum standards of materials

When manufacturers are developing improvements on existing materials, they will produce a prototype material that has properties which at least match (but generally greatly exceed) those laid down by the **International Standards Organization** (**ISO**) for each type of material. Once the prototype has been manufactured and tested, then the laboratory phase of the development is complete and the material is then ready for clinical evaluation (see website for information on ISO).

CLINICAL EVALUATION

Very often selected clinicians are invited to evaluate the new material or alternatively the company may use their own in-house dentists to use the material clinically and to monitor its performance. With any entirely new material it is quite common (but not essential) that a clinical evaluation is carried out by an independent operator or group to study the product's performance. This is not a requirement and frequently manufacturers' studies are only of relatively short duration. Long-term clinical evaluations are almost entirely carried out independent of the manufacturer, but suffer from the fact that after a relatively short period of time (for example 5 years or so) many of the materials used have been replaced by newer variants, rendering the information obsolete. New products are launched regularly in an attempt by manufacturers to keep their market share. It is therefore very difficult for the dentist to meaningfully analyse materials. It is widely acknowledged that dentists are carrying out clinical trials inadvertently by using a product for a long period of time and collecting information on their performance either formally or informally. The formally collated information may be published in the dental research literature but is more commonly discussed with colleagues. Customer opinions are fed back to dental manufacturers' sales representatives, collectively or individually.

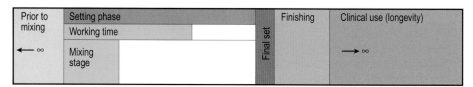

Fig. 4.22 Time line illustrating the life of a material from its constituents to its clinical use. It is important to note that the setting phase starts as soon as the components are brought together in the mixing phase. The working time is finite as setting of the material will be continuing until the material cannot be manipulated due to its increasing resistance as it is setting.

SCALE-UP

Once the material formulation has been established, it is necessary to scale up production to commercial levels. This in itself may cause difficulties as there are occasions where the scale up shows a problem that was not observed in the development phase. Fortunately, with many dental materials, the production runs are relatively small and this means that the size of the scale up does not necessarily present major problems. Recipes in a cookery book are a good analogy. If the recipe states that the quantities are intended for a number of servings then this will always work. If the cook needs to multiply or divide the quantities then the recipe will not necessarily turn out as expected.

QUALITY ASSURANCE AND CONTROL

Quality control is critical as the manufacturer needs to be able to consistently produce the material to the same standard at every production run. This process begins by monitoring the raw ingredients provided by external suppliers. These suppliers must certify that the ingredients conform to previously agreed specifications. The manufacturer will periodically verify this by carrying out analysis of the raw ingredients. The product is then synthesized according to a manufacturing specification and a sample of the material will be tested to a predetermined test programme. Once the batch has conformed to this standard, the material is placed into its packaging and labelled and stored. A small sample of each production batch is also retained so that should there be any complaint, the material can be checked. This is known as the **retained sample**. In all cases, the history of the research and development of the product together with the production programme is recorded in a design file which precisely provides all the details that any independent monitoring body can follow should the need arise.

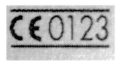

Fig. 4.23 A CE mark seen on the outer packaging of a dental adhesive product.

PRODUCT PRESENTATION AND LABELLING

Product presentation and labelling is partly the manufacturer's choice and partly a legal requirement. The product has to be defined as a **medical device** and conform to the requirements of the particular category of medical device (see 'The regulation of dental materials and the International Standards Organization' on the inside back cover of this book). Furthermore, if the manufacturer claims that the material conforms to a particular International Standard then this has to be clearly stated on some part of the packaging. Similarly if the product is sold within the European Union then it has to have a CE mark (Figure 4.23). This is a quality assurance certificate and entails an independent certifying body reviewing the documentation on the product and awarding the CE mark standard if the product complies. The documentation includes the Directions For Use (DFU) literature and the design file. Failure to get a CE mark means that the material may not be able to be sold within the European Union.

The labelling of any product is again governed by International Standards and there are certain requirements which have to be shown on the label (Table 4.1).

CE mark: this is part of the mandatory European marketing system for products which indicates their conformation to the essential requirements of a European Directive (Figure 4.23). The manufacturers have to provide proof that the product complies with these essential requirements. This process is scrutinized by what are know as **notified bodies** as part of the EU certification scheme. The guidelines for these requirements are set by national government agencies in collaboration. In the UK this 'competent authority' is the **Medicines and Healthcare products Regulatory Agency** (**HMRA**).

Table 4.1 The various warning labels found on dental materials and equipment

Information	Reason for inclusion and details	Symbol
Art Number	Code for product	Art. No **3385**
CE mark	See text for details	C€0123
Corrosive	Indication of risks attendant on the material	
Expiry date	Time from which the manufacturer determines that the material performance cannot be guaranteed	**2010-01**

(Continued)

Table 4.1 (Continued)

Information	Reason for inclusion and details	Symbol
Eye protection required/laser	Potential hazard to eyesight and that eye protection should be worn when handling equipment displaying this symbol	
Flammable	Indication of risks attendant on the material	
For dental use only	Defines the area for which the material may be used. Applications outside this area are at the user's own risk	'For professional dental use only'
Irritant	Indication of risks attendant on the material	
Lot number	For identification purposes so that the material can be compared with the retained sample made at the same time	LOT 0142296
Manufacturer's contact details	Contact for queries, etc	See Figure 4.24
Protect against water or direct sunlight	Advises storage conditions	
Recycling	Indicates material may be recycled	
Single use	These products should only be used once and then discarded	Single Use
Sterilization	Sterilized by radiation	Sterile R
Store between temperatures	Storage temperatures between which performance may be guaranteed	4–8 °C 39–46 °F 24 °C 75 °F 10 °C 50 °F

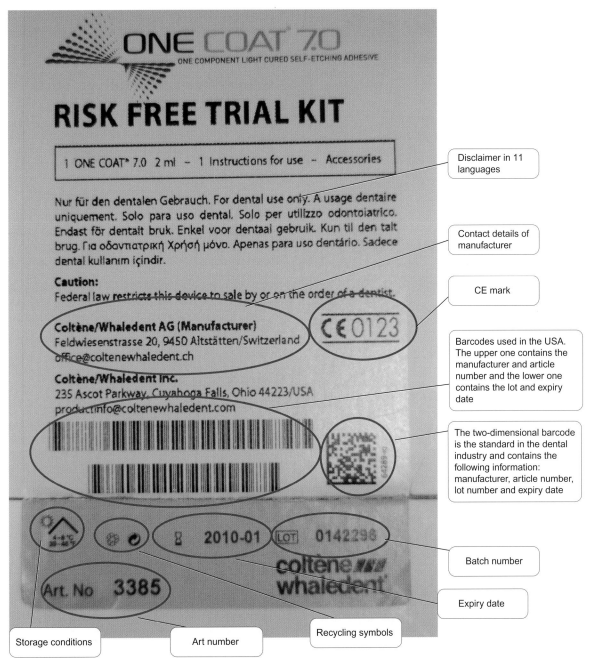

Fig. 4.24 The various warning labels found on dental materials and equipment.

Figure 4.24 shows an example of a label taken from a dental adhesive product with the salient information icons identified and explained.

TECHNIQUE CARDS

Summarized instruction guides and technique sheets are not governed by the same regulations and as such are not monitored with the same level of stringency. Technique cards (Figure 4.25) can be extremely useful as an aide memoire at the dental chairside particularly when the use of a particular material requires a number of sequential steps to achieve success, such as dentine bonding agents. The cards are frequently produced in a water-resistant form so that they can be used in the clinical environment without damage. The use of pictograms rather than text obviates the need for translation into many languages for universal comprehension. It should be said, however, that reliance on the technique sheet alone is unwise, and the DFU should be read in detail prior to using the material.

PRODUCT PROMOTION AND MARKETING

Once the material is released into the market, a range of marketing methods are used to attract clinicians to purchase the new material, for example:

- Advertising in the dental press
- Direct contact with company representatives
- By seminars organized by the company to promote the material. These are often hosted by a leading clinician who is sympathetic to the company. Such dentists are either from an academic or practice background and are known as **opinion leaders** or **key influencers (KIs)**.

Promotional literature

The amount of publicity and product promotion undertaken depends on the level of novelty and market share which the manufacturer feels the product will command. Promotional literature is produced often at not insignificant expense to achieve this. The dental team must be able to make an informed choice as to whether they understand what the product can do and they can confidently compare the new material with existing materials effectively. This will ultimately influence their decision so to whether they purchase the material.

Pitfalls in interpreting product promotional literature

Inevitably the marketing material will try to show the material in the best possible light and it should therefore be viewed with care. The end user should be aware of tactics employed in the marketing literature which may try to portray the material more favourably. While this information is true and not presented dishonestly, certain facts may be 'bent' in an attempt to flatter a particular material and perhaps play down the strengths of the rival products.

Naming other competing products

Very often, manufacturers compare their new product in a graph or table with other materials on the market to demonstrate its performance in comparison with those of the competitors. The manufacturer may choose to name their competitors' comparable products. This is done to demonstrate their product's superiority as they see it while unfavourably comparing the rival competing products. Equally, the selection of the unnamed materials to compare with may be done in such a way that the true competitors of the new material are not shown. The reason for anonymity is that if a competitor material is named then there may be legal challenge to the claims. This is likely to be on the grounds that the test methods adopted were not suitable or that the material was not handled in the correct manner.

Most manufacturers tend to use independent comparative studies, particularly when these have been published in peer-reviewed journals and show their material in a favourable light when compared with others.

Misleading graphs

Scale adjustment

By altering the scales on graphs, differences in performance can be accentuated. By producing graphs which do not have the full length axis but comparing them to full length axis graphs will show a marked difference in a particular test, which may not actually be the case.

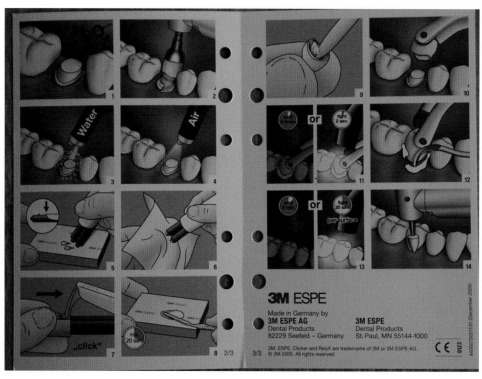

Fig. 4.25 A technique card for a cementing material for a crown (Rely X UniCem, 3M ESPE).

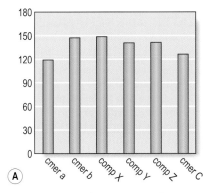 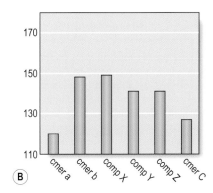

Fig. 4.26 Two bar charts illustrating the same information. One has a truncated y axis starting at 110 MPa (B) whereas the other shows the full length y axis (A). This accentuates the differences between materials where it may not be relevant.

In Figure 4.26 the two graphs of the tensile strengths of six restorative materials show the same results. In Figure 4.26B, where the y axis starts at 110 MPa, the value for compomer A appears far worst than the other materials but in Figure 4.26A, the y axis starts at 0 and the difference is not significant and would not influence clinical performance.

Error bars

Error bars indicate the **scatter** of results obtained when tests are carried out (Figure 4.27). Frequently graphs in promotional literature show no error bars, with only the average value for the results shown. This may highlight the fact that the results are quite variable with a wide scatter of values. It is wise to enquire about the variation in the results as this can give an indication of the ease of use of the material and consistency of its clinical performance. If these results were gained during laboratory testing then the situation will be much worse in the mouth where the conditions cannot be controlled to the same extent as in the laboratory. The following example illustrates this phenomenon.

Assume two materials (X and Y) are being tested for bond strength to dentine. The test is carried out 10 times for each material (see Table 4.2 for the results). The average bond strength in each case is 25 MPa (the sum of the results (250) divided by the number of tests (10)). The scatter of values for material X is between 24 and 26 MPa with very small variation in values (Figure 4.27). The other material (Y) has a similar average reading of 25 MPa. The scatter of result in this case is much greater, between 15 and 35 MPa. Although the mean bond strength values are similar, the larger variability and hence a less consistent performance is demonstrated by material Y even though higher bond strengths were sometimes gained (Table 4.2).

Table 4.2 Bond strengths (MPa) of two materials to dentine

Material X	Material Y
25	30
24	20
26	25
25	35
26	15
24	26
25	24
25	30
26	25
24	20
Mean 25 MPa	Mean 25 MPa

Company representatives – an educational resource

Dentists may have contact with a representative of the company and so may wish to question them on their products. Most company representatives are well briefed and they are able to answer any queries fully. Alternatively, specific or very technical questions may need to be referred to their scientific department for explanation. Box 4.1 suggests some questions which the clinician may wish to ask company representatives when they are presented with a new material.

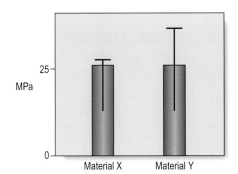

Fig. 4.27 Error bars demonstrate the scatter of results obtained during material testing.

Box 4.1 Questions for dental materials reps

- Is the chemistry of the system based on a current material? If not, how is it different and how does it work?
- What long-term studies are available to validate clinical performance? Who carried out these studies?
- What long-term laboratory studies have been carried out to evaluate ageing?
- For how long have the clinical evaluations been carried out?
- Any difficulties with manipulation and handling?
- What is the Weibull modulus?

WEIBULL MODULUS

One piece of information that is frequently missing from promotional literature is a measure of how dependable the product is. This is called the **Weibull modulus**. It was devised by a Swedish mathematician named Ernst H Waloddi Weibull and is the probability of failure versus applied stress. The higher the Weibull modulus, the more dependable is the part or material. This information is used in industry to predict when a part will fail, the weakest component being the weakness in the overall structure. A high Weibull modulus is desirable when considering aircraft parts as failure would not be desirable when flying! On the other hand, other manufacturers may wish their product to fail after a period of time in service (for example, household appliances) so that the consumer is forced to return to the market place to buy another product and hence repeat business. The Weibull modulus is becoming more recognized in dentistry. If the Weibull modulus is available for a dental material then it will give the user an indication of its likelihood of failure.

EFFECT OF THE NUMBER OF STAGES FOR PLACEMENT

A material which requires 14 stages for placement may have impressive laboratory results but will the clinician be able to achieve this in the mouth? It is highly unlikely, particularly consistently. For example, consider a new adhesive which requires eight stages to be placed. Each stage has a 95% success rate. The chance of the final result being a complete success is therefore:

$$95\% \times 95\% \times 95\% \times 95\% \times 95\% \times 95\% \times 95\% \times 95\% = 66.3\%$$

A rival product has a 90% success rate at each stage but has only three stages i.e. $90\% \times 90\% \times 90\% = 72.9\%$. The dentist would therefore be advised to select this product. Manipulation and mixing should be kept as simple as possible.

 The KISS (keep it simple stupid!) principle

Very often a material with seemingly lower success rate but a fewer number of stages will perform more consistently than a material boasting potentially higher success rates but with more stages. This should be borne in mind when the clinician is selecting materials for clinical use as it highlights the effect of operator variability on causes of failure.

MATERIAL HANDLING

The handling of the material is very much the clinician's preference and again each individual dentist will have different requirements. This means that just asking a colleague whether they are using the material is not a good way of ascertaining whether it will suit another dentist with similar experience and competence. It is the ease of handling of the material which should probably be the major influence to guide the clinician in their choice. This is one of the reasons why there are so many materials on the market. All these materials must reach a minimum standard if they claim conformity to ISO standards but equally the dentist must ask themselves 'Are they really that much different from one another?' What separates the average material from the good product is the consistency of performance. Much of this will depend on its ease of handling and manipulation, a factor that cannot be quantified as it is so personal between clinicians.

MATERIAL EXCHANGES AND PROMOTIONS

One of the frequent problems with a new material is that the clinician may well have large stocks of their currently used material which has already been purchased. If manufacturers are very keen to introduce a new material into a clinic, they may well offer to take back any unused stock and provide credit against the new purchase. Furthermore, if any new hardware is required, the manufacturer may give this away as a **loss leader** to entice the clinician into using the new material. Such marketing techniques may also retain the user's loyalty as the hardware may only be suitable for use with that particular manufacturer's products. Most manufacturers of dental materials make the majority of their profit on the sale of **consumables** and their resale time and time again. Very rarely is profit made on the hardware bought initially. Other manufacturers offer **start up (promotion packs)** piggy-backed onto a full kit so giving the dentist a no-strings-attached free trial. If the clinician does not like the product, then they can return the unopened full kit for a refund.

 If it ain't broke, don't fix it!

If a clinician is achieving good success with one particular material then why change to another?

SUMMARY

- The process from the genesis of the idea to clinical usage is a long and stringent one.
- Products must satisfy legal regulations to be sold and these may be specific to various countries and regions, for example the European Union.
- Promotional literature should be read with care and critically analysed.
- Material handling and performance are the most important criteria determining purchase by the clinician.
- It is possible that the clinician may need to identity radiographically the presence of a material in a tooth or indeed in other parts of the body. The levels of radiodensity required for comparison with other tissue must be considered.

FURTHER READING

Jacobsen, P.H., 2008. International standards and the dental practitioner. Dent. Update 35, 700–704.

SELF-ASSESSMENT QUESTIONS

1. Why may a mesial-occlusal-distal (MOD) amalgam restoration fail by fracture across the occlusal section when the patient bites together?
2. Why is it desirable that a restorative material is radiopaque?
3. What is the significance of laboratory testing on dental materials?
4. What part should clinical evaluation play in materials' development?
5. What is the role of CE marking of the material?
6. Describe the steps a manufacturer must take in order to bring a dental material to market.
7. Describe how promotional literature may mislead the reader into thinking a product is superior to its competitors.

Chapter | 5 |

Control and use of materials in practice

LEARNING OBJECTIVES

From this chapter, the reader will:
- Understand the significance of the control, storage and management of dental materials on arrival from the manufacturer before their use in the clinic
- Appreciate the importance of handling dental materials correctly prior to clinical use.

INTRODUCTION

The manufacturer is required to provide the material to the end user in an ideal condition for use. It is the responsibility of the dental team to maintain the product in this condition up to and including the time of use. In order to achieve this, a method of stock control and ordering is essential. Materials should be ordered in good time to prevent untoward absences of any material during critical procedures. Furthermore, manufacturers' instructions should be followed when using the material. Suitable methods of achieving these objectives have been set out below.

STOCK CONTROL MANAGEMENT

Economics and stock balance

Any hospital department, clinic or dental practice must hold a sufficient volume and range of dental materials which can be called on as the needs of the clinic dictate. As explained earlier, the process of getting a product to market is very costly and this significantly influences the retail price. Expensive dental products lying in stock cupboards as well as clinic drawers and cupboards represent significant capital commitment. The larger the practice or clinic, so more stock must be held. When establishing a business, the stock is a major capital investment and thereafter appears in annual accounts as current assets on the clinic's balance sheet. This is an important financial consideration as unless stock control is closely and carefully carried out, a large amount of capital will needlessly sit as stock, which may affect the profitability of the business and reduce available cash flow. This is clearly undesirable and with attention to a few factors, the volume of stock held can be minimized without impacting on the smooth running of the clinical operation. A minimum volume of stock should be held in the clinic as most operatories do not have sufficient space to store large amounts of materials. Ideally, the stock room should be situated centrally so that all clinics can easily access it. The primary objective is to have a good balance: sufficient yet not excess stock in the clinic, so obviating the need to go to the stock room for materials during a procedure. An ideal stock room carries sufficient volumes of stock so as not to run out, but not an excessive amount which will deteriorate with time, pass the usage date or ultimately, not be used and discarded.

Rationalize materials

A good working relationship and communication between the various dentists in a clinic can significantly reduce the volume of stock held. Many of the generic groups of materials are produced by more than one manufacturer as they compete for market share. There is little point in a clinic carrying more than one product of the same generic type of material from different manufacturers. For example, there is nothing to be gained by stocking two (or even more!) types of resin-modified glass ionomer lining cement. If the practice decides to use either Vitrebond Plus (3M ESPE) or Fuji Lining LC (GC) (Figure 5.1) then there is no duplication of similar materials. This rationalization between clinicians will decrease stock quantities hugely with no detriment to clinical care.

Same material, multiple indications

Some dental materials may be used appropriately for more than one indication and in different applications. This again permits the reduction in material range required by a clinic, as the dentist may use the same material for different indications. For example, the clear bite registration material (e.g. Memosil, Heraeus) can also be used as an occlusal matrix for posterior composites, obviating the need to

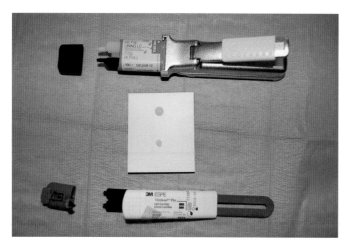

Fig. 5.1 Two similar presentations of resin-modified glass ionomer cement products (Vitrebond Plus, 3M ESPE) and (Fuji Lining LC, GC).

carry other bite registration products (Figure 5.2). Similarly, a material such as a flowable resin composite may be used in many applications (see Chapter 7).

Importance of the use-by date

With a smaller stock, a rapid turnover of materials will result in less wastage as the use-by date (following which the manufacturer will not guarantee the product will perform satisfactorily) will not be reached. Prior to use in the clinic, the use-by date of each dental material should be checked (Figure 5.3). If this date has been passed then the material should be discarded. Some of the ingredients might have degraded and the material may not perform as intended. For example, a catalyst not functioning properly will result in the material not setting fully, which in turn will impact on the material's physical properties and therefore its clinical performance. When removing materials from the stock cupboard, the material with the closest use-by date should be selected to decrease the risk of the stored stock exceeding its **shelf-life**. The shelf-life of the material may

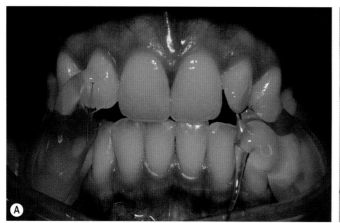

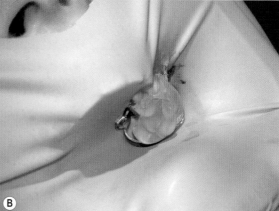

Fig. 5.2 A product (Memosil, Heraeus) being used for more than one application. (A) Use as a bite registration material and (B) as an occlusal matrix when using resin composite posteriorly.

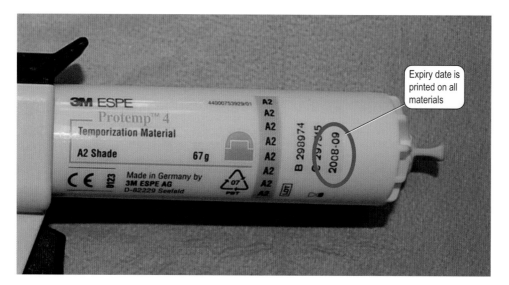

Fig. 5.3 Temporary crown and bridge material in delivery cartridge showing expiry or use-by date, in this example, end of September 2008.

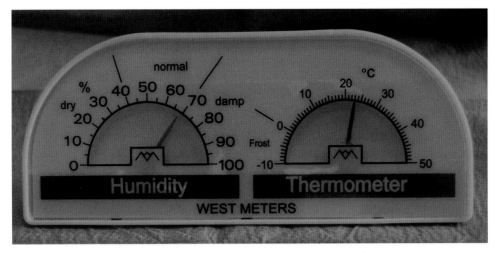

Fig. 5.4 Metering device to monitor room temperature and humidity.

play a part in influencing the dentist's selection of one material in preference to another. A longer shelf-life reduces the risk of the use-by date being exceeded and the material having to be discarded.

Use-by date: the date after which the manufacturer will not guarantee the product will perform satisfactorily.

To minimize exceeding the shelf-life of a material, place newly bought material *behind* the older material.

Stock ordering

It is apparent from the above that stock control must be well organized and carefully managed to achieve the delicate balance required. Many clinics now use a computerized stock database, and this has its advantages;

- At stock take (in many establishments an annual exercise or possibly even more frequently such as quarterly) the process can be carried out quickly by accessing the data by interrogating the computer program.
- Weekly ordering can be more quickly and easily done by determining what stocks were used since the last ordering day and therefore what needs to be replaced.

It is much more effective and efficient to carry out a regular ordering program rather than randomly ordering items from a dealer as the clinic runs out of a product. A report can be produced which can be either printed off or emailed to the dental wholesaler to order new stock, saving substantial staff time, another significant cost. For this to work effectively an ordering protocol must be devised and explained to all members of the dental team. They must all clearly understand the process. Generally the responsibility for placing orders should reside with one appointed member of staff. Most systems work by the 'one out, one in' principle, that is, when one unit of stock is removed from the stock cupboard, this is recorded and the information passed to the staff member responsible for ordering to replace it so as to maintain the stock balance.

 Efficient stock control

- Calculate accurately the minimum amount of stock needed for the running of the clinic.
- Store as much as possible in the central store cupboard and not in the clinic(s).
- Achieve agreement with all clinicians in the dental office to use the same products.
- Use materials which have multiple applications.
- Use products with earlier use-by dates first.
- Never use materials which are out of date.
- Develop an efficient computer-based system of stock control and delegate one member of staff to actively manage it.

STOCK ROOM ENVIRONMENT

The storage conditions under which the stock is kept is critical for optimum performance of the materials. The room should be at ambient room temperature and humidity as the extremes of these conditions have detrimental effects on a wide range of dental products. This can be easily and inexpensively checked by the purchase and usage of a temperature and humidity gauge (Figure 5.4). For example, if the room is too cold, then some elastomeric impression materials become stiffer. If these are then placed in an automatic mixing machine (e.g. Pentamix, 3M ESPE), the piston mechanism could be damaged. At low temperatures, some composites become very viscous and brittle in their pre-polymerized state, thus compromising their ease of handling (Figure 5.5).

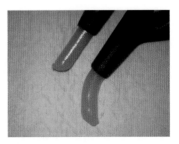

Fig. 5.5 Comparison between a resin composite stored in too cold a condition (upper compule) and another which is too warm. Note their different viscosities: the colder material is more rigid and the warmer one is more fluid.

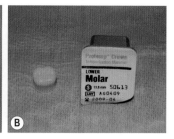

Fig. 5.6A,B Two temporary materials (GC Revotek LC, GC, and Protemp Crown, 3M ESPE) that are presented in light-tight containers to protect them from degradation before use.

Too high a temperature will result in premature ageing of products and so compromise their clinical performance even before they reach their use-by date. The temperature of the clinic is likely to be much higher than the store cupboard and show greater fluctuations in temperature, reinforcing the concept of storing a minimum amount of materials to prevent them from degrading. There may be a need to provide a small refrigerator in the stock room since there are some materials, such as some of the bonding systems, which require storage in a refrigerator to prolong their shelf-life. Other materials are photolytic and should be kept out of direct sunlight and in light-proof containers in which they are presented (Figure 5.6).

USE IN THE CLINIC

All materials come with an instruction or directions for use (DFU) book (or books as a recent European Union directive prescribed instructions to be provided in 27 languages). It is essential that this information is consulted prior to usage and the instructions are followed exactly. Frequently, when a new pack is opened all the packaging and instructions for use are discarded without thought (Figure 5.7).

This temptation should be resisted as materials can and do evolve and the manufacturer may change their recommendations for use. Failure to note and adapt to these changes may result in the material being used inappropriately, and leading to a decreased clinical performance.

Many clinics retain instructions books and arrange them in a file (Figure 5.8), which is considered to be good practice. An additional benefit is that only one set of instructions need to be kept and all staff are aware of the availability of this file, which they can readily access. It is important to note that this resource needs to be updated with any new instruction books being filed immediately as new packs are opened. The responsibility for monitoring this practice should reside with one person, preferably the person responsible for the ordering and acceptance of stock.

- When a new material is received, all clinical staff should be informed of this and the DFU should be filed in the instruction book file.
- One of the duties of the staff member ordering and receiving the goods should be to check that the new DFU is similar to that on file. There are occasions where minor changes are made by the manufacturer which require different methods of handling the material.

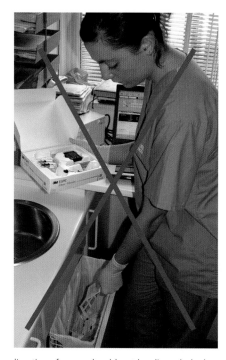

Fig. 5.7 The directions for use should not be discarded when a new material arrives!

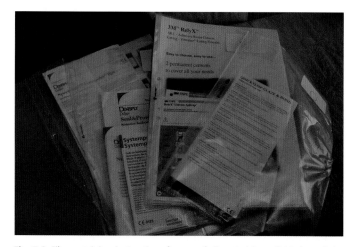

Fig. 5.8 File containing instructions for use of all materials available in a clinic.

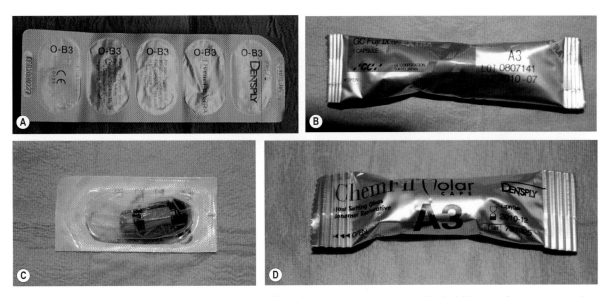

Fig. 5.9A–D Compomer, encapsulated glass ionomer and resin modified glass ionomer cements stored in their blister packs to prevent moisture ingress.

Protective product packaging

Manufacturers go to great lengths and expense to present their products so that they arrive in the clinic in optimum condition. Materials presented in foil bags or sealed dimple (blister) packs should be left in these protective coverings until required for use (Figure 5.9).

Many of these materials, for example compomers, are designed to absorb water during function. If they are exposed to moisture during storage then the material performance and setting may be compromised prior to placement in the mouth. It may seem inconvenient and a waste of precious clinic drawer space, but it is essential to store products as they are presented.

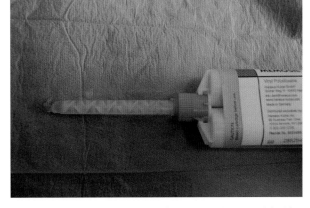

Fig. 5.10 Cartridge delivery containing bite registration material with mixing tip *in situ* to prevent cross-contamination between the two tubes leading to premature set.

Storage and care of materials

- Check the temperature and humidity of the store are always correct.
- Follow manufacturer's instructions on storage, e.g. keep in the refrigerator, dark, etc.
- Store in presentation packaging until ready for use, both in the store and the clinic.
- In the clinic, store partially used cartridges with the previously used mixing tip on; never replace the cap as it may initiate the setting reaction, *but* ensure that the external surface is decontaminated by wiping it with an alcohol wipe (Figure 5.10).
- Collate directions for use (instruction) guides and keep in a central file as a reference tool.
- Read directions for use with every new pack of material and follow these instructions fastidiously.

Cross-contamination considerations

Cross-infection is of great importance in clinical practice. All instruments that are likely to come into contact with a patient should either be disinfected, sterilized or disposed of and incinerated or otherwise safely destroyed. The presentation of some materials has been designed to facilitate this. The two most common presentations of a resin composite are a compule and a syringe (Figure 5.11).

The compule presentation has been designed to be used once on a single patient and then discarded, thus obviating the need for disinfection. This presentation is superior from a cross-infection perspective, if used in such a manner. A syringe cannot be effectively disinfected and so more care must be used when handling this

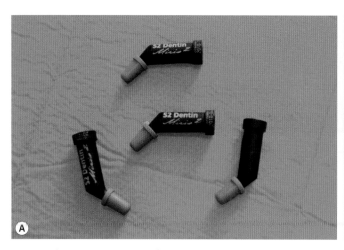
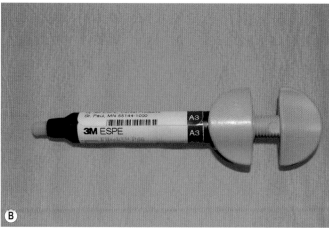

Fig. 5.11 The two presentations of a resin composite: (A) a single use compule and (B) a syringe for multiple use.

presentation. The correct amount of material required must be dispensed onto a mixing pad by either a 'clean' nurse or by the chairside ('dirty') nurse having carried out disinfection procedures namely degloving, washing and drying hands and re-gloving before re-entering the 'dirty' zone. If further material is required then this process becomes time consuming and, under the pressures of clinical dentistry, this frustrating procedure must be repeated so as not to contaminate the syringe stored in the 'clean' zone.

Clearly some products provide the clinical team with a problem as to how to disinfect them effectively after use. The cartridge with its mixing tip left in situ in Figure 5.10 will have been handled by the dentist and probably used intraorally. As such it will need to be effectively decontaminated prior to use on another patient. It would be both impractical and uneconomical for this product to be used only once as much material would be wasted. Equally it could not be autoclaved as this process would destroy the material's contents so rendering them unusable. The dental team's only solution to this dilemma would be to thoroughly wipe down the cartridge with an alcohol wipe. While this is not ideal, it is probably the only appropriate means of decontamination of the product. However, single-use disposable sheaths are now available for certain products (Figure 5.12), which obviate the need for the dental team treating the patient to touch the product during clinical use and should be used wherever possible.

Material wastage

Wastage is potentially a major problem in clinical practice and is of financial and environmental importance. The choice of compule versus syringe presentation has advantages and disadvantages from a disinfection perspective. Similarly, one presentation is superior with respect to wastage. More material may be potentially wasted by using compules whereas syringes have the advantage of minimum wastage if used with care. However, in practice there is a tendency to dispense too much material from a syringe, thus negating the theoretical advantage. The overriding factor between the amount of material wasted and effective cross-infection must be the latter, and this may be the most compelling factor to influence the clinician when choosing a material's presentation.

Another potential for wastage is the size of mixing tips in impression materials and some paste/paste composite systems (Figure 5.13). These involve an inevitable amount of material being wasted in the mixing process, particularly so when larger mixing tips are employed as more material is retained within the tip after mixing. However, with the largest mixing tips, the volume of material which goes to waste is less than 3 ml, which is much less than would be left on the mixing pad after hand mixing.

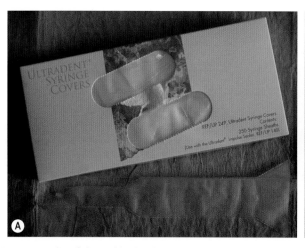
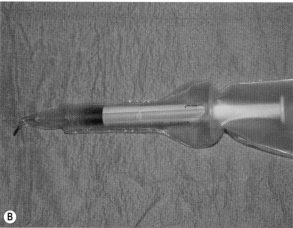

Fig. 5.12A,B Examples of disposable sheaths used to prevent the dental team from touching a product which cannot be effectively decontaminated.

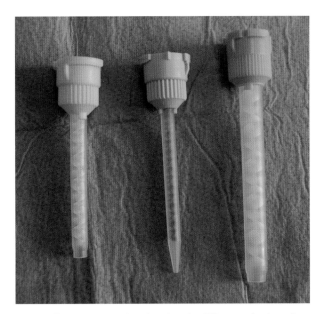

Fig. 5.13 Different mixing tubes showing the differences in the volume mixed which cannot be used and so is wasted.

The initial amount of dispensed impression material should not be used as it may not have mixed properly. However, it can be used to gauge the setting of the rest of the mix. Due to the higher temperature in the mouth, any material placed there will set more quickly than extraorally. This means that when the material on the mixing pad has set, the material in the mouth must have also set (Figure 5.14).

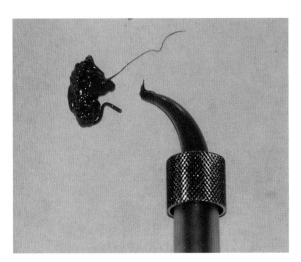

Fig. 5.14 A small amount of expressed impression material on the bracket table used as a guide to completion of set.

Additionally, less wastage means less discarded waste, and a decrease in the amount of material being placed in a landfill site or reduced carbon emissions when material has to be incinerated. While some wastage is inevitable, with thought and good management, this may be reduced to a minimum.

Minimize wastage!

- Only dispense what is likely to be used onto the mixing pad.
- Think about product presentation with respect to wastage.
- Use instruments and product presentations that are capable of being disinfected.

Material selection

The last consideration in the use of materials in the clinic is the clinician's choice and the rationale behind this. It is well documented that with the paucity of evidence-based research underpinning much of clinical dentistry, the selection of any given procedure and its associated materials is down to the dentist's clinical judgement, hunches, and experience. Pose a clinical problem to 10 dentists and they may come up with 10 entirely appropriate but different answers. Since all materials now conform to a minimum standard, the tendency is to select a material that handles in a specific way or features a presentation that the dentist prefers. However, ultimately the final choice may be determined by the cost.

It is hoped that this book may help the clinician to increase his or her knowledge and understanding of the dental materials currently available and to develop their rationale for appropriately and consistently selecting the most suitable material for any given situation. This will hopefully maximize clinical success and the patient's and dental team's satisfaction.

No dental material is ideal and no dental material is suitable for all applications. The clinician must therefore make an informed decision taking into consideration the properties and limitations of the material with regard to the clinical situation.

SUMMARY

- Efficient stock control management is important from a financial and logistics point of view.
- With careful thought, diligent management and cooperation between colleagues, the quantities and range of stock items can be minimized without impacting on the clinical operation. This reduces the amount of material wastage and capital tied up in stock.
- Materials should be stored as per the manufacturers' recommendations, so that they are in optimum condition when they are used.
- It is imperative to read the DFU, otherwise it is likely the material will not perform appropriately in clinical use.

SELF-ASSESSMENT QUESTIONS

1. Why is it important to have a stock control regime?
2. What factors would influence the purchase of compules versus syringes in the case of a resin composite?
3. How can a clinic owner reduce material wastage to a minimum?
4. Why is it essential to read the instructions prior to any given material use?
5. Why should the material be retained in its packaging during storage and prior to use?

Section | II |

Direct restorative dental materials

Chapter | 6 |

Dental amalgam

LEARNING OBJECTIVES

After studying this chapter, the reader will:

- Understand what dental amalgam is and the significance of its constituents
- Be aware of the types of alloy available, their advantages and disadvantages and the names of the currently available commercial products
- Understand the properties of dental amalgam and how they influence clinical performance
- Be aware of its manipulation and handling
- Understand the rationale behind bonding amalgam in situ
- Have an increased appreciation of how to use the material more effectively
- Understand the health and safety aspects of using dental amalgam.

DEFINITION

An **amalgam** is formed when an alloy of two or more metals is mixed with mercury. This reaction is called **amalgamation**. **Dental amalgam** is the product of the amalgamation between **mercury** and an alloy containing **silver**, **tin**, often **copper**, and sometimes other elements combined in varying amounts.

HISTORY

Dental amalgam has been used to treat teeth for many centuries. Substantial research during this time and particularly in the past 40 years has resulted in refinements of the constituents, culminating in the alloys which are used today. All this work has ensured the consistent handling, properties and clinical performance of the material. It is indeed a testimony to the material's many attributes that despite the huge advances in dental materials science, dental amalgam is still widely used today.

WHEN TO USE DENTAL AMALGAM

When placed correctly, dental amalgam has sufficient strength to withstand the high loads generated during mastication. It is therefore chiefly indicated for:

- The restoration of Class I and Class II cavities, particularly those of moderate to large size
- Core build-ups: when the definitive restoration will be a cast restoration, such as a crown or bridge retainer, as more tooth structure will need to be replaced and the tooth reinforced.

Dental amalgam is used mainly in the posterior sextants of the mouth because of its unaesthetic appearance (Figure 6.1). However, as amalgam is not tooth coloured, the core material and the tooth

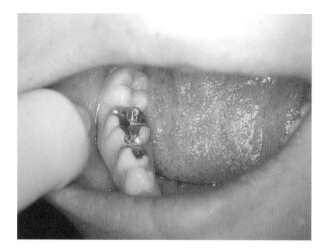

Fig. 6.1 Teeth 46 and 45 restored with dental amalgam – note the non-tooth coloured appearance of the restoration.

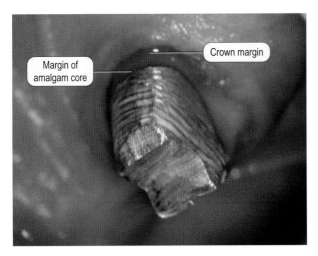

Fig. 6.2 Tooth 25 core restored with amalgam. Note the contrast between the amalgam core colour and tooth, facilitating identification of the margin of the core and of the preparation placed on tooth tissue.

Table 6.1 Constituents of dental amalgam alloy

Element	Function
Silver	Main constituent of alloy, combines with tin
Tin	Combines with silver
Copper	Increases mechanical properties, decreases creep, increases corrosion resistance, decreases the amount of the γ2 phase formation
Zinc	Acts as a scavenger of oxygen
Mercury	Sometimes added to increase the rate of reaction (pre-amalgamation)
Indium, palladium, selenium, platinum, gold	All increase corrosion resistance and improve certain mechanical properties of the final product. Decrease creep

tissue can be easily identified, ensuring that the margins of the crown are placed onto tooth tissue and not the core material (Figure 6.2).

Alloy: the by-product of the fusion of two or more metal elements after heating above their melting temperatures.
Class I cavity: a one surface preparation involving the occlusal surface of a posterior tooth.
Class II cavity: a two or more surfaces preparation that involves the proximal surface of a posterior tooth.
Sextant: One of the three sections into which a dental arch can be divided.

COMPOSITION OF DENTAL AMALGAM

The basic amalgamation reaction is that of mercury reacting with the surface of the alloy particles.

Mercury

The mercury used for dental amalgam is produced by distillation. It is distilled three times (like Irish whiskey!) to remove any impurities. This is important as contamination leads to inferior physical properties and adversely affects the setting characteristics of the amalgam. Contaminated mercury has a dull surface. Most dental amalgam products used in dentistry today are presented in encapsulated form (see p. 62). This means the dentist should have less concerns about the purity of the mercury as this is packaged in the manufacturing plant.

The alloy

Prior to 1986, all alloys, whatever their composition, were referred to as **conventional alloys**. However, work in the preceding decade evaluating the differing elemental compositions of the alloys increased the understanding of the structure and properties of the dental amalgam formed. These newer alloys produced dental amalgams which exhibited superior clinical performance.

Conventional alloys

The typical constituents of commercially available conventional alloys, their functions and clinical influence are shown in Table 6.1.

Amalgamation reaction of a conventional alloy

The mercury reacts with the outer layer (3–5 μm) of the silver–tin alloy particle in a reaction shown in Figure 6.3A. This means the bulk of the particle is left unreacted. These unreacted cores sit within a matrix of the silver–mercury and tin–mercury phases. The structure of the set material is shown in Figure 6.3B.

The role of zinc

Zinc was traditionally included in the alloy because it acts as an oxygen **scavenger** during the alloy's initial production. It preferentially reacts with any oxygen present to produce clean castings of the ingot. Alloys containing more than 0.01% zinc are called **zinc-containing alloys** and those containing less than this are termed **zinc-free alloys**.

If a zinc-containing dental amalgam is contaminated with water from saliva during the condensation process, it produces hydrogen gas, which becomes incorporated within the setting amalgam mass and leads to excessive delayed expansion. This is clearly undesirable and may cause pain and even tooth fracture. Good moisture control is therefore highly desirable when placing dental amalgam restorations (as with any other restorative material) and, in particular, those alloys containing zinc. Most modern alloys are now manufactured in an inert atmosphere so the need for zinc has been obviated.

The gamma (γ)2 phase

The γ2 (tin–mercury, see Figure 6.3) phase is the most chemically and electrically active component of the set amalgam. Its physical properties are inferior than the γ (silver–tin) and γ1 (silver–mercury) phases and its presence in conventional amalgam alloys results in:

*   Reduced strength
*   Increased susceptibility to corrosion
*   Increased creep (a conventional amalgam restoration shows about 6% creep).

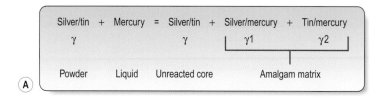

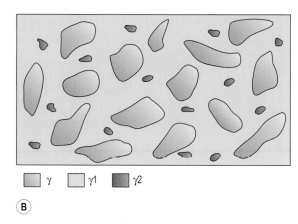

Fig. 6.3 (A) The setting reaction of dental amalgam. (B) The three major phases of set amalgam.

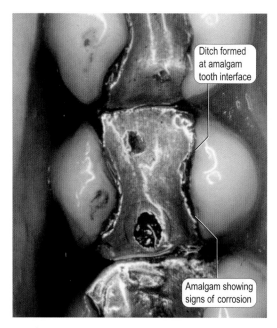

Fig. 6.4 Amalgam restoration in tooth 15 showing long-term guttering and loss of contour.

> **Creep**: gradual dimensional change under load. The clinical consequence of creep is ditching of the amalgam margin altering the marginal contour. This increases the potential for plaque retention (Figure 6.4).

High copper amalgam alloys (Figure 6.5)

More recently, attempts have been made to reduce or even eliminate the γ2 phase by increasing the copper content in the alloy to above 13%. This modification of the setting reaction has resulted in some important beneficial changes in the properties of the amalgam:

- Early full strength achieved within 1 hour of placement
- Increased mechanical properties, e.g. compressive strength
- Reduction in creep and therefore ditching (creep values of these alloys are between 0.09% and 1.8%)
- Reduced corrosion potential.

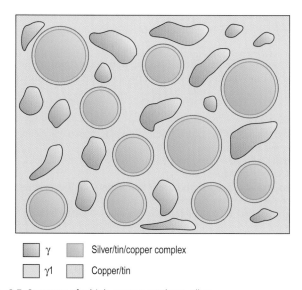

Fig. 6.5 Structure of a high copper amalgam alloy.

Setting reaction of high copper amalgam

The setting reaction of these alloys is the same as the reaction for conventional alloys (see Figure 6.3A). After the formation of the γ2 phase, there is a reaction between this and the silver–copper component, leading to the formation of a copper–tin phase and γ1. Although silver is present in the alloy particles, there is a preferential reaction between the copper and tin, thus forming a silver–tin–copper complex. The result is that little or no γ2 is left in the final amalgam.

Types of high copper amalgam alloy

There are two types of high copper amalgam alloy:

- **Dispersed phase alloys** – in these alloys, the copper is dispersed throughout the alloy and has the effect of increasing its strength. The alloy particles consist of either silver–tin or silver–copper. This means that the total silver content may be kept the same as in conventional alloys.
- **Ternary alloys** – ternary means a compound containing three elements, usually silver, tin and copper in this case. Ternary alloys are sometimes called **unicompositional** alloys as they have all three components in one particle.

Many manufacturers reduce the silver and tin content when increasing the copper content. A small amount of zinc is sometimes added to high copper amalgam to improve its clinical performance, in particular by decreasing marginal breakdown. Table 6.2 gives the general composition of the three types of alloy.

Table 6.2 Typical percentage composition of amalgam alloys by weight

Alloy type	Silver	Tin	Copper	Zinc
Conventional	63–70	26–28	2–5	0–2
Dispersed phase	40–75	0–30	2–40	0–2
Ternary	40–60	17–30	13–30	0

Implications of the composition of the alloy for corrosion

The susceptibility of the $\gamma2$ phase to corrosion offers a clinical advantage. The corrosion products fill the microgap (marginal gap) at the tooth–amalgam interface, which helps to decrease microleakage. One drawback of the high copper amalgam is that the microgap persists due to lack of the $\gamma2$ phase, and so these alloys have been associated with greater microleakage. Clinically, this may manifest as increased postoperative sensitivity with a risk of recurrent caries. It has been suggested that an intermediate bonding agent should be used in combination with these alloys to seal the dentine at the microgap (see p. 61).

> **Microleakage:** leakage of minute amounts of fluids, debris, and microorganisms through the microscopic space between a dental restoration or its cement and the adjacent surface of the cavity preparation (adapted from Mosby's Medical Dictionary, 8th edition. © 2009, Elsevier).

Types of alloy

Currently, three types of dental amalgam alloys are available: **lathe cut**, **spherical** and **admixed** (Figure 6.6). Their handling characteristics are all very different and it is important that they are manipulated correctly when used in the clinic for optimal performance of the set product (see pp. 63–65).

Lathe cut (irregular) alloys

These alloys are formed by grinding an ingot of the alloy, which produces irregular particles of varying size ranges. The different sizes of particle require different handling and their reactivity with mercury also varies. A blend of various particle sizes is used by the manufacturer to control the properties and working and setting times of the amalgam. Sometimes, after the machining process, the particles are too reactive to be used. If they are used in this state, the setting reaction would be too rapid (especially for the smaller particles as their surface area to volume ratio is higher). During commercial production, the alloys are placed in boiling water to reduce their reactivity.

Spherical alloys

These alloys are made by heating the alloy components to a molten liquid and then spraying this liquid into an inert atmosphere, usually argon. The particles coalesce as they fall, forming solidified spheres.

Admixed alloys

As the name suggests, admixed (sometimes called **blended**) alloys contain a combination of irregular and spherical particles (Figure 6.6).

The clinical ramifications of the alloy types are reflected in the different handling properties between them. Traditionally, a moderate amount of force was required to pack the amalgam in the cavity. Dentists prefer this handling characteristic and so some manufacturers have attempted to mimic this property with the newer spherical alloys by sandblasting the particles. The clinician can exert greater condensation pressure when using an admixed alloy than with other, untreated, spherical alloys.

PROPERTIES OF DENTAL AMALGAM

Strength

The dental amalgam must be strong enough to withstand forces during function, and ideally develop early strength so that it is not damaged before it is fully set. The material (as with other brittle materials) is strongest in compression and weakest in tension. The properties exhibited by the final set material depend on the structure of its various phases, their proportions and their individual strengths.

- The weakest phase is the $\gamma2$ phase so that any increase in the amount of this phase weakens the material.
- High copper and spherical alloys have higher early compressive and tensile strengths than conventional alloys.

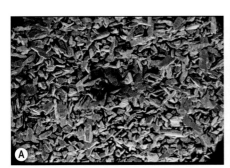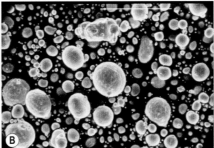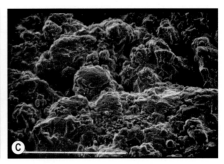

Fig. 6.6A–C Scanning electron micrographs showing the structure of (A) lathe cut (field of view 1 mm), (B) spherical (field of view 45 μm) and (C) admixed amalgam alloys (field of view 20 μm).

Thermal diffusivity and thermal expansion

As dental amalgam is metallic, it transmits heat readily (the material has a high thermal diffusivity, $9.6\,mm^2/s$). Its coefficient of thermal expansion ($22–28\times10^{-6}/°C$) is greater than that of the surrounding tooth. During thermal cycling, significant expansion and contraction may lead to:

- Microleakage
- Fracture of a tooth that has been weakened by tissue removal during cavity preparation for the treatment of dental caries
- Risk of pulpal damage in a deep cavity due to temperature rise.

Dimensional stability

When dental amalgam is setting, a dimensional change occurs. Initially the material contracts slightly as the mercury diffuses into the outer surface of the alloy particles and reacts with the silver and tin portions. The material then expands as the amalgam is setting because the ($\gamma1$) crystals expand by growth. From a clinical perspective, the combination of these two phenomena should not lead to any significant expansion or contraction:

- Excessive contraction leads to a large marginal gap between the material and the cavity.
- Expansion leads to extrusion of the material out of the cavity.

Other factors that can affect dimensional change of the amalgam are the size and shape of the particles and the type of alloy used. As previously mentioned, zinc-containing alloys expand significantly if contaminated with water at placement. The quality of the clinical condensation also affects dimensional change, so thorough condensation is important.

Working time

The working time of a dental amalgam is influenced by:

- Chemical composition
- Particle size of the alloy
- Any ageing treatments carried out during its manufacture.

Fast-, regular- and slow-set amalgams are available on the market and which of these is used is largely a matter of the dentist's preference as to the speed of set required.

Inexperienced clinicians are strongly advised to use a slow-set alloy until they have gained sufficient experience, because failure to condense the material quickly will result in an inferior restoration. If a crown preparation is to be carried out at the same appointment as placing an amalgam core, a fast-setting amalgam should be used.

Cavity design

Correct cavity design is important for the success of the final (amalgam) restoration.

- A minimum cavity depth of 2 mm is required because of the risk of fracture.
- No sharp internal line angles (Figure 6.7) should be left as this will lead to stress concentration in the juxtaposed material or lead to fracture.

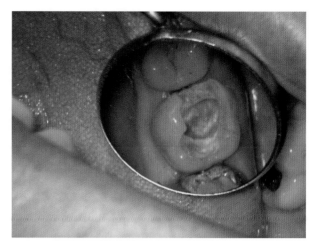

Fig. 6.7 A mesio-occlusal cavity showing no sharp line angles and appropriate cavo-surface angles.

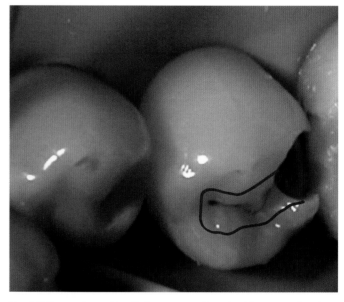

Fig. 6.8 Comparison of tooth tissue removal required for conventional (red outline) and bonded restoration (prepared cavity).

- Attention should also be paid to the cavo-surface angles (see Figure 6.7) so that neither weak amalgam nor weak unsupported tooth is left at the margin.
- If after caries removal, the cavity is not retentive, mechanical retention should be provided or preferably, the amalgam bonded in situ. Figure 6.8 illustrates the amount of tooth tissue conserved if the restoration is bonded as opposed to removing more tooth structure to create mechanical retention.

With all types of amalgam, sufficient bulk of the material needs to be used because dental amalgam is brittle and will fracture when used in thin sections.

Today, most amalgam restorations placed are due to failure of previous restorations. A method of quickly removing the existing restoration involves making two cuts in the shape of a cross, thus dividing the old amalgam into sections. These pieces can then be easily removed (Figure 6.9).

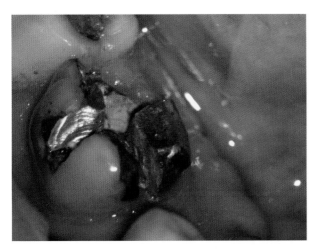

Fig. 6.9 A cruciform cut across an old amalgam, demonstrating ease of removal. Note that a quarter of the amalgam has already been lost.

BONDING OF AMALGAM RESTORATIONS

Dental amalgam does not bond to tooth structure. Thus, it cannot provide a complete seal or be retained in the cavity without some form of additional retention. If, after cavity preparation, inadequate tooth tissue remains to create a retentive cavity, mechanical retention may be created by:

- Cutting slots or grooves into the remaining tooth
- Placement of a dentine pin.

Bond: a general term that describes the technique in which attachment of a restorative material to tooth structure is attempted. These may be chemical or physical bonds between the two components.

The well-documented problems associated with the use of dentine pins may be found in operative dentistry texts. From a dental materials point of view:

- Their presence causes significantly stress concentrations in the restorative material (as well as in dentine) surrounding them
- There is also the problem of adaptation of the restorative material to the pin, particularly if the material is non-metallic
- If there is a large difference in coefficient of thermal expansion between the material and dentine pin, the material will shrink away from the pin during thermal cycling.

Instead of these mechanical auxiliary retention devices, an adhesive can be used to retain the amalgam in the cavity (Box 6.1). Many of the principles underpinning this technique are covered in

Box 6.1 Potential advantages of bonding amalgam

- Decreased microleakage
- Decreased incidence of recurrent caries
- Decreased risk of pulpal trauma and inflammation
- Decreased postoperative sensitivity
- Increased fracture resistance of the tooth
- Decreased cuspal deflection
- Bonding tooth segments together in the treatment of cracked cusp syndrome
- Conservation of tooth tissue
- Increased retention

more detail elsewhere in this text. There is a paucity of clinical evidence relating to longevity or clinical performance of bonded amalgams and for advocating this technique on a routine basis. Indeed, recent evidence questions the routine placement of bonded amalgams. Therefore, the dentist is advised to consider each case on its own merits.

Materials for bonding

Over the years, many materials have been used to fill the amalgam–tooth interface and/or improve retention by bonding, including zinc phosphate cement, polycarboxylate cement and copal varnish. Since the mid-1980s, however, resin composite adhesives, which can bond to metal both chemically and physically, have been used. It has been realized that these materials offer considerable advantages over traditional luting or lining materials in this context. Table 6.3 lists examples of contemporary products that are used to bond dental amalgam.

Since the manipulation and placement requirements differ for each group of materials shown in Table 6.3, it is imperative that the manufacturer's instructions for use are followed precisely during any restorative procedure.

Table 6.3 Materials used for bonding amalgam

Type of material	Examples on the market	Manufacturer's name
Dual-cure resin based composite	Rely X ARC	3M ESPE
Resin containing phosphonated ester of bis-GMA	Panavia 21	Kuraray
	Panavia Ex	Kuraray
	Panavia F 2.0	Kuraray
Resin-modified glass ionomer cement (used uncured)	Fuji II LC	GC
	Vitrebond Plus	3M ESPE

Good moisture control is essential for any bonding process (see Chapter 2).

Box 6.2 Advantages of encapsulation for amalgam

- Constituents are in optimum condition to react
- Precisely metered proportions
- More consistent and controlled mixing
- Easier to mix
- Easier to dispense
- Less risk of mercury spillage
- Less risk of contamination of the work environment
- Less mercury vapour released into the local environment.

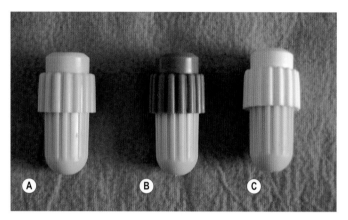

Fig. 6.10 Examples of Tytin (Kerr Hawe) colour-coded capsules containing different amounts of spills: (A) 400 mg, (B) 600 mg and (C) 800 mg.

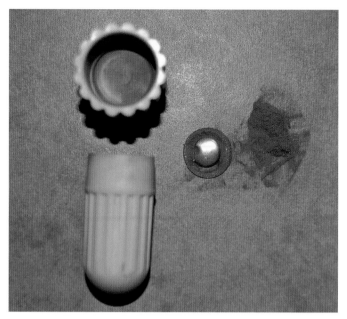

Fig. 6.11A–C A dismantled amalgam capsule (Tytin, Kerr Hawe) showing its constituents. Note the mercury-containing pillow, which ruptures to release the mercury.

Commercially available products

Table 6.4 shows representative examples of commercially available alloys and their manufacturer.

ENCAPSULATED AMALGAM

In days gone by, amalgam was mixed (**triturated**) either by hand or in a machine called an **amalgamator**, in which metered amounts of alloy and mercury were dispensed from storage reservoirs in the machine. These machines have largely become redundant as amalgam is now mainly supplied in the form of **encapsulated** amalgam, also called **precapsulation**. Box 6.2 lists its advantages.

The amalgam capsules contain different amounts of material (usually by weight), which is commonly depicted by the different colours of the top of the capsule. The capsules are usually supplied in 400 mg, 600 mg and 800 mg of alloy (Figure 6.10). The dentist can then request the mixing of a small or large amount of material depending on the amount required to fill the cavity. This reduces wastage and cost.

Manufacturers have come up with a range of modifications to simplify the use of encapsulated amalgam in the clinic:

- Capsules are generally **self-activating**, which means they may be placed directly into the mixing machine.
- Others must be activated by pressure prior to trituration. This either punctures the 'pillow' containing the mercury, thus releasing it to react with the alloy or dislodges the small plastic membrane separating the alloy from mercury
- Larger cavities may require more than one capsule to be mixed to completely fill it; this should be done one capsule at a time so that the new amalgam can be condensed onto the first amount. If too large an increment of amalgam is dispensed, condensation may be compromised.

The contents of a typical capsule are shown in Figure 6.11.

Table 6.4 Encapsulated amalgams currently available on the market

Product	Manufacturer	Amount of copper (%)	Alloy type
Amalcap Plus	Ivoclar Vivadent	11.9	Spherical
Ana 2000	Nordiska	26	Admixed
Ana 70	Nordiska	10.9	Spherical
Contour	Kerr Hawe	28	Dispersed
Dispersalloy	Dentsply	11.8	Dispersed
GS80	SDI	28.7	Admixed
GS80 Spherical	SDI	15	Spherical
Lojic+	SDI	11.8	Spherical
Megalloy EZ	Dentsply	14	Spherical
Oralloy Magicap-S	Coltène Whaledent	13	Spheroidal and spherical
Permite	SDI	15.4	Admixed
Securalloy	Septodont	13	Spherical
Tytin	Kerr Hawe	12	Spherical
Tytin FC	Kerr Hawe	13	Admixed and spherical mixture (hybrid)
Vivacap	Ivoclar Vivadent	24	Spherical

Spheroidal: A three-dimensional elliptical shape, tending towards a sphere.

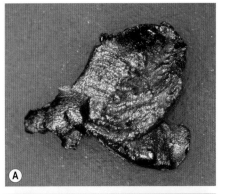

> ✓ **How to choose a dental amalgam product**
>
> The type of dental amalgam used is largely based on personal preference, and dentists should weigh the advantages and disadvantages of each amalgam product, together with their preferred handling characteristics.
> - High copper amalgam has better properties with respect to marginal integrity and strength, particularly after 1 hour.
> - Alloys with smaller particles are easier to carve. However, too small a particle size results in more alloy reacting with the mercury so more of the mercury reaction products are produced, thus rendering the final product weaker.
> - Smaller particle size accelerates the rate of set.
> - The shape of the alloy particles influences the amount of mercury used. Ratio of alloy to mercury is lower with spherical alloys than lathe-cut alloys.
> - Spherical alloys require less pressure to condense and are easier to carve.
> - Avoid zinc-containing alloys because of their propensity to expand if contaminated with moisture.
> - Alloys with spheroidal particles are easier to manipulate than those which have only spherical particles.

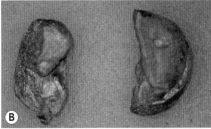

MANIPULATION OF AMALGAM

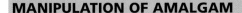

Trituration

Amalgamators

The importance of mixing the amalgam for the correct time, speed and with the correct motion and force (throw) cannot be stressed enough (see Chapter 1). Many manufacturers have attempted to address this. Some years ago, Kerr produced a machine in which programmed cards were inserted, corresponding to the alloy to be used. The machine then triturated the amalgam optimally. This machine is now obsolete as many of the cards tended to get lost or damaged during laundering of clinic clothing, as staff had forgotten to remove the cards from pockets, rendering the machine unusable.

Over/undertrituration

If after mixing, the amalgam is too wet and hot, and is difficult to remove from the capsule, it has been mixed for too long. A dry and crumbly mix indicates that the amalgam has be undertriturated. Both cases are unsatisfactory for use clinically and will result in inferior properties of the material. Undertrituration leads to:

- Low strength
- Poor corrosion resistance.

Overtrituration leads to:

- Excessive expansion
- Reduced strength.

All of the above decrease the longevity of the restoration. (See Figure 6.12.)

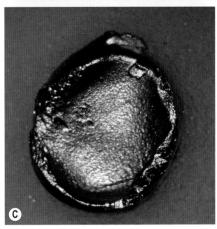

Fig. 6.12 (A) Undertriturated, (B) correctly mixed and (C) overtriturated dental amalgam.

> ✓
>
> - Ensure that hardware is compatible with the products to be used.
> - Always follow the manufacturer's instructions regarding mixing of amalgam – specifically, the time and speed.
> - Any amalgamator used in the clinic should be placed on a tray lined with aluminium foil (Figure 6.13). In the event of mercury spillage, the aluminium foil will retain the mercury and react with it. The reaction product will not, unlike free mercury, vaporize, and the risk of increased mercury vapour in the clinic is nullified.

Condensation

After mixing, the amalgam should be incrementally placed into the cavity without delay and condensed, with each increment being packed separately. The purpose of this is to remove any voids and compact the mass of the material to ensure that it is properly adapted to the cavity walls and margins.

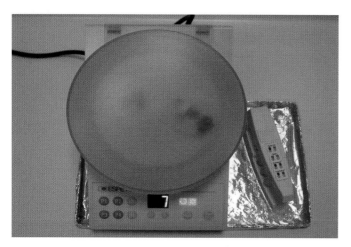

Fig. 6.13 A rotary mechanical mixer placed on an aluminium foil-lined tray.

Condensation expels excess mercury by bringing it to the surface, particularly when an admixed or lathe-cut alloy is used. There is less mercury incorporated in spherical alloys so it is generally not possible to remove excess mercury when using these alloys. Manufacturers provide less mercury with spherical alloys so that the powder to mercury ratio is optimized. Failure to remove the excess mercury will result in a weaker restoration, as more mercury will have reacted with the silver–tin (γ) phase and so increasing the silver–mercury ($\gamma1$) phase (see Figure 6.3). There are two methods of condensation:

- By hand, using a smooth-ended plugger
- With a mechanical condenser mounted on a slow handpiece coupling.

 Optimal condensation

- The diameter of the active end of the condenser is critical as sufficient force needs to be applied to the material.
- Too great a force will cause the condenser to pass through the amalgam instead of condensing it.
- A series of overlapping strokes should be made in an axial direction.
- Lateral as well as axial condensation should be carried out to ensure that the material is packed into the more inaccessible parts of the cavity.
- Spherical alloys require less force as they flow more easily, and, for this reason, mechanical pluggers are not recommended for this alloy type.
- Matrix bands should be used in Class II cavities so that appropriate force can be used to condense the amalgam. The band will resist this force and provide a support for the amalgam while it is setting.
- When bonding an amalgam restoration, a thin layer of petroleum jelly should be applied and then wiped off the matrix band using a cotton wool roll to prevent the band from being bonded in situ.
- Just prior to matrix band removal, a probe should be used to remove any thin edge of amalgam at the marginal ridge, which could break off.
- The material should be carved away from the marginal ridge using the shape of the remaining tooth to guide the instrument, thus re-creating the occlusal anatomy.

Failure to condense partially set amalgam will result in a material that will:
- Not be properly adapted to the cavity walls (Figure 6.14)
- Show poor bonding between increments
- Have inadequate mercury expressed (Figure 6.15)
- Exhibit inferior properties, in particular, strength.

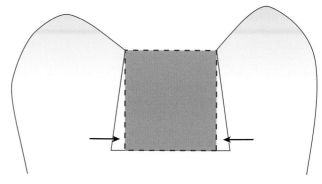

Fig. 6.14 An illustration of a Class II cavity and restoration showing the sites of poor condensation leading to voids.

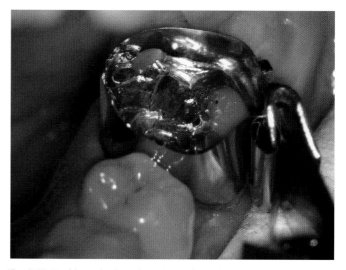

Fig. 6.15 Freshly packed amalgam in tooth 36 showing excess mercury on the surface.

It is often easier to control the initial increment of amalgam by condensing it with the larger end of the condenser, and ensuring good condensation with the smaller end thereafter. Using the smaller end first may result in the amalgam falling out of the cavity in the opposite direction! The cavity is usually overpacked, with the material condensed towards the walls of the cavity (Figure 6.16). The restoration is then carved to the desired anatomical shape, thus removing the mercury-rich surface layer.

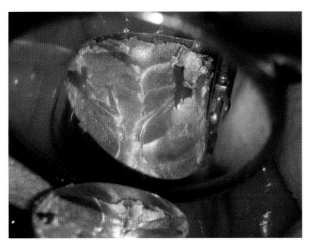

Fig. 6.16 A cavity in tooth 36 overpacked with amalgam against the cavity walls prior to carving. Note the considerable excess of material.

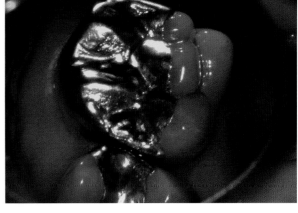

Fig. 6.17 A polished amalgam restoration in tooth 26.

 Repair of an amalgam that fractures at the time of placement

If an amalgam fractures at the time of placement (e.g. if the patient bites too heavily on it), some of the setting amalgam should be removed with a bur to create a small cavity with appropriate depth, width and shape. Then the matrix band should be replaced and freshly mixed amalgam condensed into the cavity. After removing the band, the restoration is re-carved.

While this technique will not result in as strong a restoration as one placed de novo, a strength of 75% of the original will be achieved and this should function satisfactorily. This method cannot be used with an old restoration where the setting reaction has gone to completion. Additions under these conditions will not bond and will only be retained by mechanically interlocking, unless an intermediate bonding agent is used.

Finishing

Burnishing

Once the amalgam filling has been carved, some dentists advocate burnishing the surface to adapt the material to the margins and to smooth the surface. Others advocate using a moist cotton wool pledget to remove any debris from the surface. However, neither of these steps is essential.

> **Burnish:** plastic deformation of a surface due to sliding contact with another object. Burnishing smears the texture of a rough surface, rendering it shiny.

Polishing

Polishing (Figure 6.17) an amalgam restoration renders its surface smoother and easier to keep clean. It is usually done at a subsequent appointment, when the material has fully set. The unpolished surface is rough at a microscopic level, with pits that can retain small particles of food debris and also acids. This encourages galvanic activity on the surface, leading to corrosion in extreme cases. A polished restoration undergoes less corrosion, and polishing improves marginal

adaptation of material to the tooth. A highly polished amalgam also has a more aesthetic appearance.

 Polishing an amalgam restoration

- Polish the surface to a high lustre, under copious water spray. using slow-speed stainless steel polishing burs of different shapes to access all the anatomical contours of the restoration. This avoids overheating the restoration, which can lead to release of mercury from the surface and damage to the restoration. In addition there may be thermal trauma to the pulp.
- Use the brown and then the green rubber polishing cups. These contain a fine abrasive that performs the polishing.
- Use a mix of zinc oxide powder and alcohol in a rubber cup or on a brush for a final high-lustre polish.

Some of the fast-setting alloys can be polished within 8–10 minutes from the start of trituration, as they are sufficiently set by this time to permit this. However, polishing increases the electrochemical potential of the restoration, thus releasing mercury vapour and rendering the amalgam more reactive.

> **Electrochemical potential:** measure of the energy available as a result of chemical and electrostatic charges.

Clinical trials comparing dentists' assessment of old amalgam restorations before and after polishing found that a lower proportion of dentists wished to replace the same restoration after it had been polished. Since every time a restoration is replaced more sound tooth is lost, it may be more preferable to polish the restoration rather than replacing it, if that is possible.

AMALGAM DISPOSAL

Any waste amalgam, amalgam capsules and contaminated matrix bands must be disposed of correctly. Bespoke amalgam disposal

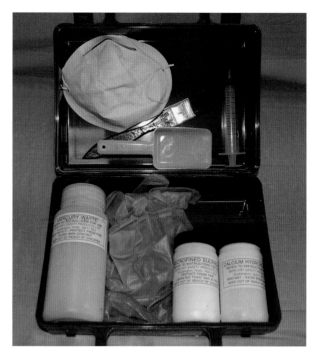

Fig. 6.18 Bespoke amalgam disposal vessels provided by MerCon. The tub on the left is used for disposing amalgam capsules etc., while the vessel on the right is used for directly contaminated amalgam waste.

vessels are available (Figure 6.18), which are collected by a specialist company to be safely disposed of. Spent amalgam capsules, disposable dappen dishes and disposable amalgam carrier tips should be placed in the tub provided for the purpose. Directly contaminated waste, such as waste amalgam and matrix bands that have been used during amalgam placement, should be deposited in the tub provided for this purpose. Matrix bands cannot safely be decontaminated and are now considered to be for single use only.

MERCURY SPILLAGE

With the advent of encapsulated amalgam, mercury spillages should be a rare occurrence, but every clinic or practice should have a mercury spillage kit (Figure 6.19) and protocol in case of an accident.

	Dealing with a Mercury spillage

- Wear protective gloves and a mask.
- Ensure there is increased ventilation by opening windows.
- Try to contain the spillage to as small an area as possible.
- Use a brush to move the globules of mercury to form one large pool.
- Pick up as much as possible using a syringe.
- Mix equal amounts of microfine sulphur and calcium hydroxide with a little water.
- Spread this onto the spillage area using the brush provided in the spillage kit.
- Brush the contaminated material into the scoop and place in the waste container.
- Dispose of all the waste using a recognized amalgam disposal container.

Consideration should be given to the floor covering when designing a dental clinic. Should mercury spillage occur, a floor covering

Fig. 6.19 Commercially available mercury spillage kit.

with a smooth surface will facilitate its recovery. It is extremely difficult, if not impossible, to retrieve any spilt mercury from carpeting and wooden floorboards. A vacuum cleaner or aspirator should never be used to deal with mercury spillage as these will re-release the mercury vapour into the atmosphere.

It has been suggested that a mercury decontamination procedure of the clinic should be carried out from time to time (perhaps monthly) and after a spillage to reduce the background exposure. This can be done by mixing two teaspoons of the microfine sulphur with equal amounts of calcium hydroxide and a little washing-up liquid in a plastic bucket with approximately 2 litres of water, and the resulting solution mopped over the clinic floor. Normal detergent can be used thereafter and the resulting contaminated solution can be safely disposed down the drain.

MERCURY TOXICITY

Much has been written about the toxicity of elemental mercury as it is widely recognized to be one of the most toxic elements on the planet. It is reasonable to suppose that had amalgam been proposed for dental use today, a product licence would not be forthcoming. While lots of anecdotal reports exist, there is, to date, no robust scientific evidence linking dental amalgam with detrimental health effects. Millions of patients have had dental amalgam placed and those restorations have been in situ for a number of years without problems. Furthermore, many dental professionals have spent years working with the material without a problem. Of course, if used incorrectly, mercury toxicity may be an issue, but an awareness of health and safety recommendations has all but eliminated this. Some precautions must be adhered to during clinical use.

- Avoid skin contact with free mercury (skin readily absorbs mercury – practice good mercury hygiene).
- Use high-volume aspiration during amalgam removal – mercury vapour can be inhaled and absorbed by the lungs.
- Ideally, use rubber dam during amalgam removal and placement. This prevents unnecessary ingestion as the gut can also absorb mercury.
- Do a risk assessment of staff using amalgam.
- Have in place a screening programme to monitor mercury levels. It is recommended this is done at least annually for each 'at risk' worker
  - This involves sending a sample of urine, pubic hair or nail pairings for analysis.
  - It may not be necessary to test each member of staff working with amalgam every 6 months. For example, half the staff liable to mercury exposure may be tested in the summer and the others in the winter.
  - If a positive result is gained, the other group should be tested.

Mercury vapour release

A minute amount of mercury vapour is released during intraoral function but this is not considered significant. More is released if the amalgam is heated over 80°C and during amalgam removal. This highlights the importance of using copious water spray during any removal process. As mentioned above, rubber dam should also be used when amalgam is being removed.

Free mercury is also released as a product of the corrosion reaction that occurs during a restoration's life. This is particularly the case in high γ2-containing amalgam. Production of free mercury allows further reaction, forming more γ1. As this phase is weaker than the γ phase, the material's mechanical properties decrease with time. In an attempt to reduce the problem, other similar materials were introduced to the market (gallium was substituted for mercury) in the past. These materials showed greater corrosion and their strength was lower that conventional dental amalgam, hence they were withdrawn.

Dental amalgam and legislation

In 1998 in the UK, the use of dental amalgam in pregnant women was banned by the Department of Health, and this ban is still in force. However, there remains a lack of evidence for the rationale for this decision. Concern has recently been voiced about the use of amalgam in children, as they have a higher metabolic rate and systemic absorption may be quicker. Other countries (e.g. in Scandinavia and Japan) have also banned amalgam, not for concerns over health but in an attempt to reduce environmental mercury levels.

Samples of soil from around crematoria have shown higher levels of mercury, and some countries have gone to the lengths of fitting mercury filters or removing those teeth in cadavers which had previously been restored using dental amalgam. The UK government may pass legislation in the future to reduce crematoria emissions of mercury and to ban the use of amalgam in dentistry. However, this would have major financial implications for the National Health Service (NHS), because amalgam is a cheaper material to use than many other alternative restorative materials used in commensurate sites in the teeth. The decrease in amalgam use in developed countries is probably more due to patient preference for tooth-coloured restorations. However, in other countries, for example in the former Eastern block, amalgam sales are still increasing because the material is cheaper and effective.

CONTRAINDICATIONS TO THE USE OF DENTAL AMALGAM

Dental amalgam is contraindicated in a limited number of situations:
- Pregnant women only in the UK, see previous section
- Allergy to any of the constituents
- Where aesthetics are of paramount importance
- In patients who object to amalgam use.

Of course, in the last category the advantages and disadvantages of the alternative materials that could be used should be fully discussed with the patient to permit them to make an informed decision.

ADVERSE EFFECTS OF DENTAL AMALGAM USE

Enamel discolouration

Since the dentine structure is permeable, it is not uncommon for a tooth to discolour when it has been restored with amalgam, particularly when the restoration has been in situ for some time. The by-products of the corrosion process in the material can migrate into the dentinal tubules causing the discolouration. This may be unsightly, particularly in the anterior sextants of the mouth and also in the upper premolar region (Figure 6.20). Figure 6.20 also shows an upper first premolar, where there is an unsightly amalgam in situ, due to the buccal extension of the cavity. The use of an aesthetic material would have been more appropriate in this situation.

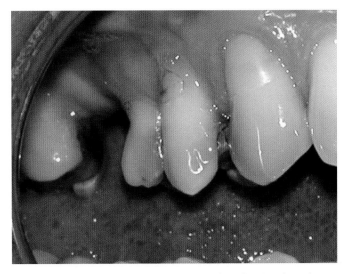

Fig. 6.20 Amalgam restorations in teeth 14 and 15 showing through the buccal tooth tissue. Tooth 14 also shows the buccal extension of the amalgam restoration, which is unsightly.

Amalgam tattoo

Occasionally, some fine particles of the material can migrate into the soft tissues, giving rise to an amalgam tattoo (Figure 6.21). This is a benign lesion but some patients may be concerned as it can mimic

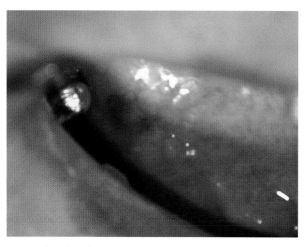

Fig. 6.21 A dental amalgam tattoo on the right lateral border of the tongue.

melanoma. If the patient is concerned or indeed if the lesion is at all suspicious, the diagnosis should be confirmed by biopsy.

Galvanic cell

The use of two dissimilar metals intraorally can set up a **galvanic cell** as saliva acts as a transporter of ions. An amalgam restoration that is placed in juxtaposition to a restoration with a dissimilar amalgam alloy or, more commonly, a gold alloy, may cause a galvanic cell to be established. The patient may experience a mild electric shock and a feeling of having 'silver paper' in their mouth. With time these effects are reduced, but it is sensible to advise the patient against having restorations with dissimilar metals where they may come in contact in the mouth. A gold crown will often become 'silvered' because of contact with amalgam as the former acts as the cathode in the equivalent of a wet cell battery.

Lichenoid reaction

Some patients have developed a lichenoid reaction to dental amalgam, and this is believed to be caused by electrochemical reactions and a type IV hypersensitivity reaction. In these situations it may be appropriate to change the restorative material after ensuring that the replacement material will not also cause such a reaction.

> **Type IV hypersensitivity reaction:** a delayed cell-mediated immune response, of which contact dermatitis is a good example.

SUMMARY

- Dental amalgam has a proven track record as an excellent dental restoration and is still widely used, particularly where economic factors are paramount as it is a relatively cheap material.
- Dental amalgam is a very 'forgiving' material, and even when placed in non-ideal conditions it will perform better than most other dental materials.
- Concerns have been raised as to the toxicity of dental amalgam and its detrimental effects on health. To date no robust scientific

work has demonstrated a relationship between dental amalgam and systemic disease.
- Environmental concerns in some countries have led to dental amalgam being banned, although the availability of newer alloys and their presentation in encapsulated form has reduced the potential environmental impact.
- Many patients now request the placement of tooth-coloured restorations, and this has led to a decreased use of dental amalgam internationally and may lead to the discontinuation of its use in the long term.

FURTHER READING

Bonsor, S.J., Chadwick, R.G., 2009. Longevity of conventional and bonded (sealed) amalgam restorations in a private general dental practice. Br. Dent. J. 206, E3.

Eley, B.M., 1997. The future of dental amalgam: a review of the literature. Br. Dent. J. 182, 247–249, 293–297, 333–338, 373–381, 413–417, 455–459.

Eley, B.M., 1997. The future of dental amalgam: a review of the literature. Br. Dent. J. 183, 11–14.

Ilhan Kal, B., et al. 2008. An unusual case of immediate hypersensitivity reaction associated with an amalgam restoration. Br. Dent. J. 205, 547–550.

Jones, D.W., 2008. A Scandinavian tragedy. Br. Dent. J. 204, 233–234.

McCullough, M.J., Tyas, M.J., 2008. Local adverse effects of amalgam restorations. Int. Dent. J. 58, 3–9.

Mitchell, R.J., Koike, M., Okabe, T., 2007. Posterior amalgam restorations – usage, regulation and longevity. Dent. Clin. North Am. 51, 573–589.

van Noort, R., 2007. Introduction to Dental Materials, third ed. Mosby Elsevier, Edinburgh (See Chapter 2.1).

Setcos, J.C., Staninec, M., Wilson, NH., 2000. Bonding of amalgam restorations: existing knowledge and future prospects. Oper. Dent. 25, 121–129.

SELF-ASSESSMENT QUESTIONS

1. A patient has recently had a Class II amalgam restoration placed. The restoration has an excellent contact area with the adjacent Class II restoration, which is cast gold. The patient complains of pain and says 'it feels like silver paper' in their mouth. What is the diagnosis and how can it be treated?
2. A capsule of amalgam is mixed in an amalgamator. At the end of the mixing cycle, the material is hot, wet and sticking to the sides of the capsule. What is the problem and what parameters could be changed?
3. A patient brings a folder full of papers printed off from the internet, of 'evidence' that dental amalgam is harmful. What points should the clinician make to reassure them that the material is safe to use clinically?
4. When using an admixed alloy, which condensing instrument would be the most appropriate? How would the clinician's choice differ when using a spherical alloy?
5. What is the rationale for polishing an amalgam restoration?
6. Small restorations in Class II cavities fail by fracturing across the narrowest part of the occlusal surface (isthmus). What are the causes of this?

Chapter | 7 |

The tooth-coloured restorative materials I: Resin composites

LEARNING OBJECTIVES

From this chapter, the reader will:

- Understand what resin composites are
- Understand the influence their constituents have on the material's handling and its clinical applications
- Understand the properties of these materials and the significance of these on clinical manipulation and performance
- Understand their indications, contraindications and limitations
- Have an increased appreciation of how to use these materials to their best effect
- Know the names of currently available commercial products.

INTRODUCING THE TOOTH-COLOURED RESTORATIVE MATERIALS

There is a range of directly placed tooth-coloured restorative materials available to the dentist. These materials form a continuum that links resin based composites to glass ionomer cements, with resin composite at one extreme and glass ionomer cement at the other and two hybrid materials in between (Figure 7.1).

Resin composites are hydrophobic materials consisting of an inert glass and a polymerizable resin. Glass ionomer cements are hydrophilic cements which are based on the reaction between glass with an acid to form a polysalt matrix in which the unreacted glass is sheathed. They contain no polymerizable resin. Compomers (or polyacid-modified resin composites) are primarily resin based

and are closer in behaviour to the resin composites than the glass ionomer cements. The reactive glasses used as the filler in these materials is similar to that used in glass ionomer cements, but the resin system uses two methacrylate based resins. Setting is achieved by a polymerization reaction, with no water being present in the material before placement. Resin-modified glass ionomer cements are glass ionomer cements to which a resin component has been added by grafting methacrylate groups onto the polyacrylic acid chain. A water soluble methacrylate resin is also added. The cement still requires water as an intrinsic part of the setting reaction. This material is closer in nature to glass ionomer cements than resin composite.

THE RESIN COMPOSITES

Resin composites are widely used in dentistry and their applications are increasing as technology advances. As already mentioned in Chapter 6, dental amalgam is not necessarily the automatic material of choice for restoring posterior teeth in contemporary practice. The market is patient driven as most patients wish for the excellent aesthetics afforded by tooth-coloured restorations. Resin composite is the directly placed material of choice when the best aesthetic result is required. The early composite materials did not have long-term durability as they had a tendency to wear and showed staining. However, as materials and techniques have improved the longevity of resin composite restorations has increased. This chapter describes resin composites in detail and their applications and clinical manipulation.

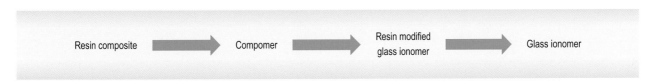

Fig. 7.1 The spectrum of tooth-coloured restorative materials.

The original tooth-coloured restorative materials (Table 7.1), the silicate cements and the acrylics, exhibited several shortcomings. The development of resin composite materials was aimed at overcoming these factors. As their properties have improved with time, they have tended to become ubiquitous materials, being used increasingly at the expense of other traditional materials.

> **Silicate cement:** cement formed from reaction between alumino-silicate-glass and phosphoric acid (see Chapter 12).

DEFINITION

A **composite** material is one that is composed of more than one different constituent. There are many composite materials in use in dentistry of which **resin composites** are one example. These materials are composed of a **chemically active resin** component and a **filler**, usually a **glass** or **ceramic**. The resin and the filler are bound together by a **silane coupler**. The structure of resin composite is illustrated in Figure 7.2, and the constituents of resin composite materials are shown in Table 7.2. The many component parts of a resin-based composite material are shown in Figure 7.3.

Table 7.1 Shortcomings of acrylics and silicate cements

Acrylics	Silicates
High water sorption	Low strength
High coefficient of thermal expansion	Wash out
Large polymerization shrinkage	Low pH
Considerable microleakage	Pulpal irritation
Extrinsic and intrinsic staining	
Highly exothermic on curing	
Wear	
Poor colour stability	

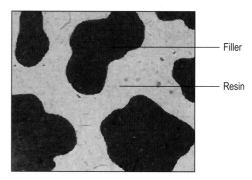

Fig. 7.2 The structure of a resin-based composite material.

Table 7.2 Chemical constituents of resin composite materials

Ingredient	Examples	Reason for use
Filler (inorganic)	Glass Ceramic	Provides strength Influences the optical properties of the material
Principal monomer	Bis-GMA Bis-EMA UDMA	Forms polymer matrix Used as a primary monomer
Diluent monomer	TEGDMA UDMA	Reduces the viscosity of the main resin so that the material can be used clinically
Silane coupling agent	γ-methacryloxypropyl-trimethoxysilane	Bonds the filler to the resin
Photo-initiators	Camphorquinone PPD Lucirin TPO	Initiator of polymerization reaction
Other chemicals for the curing process	Tertiary amine such as N,N-dimethyl-p-toluidene	Accelerator of polymerization reaction
Ultraviolet stabilizers	2-hydroxy-4-methoxybenzophenone	Prevents shade change over time due to oxidation
Polymerization inhibitors	Monomethyl ether of hydroquinone	Prevents premature curing of the composite prior to use
Radiopaque materials	Barium, strontium and lithium salts	Permits the material to be seen on radiographs (see Chapter 4)
Pigments and opacifiers	Iron and titanium oxides	Varies the optical properties and the colour of the final material to achieve a good shade match

UDMA, urethane dimethacrylate; TEGDMA, tri(ethylene glycol) dimethacrylate; PPD, phenylpropanedione; Lucirin TPO, ethyl 2,4,6 trimthylbenzoyldiphenyl-phosphine oxide.

made up of aliphatic components. UDMA is now used quite frequently as an alternative to bis-GMA.

> **Molecular weight:** the mass of one molecule of a substance.
> **Aliphatic:** compounds containing carbon atoms which are joined in straight or side chains. They do not contain any ring structures.

Although manufacturers may claim that they use the same generic resins e.g. bis-GMA, the synthesis of this molecule can vary from manufacturer to manufacturer. Likewise the molecular weight and reaction products in the resin will vary. It is essential that different commercial materials used in one restoration are sourced from the same manufacturer. Mixing and matching materials from different manufacturers will produce a substandard material with poorer mechanical properties.

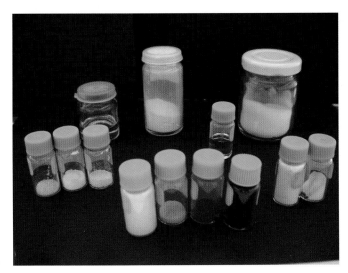

Fig. 7.3 The constituents of a resin composite material (with thanks to Coltène Whaledent).

CONSTITUENTS OF A RESIN COMPOSITE

Resin component

Principal and diluent monomers

The main **resin** component is based on the chemical reaction of two resins, namely **bisphenol A** and **glycidyl methacrylate**, which form a chemical called **bis-GMA (bisphenol A diglycidyl ether dimethacrylate)**, also known as **Bowen's resin** after its inventor. It is a long chain **monomer** with a methacrylate group at either end of an aromatic spine. This chemical is highly viscous due to its high molecular weight and aromatic spine, which reduces mobility of the monomer so that it cannot be manipulated clinically (Figure 7.4).

> **Aromatic:** a hydrocarbon with phenolic component included in the chain.

It is necessary therefore to add other monomers to the bis-GMA to permit clinical handling and proper mixing with the inorganic components. These lower-molecular-weight monomers are called **diluent monomers** and have also been termed **viscosity controllers**. Examples of these chemicals are:

- Methylmethacrylate (MMA)
- Ethylene glycol dimethacrylate (EGDM)
- Tri(ethylene glycol) dimethacrylate (TEGDMA)
- Urethane dimethacrylate (UDMA).

Chemicals such as methylmethacrylate have low molecular weights and have only one reactive group. This leads to greater shrinkage. The disadvantages of the single methacrylate group materials are as follows:

- Wear resistance is poor
- Strength is poor
- Shrinkage is marked on polymerization.

The dimethacrylates have active methacrylate groups at either end of a backbone. The longer the backbone, the smaller the shrinkage as the reaction only occurs at the active methacrylate groups. Bis-GMA is an example of this, having a long backbone made up of phenolic aromatic rings. UDMA also has a long chain backbone, but in this case it does not contain phenolic groups with the backbone being

Filler component

The resin, if used alone, shows a number of shortcomings:

- Inadequate wear
- High shrinkage
- Increased exothermic reaction.

The incorporation of an inorganic filler into the system compensates for these shortcomings. By implication, when a filler is added, the amount of resin present decreases. The material thus created should exhibit:

- Increased strength
- Increased wear resistance
- Reduced polymerization shrinkage
- Improved optical properties such as colour, fluorescence and translucency
- Radiopacity as heavy metals (such as barium) may be added as salts to the glass constituents before firing to produce the glass
- Less heat production during polymerization: the filler acting as a heat sink
- Reduced thermal expansion (closer to tooth).

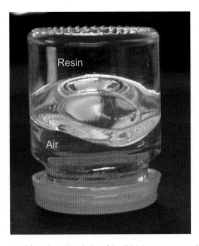

Fig. 7.4 An inverted bottle containing bis-GMA monomer. Note that the resin stays in the lower part of the bottle, defying gravity due to its high viscosity. It will take in excess of 14 days for the resin to slump to the bottom of the bottle.

One of the consequences of filler addition is that the resin composite material takes on the properties of the main constituent, and thus it becomes more brittle in nature. As its elastic modulus is increased, the material has a decreased capacity to withstand flexion encountered during function. This will occur in any dental restoration and is of particular significance with the flowable resin composite presentation as explained later.

Filler types

Resin composites have been classified by:

- Type of resin
- Filler type
- Size and the distribution of filler particles within the resin.

The next two sections deal with the composition of the filler and the influence of the size and distribution of the filler particles on the resin composite. The fillers include both **glasses** and **ceramics**.

Glasses

A glass is an amorphous (non-crystalline) solid material. While there are many different chemical compositions of glass, the formulations used in resin composites are quite limited. Those which are used in these materials are listed in Table 7.3.

The formulation of the glass is important as it has a major effect on the appearance of the final composite. It also in part influences the mechanical properties. Quartz is the hardest material but is not radiopaque. The silicate glasses produced for resin composite contain heavy metals such as barium but are slightly softer and also degrade very slowly when exposed to water. Those materials containing barium, strontium and lithium are easier to finish and exhibit an improved surface finish. Of the three, strontium-containing glasses degrade the fastest in water, which is why they are used in only a small percentage of the overall glass content. Colloidal silica is also frequently found in many of the modern composites. However, the behaviour of the product will be determined by the volume fraction of filler particles in the material. Some resin-based composites release very small amounts of fluoride. This fluoride is leached from the glass and so depends on the formulation of the filler used. The loss of fluoride will also accelerate the degradation process as the glass is weakened.

Table 7.3 Commonly used glasses as fillers in resin-based composite materials

Generic name	Chemical composition	Average particle size	Notes
Quartz	Crystalline silica (silicon dioxide)	Fine	Neither opaque or radiopaque
Silica-based glasses	Lithium-aluminium silicate glass	Fine	Not opaque but radiopaque
	Barium-aluminium silicate glass	Fine	Radiopaque
	Barium aluminoborate silicate	Fine	Radiopaque
	Borosilicate glass containing zinc or strontium or lithium	Fine	Radiopaque
Amorphous silica (Aerosil, Evonik Industries)	Colloidal silica (silicon dioxide)	Microfine	Swells if exposed to water
Ytterbium fluoride	Fluoride salt	–	Fluoride release

It must be borne in mind that the density of all these glasses is about four times that of the resin. Many manufacturers often quote the filler loading by weight. The more significant value is the volume of the filler because of the disparity between the densities of the resin and the glass – then the volume fraction is always less than the weight fraction of filler present.

Once the glass has been produced by firing the various components of the glass together, the resulting solid mass is ground to the desired size of particle. Figure 7.5 shows a block of glass as supplied by the glass manufacturer and after it has been **milled** (ground).

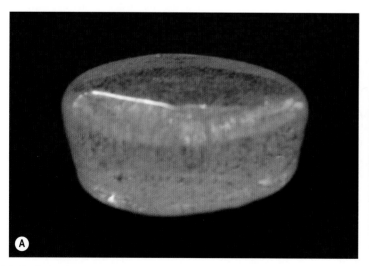
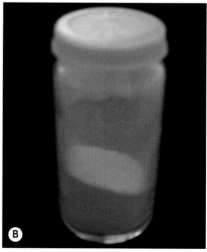

Fig. 7.5 A block of glass (A) prior to milling and (B) the ground glass product.

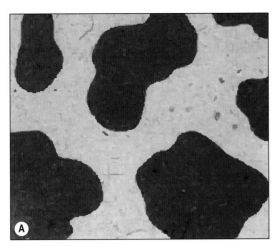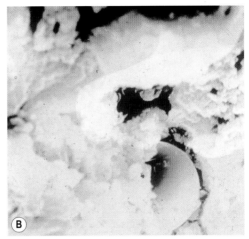

Fig. 7.6A,B (A) Diagram of surface of macrofilled composite showing the particle size and distribution. (B) Photomicrograph of surface. Note the large areas of resin.

Ceramics

The other family of materials which has been incorporated as a fraction of the filler in resin composite materials are the **ceramics**. A ceramic is an inorganic, non-metallic solid prepared by the action of heat and subsequent cooling. The ceramics used in dental resin composites include synthetic materials such as:

- **Zirconia-silica** filler. This is manufactured in a sol-gel process. The particles have round edges and so more filler is able to be incorporated into the material. It is claimed to have very good translucency.
- **Zirconium oxide**. Groups of materials based on this oxide have the advantage that the composition can be finely controlled and may be varied by the manufacturer. Other benefits of this type of filler are limited at present and cost of production is considerably greater than the conventional filler production.

Sol-gel process: This is a process of glass or ceramic manufacture from the constituent oxides components and suitable volatile solvents. Once the volatile solvent has been removed the structure which is formed is known as a **xerogel**. On further heating, this structure consolidates into a form where it may be used as a filler. The resulting product is better in that it is more consistent in quality.

Effect of filler particle size and shape

The size and shape of a resin composite filler has an important influence on the properties of the material together with the amount of filler (**filler loading**) in the product. The particle size and shape determines the amount of filler that can be added to the resin. Furthermore, a large discrepancy between the hardness of filler and the resin will affect the surface finish and wear. Classification of resin composites by the size of their filler particles is in part historical as it chronicles the development of each material.

Macrofilled

The macrofilled composites were the first to be developed. The large size of the filler particles (range 15–35 μm maximum and minimum, 5–100 μm) meant that although the materials displayed good mechanical properties (high strength), they were notoriously difficult to finish to an acceptable level. This was because the particles would protrude above the surface in the resin and when the surface was polished these particles were displaced and a satisfactory polish was never achieved (Figure 7.6).

The rough surface of these composites attracted plaque and during clinical use the surface became rougher because of preferential wear of the resin matrix. The wear resistance of the material is therefore relatively poor. The only way to get a good surface finish is to cure the material using a matrix strip and leaving it unpolished. The strip forces the filler particle below the surface and the resin layer produced is smoother. This resin-rich surface, however, wears away with time. Larger particles can support higher loads as they have a lower surface area to volume ratio. These materials are on average approximately 70% filled by weight or about 55% by volume.

Fine particle

Reduction in the particle size leads to better packing of the filler and the reduction in the inter-particular distance which is filled with resin. This reduction in exposed resin surface will reduce wear to some extent. The reduction in size achieved by grinding means that the particles approximate more in shape to spheres. This confers a number of benefits including easier finishing and a smoother surface. The increase in filler load to between 75% and 80% by weight means that the mechanical properties are enhanced. While a filler loading of 75–80% by weight sounds very impressive, it is important to remember that glass is a much denser material than the resin. This means that the volume of the filler is always less than the weight fraction mentioned. Often the volume of filler in the restoration does not exceed 60% of its total volume.

Microfilled

The failure to achieve an acceptable finish led the manufacturers to consider microfine fillers. The most acceptable material to use was **colloidal silica**. The particles of this material are sub-micron in size (0.04 μm). This type of material is most commonly used as a thickening agent. The particle has an affinity for water and if uncoated, takes up water leading to hydrolytic degradation. To overcome these problems and to produce a resin composite, the manufacturer takes the base resin and warm the mixture to below the glass transition temperature. The resin mixture becomes more fluid and at this point colloidal silica is introduced to the resin mass and a volume added until the resin is almost solid.

Glass transition temperature: the temperature above which a glassy material starts to become rubbery.

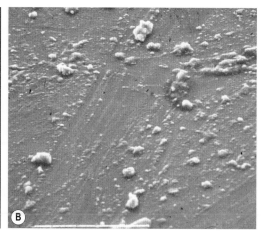

Fig. 7.7 (A) The distribution of the fine particles within the microfine resin (B) Photomicrograph showing the surface of a microfine material. The field of view is 30 μm and there is no evidence of filler at the surface. The debris observed is from the matrix strip used to make the sample.

The semisolid mass is then heated to polymerize it and the result is a resin block with 'seeds' of colloidal silica embedded in it (Figure 7.7). This resin mass is then ground up to form 'filler' particles which are then mixed with unpolymerized resin to form the paste provided to the dentist. The inorganic phase, colloidal silica, in these materials does not exceed 45% by volume. However, the presence of already polymerized resin means that the polymerization shrinkage observed is not greatly above that for the other types of resin composite.

One of the consequences of retaining more resin is that the water uptake of the material is increased. This is not as bad as might be expected since the pre-polymerized blocks of resin have a very high conversion rate which reduces the water uptake. It should be stressed that the water uptake is a slow process and the amount involved is relatively small.

The type of 'filler' and the nature of the resin means that the inorganic filler loading in these materials is substantially lower than that found in other resin composites, in the range of 40–45% by weight. Any attempt to increase this usually results in the resin not coating all the particles and particles agglomerating. Substantial amounts of time, research and money have been spent on this during the development of these resin composite materials with relatively limited benefits.

The strength of these materials is not as high as that of conventional resin composites. Cases have been reported of marginal ridge or incisal tip fracture. However, over time observed wear with these materials is no better or worse than a conventional resin composite.

Hybrid

As the term suggests, a hybrid composite contains particles of various sizes and shapes. They were developed to try to gain all the benefits of the microfine and macrofilled resin composites. These products offer a higher filler density as the particles can get closer together and fit into each other so interlocking. This means that there is a decreased amount of resin. The structure of a hybrid resin composite can be compared with crazy paving (Figure 7.8 and Figure 7.9), with the stone paving slabs representing the particles and the cement grout the resin. It can be seen that they are remarkably similar although the hybrid has slightly more space between the particles. This is one of the limitations of the hybrid in that the resin viscosity tends to prevent the close apposition of the particles unlike the cement in the crazy paving which can be a much lower viscosity.

Under ideal conditions packing can be improved substantially with the resin acting as a binder. Figure 7.10 shows the ideal distribution of packing to achieve an optimum filler loading (a **trimodal distribution**). Here the large particles form the bulk of the restorative. In the spaces between them are smaller spheres of intermediate size. There still remain even smaller spaces between the larger and small spheres. If even smaller spheres are then used to fill those gaps, a trimodal distribution of particle sizes (large, medium and small) is

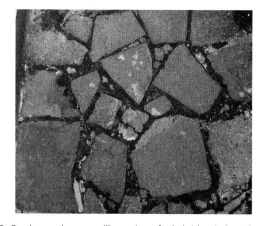

Fig. 7.8 Crazing paving as an illustration of a hybrid resin-based composite. The differing sizes and shapes of the stones (filler particles) reduce the amount of cement (resin) as they are able to pack more closely together.

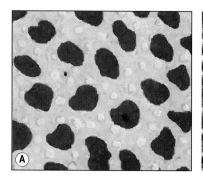
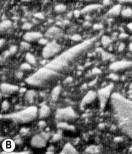

Fig. 7.9A,B The structure of a hybrid resin composite.

established. The filler distribution in Figure 7.10 is 15 large (green), eight small (blue) and 32 smallest (red). These fillers form the bulk of the restorative. Manufacturers attempt to produce this type of distribution but are limited by the variable particle size within each category. It is also difficult to ensure that the distribution is uniform through the material.

The size range of particles is generally between 5- and 10 µm for the larger particles with the small particles being made up of colloidal silica. The amount of filler incorporated is a compromise between the stiffness (viscosity) of the paste and the handling

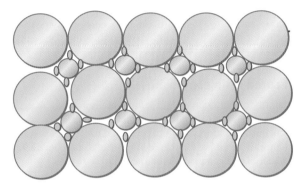

Fig. 7.10 Trimodal distribution of particle sizes and the ideal packing scenario.

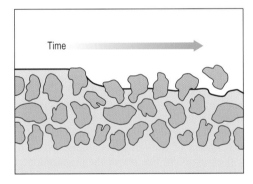

Fig. 7.11 The effect of finishing a composite. The resin matrix is preferentially removed and excessive trimming will mean a loss of filler, as the greater diameter of the filler is exposed and the filler particles are plucked out.

characteristics required by the clinician. Maximum filler loading is in the region of 82–84% by weight of filler. This increase in the bulk of the filler has benefits in that the coefficient of thermal expansion is slightly reduced and the mechanical properties of the composite are enhanced. The materials can, however, become more brittle. The increase in filler loading may also lead to larger volumes of diluent monomer being used with the resulting material being prone to greater polymerization shrinkage.

Hybrid resin composites are often termed universal resin composites as they may be used in all sites within the mouth for all applications. Several varieties of hybrids with varying particle sizes and distributions are available. As the particle size is reduced, manufacturers have applied stylized names to these minor differences. These include 'fine' and 'micro' hybrid, which refers either to the average particle size or a blend of particles being included with an increased proportion of sub-micron sized particles.

As the particle size decreases, a further complication arises in that light is not reflected within the restorative and more shades and tinting agents are required to make the materials aesthetically pleasing. Modern resin composites are close to the maximum filler loading that is achievable, this being about 86% by weight (70–72% by volume). These heavily filled materials provide a reasonable surface and can be finished using fine diamonds burs, sanding discs and abrasive stones to produce a relatively smooth surface. The long-term performance is not ideal as the resin surface soon starts to wear away (Figure 7.11).

Nanofilled

Nanomers are discrete non-agglomerated and non-aggregated particles of between 20- and 70 nanometres. To put this size into perspective, one human hair is 80 µm in diameter, which is 80 000 nm, a nanomer being 1/1000 of a micrometre (micron).

The **nanoparticles** coalesce into **nanocluster** fillers, which are loosely bound agglomerates of these particles. Agglomerates act as a single unit, enabling high filler loading and high strength. These materials have the strength of a hybrid material but are easier to polish as the individual filler particles are much smaller. There are some materials which are conventional hybrid materials to which nanoparticles have been added to fill inter-particular space (see Figure 7.12).

Effect of filler loading

The aim of increasing filler loading is to make the mechanical properties of the resin composite closer to those of the filler. This means that the strength in compression goes up but that the material

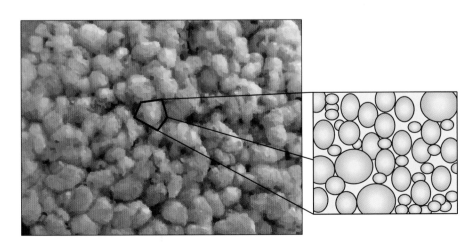

Fig. 7.12 An example of a nanomer with agglomerated particles approximately 0.6–1.4 µm using a rice cake as an example. These are made up of much smaller particles (1–10 nm, maximum 75 nm) which are clustered together.

becomes more brittle. The resistance to wear is potentially increased but overfilling may lead to surface breakdown as there is inadequate resin to bind the filler together. The more filler that is added, the stiffer and more viscous is the paste, and manipulation can become much harder. Sometimes adaptation to the cavity margin and wall is compromised.

Silane coupler

When the filler is added to the resin, the resultant product actually becomes weaker than the original resin component alone, which clearly negates the objective of adding the filler. This is because no bonding occurs between the filler and the resin. Manufacturers therefore have to chemically coat the surface of the filler particles to facilitate their bonding with the chemically active resin. This chemical is called a **silane coupler**. The silane molecule facilitates the formation of a chemical bond between the resin and the filler. The principle is similar to **silanation** treatment, when ceramics are to be bonded to the tooth using a resin composite bonding system, for example in the bonding of ceramic restorations such as veneers (see Chapters 11 and 22). One example of a silane coupler in glass-filled resin composite is **γ-methacryloxypropyltriethoxysilane (γ-MPTS)**, a vinyl silane compound. The silane molecule is bifunctional with groups that react with the inorganic filler and others that react with the organic resin, hydrophilic and hydrophobic groups, respectively. The γ-MPTS is acid activated and when reacted with the filler, the methoxy- groups hydrolyse to hydroxyl groups, which in turn react with hydroxyl groups on the filler. There is also a condensation reaction with the hydroxyl group of the hydrolysed silane. The silane coupler then bonds via its carbon double bond to the resin. The bond can be degraded by water absorbed by the material during clinical function.

> **Bifunctional molecule/monomer:** a bifunctional monomer is a monomer unit with two active bonding sites.

The bond between the filler and the resin needs to be durable and strong. If this is not the case, stresses applied to the set material will not be equally distributed within the material and the resin will have to absorb more. This will lead to creep and wear of the restoration, further leading to fracture. Stress concentrations will also occur at the interfaces between the filler and resin, so leading to the formation of crack initiation sites. Fatigue fracture will occur as the resin does not have a high resistance to crack propagation. Stress can therefore be transferred from the strong filler particles to the next through the lower strength resin.

However, there is a major problem in that the resin is hydrophobic while the modern glasses used in composite will take up water and can undergo slow hydrolytic degradation. Once water ingress occurs, these materials start a very long and slow process of degradation, which leads to surface disruption with time.

Chemicals required for the curing process

Historically, resin composites set by chemical means and it was only in the late 1970s that light curing became more prominent. This led to a step change in performance of these materials. The resin composites can therefore be divided conveniently into:

- Chemically cured (sometimes referred to as self-cured)
- Light cured
- Dual cured, materials that are activated both by light and chemically.

The chemicals necessary to initiate and then complete the setting reaction are contained in the unset material. The reaction in both chemical and light curing materials is a **free radical polymerization**.

Chemically cured resin composites

Chemically cured resin composites are supplied as a two-paste system with the setting reaction commencing when the two pastes are blended. The base paste contains monomer and filler together with a tertiary amine such as **N,N-dimethyl-p-toluidene** and the catalyst paste contains monomer and filler, but in this case there is the extra addition of benzoyl peroxide dispersed in a phthalate. The chemical reaction is sometimes referred to as a **dark cure**, implying that it will occur without the need for light energy unlike the light cured resin composites.

Light cured resin composites

The majority of light cured resin composite restorative materials are cured only when the material is exposed to light energy, which initiates a chemical reaction within the material to form the set material. The chemicals required for the curing process are contained in the unset material and can be divided into:

- A **photo-initiator**, usually a **peroxidase** or a **diketone** such as camphorquinone. More recently, novel photo-initiators have been considered such as phenylpropanedione (PPD) and Lucirin TPO (ethyl 2,4,6-trimethylbenzoylphenylphosphinate) (see Chapter 2).
- An **accelerator**, a tertiary amine such as that used in the chemically activated two-paste systems.

Mechanism of cure

On exposure to a sufficient amount of light energy at the correct wavelength of light, the monomers will polymerize to form a rigid cross-linked polymer, the various polymer chains linking via the methacrylate groups. The process of light curing is explained in detail in Chapter 2.

It is possible to accelerate the polymerization reaction by increasing the concentration of the camphorquinone. While the material sets quickly, the penalty for this is that the propagation phase of the polymerization process is shortened such that there are shorter chain lengths formed and the material is not as strong. Additionally, the material may be more susceptible to ambient light and can start to set if exposed to the dental operating light.

Once the activating light is switched on, the reactive groups on each resin chain start to polymerize. The reaction goes through two stages:

- An initial **pre-gelation phase** where there is considerable mobility of the polymer chains. This occurs during the first 8 seconds of a 10-second curing cycle. During the last 2 seconds of the curing cycle the material goes through the gel stage and become much stiffer. This is known as the **post-gelation phase**. About 85% of the conversion that will be achieved occurs in this period. After the material is considered to be clinically set some post-curing continues but this is very limited – not exceeding 15% – and the bulk of which is generally complete within 2 hours. Little change occurs after 24 hours.

It should be remembered that the polymerization reaction is **anaerobic**, that is, in the presence of air the material will only be partially cured. This explains why if no matrix is used to cover the surface of the restoration the surface will remain tacky and is then called the **oxygen inhibition layer**. This partly cured layer should be removed and the restorative trimmed back to the fully set material.

Dual cured

These materials give the dentist the advantages of setting the cement when they are satisfied with the placed restoration as well as peace of mind should insufficient light energy reach any inaccessible regions so the cement will cure by the dark or chemical cure. To permit this to occur, these products contain both chemical accelerators and light activators.

Ultraviolet stabilizers

When exposed to natural light, the material will, over time, change colour due to oxidation. This is prevented by the addition of **ultraviolet absorber** such as **2-hydroxy-4-methoxybenzophenone**, which works by absorbing **electromagnetic radiation**.

Polymerization inhibitors

Even though resin composites are solely light cured, dimethacrylate monomers will polymerize on storage because they invariably contain small amounts of chemical catalyst from the manufacturing process, which will eventually decompose initiating polymerization. Chemical inhibitors are also added to resin composite to prevent premature setting and to increase the material's shelf-life. **Hydroquinone** was used in a few parts per million but it tended to cause discolouration of the material so a **monomethyl ether of hydroquinone** is now used.

Radiopaque materials

The need for restorative materials to be radiopaque was discussed in Chapter 4. In many cases the filler particles contain heavy metal derivatives which are inherently radiopaque, such as barium, zinc, strontium and ytterbium. In those materials containing radiolucent filler, particles such as quartz or lithium aluminium silicate, and barium salts, can be added to convey radiopacity to the material. There is an ISO requirement (see 'The regulation of dental materials and the International Standards Organization' on the inside back cover of this book) that the radiopacity of these materials is equivalent to 2 mm of aluminium. However, there is variation in the radiodensity of materials above this which depends on the volume of radiopaque filler used.

Pigments and opacifiers

Clearly the material must exactly match the tooth tissue it is being used to restore. A range of shades must therefore be available. Inorganic oxide compounds such as **iron oxides** are added in very small quantities to the resin to vary the shade and other optical properties such as opacity and translucency.

PROPERTIES

Polymerization shrinkage

Polymerization shrinkage of resin composites has been cited as one of the most important shortcomings of this family of materials.

- A material which shrinks markedly will leave a gap at the tooth–restoration interface, thus allowing the passage of bacteria and oral fluids. This is termed **microleakage** (Figure 7.13).
- As is discussed in greater detail in Chapter 11, the bond achieved between the material and tooth is very good indeed. During curing, a large amount of shrinkage will cause high levels of stress to be built up in the remaining tooth structure, the tooth–restoration interface or the restorative material itself.

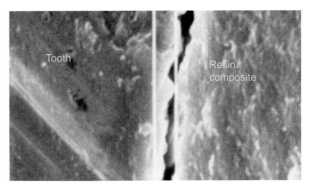

Fig. 7.13 Interface between the tooth and restorative after polymerization shrinkage. The gap is approximately 30 μm wide.

- It is also more difficult to manipulate the material to form good contact areas and stable occlusal relationships when the material will shrink (Figure 7.14).

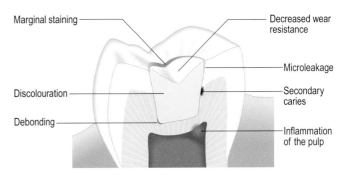

Fig. 7.14 The sites where polymerization shrinkage can affect a restoration: marginal staining; microleakage down the wall with risk of recurrent caries; microleakage causing pulpal irritation; and pull away and debond from floor of cavity.

The advantages of decreased shrinkage are summarized below:

- Reduced postoperative sensitivity
- Reduced stresses within the tooth tissue, at the tooth–restoration interface and within the material
- Reduced bulk or microfracture of tooth tissue
- Reduced microleakage
- Reduced secondary caries
- Improved bonding between the resin, adhesive and the tooth due to greater dimensional stability.

Some manufacturers have changed the resin chemistry by changing the constituents of the resin. By attempting to eliminate the lower molecular weight monomers that exhibit greatest shrinkage on polymerization, the overall shrinkage of the resin can be reduced. Many products have as their resin component a mix of bis-GMA with **bisphenol A polyethylene glycol diether dimethacrylate** (bis-EMA) and UDMA, which shrink much less on curing that the original bis-GMA/lower molecular weight systems. By using this system, there is virtual elimination of TEGDMA and the higher polymerization shrinkage values seen with it. This resin is more hydrophobic and a slightly softer resin matrix is created, which may influence wear resistance. The resin base colour is lighter and the higher molecular weight leads to less shrinkage as there is greater distance between the methacrylate groups on the monomer chain.

Of the methacrylate-based resin composites currently available, the lowest shrinkage is of the order of 2.2% by volume while the average value is between 2.5% and 3%. This is seen in products using the bis-EMA/UDMA resin combination and not bis-GMA resins alone and occurs when the monomer matrix converts to the polymer state. This figure while low, still represents a significant problem clinically and so manufacturers have attempted to further reduce it in a number of ways to reduce the effect of this shrinkage.

Strategies to overcome polymerization shrinkage

In general when a polymer sets it shrinks toward the centre of its mass. If it is in the form of a sphere, the diameter of the sphere is reduced. In a cavity the problem is more complex but the basic principle is the same. When placing these materials the dentist can reduce the effect of shrinkage of the overall restoration in a number of ways. Firstly, if the material is placed in increments and each increment is cured prior to the placement of the next increment, the shrinkage is minimized and compensated for to some extent. This technique is termed **incremental build-up**.

The magnitude of stress depends on the composition of the composite and its ability to flow before gelation occurs. This is influenced by the shape of the cavity and can be overcome by the way the dentist places the material into the cavity. This has been termed the **configuration factor (C factor)** and is the ratio of bonded to unbonded surfaces. The higher the ratio the more stress is potentially incorporated into the situation. A Class I cavity has the highest C factor as there are five bonded surfaces (four axial walls and the cavity floor) and only one unbonded surface where stress relief can occur (the occlusal surface). Compare this with a Class IV cavity or a cuspal replacement where the converse occurs. Techniques have been advocated for the placement of resin composite so that only one or two surfaces are contacted by the material at any one time, which decreases the C factor to eliminate stress. This will also allow for compensation of the polymerization shrinkage, with each subsequent increment offsetting the effects of this shrinkage. Unfortunately, the recommendation to keep cavities small tends towards having cavities with high C factors, which means that greater stress is set up with the inherent risk of interface failure.

Class IV: cavity which involves the incisal tip of an anterior tooth.

Incremental build up allows for more effective and uniform polymerization and reduces total polymerization shrinkage (Figure 7.15), which may decrease stress generated at cavity walls and so reducing potential for debond gaps and cuspal deflection. It has, however, been shown that even with incremental build-up, once the final increment is placed the risk of cuspal flexure still exists. Proper placement of the first increment is the most important step and the dentist should ensure that it is fully polymerized as this increment is the furthest from the light.

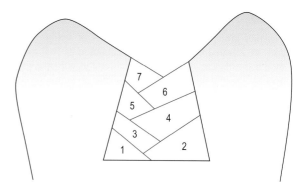

Fig. 7.15 The herring bone incremental build-up for resin composite placement in a posterior cavity.

Stresses within teeth will also depend on the **compliance** of the tooth. This is the ability of the tooth to withstand flexure and is dependent on the amount and quality of the remaining tooth tissue and its position. Furthermore, how each increment is placed in the cavity and polymerized can influence the stresses built up within the tooth, at the tooth–restoration interface and within the resin composite material itself. When the composite shrinks, various effects can occur in the cavity:

- If the tooth tissue is of sufficient bulk that it is stiff and inflexible, all the stresses will be concentrated at the interface between the tooth and the filling.
- If these forces exceed the bond strength at the interface, a gap will develop. As has been seen above, this is associated with a potential risk of failure of the restoration.
- Shrinkage occurs towards the wall of the preparation to which the composite is most strongly bonded. Separation at the interface may occur if the contraction force exceeds the bond strength.
- Fracture of enamel and dentine may occur causing fracture of thin enamel margins, cuspal flexure or cracked cusp.

Stresses also occur within the composite material itself. If, however, the remaining tooth tissue is less bulky and can flex, when the polymerization shrinkage takes place, the stresses are dissipated through the remaining tooth tissue and the interface between the tooth and restoration. In this case some flexure of the tooth can occur. Partial or total bond failure will allow bacteria to penetrate the tooth–material interface, causing caries, staining and postoperative sensitivity. The restoration may also be lost.

Polymerization stress is mainly determined by three factors:

- Polymerization shrinkage
- Internal flowability of the materials
- Polymerization kinetics (speed of cure).

Sensitivity to ambient light

Resin composite materials are **photophilic**. This can work in two opposing ways for the dentist. It is an obvious advantage to be able to cure the material at will when the clinician is happy with the form of the restoration placed. However, due to the strength and amount of ambient light in the clinic, the material can start to set prematurely with consequential clinical problems. Thus it may be necessary to reduce the light that the unset material is exposed to by either angling the operating light away from the area being worked on or by using an orange shield to filter light of the photo-initiator's wavelength (Figure 7.16). The manufacturer can also play a part in the control of this by varying the amount of tertiary amine included in the paste.

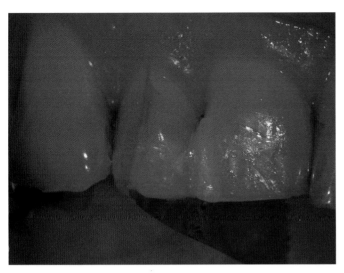

Fig. 7.16 An orange filter being used when the dentist is manipulating unset resin composite. This filter reduces light to the optimum wavelength so preventing premature set of the material and allowing the dentist to work with the material until it is desirable to light cure.

Fig. 7.17 Change in composite volume with respect to time after polymerization and then immediate immersion in water. Immediately on polymerization there is a 2.3% reduction in volume which by 10 weeks has reduced to 1.9%. The composite restoration remains smaller than the cavity that it was designed to obturate.

Sensitivity to water and water uptake

All resin-based composites are inherently **hydrophobic** (sensitive to water contamination) due to their chemical nature and so excellent moisture control is essential during placement and prior to curing to optimize placement and longevity. During clinical use, water from oral fluids may be taken up into a dental material. This is termed **water sorption** and occurs in resin composite materials. It can cause irreversible degradation of properties of the resin composite, affecting its wear resistance and colour stability as staining can occur. The water is **absorbed** by the resin. The filler particles will not absorb water but **adsorb** it on its surface. In the long term this will also mean filler degradation.

Rubber dam, which is the most effective means of achieving a dry field, has been strongly advocated when resin-based composites are being used clinically. If the tooth to be worked on cannot be properly isolated or if the cavity extends into an area where good moisture control cannot be gained then consideration should be given to using an alternative material.

The amount of water taken up primarily depends on the resin content of the resin composite and the durability of the bond between the filler and resin. In general, the greater the resin volume in the composite, the greater the water sorption. As water sorption occurs, the material will swell due to **hygroscopic expansion**. This phenomenon starts about 15 minutes after initial polymerization and continues for up to 10 weeks, depending on the size of the restoration. It has been postulated that this expansion helps to offset the effects of polymerization shrinkage. However, this fluid exchange is a slow process so it cannot prevent the instantaneous shrinkage seen on setting. The volume uptake is also substantially less than the volumetric shrinkage, so this can never compensate for the initial shrinkage (see Figure 7.17).

Coefficient of thermal expansion

Resin composites generally have a coefficient of thermal expansion relatively close to that of tooth tissue. Again the expansion is usually greatest with those resin composites that have a large volume fraction of resin. The significance of this is that during normal use on ingesting cold food the restoration shrinks more than the tooth, stressing the tooth–restoration interface. When hot liquids and food are ingested the restoration expands more than the tooth, causing the restoration to become larger than the cavity and compressing the tooth tissue with which it is in contact.

Biocompatibility

Many millions of resin composite restorations have now been placed worldwide with no adverse biological effects. However, a number of potential problems have been attributed to this family of materials.

- Bisphenol A is known to mimic the hormone oestrogen in vitro and has been linked with male infertility, and prostatic and breast carcinomas. This is primarily when in monomeric form. After polymerization the risks are reduced.
- Bis-GMA, TEGDMA and UDMA are cytotoxic in vitro in their pure form. There is concern about the biological effects of these chemicals eluding from resin composites restorations after curing. The amount of chemical released depends on the type of the resin composite and the method and efficiency of its cure. There is evidence of mild pulpal inflammation when the material is placed directly on the pulp. This response continues for some time.
- Hydroxyethylmethacrylate (HEMA) is contained in many resin composite products and bonding agents. Its potentially harmful effects are discussed in Chapter 10.

For these reasons the use of resin composites on pulp tissue or where micro exposures may be present is contraindicated.

Durability

The longevity of these materials is still not as good as other materials such as amalgam. The number of restoration surfaces has a directly proportional influence on survival outcome. This at first sight is a surprise as the vast majority of the mechanical testing values for the resin composites are as good as those for amalgam. However, the Achilles heel of the composites is that the resin is relatively much weaker than the filler. The detrimental effects of water sorption and solubility linked to the less than ideal level of conversion often obtained in the mouth means that the results will always be more variable, and any restoration will undergo a slow but steady degradation after placement. This is compounded by the wear that can occur as a result of the problems at the interface between the resin and the filler.

RESIN COMPOSITE CATEGORIES

As mentioned on page 76, the resin composites can be divided conveniently into:

- Chemically cured (sometimes referred to as self-cured)
- Light cured
- Dual cured.

Chemically cured resin composites

The setting of chemically cured materials started as soon as the two pastes are blended together by hand mixing. Disadvantages of these materials are:

- They have a finite working time prior to their setting.
- Air can be incorporated into the mixed mass during mixing so causing porosity and failure due to internal stress concentrations as a result of air inhibition of the setting reaction (Figure 7.18).
- Their presentation makes their clinical manipulation more difficult.

- Inferior colour stability due to the increased amount of tertiary amine needed to chemically catalyse the reaction. These materials tended to become yellow over time (Figure 7.18).
- Their abrasiveness damages the stainless steel instruments used to mix them.
- There is lower conversion of monomer to polymer.

As a result, chemical cured composites have largely fallen out of favour since the development of light (command) curing.

Commercially available products

Some materials are still available on the market (see Table 7.4).

Table 7.4 Some chemically cured resin composites still available on the market

Product	Manufacturer
Adaptic	Dentsply
Chemical Cure Composite	Sci-Pharm
Clearfil Core New Bond	Kuraray
Clearfil FII	Kuraray
Clearfil Posterior 3	Kuraray
Concise	3M ESPE
LuxaCore	DMG

Mixing

Two equal-sized portions of paste (one catalyst, the other base) are dispensed onto the mixing pad. These portions should be rapidly mixed with a plastic spatula and the blended paste applied quickly

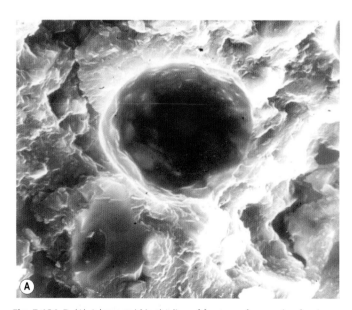
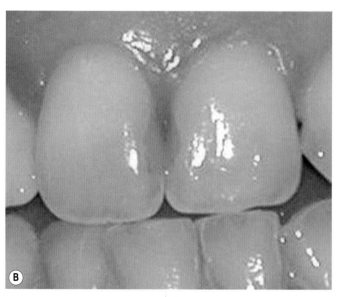

Fig. 7.18A,B (A) A large void in the line of fracture of a sample of resin composite, which was formed as a result of air incorporation during mixing. (B) A chemically cured composite which has discoloured in bulk due to the decomposition of the tertiary amine.

to the cavity to be restored. The material should then be left undisturbed for 4–5 minutes to allow it to achieve its full set.

Light cured resin composites

Generally speaking, light cured materials are more convenient and these days the majority of the resin composite products available involve some exposure to light energy to effect their cure. The mechanism of light curing is described in detail in Chapter 2.

Dual-cured resin composites

As the name suggests these materials have the ability to set chemically without exposure to light energy or can be cured by command with a curing light. These materials tend to be used as core build-up materials or for bonding indirect restorations (see Chapter 11).

Commercially available products

Representative examples of dual cured resin composites are shown in Table 7.5.

Table 7.5 Some dual-cured resin composite core build-up materials currently available on the market

Product	Manufacturer
Clearfil DC Core Automix	Kuraray
Core Restore 2	Kerr Hawe
CromaCore Twix	Morita
LuxaCore Dual	DMG
MultiCore HB	Ivoclar Vivadent
ParaCore	Coltène Whaledent
Rebilda DC	Voco

Core build-up materials need to be strong by definition. It is advantageous that their hardness is such that they cut like dentine during the subsequent crown or bridge abutment preparation. Many products are used with core forms to facilitate their placement. Some products are advocated to cement posts in situ as well as being used as the core build-up material which is clearly convenient in that the clinician need only use one material, simplifying the procedure. Care must be taken to ensure that the margin of the definitive cast restoration extends beyond the margin of the resin composite core, otherwise there is a risk of failure as the resin composite degrades.

ADVANTAGES AND DISADVANTAGES OF RESIN COMPOSITES

The advantages and disadvantages of using resin composite as restorative materials are set out in Table 7.6.

Table 7.6 Advantages and disadvantages of resin composite materials

Advantages	Disadvantages
Excellent aesthetics	Time consuming to place so more expensive
More conservative cavities	Hydrophobic
Command set	Photophilic
Multiple applications	Polymerization shrinkage
Can be repaired adequately	Technique sensitive, more difficult to place
May be bonded to enamel and dentine using adhesive systems	Decreased longevity with increased number of restored surfaces compared with amalgam
Reduced microleakage when compared with amalgam	Attract greater number of bacteria than amalgam restorations unless well polished
Low thermal conductivity	Difficult to finish adequately

INDICATIONS AND CONTRAINDICATIONS

The indications and contraindications for resin composites are set out in Table 7.7.

GENERAL SUBTYPES OF RESIN COMPOSITE MATERIALS ON THE MARKET

Resin composites can also be classified into three groups defined by their handling characteristics:

- **Universal**: used for general work, having been available for the longest time. Can be used for all applications but there may be some compromise in specific uses.
- **Flowable**: more fluid composites used especially for the ultraconservative restoration of teeth.
- **Packable**: more viscous materials generally only used in posterior situations.

The handling characteristics are manipulated by the manufacturers by varying the constituents of the materials. Generally, the stiffer materials have higher filler loading with the opposite being true for the flowable materials. Figure 7.19 illustrates the varying viscosities of flowable, universal and packable resin composite materials, all manufactured by the same company.

Build-up or layering techniques have become popular with those clinicians and patients desiring the highest quality of aesthetic restoration. These are mainly used anteriorly but their use in the posterior segments is increasing. The materials appropriate for this technique have been termed **layering** or **build-up composites**. The materials have varying levels of filler opacifiers and tints to alter translucency, opacity and shade of the material. The selection of the appropriate materials for a particular use is therefore of some importance if an optimum result is desired.

Table 7.7 Indications and contraindications of resin composite materials

Indications	Contraindications
Conservative repair of direct and indirect restorations	Poor oral hygiene
Direct restorations where aesthetics are of prime importance	Where excellent moisture control cannot be guaranteed
Patient preference	Extensive cavities
Core build-ups	Operator inexperience
Splinting of periodontally compromised teeth or replacement of exfoliated teeth	When any cavity margin is not in enamel
Treatment of non-carious tooth surface loss (NCTSL) lesions	High occlusal loads/unfavourable occlusion
Restoration of small- and medium-sized Class I and II cavities and perhaps larger cases depending on the clinical situation	With dentine pins
Allergy to other materials (such a metals)	Proven cases of sensitivity to any of the materials contained therein or their adhesives
Treatment of fractured cusp	High caries rate
Ultraconservative treatment of carious lesions (preventive resin restoration)	Insufficient time available to complete the procedure
Minimally invasive techniques	Use with a eugenol-containing dental material, e.g. lining or temporary luting agent
Bonding of indirect restorations	
Restoration of Class III and IV cavities	
Restoration of cavities in patients opposed to amalgam use	
Where it is not possible to obtain retention form for a non-adhesive restoration	

✓ Which resin composite should the dentist choose to use?

As with any dental material, the ease of which the clinician can use and manipulate the material is an important factor; therefore personal preference is a significant factor. Other criteria which should be considered when selecting a resin composite material are:

- The intended use; anterior, posterior or highly aesthetic restoration. Can one material have multiple uses clinically?
- An adequate range of shades available for the intended situation.
- The resin composite consistency:
  - The ease of removal from the compule or syringe
  - Adhesion to instruments
  - The ease of placement in the cavity
  - The ease of adaptation to the cavity
  - The ease of manipulation and sculpturing
  - The ability to retain shape during manipulation (i.e. its resistance to **slump**)
  - Incremental adaptation to bulk without voids being created.
- Sensitivity to ambient light, i.e. premature polymerization under normal clinic lighting during placement.
- Curing efficiency of light polymerizing unit: will the selected light cure the selected material effectively?
- Ease of polishing and the ability of the material to retain this in clinical use.
- Cost effectiveness. Very often cheaper materials will not perform well, necessitating their replacement at extra financial cost to the dentist. Frequently there will be a biological cost to the tooth as more tooth will be lost with each subsequent replacement. The prudent dentist will insist of using good-quality materials which may be more expensive initially but whose performance and longevity have been proven to be superior.

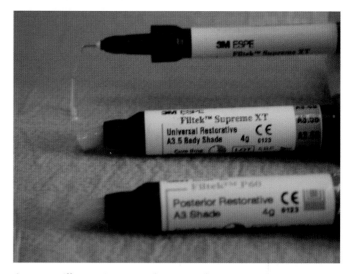

Fig. 7.19 Difference in viscosity between a flowable (Filtek Supreme Flow), universal (Filtek Supreme XT), and a packable resin composite (Filtek P60) (3M ESPE).

Universal resin composites

The universal resin composites are the conventional presentation and 'work horse'. They perform satisfactorily in many situations and often provide a clinically acceptable result (Table 7.8 and Figure 7.20). However, their properties limit their application in the specialized practice where more complex and challenging aesthetic treatments are being carried out.

Table 7.8 Indications for the clinical use of universal resin composite materials

Indications	Contraindications
Restoration of Class III and Class IV cavities where aesthetics are important but not paramount	Where aesthetics are critical
Repair of incisal non-carious tooth surface loss (NCTSL) lesions	Too conservative a cavity
Use with reinforcing fibres for splinting	Where inadequate enamel surface is available for etching
Class V to restore carious lesions where retention is by an undercut	
Restoration of small Class I and II cavities	

Table 7.9 Some regular viscosity resin composite materials

Product	Manufacturer	Type of composite
Amaris	Voco	Hybrid
Brilliant Esthetic Line	Coltène Whaledent	Fine hybrid
Ceram.X Mono	Dentsply	Nanofilled
Charisma	Heraeus	Microhybrid
Clearfil Majesty Esthetic	Kuraray	Nanofilled
Durafill VS	Heraeus	Microfilled
EcuSphere	DMG	Microfilled
EcuSphere Carat	DMG	Microhybrid
EcuSphere Shape	DMG	Microhybrid
Filtek Supreme XTE Universal Restorable	3M ESPE	Nanofilled
Filtek Z250	3M ESPE	Microhybrid
GC Gradia Direct	GC	Microhybrid
Glacier	SDI	Microhybrid
GrandioSO	Voco	Nanohybrid
Helio Progress	Ivoclar Vivadent	Microfilled
Herculite XRV	Kerr Hawe	Microhybrid
Ice	SDI	Nanohybrid
N'Durance	Septodont	Nanohybrid
Photo Clearfil Bright	Kuraray	Microfine
Point4	Kerr Hawe	Microhybrid
Polofil Supra	Voco	Microhybrid
Premise	Kerr Hawe	Nanofilled
Prodigy	Kerr Hawe	Microhybrid
Spectrum TPH 3	Dentsply	Microhybrid
Synergy D6	Coltène Whaledent	Nanohybrid
Synergy Nano Formula Duo Shade	Coltène Whaledent	Nanohybrid
Tetric	Ivoclar Vivadent	Microhybrid
Tetric EvoCeram	Ivoclar Vivadent	Nanohybrid
Venus	Heraeus	Microhybrid
Z100MP	3M ESPE	Microhybrid

Commercially available products

See Table 7.9 for products currently on the market. Some are available in shades which correspond to gingival tissue (for example GC's Gradia Gum). This is useful if the clinician wishes to mask an area in the cervical region of a tooth to make it look like gingival tissue.

For many of the products in this universal resin composite category, the manufacturers claim that they may be used in the posterior segment. The clinician should be careful with this indication as the durability of these materials is still being questioned and results of existing long-term studies are equivocal.

Flowable composites

Flowable resin composite materials have been available since the mid-1990s. They complement the universal resin composites as they have a much lower viscosity with different handling characteristics. They are chemically similar to conventional resin composite materials but with a substantially lower filler loading. In some products the filler particle size has been increased to compensate

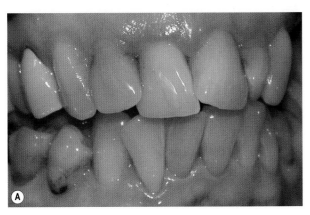
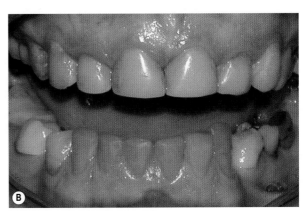

Fig. 7.20 A universal resin composite being used for two different indications: (A) a distoincisal Class IV restoration in tooth 11 and (B) build up of incisal edges of the lower incisors and canines affected by non-carious tooth surface loss. Note that while the aesthetics are acceptable they are not as good as they could have been had a layering resin composite been used.

for this. When compared with universal resin composite materials they:

- Are not as strong in compression
- Are not as wear resistant
- Exhibit greater polymerization shrinkage upon curing.

They behave more like the resin component of the composite. Table 7.10 lists the indications and contradictions of flowable composite products and two examples of small Class I cavities filled with flowable composite are illustrated in Figure 7.21.

Commercially available products

A representative examples are shown in Table 7.11. The flowable resin composite materials currently on the market are presented in a variety of shades and opacities, including a pink shade to mimic gingival tissue. Some of the newer products on the market are self-etching (Vertise Flow, Kerr Hawe) and provide a means of enhanced micromechanical attachment due to etching of the enamel. There may be some chemical interaction but to date this has not been demonstrated conclusively. The handling of these materials varies between products but generally their thixotropic characteristics are such that they hold their shape when they are placed and do not 'run', drip or slump.

> **Thixotropy:** certain gels or fluids are thick and viscous under normal conditions, but can flow, becoming thinner and less viscous, when shaken, agitated, or otherwise stressed. In the dental arena, stressing by manipulating the material will allow it to thin and once manipulation ceases it will thicken again.

Table 7.10 Main indications and contraindications of flowable resin composite materials

Indications	Contraindications
Small Class I cavities particularly involving enamel only or a small amount of dentine in permanent or deciduous teeth	High stress bearing situations, for example, the restoration of tooth wear on the incisal edges of anterior teeth
Class V cavities especially caused by non-carious tooth surface loss (NCTSL)	Restoration of anything larger than small Class I cavities.
Repair of deficient amalgam margins where the restoration is otherwise sound	Where good moisture control cannot be achieved
As a lining material especially when a packable composite is to be used to restore the cavity	Restoration of any Class II cavities
Blocking out of undercuts in inlay preparations	
To enhance the bond between the enamel margin and a more heavily filled (i.e. packable) resin composite at the bottom of a Class II box	
Ceramic repairs in non-stress-bearing situations	
Repair of bisacryl composite temporary restorations (Chapter 14)	

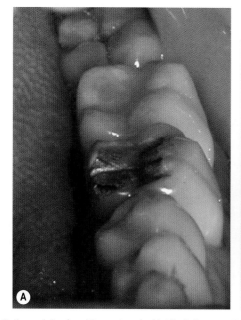 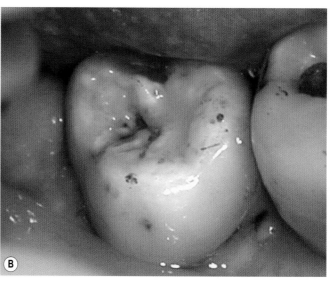

Fig. 7.21A,B Two minimal cavities restored with Filtek Supreme XT Flow (3M ESPE) (A) Tooth 37, the material is covering the whole of the occlusal surface. (B) The restored mesial part of the occlusal fissure in tooth 48.
(Photo on the right courtesy of Dental Update.)

Table 7.11 Some flowable resin composite materials currently available on the market

Product	Manufacturer	Type of composite
Clearfil Majesty Flow	Kuraray	Microhybrid
Durafil Flow	Heraeus	Microfilled
Filtek Supreme XTE Flowable Restorative	3M ESPE	Nanofilled
G-ænial Flowable	GC	Nanohybrid
GC Gradia Direct Flo	GC	Nanohybrid
GC Gradia Direct LoFlo	GC	Microhybrid
Grandio Flow	Voco	Nanohybrid
Heliomolar Flow	Ivoclar Vivadent	Microfilled
N'Durance Dimer Flow	Septodont	Nanohybrid
Premise Flowable	Kerr Hawe	Nanofilled
Revolution Formula 2	Kerr Hawe	Hybrid
Smart Dentine Replacement (SDR)	Dentsply	Microfilled
Synergy D6 Flow	Coltène Whaledent	Nanohybrid
Synergy Flow	Coltène Whaledent	Nanohybrid
Tetric EvoFlow	Ivoclar Vivadent	Nanohybrid
Vertise Flow	Kerr Hawe	Nanohybrid
Venus Flow	Heraeus	Hybrid
Wave	SDI	Nanofilled
X-Flow	Dentsply	Nanofilled

Applications

Non-carious tooth surface loss lesions

A restorative material with a lower modulus of elasticity such as a flowable resin composite has an increased ability to flex during function, and is thus better able to withstand flexural forces. This is also dependent on the bonding between the tooth and restoration (see Chapter 11). Lower modulus of elasticity is particularly useful when the clinician wishes to restore **non-carious tooth surface loss** lesions as stresses are concentrated in the cervical region of a tooth. This has been termed abfraction. Universal resin composites should be used with caution in this situation as unlike flowable resin composites, their high filler loading makes them more rigid and more prone to marginal disruption. Flowable composite materials have the advantage of better aesthetics when compared to the glass ionomer cements which have also been advocated for use in these sites (Figures 7.22 and 7.23).

Abfraction: During function, flexion occurs in the teeth and this flexion is concentrated at the cementoenamel junction. The enamel crystals in this region suffer microfractures and the defect is born as the enamel and dentine break away. The lesion can be exacerbated by the effects of **abrasion** (foreign body to tooth wear e.g. tooth brushing) and also by chemical means (**erosion**).

Preventive resin restoration

Flowable resin composite materials may be used to provide a thin covering on the occlusal surface of molars and premolars where early fissure caries has been removed.

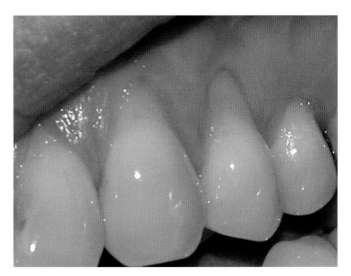

Fig. 7.22 Preoperative view of buccal (Class V) non-carious tooth surface loss lesions on teeth 23 and 24.
(Photo courtesy of Dental Update.)

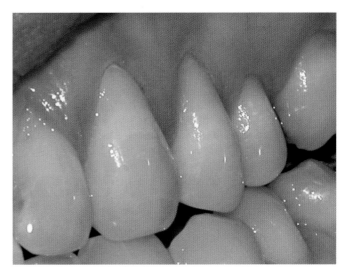

Fig. 7.23 The non-carious tooth surface loss lesions shown in Figure 7.22 restored using a flowable resin composite material (Filtek Supreme XT Flow, 3M ESPE).
(Photo courtesy of Dental Update.)

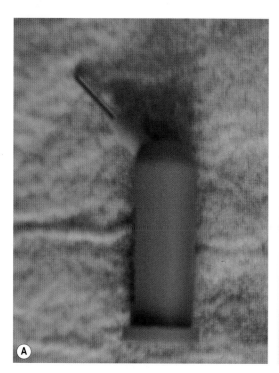 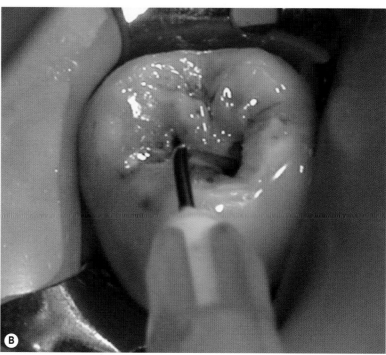

Fig. 7.24 (A) A compule containing a flowable resin composite material (X-Flow, Dentsply) and (B) a thin metal cannula directing a flowable resin composite material into a small occlusal cavity.
(Photo on the right courtesy of Dental Update.*)*

Many flowable resin composite materials are presented in compules or syringe presentation with a blunt-ended needle. This facilitates clinical placement as the material can be precisely directed into the area into where it is required (Figure 7.24). This blunt tip may also be used to 'sweep' the material into the desired position, or, alternatively, an instrument with a broad tip such as William's periodontal probe could be used (Figure 7.25).

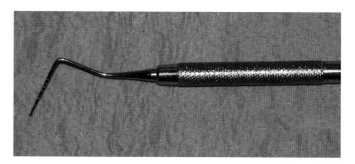

Fig. 7.25 The blunt end of William's periodontal probe can be used to sweep flowable resin composite into the fissure system or small occlusal cavity.

Where the lesion is deeper, the bulk of the cavity is restored with either a glass ionomer cement or a universal composite and then covered with the flowable composite to give a smooth surface. This technique is used primarily in paediatric dentistry.

Fissure sealants

Fissure sealants are placed on the occlusal surface of newly erupted molar teeth to occlude the fissure pattern and thereby delay or prevent the onset of fissure caries (Figure 7.26). These materials were probably the precursor to flowable composites. The initial materials had no filler but more recently a low loading of filler particles has been added to aid manipulation and as a means of identifying the sealant once it has been placed. The absence of filler in some sealants means that the products are transparent. This permits the examination of the tissue underneath them to detect recurrent caries. The yellow colouration of the resin makes diagnosis of a recurring lesion difficult unless it is extensive. Some products are coloured pink initially to aid in the application and, like some ceiling paints, change colour when light cured to facilitate their placement. Some resin systems are claimed to release fluoride.

There has been concern that materials predominantly based on bisphenol A may potentially mimic oestrogen. This concern is based on the effect of the unpolymerized bisphenol A, which may remain on the surface of the fissure sealant as a result of the inhibition of the polymerization by oxygen.

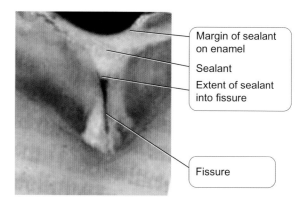

Margin of sealant on enamel

Sealant

Extent of sealant into fissure

Fissure

Fig. 7.26 Cross-section through a tooth showing the extent of a resin sealant over its occlusal surface and into the depth of the fissure.

Commercially available products

A selection of the commercially available materials are listed in Table 7.12. Other materials available which have been used for fissure sealing include glass ionomer cements and compomers.

Table 7.12 Some fissure sealant products currently available on the market

Product	Manufacturer	Notes
Clinpro Sealant	3M ESPE	Changes from pink to white when cured
Concise	3M ESPE	White
Conseal F	SDI	Releases fluoride
Delton	Dentsply	Available in white or transparent
Fissurit	Voco	Available in white or transparent
Fissurit F	Voco	White with fluoride release
Fissurit FX	Voco	White with increased filler loading
Fuji Triage	GC	This is a glass ionomer cement
Grandio Seal	Voco	White nanohybrid resin sealant
Guardian Seal	Kerr Hawe	Can be seen yet allows caries detection
Helioseal	Ivoclar Vivadent	White in colour
Helioseal Clear	Ivoclar Vivadent	transparent
Helioseal Clear Chroma	Ivoclar Vivadent	Transparent with reversible colour change
Helioseal F	Ivoclar Vivadent	White with fluoride release

Packables

This presentation was developed to be used in posterior situations. The more viscous nature of packable resin composites necessitates increasing the force the clinician must apply to place the material into the cavity. Their handling on placement is more like dental amalgam, in that it requires force to condense the material into the cavity. Indeed one reason that packable resin composites were produced was to mimic this property of dental amalgam. Dentists subconsciously compare all materials to the handling of dental amalgam, however, unlike amalgam, the molecules in the materials are not condensed closer to each other and so the term 'packable' is more correctly used than 'condensable'. The increased viscosity is usually gained by a higher volume of filler (in excess of 60%) incorporated into the resin matrix. The majority of these materials are hybrid materials to achieve good filler packing. The effect of a higher filler load increases the fracture resistance of the material which is required in the posterior region of the mouth to withstand forces during function. Manufacturers expend much time in achieving a homogeneous paste at these filler loadings and ensuring that there is sufficient resin to bind the filler particles together. The high viscosity of packable composites can potentially increase the tendency to create voids along the cavity walls and between each increment of

material. Figure 7.27 shows a molar restored using a packable resin composite material.

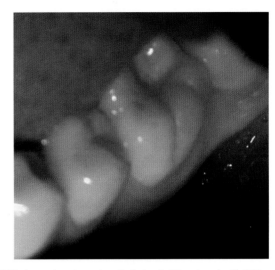

Fig. 7.27 An occluso-buccal cavity in tooth 36 restored with P60 (3M ESPE).

Commercially available products

Table 7.13 lists some of the currently available commercial materials. Materials such as GC Gradia Direct X contain **pre-polymerized filler** to further reduce the amount of resin and with it the amount of polymerization shrinkage.

Table 7.13 Some packable resin composite materials currently available on the market

Product	Manufacturer	Type of composite
Clearfil Majesty Posterior	Kuraray	Nanofilled
Clearfil Photo Core	Kuraray	Core build-up material
Clearfil Photo Posterior	Kuraray	Nanofilled
Filtek P60	3M ESPE	Hybrid
G-ænial Posterior	GC	Nanohybrid
GC Gradia Direct X	GC	Nanofilled
GC Gradia Posterior	GC	Nanofilled
Heliomolar	Ivoclar Vivadent	Microfilled
Heliomolar HB	Ivoclar Vivadent	Microhybrid
Premise Packable	Kerr Hawe	Nanohybrid
Prodigy Condensable	Kerr Hawe	Hybrid
QuiXfil	Dentsply	Hybrid
Rok	SDI	Hybrid
Solitaire 2	Heraeus	Hybrid
SureFil	Dentsply	Hybrid
Synergy Nano Formula Compact	Coltène Whaledent	Nanohybrid
Tetric Ceram HB	Ivoclar Vivadent	Microhybrid
X-Tra Fil	Voco	Hybrid

Layering resin composites

With the increasing patient demand for aesthetics of a high order, dental materials manufacturers have responded by developing resin composite materials to produce as good an aesthetic result as possible. These materials have been on the market for over 10 years and are composed of composites of differing shades, opacities and translucencies within the same kit akin to an artist's palate. The dentist must create the restoration by building up the tooth in layers using the appropriate dentine and enamel shades. The method adopted is to incrementally build up the tooth using the appropriate shade, opacity and amount of materials to characterize the tooth rather than using one shade packed to excess and cutting back. Placement of the material can be facilitated by utilizing a matrix technique. This can be either a silicone putty index anteriorly or an occlusal index using a translucent bite registration material. Layering results in minimal finishing.

With the layering resin composite materials, the correct amount of composite should be placed in the right place and not cut back! The use of indices facilitates this.

The use of layering resin composites requires much time and perseverance to become fully accustomed, comfortable and competent in their use. It is strongly recommended to attend a course and then practise on a manikin head prior to attempting to use these products in the clinic. There is a long learning curve but practice makes perfect!

Younger teeth are more translucent, the dentine being lighter in shade. As the tooth ages, the dentine darkens, turning almost ivory. Similarly the enamel surface wears and surface detail is lost. Layering resin composite systems permit matching the restoration to tooth under these varied conditions. Thus their main indication and usage is when the best possible aesthetic result is required, particularly in the anterior region. Figure 7.28 shows the enhanced aesthetic results which can be achieved by using this technique with the appropriate materials.

While optimized aesthetics are of great importance in the anterior sextant of the mouth, in the posterior region a slight mismatch of material with tooth aids in restoration removal if necessary and tooth conservation. In addition, the clinician should check that the material is suitable for posterior use with respect to parameters such as shrinkage and wear resistance as many of these materials have inappropriate filler loading for posterior applications.

Commercially available products

A selection of the currently available aesthetic layering resin composites are shown in Table 7.14.

Table 7.14 Some aesthetic layering resin composite materials currently available on the market

Product	Manufacturer	Type of composite
Ceram.X Duo	Dentsply	Nanofilled
Clearfil AP-X	Kuraray	Microhybrid
Direct Venear & Composite System	Edelweiss Dentistry	Nanohybrid
Esthet-X	Dentsply	Microhybrid
Filtek Supreme XT	3M ESPE	Nanohybrid
G-ænial Anterior	GC	Nanohybrid
Gradia Direct Anterior	GC	Microhybrid
Herculite XRV Ultra	Kerr Hawe	Nanohybrid
IPS Empress Direct	Ivoclar Vivadent	Nanohybrid
Miris 2	Coltène Whaledent	Nanohybrid
Premise	Kerr Hawe	Nanohybrid
Tetric Color	Ivoclar Vivadent	Microhybrid
Venus	Heraeus	Microhybrid
Venus Diamond	Heraeus	Nanohybrid
Venus Pearl	Heraeus	Nanohybrid

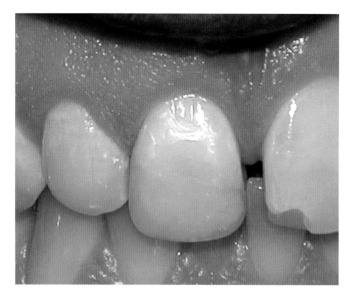

Fig. 7.28 A Class IV cavity in tooth 11 restored using a layering resin composite. Note the excellent aesthetics, the restoration is almost imperceptible.

Patients would prefer to have an imperceptible posterior resin composite restoration, however, the dentist should view this with caution. Although longevity of composite restorations has increased as the materials and techniques improve, the restoration will still have to be replaced at some point in the future. The clinician should plan for this. If the shade match of the restoration is exact, it will be difficult or impossible to differentiate between the material and the surrounding tooth during its subsequent removal. This could lead to excessive tooth tissue removal. It is therefore considered advisable to mismatch the shade slightly when used posteriorly (Figure 7.29).

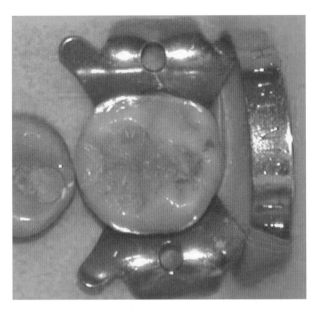

Fig. 7.29 A Class II cavity in tooth 37 restored using Miris (Coltène Whaledent), whose shade is appropriate for the case as there is a slight mismatch, which is considered ideal for a posterior restoration.

The dentist should be consistent when using resin composites and never be tempted to mix and match different manufacturer's products in an attempt to alter the shade. This will result in the final mass becoming grey in appearance. In addition, the differing chemistry of the different composites will affect the properties of the final restoration. It is essential that the same manufacturer's composite should be used for any one restoration.

Tints and characterizations

Some products (Figure 7.30) provide tints, coloured unfilled resins, which may be used to enhance opacity or translucency, increase or decrease chroma or to include features such as fracture lines or hypoplastic spots. Their wear resistance is poor and so to prevent their loss due to occlusal wear, they should not be placed on the surface but

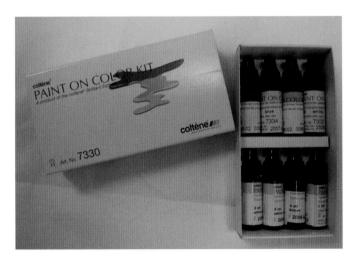

Fig. 7.30 Coltène Whaledent's Paint on Color Kit used to characterize resin composite restorations.

within the mass of the restoration. The covering resin composite will then protect against wear while the translucency of the 'enamel' composite will permit the tint to be seen through it.

Chroma: the perceived intensity of a specific colour.

Resin-based composites and tooth whitening treatments

There has been a huge increase in the number of patients requesting tooth whitening treatments. Many of the currently available resin composite materials (designed for general and aesthetic use) are thus now being supplied with bleach shades. This allows a good shade match being gained between the restoration and bleached tooth. This shade match may be achieved using a different photo-initiator, which may work at a different wavelength. As previously discussed (see Chapter 2), the clinician should ensure that the curing light they are using is compatible with the material being cured. For more information on tooth whitening systems and the effects of tooth whitening ingredients on dental materials, see Chapter 18.

Delay bonding resin composite to teeth which have undergone a bleaching procedure for at least 2 weeks (and preferably longer if possible) postoperatively as the bleaching process has an effect on the tooth tissue.

Non-methacrylate-based resin composites

Dental manufacturers are always thinking of ways of improving their products as new information and knowledge becomes available. With a resin composite, there are two (major) components of the material which could potentially be modified: the filler or the resin. As has been discussed earlier, the filler has been modified extensively and manufacturers are at a point where not much more could be done. As a result, some manufacturers are now looking at ways of modifying the resin component.

One company (3M ESPE) has produced a novel resin with the intention of decreased polymerization shrinkage and the problems associated with it. The product (Filtek Silorane) was first launched in October 2007 and claims to have a shrinkage of 1%, which was considered to be sufficient as this resin system's longer-term expansion due to water sorption appears to be relatively close to the shrinkage value. This compensation assumes that the shrinkage is uniform throughout the restoration but this is not necessarily the case. Although the approach is simplistic, it does at least attempt to take account of the longer-term behaviour of the resin composite in function in the mouth.

The resin employed in this material is non-methacrylate based and instead utilizes a resin produced by reacting a **siloxane** with an **oxirane**. Siloxanes are already used in dentistry in addition silicone impression materials (see Chapter 15) and confer hydrophobicity on the resin. Besides imparting lower water uptake, this also confers greater longer-term stability to the resin phase of the composite. The oxiranes have been used industrially in applications where they are subjected to high loads and where the physical environment can be harsh, such as the construction of skis and in aviation. The oxirane polymers are known for their low shrinkage and they have high

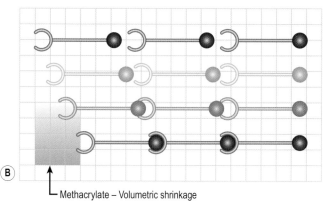

(A) └── Silorane – Volumetric shrinkage <1%

(B) └── Methacrylate – Volumetric shrinkage

Fig. 7.31A,B The difference in the shrinkage with (A) silorane molecule compared with (B) a methacrylate resin.

stability. The siloxane molecules form a core to which the oxirane molecules are attached.

The oxirane components of the molecule undergo a ring-opening reaction during polymerization so connecting the monomers together. As the rings opens its length increases linearly and the molecules then extend towards each other, as compared with methacrylate-based resin where the linear molecules contract towards each other during polymerization so the material is seen to shrink (Figure 7.31). The filler is a silane-coated fine quartz and ytterbium fluoride. Quartz was selected as:

- The surface chemistry and refractive index of the quartz matches the resin
- Zirconium oxide fillers cannot be used as the epoxy resin is incompatible with the silanization process required to bond the resin with the fillers.
- Yttrium fluoride is added to impart radiopacity to the material.

The material is categorized as a microhybrid. The material uses camphorquinone as its initiator together with light at the peak excitation wavelength (470 nm). This combines with an iodonium salt and an electron donor, which generates reactive cationic species that initiate the ring-opening polymerization process. The silorane resin has a threshold for activation requiring an extended cure time of 20 seconds, because a critical mass of initiating active cationic species must be present before polymerization will commence. Increased intensity of light does not shorten this period so that high-intensity lights and plasma light will:

- Not shorten the curing time
- Generate heat which could damage the tooth.

Indications and clinical use

Non-methacrylate-based resin composites materials are indicated for restoration of Class I and Class II cavities. As with many bespoke posterior resin composites, they are only available in a few shades (Figure 7.32).

Although chemically different, epoxy resin-based composite is compatible with traditional materials such as resin-modified glass ionomer cements and glass ionomer cements. They can therefore be used as linings in sandwich techniques. However, flowable resin composites and compomers cannot be used with epoxy resin-based composites as the composite and the (conventional) adhesive required for bonding are incompatible. Methacrylate composites can be used to repair cured epoxy resin-based composites.

!
- The dedicated self-etch adhesive provided with Filtek Silorane (Figure 7.33) should only be used with this product. No other adhesive should be used as the epoxy resin in this resin composite and traditional methacrylate bonding systems are incompatible. Similarly this adhesive should not be used with traditional (methylmethacrylate-based) composites (Chapter 11).
- Finishing of Filtek Silorane can be difficult due to its toughness. It is therefore recommended that an index technique (see later) is used to minimize finishing so that only final polishing is required after curing.

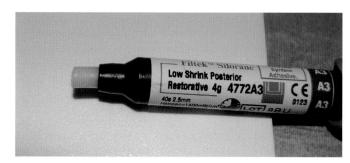

Fig. 7.32 Filtek Silorane (3M ESPE), a non-methacrylate-based composite.

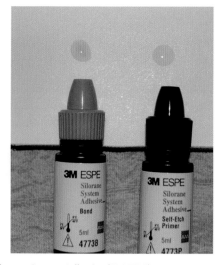

Fig. 7.33 Silorane System Adhesive (3M ESPE).

Ormocers

Ormocer is the acronym for **O**rganically **M**odified **Cer**amics. Ormocers are methacrylate substituted alkosilanes and were introduced to the market approximately 10 years ago. They are **inorganic-organic copolymers** and are synthesized from multifunctional urethane and thioether(meth) acrylate alkoxysilanes. Alkoxysilyl groups of the silane permit the formation of an inorganic (silicon-oxygen) cross-linked network by hydrolysis and condensation polymerization reactions. Ceramic filler particles (apatite and barium glass) are embedded into this network.

The inorganic backbone is based on silicon dioxide (such as quartz or ceramic) and this influences thermal expansion, thermal and chemical stability, and elasticity. The methacrylate units allow photochemical polymerization as well as the hardness and the material's (tooth-coloured) optical properties. Other molecules are added to the material to improve the bonding abilities of the material by chemically attaching it to tooth tissue via calcium complexing groups. The material is claimed to be biocompatible, exhibits low polymerization shrinkage (under 2%) and its properties such as abrasion resistance, stable aesthetics equally favourable to those of composite materials.

Voco's Admira is an example of an ormocer and this product is presented is a regular and flowable material. Its indications are similar to those of a regular or flowable resin composite, respectively, with similar handling properties to the commensurate presentation. Admira Bond is recommended for use in conjunction with the restorative material to bond to tooth tissue.

Laboratory composites

Attempts have been made to overcome the primary disadvantages of resin composites, polymerization shrinkage and wear. This has entailed the use of an **indirect** technique to produce intracoronal restorations, which can be designed as either inlays or onlays.

> **Inlay:** a fully intracoronal restoration constructed either in a dental laboratory or in the cavity to be restored before being cemented in situ.
> **Onlay:** a restoration constructed either in a dental laboratory or in the cavity to be restored which is partially intracoronal but also covers part or all of the occlusal surface, usually with the intention of affording the underlying tooth some resistance to fracture during function.

More effective polymerization may be achieved in the dental laboratory. By increasing the level of conversion the mechanical properties of the material are enhanced and the total shrinkage while being greater is uniform throughout the mass of the restoration. The defect between the cavity wall and the inlay caused by the shrinkage can then be filled with a resin during the cementation process where the volume of cement used is small and shrinkage is less significant. This process can be achieved by light and additionally by heat.

A large restoration can be more easily constructed on the laboratory bench in close to 'ideal' conditions. Here, the technician can produce a good contour, approximal contacts and achieve the correct occlusal anatomy more easily than the clinician working in the mouth where the conditions are more challenging. There is also the benefit of reduced costly chairside time although an extra appointment is required to cement the restoration.

The final restoration is cemented in place using a resin luting cement. The luting phase is the weak link in the system, as the luting resin itself has a lower viscosity because of reduced filler loading. This results in greater shrinkage of the cement lute, which may be sufficient to cause shrinkage stresses leading to failure of the bond, especially to dentine (Figure 7.34). The union between the inlay and the resin lute may also be reduced as the high level of conversion means that there are fewer available unreacted methacrylate groups left on the surface with which the luting cement can react. The majority of laboratory resin composites are similar to their clinical counterparts and therefore have the same advantages and disadvantages.

Commercially available products

Some of the commercially available laboratory composites are listed in Table 7.15.

Table 7.15 Some laboratory resin composite materials

Product	Manufacturer
Adoro	Ivoclar Vivadent
Artglass	Heraeus
GC Gradia	GC
Premise Indirect	Kerr Hawe
Sinfony	3M ESPE
Solidex	Shofu
SR Chromasit	Ivoclar Vivadent
Tescera ATL	Bisco

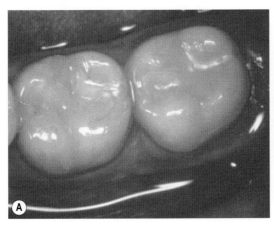

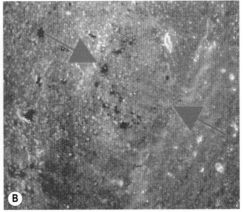

Fig. 7.34A,B (A) Two occlusal composite inlays in teeth 36 and 37. Note the white line that is developing on the mesial margin of 37 where cement is washing out. (B) Cement lute between inlay and tooth structure. Distance between the arrows is 300 μm and denotes the cement thickness.

Fibre-reinforced resin composite

A number of systems have been developed for the reinforcement of composites and resins. The use of fibres as a reinforcement is a benefit if there is only one surface which is under stress since the orientation of the fibres is critical. The other problem is the union between the fibres and the resin. This has proved to be a technology which is difficult to adapt to the dental arena and only one glass-impregnated resin system has been used to any great extent. The fibres may exist as mesh, woven mat or single fibres depending on the application. The best results are achieved if the fibres are impregnated with the resin forming a continuum which is difficult to rupture. The technology may have greater applications in the future.

Commercially available products

Some of the currently available fibre-reinforced resin composites are shown in Table 7.16.

Table 7.16 Some fibre-reinforced resin composite materials

Product	Manufacturer	Fibre type	Fibre form
Connect	Kerr Hawe	Polyethylene	Braid
Construct	Kerr Hawe	Polyethylene	Fibres
Everstick C&B	Sticktech	Glass	Unidirectional fibre bundle
Everstick Net	Sticktech	Glass	Mesh
Everstick Perio	Sticktech	Glass	Unidirectional fibre bundle
Everstick Post	Sticktech	Glass	Unidirectional fibre bundle
Fiber-Splint	Polydentia	Glass	Fibre layers
Fiber-Splint	Nulite	Glass	Fibre layers
Fiber-Splint ML	Polydentia	Glass	Multiple layer
Fibrebind	Nulite	Glass	Fibres layers
Ribbond	Ribbond Inc.	Polyethylene	Weave
Vectris	Ivoclar Vivadent	Glass	Mesh
Vectris pontic	Ivoclar Vivadent	Glass	Unidirectional

Indications of fibre reinforced composites

- Bite splint repair and reinforcement
- Denture repair and reinforcement
- Orthodontic retainers
- The splinting of periodontally compromised teeth
- Provisional composite and acrylic crowns and bridges
- Reinforcing for composite crowns and bridges
- Single tooth stress-bearing restorations.

CLINICAL PLACEMENT OF RESIN COMPOSITE MATERIALS

While resin composites have many applications, their handling and placement is more demanding than almost any other restorative material. Failure to determine the appropriate use or to manipulate them in the correct manner will lead to early restoration failure and non-optimization of the properties of the material. The following aspects should be considered for each resin composite placement in order to ensure that the material performs as well as possible.

Occlusion

The occlusion should always be examined in centric occlusion and all excursions prior to isolation with rubber dam. The cavity outline should be determined in relation to the occlusal contact with the opposing teeth to reduce the risk of direct contact with opposing cusps and thus the occlusal load on the restoration, and such that the remaining tooth tissue is used to support the restoration. Occlusal contacts should be placed on enamel if possible, and heavy occlusal contacts at cavity margins should be avoided. An impression reproducing the occlusal configuration may be taken to act as a template for the final occlusal surface. This will reduce finishing time.

Cavity design

To reduce risk of failure due to fracture, a rounded internal cavity form is desirable. This will also reduce stress concentration and aid adaptation of the material to the cavity walls during placement (Figure 7.35). Current thinking is that only the area that needs to be restored should be prepared and not the uninvolved fissure system. Maximal retention of tooth tissue by only removing diseased tissue,

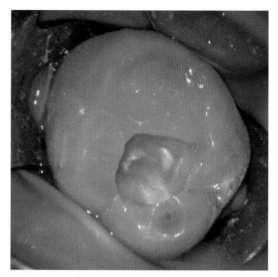

Fig. 7.35 An occlusal cavity in tooth 26 being restored under rubber dam using a resin composite.

that is minimizing the cavity size, reduces the risk of wear to the restoration. However, the minimal cavity design may need to be modified to permit adequate access and visibility. In addition,

- It is necessary to extend through the contact area cervically (so that any caries which is found under the contact area can be identified and removed), but there is no need to remove the axial margins unless these are compromising matrix placement.
- While some unsupported enamel may be retained, there is a risk that retention of excessive unsupported material may lead to fracture. A white line at the margin is indicative of this phenomenon.

The resin composite can, however, be mechanically bonded to the enamel, providing some support. The amount of enamel that may be retained must be judged in the light of the stress which will be placed on the restoration–tooth complex.

While bonding of resin composite to tooth tissue may be achieved using an intermediate bonding layer (see Chapter 11), this should not be relied on to retain the restoration. Additionally, mechanical retentive features such as undercuts should be incorporated in any cavity design. The use of dentine pins is inadvisable as adaptation round the pins is poor and there is a risk of thin sections of composite fracturing away from the pin surface.

- The final choice of restorative material should be delayed until after the cavity preparation is complete.
- Peripheral staining should be removed as this may show through the composite restoration. This would compromise the aesthetic result.

Marginal seal

Resin composites do not bond directly to enamel and dentine. An intermediate material must be used and the best results are usually obtained when bonding to enamel. It is thus desirable that all margins are within the enamel, especially in the posterior region. If enamel is not present along the entire cavity margin, the dentist should reconsider whether resin composite is the best material for the situation.

Bevelling has been advocated to enhance the bonding of resin composites to tooth tissue by altering the angulation of the enamel prisms. This should be considered on a case-by-case basis, as there are some contraindications:
- Occlusal margins. Bevelling may leave a thin margin of composite and render it more susceptible to cracking especially if placed in an unfavourable occlusal scheme.
- Base of the gingival box. Bevelling in this situation may well remove any small amount of peripheral enamel so compromising the bond gained.
- Proximal wall. Pooling of the bonding agent by capillary action will lead to a weakened bond that is more liable to breakdown. Bevelling in this region may also be difficult to do without damaging the adjacent tooth.
In anterior cavities, bevelling is generally considered to be advantageous as the bond strength is improved and outweighs the most significant drawback that the resin composite is difficult to finish to an oblique margin.

Moisture control

As these resin composites are hydrophobic in nature, excellent moisture control is essential. If the material is contaminated with moisture, the final restoration will have inferior properties, and bond strength between the resin composite and the tooth and the longevity of the restoration will be decreased. Moisture control is best achieved by use of rubber dam. The dam may also retract the gingivae, preventing any fluid seepage into the cavity which can further contaminate the material. Other methods of moisture control such as the use of cotton wool rolls and high volume aspiration may be sufficient but are not as effective as the operating conditions gained when rubber dam has been placed properly. If it is not possible to isolate the operating site from water, the dentist should reconsider the choice of material for the restoration.

Ideally rubber dam should be used for the whole procedure of resin composite placement, including preparation of the cavity. This will prevent gingival damage due to retraction of the soft tissues. A cleaner, drier environment is gained, aiding the subsequent restorative procedure.

 Linings

Any lining material may be used under resin composites with the exception of those containing eugenol. Eugenol interferes with the polymerization process, which means that the resin mass is plasticized and the restoration will have inferior mechanical properties. Materials containing eugenol should therefore not be used either in conjunction with resin-based materials or prior to their use, as they may contaminate the tooth tissue which subsequently may come contact with resin composite. This will adversely affect the set of the resin.

Etching and bonding

These steps are crucial for clinical success. It is imperative that the dentist carefully reads the instructions supplied with each kit and follows them fastidiously. Bonding systems should be consistent and therefore compatible with the composite materials being used. Under no circumstance should adhesives and bonding systems be mixed and matching. Etching and bonding are covered in more detail in Chapter 11.

Clinical placement

It is essential to use the right instrumentation to place these materials, including the matrices for posterior restorations and placement instruments designed for use with resin composites.

Matrices

One of the most challenging aspects when placing a posterior composite is to achieve a good contact area, and the use of the correct matrix system is vital. Matrices need to incorporate some form of luxation force to open the interproximal region and allow the thin matrix to be burnished against the adjacent tooth. This will provide both a tight contact area and improved contour, facilitating oral hygiene. On removal of the matrix, the teeth will spring back towards each other, helping to offset the effect of polymerization shrinkage

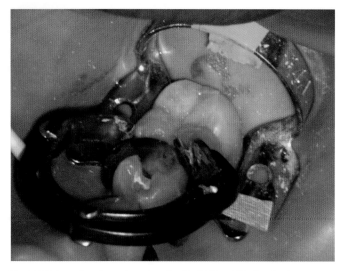

Fig. 7.36 A sectional matrix system in situ (V-Ring, Trio Dent) where a Class II resin composite restoration is to be placed in tooth 35.

and creating a tight contact. An example of a sectional matrix system is shown in Figure 7.36 and such systems available on the market include the products listed in Table 7.17. In addition, correctly placed wedge(s) will prevent the formation of an overhang.

Overhang: cervical extrusion of restorative material leading to a non-confluent restoration margin with the adjacent surrounding tooth. Overhangs compromise cleaning and thus lead to accumulation of plaque.

With larger cavities, there may be insufficient tooth tissue to allow the placement of a sectional matrix initially. In this case, the dentist should first build up any missing buccal or lingual walls to permit placement of the sectional matrix. Alternatively, a circumferential matrix system also designed for the placement of resin composite may be considered.

Flexible wedges (Figure 7.37) can be used in cases with concavities of the cervical margin so preventing the formation of an overhang.

Table 7.17 Sectional matrix systems indicated when Class II resin composites restorations are being placed

Product	Manufacturer
Composi-Tight	Garrison Dental Solutions
Palodent System	Dentsply
V-Ring	Trio Dent

When restoring a Class II cavity, it is advisable to restore the proximal surface first as this effectively creates a Class I cavity which is easier to restore and gives best results with respect to contact areas. Once this wall has been constructed the matrix system may be removed to improve access. However, gingival haemorrhage may result when the matrix is removed so compromising the operating area. It is therefore advisable to leave the matrix system in situ until all of the restoration has been placed.

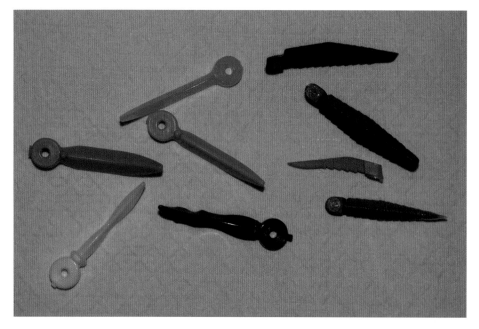

Fig. 7.37 A selection of flexible wedges: Flexiwedges (Optident) on the left and Wave Wedges (Trio Dent) on the right.

Placement into the cavity

Resin composites have a tendency to adhere to instruments, particularly if the instruments have scratches or have been abraded when being used for other applications. Ideally, instruments should be earmarked for sole use with composites (Figure 7.38) to prevent damage to them. Bespoke instruments are available in highly polished stainless steel, titanium nitride or are Teflon coated to overcome these problems. All instruments for use with composites should be decontaminated carefully, ensuring that they do not become scratched.

Over-manipulation of the unset material will lead to air incorporation and porosities within the restoration mass, causing localized air inhibition of the setting reaction and stress within the material, leading to early failure. These problems are of greatest significance with layering techniques. Matrices may be used to minimize handling, such as polyester or cellulose acetate strips and crown forms or matrices made from addition silicone. Matrices also exclude oxygen so the resin is fully cured up to the surface.

Some clinicians advocate warming resin composite to soften it, so facilitating its placement, as they prefer working with a more malleable material. This is not advisable as heating the material may cause certain components to evaporate and may initiate the setting reaction.

Index techniques to enhance surface contour

With all aesthetic restorative materials, finishing a restoration is an exercise in damage limitation as the material has to be ground away. This places stresses on the material and frequently reduces the aesthetic result of the final restoration. Minimal finishing is the objective so that there is no detrimental effect on the mechanical properties of the final composite. To this end, the dentist may choose to use an index technique which copies the existing functional palatal or occlusal surface and is then used to transfer this information to the new restoration. In other words the index helps copying the surface contour precisely. If the surface contour needs to be modified, this may be achieved prior to preparation by adapting the surface with wax or resin composite. An index may then be taken in an impression material and retained for later use. This technique permits:

- Reduction in the need for finishing as only minimal adjustments are required
- More predictably shaped restoration that will function better with respect to the occlusion.

Filling to excess and then trimming back the restorative will, as well as damaging the restoration, also mean that the restoration is in many cases overcontoured and occlusal stops are lost. While an index technique will not eliminate this, it will make restoration of this surface easier.

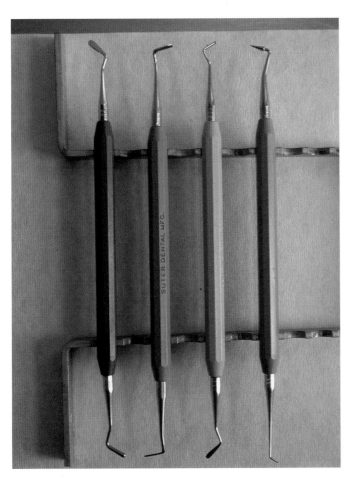

Fig. 7.38 Bespoke resin composite placement instruments in various shapes and sizes made of stainless steel (Suter Dental Instruments).

Separating media

Unfilled resin can be used as a separator. This must be used with caution as too much may dilute the resin composite material, altering its properties. Alcohol wipes should not be used as a separating medium or to wipe instruments during resin composite placement. Alcohol acts as a plasticizer so weakening the resin composite. Clean, dry paper tissues (Figure 7.39) are preferred should excess material be needed to be removed from instruments.

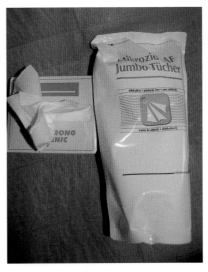

Fig. 7.39 Paper tissues are preferred to alcohol wipes to remove excess unset and other dental materials from instruments used for manipulating resin composites.

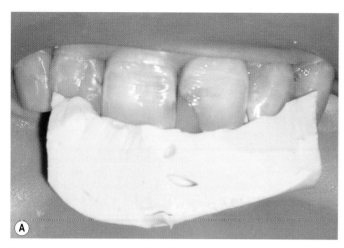 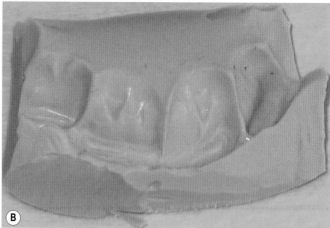

Fig. 7.40A,B A preoperative index of the palatal surface of tooth 21 made using an addition silicone putty.

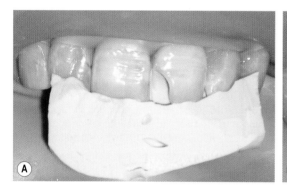 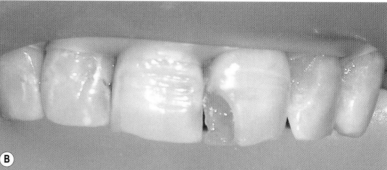

Fig. 7.41A,B After the mesio-incisal cavity in tooth 21 has been prepared, lined, etched and bonded, the putty index is replaced and the palatal surface laid down in resin composite.

Index construction

Different materials are used to construct the index, depending on whether the cavity to be restored is located anteriorly or posteriorly. Anterior indices are best constructed with a matrix made out of putty whilst a transparent bite registration material can copy the occlusal surface of posterior teeth.

The technique for anterior index construction is as follows:

1. A preoperative index of the palatal surface is made using an addition silicone putty such as Affinis (Coltène Whaledent) (Figure 7.40). Any deficiencies in the palatal surface are made good prior to index construction or by a diagnostic build up. The index should be trimmed to ensure that it will reseat onto the palatal surfaces accurately.
2. After removal and trimming, the index is put to one side. The cavity is then prepared, lined (if necessary), etched and bonded. The index is replaced and the palatal surface laid down in resin composite (Figure 7.41). This is then light cured and the matrix is removed, so creating another index into which the rest of the restoration may be constructed.
3. The rest of the restoration may be constructed, finished and polished (Figure 7.42).

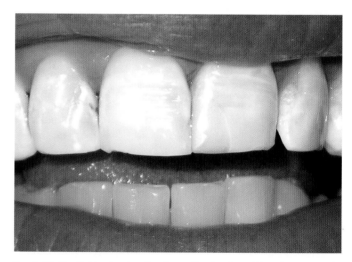

Fig. 7.42 The finished restoration immediately after rubber dam removal and polishing.

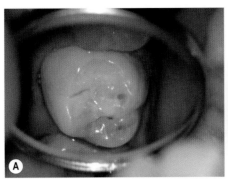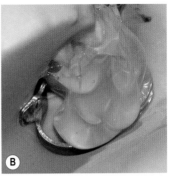

Fig. 7.43A,B Preoperative view of the occlusal surface of tooth 16. Transparent silicone matrix has been syringed onto the occlusal surface of the tooth.

The sequence for use in the posterior regions is similar namely:

1. A preoperative index of the occlusal surface is made using a transparent addition silicone such as Memosil (Heraeus) (Figure 7.43). Any deficiencies in the occlusal surface are dealt with prior to index construction. The index should be trimmed to ensure that it will reseat onto the occlusal surface accurately.
2. After removal and trimming the index is put to one side. The cavity is then prepared, lined (if necessary), etched and bonded. The resin composite is placed and cured incrementally until the final uncured increment is placed. The index is then firmly seated on top of the uncured material. Any excess is removed and the final increment is then light cured (Figure 7.44).
3. The matrix is then removed and the restoration is finished and polished (Figure 7.45).

Light curing

Chapter 2 deals in great detail with the light curing of resin composites. It is essential that the clinician appreciates that the material will only cure satisfactorily when it is exposed to sufficient light energy at the correct wavelength. The resin composite should be placed incrementally, and each increment cured prior to placement of the next. Resin composites do not fully cure in the presence of oxygen, and the **oxygen inhibition layer** has inferior mechanical properties, which will have detrimental clinical effects. When a resin composite is being placed posteriorly, the clinician should consider applying a coat of unfilled resin (for example bonding resin or bespoke products such as G-Coat Plus, GC or Biscover, Bisco) to the outer surface of the restoration and then cure again for 40 seconds. This technique will ensure full cure of the composite beneath and the composite surface will be unlikely to fail due to inadequate polymerization. The

unfilled resin application to the surface will additionally seal surface defects so improving the appearance and stain resistance.

Even after full polymerization the level of conversion of the resin composite is never more than 70%. After light curing has been completed, there is some further polymerization and it is estimated that a further 10% cross-linking occurs in the subsequent hour after the restoration as been completed. This is termed **post cure** and is the reason for minimal finishing immediately after placement as the restoration is still undergoing its final setting phase. Disruption of the polymer during this stage will weaken the final restoration and reduce durability.

Finishing

It is good practice to delay finishing as long as possible (ideally 24 hours). Excessive cutting back and finishing is likely to lead to white line fracture around the restoration as the interface between the tooth and restorative is disrupted.

The many instruments available to finish resin composites range from high speed diamond or tungsten carbide burs to aluminium oxide polishing discs, silicone points, cups and discs of various shapes and sizes and diamond impregnated brushes. Various **lustre pastes** are also available. See Chapter 19 for more information on the range of instruments available and how to achieve the desired result.

Wherever possible dentists are strongly advised to finish restorations under magnification and with the use of water spray and intermittent light pressure.

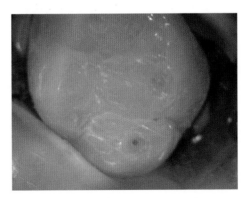

Fig. 7.44 The matrix is replaced and the final increment of resin composite and cured through the matrix.

Fig. 7.45 The (occlusal) resin composite restoration after matrix removal. It is essential that the material from which the index is constructed is rigid enough so that it does not deform under pressure, otherwise the exercise will be fruitless.

Polishability

The degree of polishability of any given resin composite material depends on its constituents, in particular, its particle size as has already been described earlier in this chapter. Microfilled materials are easier to polish than macrofilled materials.

With the introduction of the build-up resin composite products, emphasis is on correct placement of the correct amount of the material so post placement finishing is minimized. The optimal mechanical properties of the resin composite occur just under the oxygen inhibition layer. Excessive trimming will remove this outer thickness, so exposing material with inferior properties. Gross finishing can also lead to collateral damage on the adjacent enamel, which is clearly undesirable. Where dual-curing composites are used, it is wise to delay finishing for a longer period of time as the chemical curing phase is slower to complete than the light cured phase.

When finishing resin composite restorations, copious water spray should be used with rotary instruments to prevent overheating of the restoration. Absence of coolant can lead to hot spots and the resin temperature will rise above the glass transition temperature, leading to melting alterations in resin form.

LONG-TERM FAILURE

The possible reasons for failure of resin composite restorations have been discussed previously. However, an inadequate clinical technique is frequently a cause of the long-term failure of resin composite restorations due to:

- Leakage: this may result from inadequate placement of the material into the cavity. It is associated with failure at the interface between the tooth and the resin composite/adhesive. It is often associated with polymerization shrinkage, stressing the bond and leading to failure. Percolation of oral fluid at the interface will then lead to leakage of fluid down the interface.
- Recurrent caries. This is linked to the microleakage at the restoration and tooth interface. It may also occur due to failure to remove the carious lesion completely or as a result of leakage as above.
- Tooth flexure. This may occur during function particularly with excessive tooth tissue removal. Any movement of the tooth complex will stress the union between the restorative and the tooth. The resin composite bond will slowly fatigue and fail leading to microleakage along the interface. Tooth fracture may also result.

When incisal non-carious tooth surface loss lesions are being restored, a sufficient bulk of resin composite material should be provided. If these restorations are done as thin sections, they tend to debond due to the occlusal stresses placed on them (see Figure 7.20, p. 83).

RESTORATION REPAIR

One of the advantages of resin composite materials is that restorations may be repaired without the need for total removal of the existing restoration. However, the strength of the union between the old and new material is less than 60% of the full strength of the material. This is in part because there are limited methacrylate groups available for reaction with the new material. Much of the union is probably micromechanical. However, evidence of adhesive failure in laboratory testing of composite repairs suggests that there is some chemical interaction between the two components old and new. The epoxy resin systems now on the market only form a small oxygen inhibited layer and so this may present a problem when the material needs to be repaired.

SUMMARY

- Resin composites are one of the commonest restorative materials used today.
- These are glass and silica filled resins that set by light polymerization.
- Shrinkage occurs during the polymerization process.
- Their mechanical properties are relatively close to amalgam except in flexure.
- Alone they do not bond to tooth tissue.
- Variations in filler loading allow them to be adapted to a variety of uses.
- The greater the filler loading the more brittle the material is and likely to fracture.
- The manipulation and polymerization must be carried out in a dry field.
- They may be used as preventive materials, for example as fissure sealants.

FURTHER READING

Bonsor, S.J., 2008. Contemporary use of flowable composite materials. Dent. Update 35, 600–606.

Burke, F.J., Shortall, A.C., 2001. Successful restoration of load-bearing cavities in posterior teeth with direct-replacement resin-based composite. Dent. Update 28, 388–398.

MacKenzie, L., Shortall, A.C., Burke, F.G., 2009. Direct posterior composites: a practical guide. Dent. Update 36, 71–95.

Powers, J.M., Sakaguchi, R.L., 2006. Craig's Restorative Dental Materials. Mosby Elsevier, St Louis. (See Chapter 9)

van Noort, R., 2007. Introduction to Dental Materials, third ed. Mosby Elsevier, Edinburgh. (See Chapter 2.2)

SELF-ASSESSMENT QUESTIONS

1. Outline the key points in the placement of a Class II resin composite restoration.
2. Following restoration of incisors using resin composite material, unfortunately some of the restorations have debonded quite quickly after their placement. What could be the possible causes for this?
3. A Class IV resin composite restoration has been placed under rubber dam and the shade match is excellent immediately postoperatively. Unfortunately, the patient returns the next day as the shade is now too light. What mistake has the clinician made?
4. What is a hybrid resin composite? Why is this advantageous clinically?
5. What are the major shortcomings of composite resins? How may these be reduced during the manipulation of the material?
6. Why should the finishing of composite be delayed for 24 hours? What may happen if the material is finished immediately?

Chapter 8

The tooth-coloured restorative materials II: Compomers

LEARNING OBJECTIVES

From this chapter, the reader will:

- Understand what compomers are
- Appreciate the significance of their constituents and how these influence the properties of the material
- Understand how the constituents affect the material's clinical performance
- Have an increased appreciation of how to use this type of material more effectively
- Be aware of the wide spectrum of usages and know the names of currently available commercial products.

INTRODUCTION

Compomers first appeared in the early 1990s in an attempt to combine the potential advantages of fluoride release as seen with the glass ionomer cements, with the many advantages of the resin composites. The aim was therefore to produce a resin composite which exhibited a sustained and effective release of fluoride. Previous attempts to achieve this had involved adding various fluoride salts to conventional resin composite formulations, but this proved to be less than successful. The mechanism of fluoride release relies on water being absorbed by the resin composite which then dissolves fluoride salts such as ytterbium fluoride followed by diffusion of fluoride ions out of the material. However, the nature of the resin composites meant that only the fluoride in the subsurface layers was released by this process because of the difficulty encountered by the fluoride ions in diffusing through the bulk of polymerized resin. Small amounts of fluoride were released initially but this was not sustained in the longer term. Unfortunately, another effect of these additions was to reduce the resin composite's longevity because of degradation of the methacrylates.

The material finally developed lies closer to the resin-based composites in the continuum of materials than to the glass ionomer cements. It is primarily a resin system and is manufactured without the addition of any water. Instead an additional resin is incorporated which is difunctional.

> **Difunctional monomer:** a resin monomer with two modes of chemical reaction that are made possible by the presence two separate reactive groups on the resin molecules. The word **bifunctional** is synonymous.

NOMENCLATURE

The commonly accepted name for these materials is 'compomer', which was coined by Dentsply, the manufacturer of Dyract, the first material of this type (Figure 8.1). However the generic name for this material is **polyacid-modified resin composite**, which effectively describes their composition and, by implication, their setting mechanism.

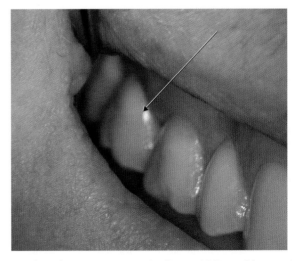

Fig. 8.1 A buccal compomer restoration (Dyract AP, Dentsply) on tooth 16 after having been in service for 8 years.

COMPOSITION

The material is essentially a composite in nature, in that it is composed of a resin components and a filler (Table 8.1).

Table 8.1 Components of compomer materials

Component	Chemical example	Reason for inclusion
Filler	Fluoro-alumino-silicate glass	Imparts strength
		Source of fluoride ions for use in the secondary reaction
Dimethacrylate monomer	Urethane dimethacrylate (UDMA)	Primary monomer forming the resin matrix
Difunctional resin	**TCB** resin: the reaction product of **butane tetracarboxylic acid** and **hydroxyethyl methacrylate**	Cross-linking agent in the primary reaction
		Source of carboxyl groups for secondary reaction with glass
Photo-activator and initiator	Camphorquinone	Required to effect light polymerization
	Tertiary amine	
Hydrophilic monomers	Glycerol dimethacrylate	Enhances water diffusion within resin matrix

Resin component

The resin part has two monomeric components:

- A **dimethacrylate**, usually urethane dimethacrylate (UDMA) and
- A **difunctional resin monomer**, which has both carboxyl and methacrylate groups. Another type of resin which may perform in the same way is the methacrylated polycarboxylic acid found in some resin-modified glass ionomer cements (see Chapter 10).

Filler

The principles of resin-based composite manufacture hold true for compomers in that a filler is added to decrease the amount of resin and to improve the mechanical properties and influence the material's appearance.

The filler is a fluoro-alumino-silicate glass, which is similar to that found in a conventional glass ionomer cement, to provide a source of fluoride ions and form a salt matrix with carboxylate groups. This fine glass powder is in the sub-8 μm size range with a filler loading volume of between 42% and 67%. The glass usually contains lithium or strontium to convey radiopacity to the material.

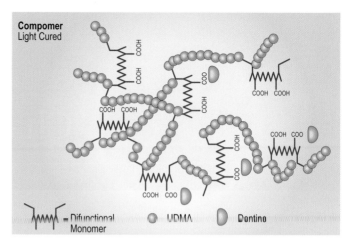

Fig. 8.2 First stage in the setting reaction of compomer materials. The initial cure is by light polymerization.

Photo-activators and initiators

Setting is initiated by the same photo-activator usually found in resin composites, such as **camphorquinone** and a **tertiary amine** (see Chapters 2 and 7).

SETTING REACTION

The setting reaction is a two-stage process.

Stage 1

When the clinician is satisfied with the material's placement in the cavity, the initial setting reaction is initiated by light as with the composite resins. This is a **free radical polymerization** reaction that leads to **cross-linking** of the end groups on the UDMA and the methacrylate groups on the difunctional resin to form a resin polymer matrix in which the glass is trapped (Figure 8.2).

Polysalt matrix: matrix formed of a range of salts derived from the acid and base in the cement.

Stage 2

A secondary reaction occurs between the glass and the carboxylate groups of the difunctional resin. This requires the restoration to be bathed in saliva. When it becomes wet, water is taken up by the resin system. The acid side groups (hydrogen ions) start to dissolve the outer surface of the glass and release the fluoride ions, which will diffuse out of the material. A polysalt matrix is formed around the glass as in a conventional glass ionomer cement. This is an acid/base reaction that is aided by additions of small percentages of hydrophilic resin (such as **glycerol dimethacrylate**) to the resin mix to encourage diffusion of water within the resin and fluoride out of it. The diffusion process takes several weeks and there is a slow but steady release of fluoride from the restoration once this process commences (Figure 8.3).

It is important to note that the setting reaction is primarily a polymerization reaction which is complete on exposure to the curing light energy.

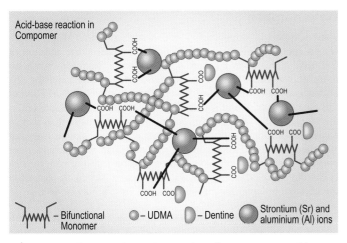

Acid-base reaction in Compomer

- Bifunctional Monomer
○ - UDMA
- Dentine
● Strontium (Sr) and aluminium (Al) ions

Fig. 8.3 Second stage in the setting reaction of compomer materials. The secondary (acid/base) reaction occurs after the restoration comes into contact with water.

PROPERTIES

Mechanical properties

The mechanical properties of compomers lie within the range for most composite materials although they generally have lower compressive and flexural strengths (Table 8.2) and lower elastic moduli. Comparison of the properties of the same manufacturer's resin composite and compomer products generally reveals that the resin composite has higher mechanical properties. Compomers should therefore not be used in situations where higher stresses are anticipated. For further details of these values for all materials (see Representative values of various mechanical and physical properties of generic dental materials on prelims page ii).

Table 8.2 Comparison of some mechanical properties of compomers and resin composites

	Compomer	Composite
Compressive strength	Lower	Higher
Tensile strength	Lower	Higher
Flexural strength	Lower	Higher

Physical properties

Polymerization shrinkage

The presence of a resin component in the paste means that the material will shrink on polymerization. The shrinkage is similar to that observed for composites (Table 8.3), being between 2% and 3.5% by volume and occurs immediately on light curing. This can disrupt any bonding that is being attempted at this stage, since once the resin has polymerized migration of any ions which have been released is very limited. The clinician should be mindful of the significance of polymerization shrinkage and consider what they can do to minimize its detrimental effects on the restoration as detailed in Chapters 2 and 7.

Adhesion

As already discussed, a resin-based composite has no inherent ability to bond to tooth tissue. It requires an intermediate bonding system to achieve adhesion to tooth tissue. Since compomers are primarily resin-based systems, they too require the use of a bonding system. Many products are available for this.

There is little or no adhesion as a result of the secondary setting reaction, even though there may be a number of carboxylate groups available for chelation with calcium in dentine. This is because unless the carboxylate groups are in close proximity to the tooth surface, no chelation reaction will occur. These groups may also be bound up in the resin matrix which has already formed, so rendering them unavailable.

> **Chelation:** the process of formation of stable complexes with metal ions.
> **Chelating agent:** A chelating agent is a compound that forms stable complexes with metal ions, such as calcium.

Table 8.3 Comparison of the physical properties of compomers and resin composite materials

	Compomer	Composite
Wear resistance	Lower	Higher
Polymerization shrinkage	Greater	Smaller
Opacity	Higher	Lower
Depth of cure	Smaller	Greater
Polishability	Same	Same
Fluoride release	Slight	Negligible
Water sorption	Higher	Lower
Stain resistance	Lower	Higher

✓ Compomers: to etch or not to etch?

There has been much controversy since compomer materials were launched to market as to whether the clinician should etch the tooth with phosphoric acid prior to application of a bonding agent. Compomers may be placed without acid etching and this is recommended by some manufacturers in an attempt to simplify the bonding process. However, omission of this step will result in reduced bond strengths. As compomer materials are similar to resin composites, most restorative dentists advocate etching prior to bonding to maximize adhesion.

Fluoride release

The release of fluoride from compomers is reliant on the secondary setting reaction which occurs after placement. The pattern of release is a slow steady release with respect to time. There is little or no fluoride burst or washout initially and the rate of release is substantially slower and in smaller amounts than that observed for glass ionomer cement and resin-modified glass ionomer cements. This is primarily because the process is one of diffusion of the fluoride ions into the surroundings, which is dependent on a concentration gradient between the external environment and the restoration surface. If the surface of the restoration has a greater fluoride ion concentration than the surroundings then the ions will migrate out into the saliva or into the surrounding tooth tissue.

The concentration of fluoride within the restoration is determined by the rate of the secondary reaction of the glass with the pendant carboxyl groups, which in turn is determined by their proximity to the reactive glass surface. Since the resin phase of the system has already set there is limited ability for reaction between the glass and the carboxyl groups. This further limits the amount of fluoride ions released. The fluoride ions have to migrate through the material in order to achieve any release.

> **Pendant group:** group hanging off the side of a polymer chain and available for reaction.

Uptake from the surroundings does not occur in contrast to the glass ionomer cements or resin-modified glass ionomer cements (see Chapters 9 and 10). Also note that there is a difference of availability of fluoride ions between products. Measurement of fluoride release into water shows that there is a slow, steady release of fluoride (Figure 8.4).

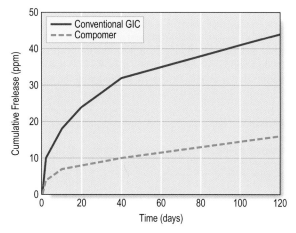

Fig. 8.4 Comparison of the amount of fluoride released from a glass ionomer cement and a compomer.

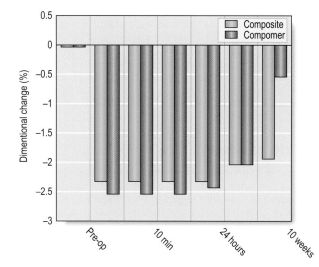

Fig. 8.5 Change in dimensions of a compomer with respect to time in comparison with a conventional resin composite. Note that although the compomer shrinks more, at the end of 10 weeks the water uptake of the compomer has reduced the percentage shrinkage to 0.5% whereas the composite is still nearly 2% by volume smaller than originally.

Water sorption

Water sorption is a characteristic which adversely affects most hydrophobic resin systems. In the case of the compomers, the addition of hydrophilic resins can facilitate uptake of water. Compomer restorations are not fully set until water sorption has occurred and the secondary glass filler/carboxyl reaction has been completed. Saturation of this type of material will usually occur within a week of placement in the mouth as the rate of diffusion of the water is greater than that of conventional resin composites. The amount of water uptake is greater and there has been some concern that this is an uncontrolled reaction that may lead to excessive expansion of the material with the risk of damage to the tooth. That said, this expansion may in part offset the effect of polymerization more quickly and so may be seen as an advantage.

Figure 8.5 shows the change in dimensions of a compomer with respect to time in comparison with a conventional resin composite. While the resin composite shrinks after polymerization and shows very little dimensional change thereafter, the compomer shows initial shrinkage. This is compensated by expansion due to water uptake, and may be a way of eventually achieving a seal, but the expansion is not controlled.

Stain resistance

It is well accepted that the uptake of oral fluids may lead to discolouration of the restoration as was frequently seen in the older composite resins. This is particularly the case for compomers, as the uptake of oral fluids leads to some of these materials showing staining relatively shortly after placement (Figure 8.6). Manufacturers of newer products have attempted to overcome this disadvantage by improving the bonding between the filler and resin.

Wear resistance

The original materials showed very variable amounts of wear in the studies conducted by the manufacturers to investigate this phenomenon. In all cases, wear was observed quite quickly after placement. Re-formulation of a number of materials has led to a reduction in the

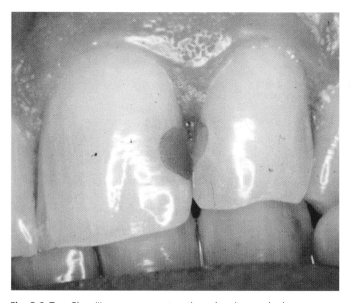

Fig. 8.6 Two Class III compomer restorations showing marked discolouration after some time in clinical use.

Table 8.4 Indications and contraindications of compomer materials

Indications	Reason	Contraindications	Reason
Class III cavities	Material strong enough for purpose Aesthetics acceptable	Where aesthetics are of critical importance	Composites are better aesthetically and do not stain as much as compomers
Class V cavities	Matrix more flexible so is able to be retained in abfraction lesions	Core build-ups	Material not strong enough Water uptake is needed to fully cure material, which is impossible to achieve when covered by a cast
Fissure sealants	Available in flowable form	With dentine pins	No adaptation to dentine pin Stress concentrations within material and around dentine pin
Luting of metal based indirect restorations and orthodontic brackets	Available in luting form	Luting of all ceramic crowns	May be a slight risk of fracture due to dimensional change in function
Restoration of deciduous teeth	Bonds to tooth tissue	Class I, II and IV cavities	Material not strong enough
		Inter-visit restoration of endodontic access cavities	Poor ability to seal as demonstrated by microleakage studies

rate of wear but these materials still show less wear resistance than resin composites. The clinical significance of this is the restriction of use of these materials to non-load-bearing areas.

INDICATIONS AND CONTRAINDICATIONS

The lower mechanical properties and the nature of the water uptake tends to make compomers unsuitable for restorations which are load-bearing. One product has been launched for use in Class I and Class II restorations in adults but this is not to be recommended. Compomers are suitable for use in the deciduous dentition where lower loads are experienced. They are also available in a flowable form when a material of this presentation is preferred (see indications of flowable resin composites in Chapter 7). However, the choice of a flowable resin composite versus a flowable compomer would tend to favour the use of the resin composite as no advantage is gained by using the compomer.

While their aesthetics are satisfactory, they are not as good as resin composites. If aesthetics are of prime concern, then resin composites should be chosen in preference to compomers. As mentioned previously, compomer luting cements are also available on the market (Table 8.4).

PRESENTATION

The materials are normally supplied as a paste in light-tight compules (Figure 8.7). This paste contains no water and is presented in foil blister packaging to prevent absorption of water from the atmosphere, which would cause premature setting and degradation of the material.

Compomers should always be stored and placed in a water-free environment. The material is presented in foil blister packs, which prevents moisture from the air contaminating the material (Figure 8.8).

Good moisture control during placement (preferably under rubber dam) is very important. Failure to do this may result in premature setting of the material.

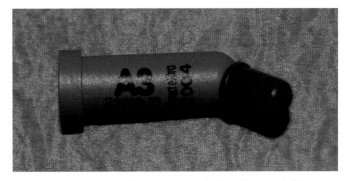

Fig. 8.7 Compomer material presented in a light-tight compule (Dyract, Dentsply).

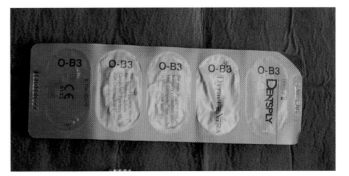

Fig. 8.8 Compomer compules presented in foil blister packs to prevent moisture in the air from contaminating the material prior to clinical use.

Table 8.5 Some compomers currently available on the market

Product	Manufacturer	Indications				
		Class III	Class V	Fissure sealants	Luting	Restoration of deciduous teeth
Compoglass F	Ivoclar Vivadent	√	√	X	X	√
Compoglass Flow	Ivoclar Vivadent	X	√	√	X	X
Dyract Cem Plus	Dentsply	X	X	X	√	X
Dyract eXtra	Dentsply	√	√	X	X	√
Dyract Flow	Dentsply	X	√	√	X	X
F2000	3M ESPE	√	√	X	X	√
Freedom	SDI	√	√	X	X	√
Glasiosite	Voco	√	√	X	X	√

HANDLING AND MANIPULATION PRIOR TO CURING

These materials require handling in a similar way to resin composites as their major constituents are similar. Some products do have a tendency to slump as they are of a slightly lower viscosity than resin composites counterparts. They also tend to be stickier, with the result that they 'cling' more to instruments making their manipulation more difficult.

Due to their stickier nature and the difficulty in handling and manipulating compomers, the clinician may find it easier to place the material and then adjust the restoration's contour after light curing with rotary instrumentation. Alternatively polyester matrices may be used.

Commercially available products and their indications

Table 8.5 shows representative examples of commercially available products.

SUMMARY

- Compomers have two setting reactions; they are polymerized by light curing but have a secondary reaction that permits fluoride release.
- Their properties are slightly inferior to resin composites but they offer a low, steady release of fluoride .
- Polymerization shrinkage is partly compensated for by water uptake.
- Compomers are not as easily manipulated as resin composites.
- They have a relatively limited area of applications.

FURTHER READING

Powers, J.M., Sakaguchi, R.L., 2006. Craig's Restorative Dental Materials. Mosby Elsevier, St Louis. (See Chapter 9).

van Noort, R., 2007. Introduction to Dental Materials, third ed. Mosby Elsevier, Edinburgh. (See Chapter 2.2).

SELF-ASSESSMENT QUESTIONS

1. What are the similarities and differences between compomers and resin composites?
2. List the indications of compomers and the advantages and disadvantages for each application.
3. Why should compomers not be used as a core build-up material prior to the provision of a full crown?
4. Describe how water uptake may be both advantageous and disadvantageous for compomer restorations.
5. Describe the setting mechanisms of compomers and their clinical relevance.

Chapter | 9 |

The tooth-coloured restorative materials III: Glass ionomer cements

INTRODUCTION

The next group of tooth-coloured restorative materials are the **glass ionomer cements**. This generic group of materials is distinguished by setting involving an acid–base reaction, requiring the presence of water. All commercially available glass ionomer materials involve a reaction of an acidic liquid with a basic glass. From a chemical and ISO terminological perspective, the term **glass polyalkenoate cements** is strictly speaking more correct when referring to this group of materials. The original term (glass ionomer cements) excludes some of the acids being used in the currently available products.

> **Acid–base reaction:** a chemical reaction in which an acid reacts with a basic oxide to form a salt plus water.

HISTORY

The original glass ionomer cement produced in the 1970s was derived from dental **silicate cement**. This was the restorative material of choice for use in the anterior segment of the mouth in the

The term a **light-cured glass ionomer** is often used by dental manufacturers in promotional literature. It is important to stress that this refers to materials which are *not* true glass ionomer cements. Light curing is required because of the addition of a resin to the material (together with the chemicals needed to effect light polymerization of the material). These materials should be referred to as resin-modified glass ionomer cement. Chapter 10 deals with these materials.

1930s–1950s because it had better aesthetic properties than any of the other materials available at that time. It was based on a fluoro-alumino-silicate glass combined with phosphoric acid. It had limited applications as:

- The material was soluble in saliva.
- It had insufficient strength to withstand occlusal loading.

However, silicate cement did have certain advantages in that it released fluoride ions, which was considered to provide some resistance to the development of recurrent caries. The initial objective underpinning the development of glass ionomer cements was to overcome the inherent disadvantages of silicate cement while retaining the perceived advantage.

> **Cariostatic:** the property of prevention of the spread of dental caries. A lesion is unlikely to regress, but will not spread in the presence of a cariostatic agent.

COMPONENTS OF A GLASS IONOMER

The material is the product of the chemical reaction between the **glass** and an **acid** when the two components are mixed together. There is an initial dissolution of the surface of the powder. The soluble components of the glass react with the **polyacrylic acid** to form a matrix. After setting, the residual unreacted material is encased in

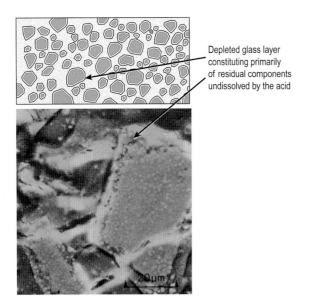

Depleted glass layer constituting primarily of residual components undissolved by the acid

Fig. 9.1 Composition of a glass ionomer cement: the depleted glass layer is surrounding the remaining unreacted glass core.

this salt matrix, which holds the cement together (Figure 9.1). The set material is therefore a cored structure in which only the surface of the glass has reacted to permit the binding of the glass particles together.

> **Salt matrix:** the part of the glass ionomer structure which is formed from the reaction of the acid and the glass surface. This salt structure binds the glass particles together.

Glass

The glass is relatively similar to that used in silicate cement, being based on a combination of fluoro-alumino-silicate glasses. Different properties can be given to the final cement by the manufacturers by varying the composition of the glass, such as:

- Adding additional elements, e.g. strontium and lithium, to impart radiopacity
- Making the cement more translucent by altering the aluminium/silica ratio
- Altering the rate of ion release, an important factor in determining solubility, setting characteristics and release of fluoride.

The glass has a formulation based on the firing of a combination of chemicals (Table 9.1). Figure 9.2 shows some typical glass

Table 9.1 Compounds contained in the glass of a typical glass ionomer cement

Compound	Percentage composition
Alumina (aluminium oxide)	14.2–28.6
Silica (silicon dioxide)	30.1–41.9
Calcium fluoride	12.8–34.5
Aluminium fluoride	1.6–11.0
Aluminium phosphate	3.8–24.2
Sodium fluoride	3.6–12.8

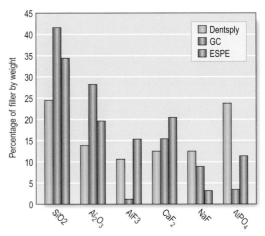

Fig. 9.2 Typical glass formulations of glass ionomer cements in commercial use.

formulations for commonly available cements and highlights the substantial variation in the formulations of glass which may be used to produce a glass ionomer cement.

Manufacturing process for the glass component

The glass mixture is heated to a temperature between 1150°C and 1450°C. The molten mass is then poured onto a metal plate and then into water, a process termed **shock cooling**. The glass is then broken up to form a glass frit (Figure 9.3). All the glasses for the currently available cements are then either wet or dry milled to produce small particles of glass. Various ranges of particle size are used depending on the requirements and usage of the cement. The larger glass particle sizes are used in those cements intended as restorative materials (up to 20 μm) while the smaller particle sizes (<5 μm) are used for luting cements.

> **Frit:** This is the product of pouring molten glass into water. It usually consists of small particles of glass which will be ground up to smaller size later in the glass preparation process. The size of the glass particles is determined by the use or application.
> **Wet milled:** The glass particles are placed in a cylindrical ceramic vessel with a volume of water and a number of ceramic balls. The whole assembly is then rotated. The ceramic balls tumble around the vessel grinding the glass frit down in size. The longer the tumbling process the finer the particles of glass.
> **Dry milled:** as for wet milling but with the exclusion of the water.

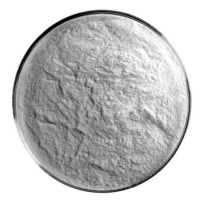

Fig. 9.3 Glass frit produced after firing.

If the glass is mixed with a polyacid at this point, it would set very rapidly with too short a working time for clinical use. The manufacturers all now adopt a **passivation** treatment to reduce the reactivity of the glass. The glass is washed in **acetic acid** for up to 24 hours and then dried. This process leads to ion depletion of the glass surface, resulting in fewer ions being immediately available to form the salt matrix when mixing starts. Passivation of the glass is of greater significance when the particle size of the cement is reduced, as the smaller the particle the more rapid the set.

Acid

The acid used is part of a series of **polyacids**, including **polyacrylic acid**, **polymaleic acid** and a number of **copolymers** of **polyacrylic acid**. The combination of polyacids that are suitable for copolymerization can be varied widely so conveying different properties to the final product. The acid in the glass ionomer cement is a variant of either the homopolymer of acrylic acid, its co-polymer or maleic acid, depending on the manufacturer. The functional group which all these acids contain and which plays a part in the chemical reaction is a carboxylate group – which in water ionizes to carboxyl and hydrogen ions. A small number of cements also include a **polyphosphonic acid**. This is thought to provide a short sharp set but does not appear to enhance the physical properties to any great extent.

> **Homopolymer:** a polymer that contains one single monomer type.
> **Ion:** An ion is an atom or molecule where the total number of electrons is not equal to the total number of protons, giving it a net positive or negative electrical charge.
> **Copolymerization:** the method of chemically synthesizing a copolymer.

The performance of the cement is related to the **molecular weight** of the acid used and this explains why two cements with apparently similar compositions can behave differently. It is generally considered that the higher the molecular weight of the acid used, the better the mechanical properties. However, this benefit is offset by the increase in viscosity of the aqueous acid solution with increasing molecular weight. To overcome this, some manufacturers vacuum dry the acid solution and then mix the anhydrous powder so formed with the glass. Activation of the cement is achieved by adding water. This addition from a dropper bottle starts the chemical reaction as the vacuum-dried acid starts to go into solution, which then is followed by the initial dissolution of the glass surface.

> **Anhydrous:** a material which does not contain water. The term anhydrous refers to the presentation of some glass ionomer cements in which the powder has been dried.

Maleic acid, one of the alternatives to polyacrylic acid, is a less viscous aqueous solution and this has permitted one manufacturer (3M ESPE) to use the acid in aqueous form in the encapsulated presentation more easily.

Changes in molecular weight will also influence the working and setting time of the cement. The higher the molecular weight (and so the viscosity), the shorter the working and setting times. A small amount of **tartaric acid** is added to all materials to accelerate the setting phase of the reaction while maintaining the working time (Figure 9.4).

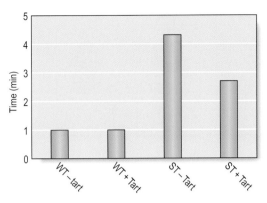

Fig. 9.4 Bar graph illustrating the effect of the addition of tartaric acid on working times (WT) and setting times (ST) of a glass ionomer cement. There is no change in working time but there is a marked reduction in setting time on addition of 2% tartaric acid.
(Data from Wilson AD, Nicolson J Acid-Base Cements: Their Biomedical and Industrial Applications. Cambridge University Press, Cambridge, 1993 (Chapter 5).)

PRESENTATION

Two typical presentations of glass ionomer cements commonly exist: **encapsulated** and **hand mixed**. The chemical constituents of each are described in Table 9.2.

Table 9.2 Typical composition of encapsulated and hand-mixed glass ionomer cements

	Encapsulated	**Hand mixed (anhydrous)**	**Conventional hand mixed**
Powder	Glass	Glass A vacuum-dried poly(acrylic acid) Tartaric acid (vacuum dried)	Glass
Liquid	Polyacid Tartaric acid	Water	Polyacid Water Tartaric acid

Conventional hand-mixed materials usually use a much lower molecular weight polyacrylic acid.

SETTING REACTION

The setting reaction of a glass ionomer cement involves many stages (Figure 9.5). On mixing the cement paste:

1. The glass is attacked by hydrogen ions from the acid, liberating aluminium and calcium ions. Fluoride and sodium ions are also released.
2. The pH of the aqueous phase rises and leads to a further ionization of the polyacrylic acid.
3. This leads to migration of aluminium and calcium cations into the aqueous phase.

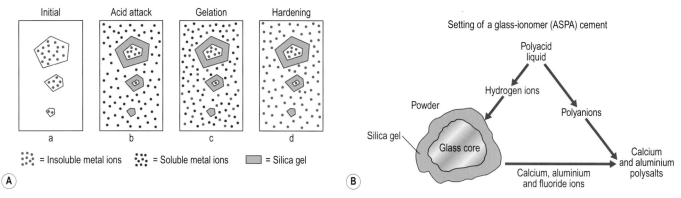

Fig. 9.5 (A) The stages of a setting reaction in a glass ionomer cement: (a) Initial stage with glass alone and insoluble (blue) metal ions in the glass; (b) Acid attack causes some metal ions to dissolve in the acid (red). The surface of the glass from where these ions have migrated is now an ion depleted zone primarily consisting of silica gel. (c) At the **gelation stage** sufficient metal ions are present in solution hence a number start to reprecipitate as the salt matrix. (d) During the hardening process this reprecipitation continues until the matrix is completely formed. (B) The ions released during the matrix formation in a glass ionomer or alumino-silicate polyacrylate (ASPA) cement.

4. Ionization of the polyacrylic acid leads to unwinding of the polymer chain. This causes the viscosity of the paste to increase, and the cation concentration also increases.
5. The cations then condense on the polymer chain.
6. This leads to the formation of an insoluble salt.

The condensation process occurs more rapidly with the calcium ions. Within a minute of the commencement of the reaction, **calcium polyacrylate gel** is formed. **Aluminium polyacrylate** formation takes substantially longer. These salts do not appear until about an hour after the start of mixing. This is attributed to the fact that the aluminium ion is triple charged and less mobile. Complexes are also formed with the fluoride ions in the solution.

The cement then goes through a period of maturation. Further cross-linking of the matrix occurs and more cations become bound onto the polyanion chain. This maturation phase may be extended in time. This also has the effect of increasing the mechanical properties of the material substantially. The maturation phase can continue for some months.

> **! Etching glass ionomer cements**
>
> The etching of glass ionomer cements has been recommended in some restorative procedures to enhance the union between the two materials such as in the sandwich or laminate technique, where a resin composite forms the surface of the restoration and the glass ionomer acts as a base. The etching may, however, damage the cement structure. The earlier the etching process is performed in the glass ionomer cement setting reaction, the more likely it is that the salt matrix will be damaged as it has not matured. If etching is carried out within 5 minutes of placement, the matrix is completely removed within 15 seconds of applying the 37% phosphoric acid etchant (Figure 9.6). Successful etching of the glass ionomer cement can only be achieved after the matrix has matured, that is, after 24 hours. After this time the rate of removal of the salt matrix is much slower and a partial surface removal of the salt matrix will occur.
>
> Placement of the resin composite will lead to the glass particles being pulled away from the underlying cement during the polymerization process, leaving a void between resin and underlying cement.

Anion: an ion carrying a negative charge
Cation: an ion carrying a positive charge.
Cross-linking: bonds which link one polymer chain to another.
Polyanion: a molecule carrying a large number of negative charges. In the case of a glass ionomer cement, there may be a number of carboxyl groups on one polymer chain and these will individually react with metal ions which are in solution.

SETTING TIME

One of the major limitations of the conventional glass ionomer cements is the time to full set after commencement of mixing. This is quite lengthy and it is in direct contrast with the rapid setting of resin-based composites when light activated. The ability to reduce in setting time is limited as any shortening of the set time usually results in a shortened working time.

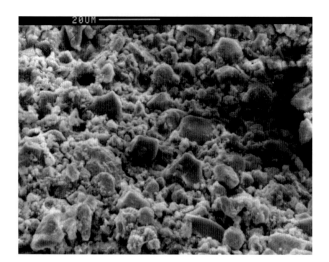

Fig. 9.6 Glass ionomer cement after etching with 37% phosphoric acid for 15 seconds.

Open sandwich: A restoration in a tooth in which two restorative materials are used. They are generally mechanically and/or chemically bound together. The open sandwich technique is usually used for Class II restorations where the underlying material forms part of the axial wall and is exposed to the oral environment (Figure 9.7).

Closed sandwich: in a closed sandwich restoration the underlying material does not come into contact with the oral cavity (Figure 9.8).

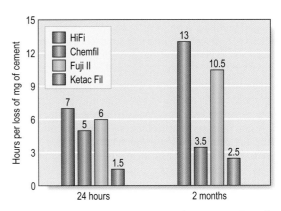

Fig. 9.9 The rate of cement loss decreases with respect to time of exposure to water. At 2 months, for all the cements, it takes a much longer time for the same amount of material to be lost.

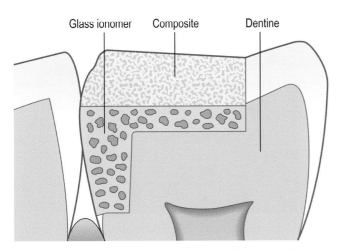

Fig. 9.7 A Class II open sandwich restoration. The glass ionomer is extending to the approximal surface of the restoration.

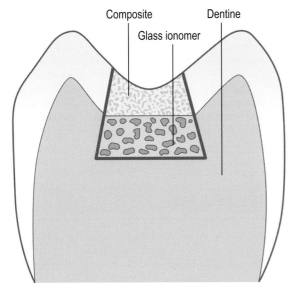

Fig. 9.8 A closed sandwich restoration. The glass ionomer is completely covered by the composite and not exposed to the oral environment.

MECHANICAL PROPERTIES

The mechanical properties of conventional glass ionomer cements are not ideal.

- The compressive strength of the cement is adequate, just below that of dentine.
- The flexural strength is relatively low compared with other restorative materials. However, in most cases under load it is protected by the restorative.
- The compressive and flexural strengths increase with time as the cement matures.
- The solubility varies with time of exposure to the oral environment after mixing.
- The longer the restoration is protected from moisture, the better the resistance is to erosion (Figure 9.9).

Any protective layer placed on the restoration will extend the time before the restoration is attacked by oral fluids.

ADHESION

One of the advantages of glass ionomer cements is their ability to chemically bond to tooth tissue without the use of an intermediate material. There are two recognized mechanisms:

- An ion exchange process where the polyacrylic acid displaces surface phosphate and calcium, enters the hydroxyapatite structure and forming a calcium polyacrylate salt. Thus an intermediate layer of calcium and aluminium phosphates and polyacrylates are formed at the tooth/restoration interface.
- A secondary bond, which is thought to occur with the collagen within the dentine, possible via hydrogen bonding.

The bond strength is relatively low (5 MPa) but appears to be durable and fit for purpose. There is considerable evidence that the bond can re-form if broken, thus it can be termed **dynamic**. This is due to the polyacrylate and calcium ions being in close proximity to each other.

The reliability of the bond is improved by **preconditioning** the surface of the tooth by the use of an acid **conditioner**. This is primarily to remove smear layer and debris from the surface of the tooth. Both citric and polyacrylic acids have been used as conditioners. The best results are obtained using polyacrylic acid as this acid is not so highly ionized. This step may be included in a clinical protocol when using glass ionomer cements. However, evidence does exist that although restorations whose cavities were conditioned lasted longer, there was no statistically significant difference in longevity between those restorations placed without conditioning. It is likely that other factors will affect the performance to a greater degree.

Glass ionomer cements have been advocated in the treatment of non-carious tooth surface loss and, in particular, **abfraction** lesions as the material has the ability to re-form broken bonds so contributing to its retention. This is in contrast to resin-based systems where the polymerization shrinkage lead to pull away from one margin, usually the cervical, and microleakage then occurs (Figure 9.10).

Smear layer: layer of organic and inorganic debris found on a surface of a tooth.

! Conditioning and etching – what's the difference?

Conditioning uses a less ionized acid (usually polyacrylic acid) to remove the smear layer and so priming the dentine to accept the restorative material which forms **chemical** bonds. The acid makes the surface chemically active. Little or no tissue is removed.

Etching requires a stronger acid such as phosphoric acid which preferentially dissolves the dental hard tissue, in particular enamel, to create pits in its surface. The restorative material (usually containing resin-based composite) is retained **micromechanically**. Etching affects the subsurface of the tooth tissue while conditioning is primarily a surface treatment (see Chapter 11).

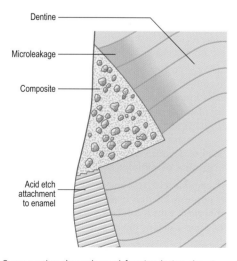

Fig. 9.10 Cross-section through an abfraction lesion showing where failure occurs when resin composites are used.

Dentine

Microleakage

Composite

Acid etch attachment to enamel

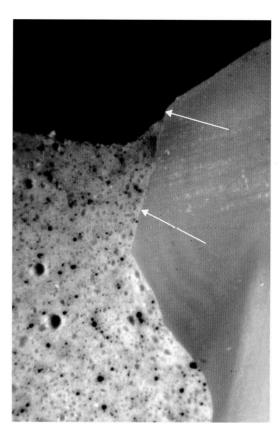

Fig. 9.11 Micrograph showing the good adaptation of glass ionomer cement with tooth tissue. Note that a (red) dye marker has only tracked down the outer third of the enamel thickness, denoted by the arrows.

SEALING CAPACITY

Leakage around glass ionomer cement (if mixed and placed in the recommended manner!) will be relatively low (Figure 9.11). Therefore a glass ionomer cement is an excellent choice as the restorative material between visits when an endodontic procedure is being undertaken. The cement seals the access cavity effectively thus preventing the ingress of microorganisms and reinfection of the root canal system. Furthermore, the stability of the cement with little or no dimensional change means that the bond between tooth and restoration is unstressed.

FLUORIDE RELEASE

One of the most important clinical considerations of glass ionomer cements is their ability to release fluoride from the bulk of the restoration. This was also observed with the original silicate cements and is the result of the leaching of fluoride ions from the matrix into the surrounding environment. The ions are released from the glass during the setting reaction and lie within the matrix but are free to migrate. The factors that influence the migration are the relative concentrations of ions in the cement and in the surrounding environment as well as the pH of the environment.

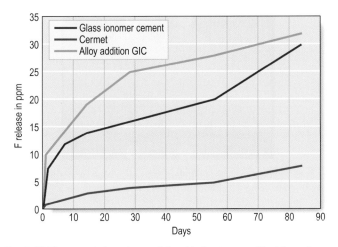

Fig. 9.12 The cumulative release of fluoride (parts per million) from three types of glass ionomer cement with respect to time.

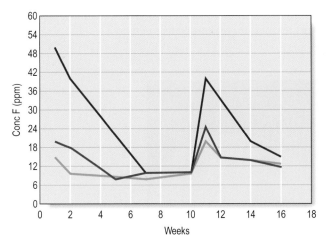

Fig. 9.13 Initial release of fluoride ions into saliva from three different types of glass ionomer cements in patients using a non-fluoridated toothpaste for 10 weeks. Over this time the release of fluoride slowed and levelled off between weeks 6 and 7. At week 10 all participants in the study were provided with a fluoride toothpaste for use over the next week. At week 11 they returned to the use of a non-fluoridated toothpaste. During that week the fluoride in saliva went up substantially. However, from week 11 it showed a slow decline and even at week 15, at the end of the study, the fluoride release was above that at the beginning of week 6.
(Data from Hatibovic-Kofman S, Koch G. Fluoride release from glass ionomer cement in vitro and in vivo. Swedish Dental Journal 1991;15:253–8.)

Fluoride release follows a similar pattern for all glass ionomer cements. There is an initial washout phase which is associated with the maturation phase of the setting reaction of the cement. Following this, the release rate slows and follows a normal diffusion pattern. The duration of this diffusion-related release has not been defined but appears to go on for a period of years (Figure 9.12).

It has been established that these restoratives also have the capability of taking up fluoride ions from the surroundings if the concentration externally is higher than that in the surface of the cement. This **recharge** mechanism has been demonstrated with fluoride toothpaste solutions and gels. The re-release of the retained fluoride occurs when the external concentration drops below that of the restoration (Figure 9.13). Thus, these materials act as a **fluoride sink** that provides a source of fluoride ions for many years. The fluoride ion concentration may be sufficient to inhibit bacterial growth and plaque build-up (Figure 9.14).

> **Biofilm:** a community of microorganisms surrounded by a self-formed polymer matrix which adheres to both living and inert surfaces. Dental plaque is regarded as a classic example of a biofilm.

There is also a long-term exchange of ions between the tooth surface and the restoration. It has been shown that in artificial caries media, the level of demineralization around a glass ionomer restoration is substantially less than that observed around a composite. While there is some disagreement as to the long-term effect of the fluoride release, it is fair to say that studies on this effect are retrospective and very heterogeneous in their use of criteria for judging the benefits. Some studies have shown the ability of fluoride to prevent recurrent caries whereas others have demonstrated no difference in recurrent caries levels when compared with other non-fluoride-leaching restorative materials.

AESTHETICS

Glass ionomer cements have had a chequered history with regard to their aesthetic properties. The early materials were opaque and showed a poor match with the tooth tissue as there was no reflection from the surrounding tooth tissue. More translucent glasses have been produced, which have improved this, but there is still a

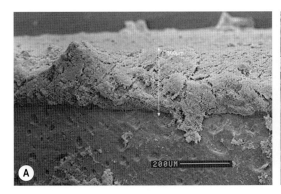

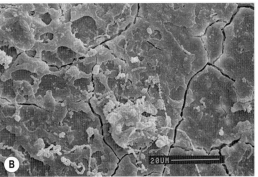

Fig. 9.14 (A) Photomicrograph showing a thick biofilm growing on a hydroxyapatite disc. (B) Photomicrograph showing limited bacterial activity on the surface of a glass ionomer cement which releases fluoride.

period after placement where the shade match is not always as good as that achieved after 2–3 days. This is due in part to the maturation of the matrix and is very much material dependent (Figure 9.15). While the colour match is not particularly good, glass ionomer cements exhibit much greater resistance to changes in colour when compared with resin-based composites over the restoration's life (Figure 9.16).

Although the modern glass ionomer restorative cements exhibit acceptable aesthetic properties, if aesthetics are of paramount importance then a resin composite material would be the material of choice.

WEAR

Glass ionomer cements show variable rates of wear and can perform very well if allowed to mature fully protected from washout by saliva. However, they frequently show rapid wear during the first 10 days, after which the wear rate slows down to comparable values for other restorative materials. The mode of wear is the loss of glass particles from the matrix particularly in load-bearing areas. Although the glass

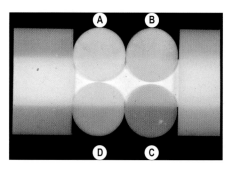

Fig. 9.15 Four discs made of different materials: (A) a composite, (B) a glass ionomer cement just after mixing (C) the same material 24 hours after mixing, and (D) a compomer. Note the change which can occur in translucency over the 24-hour period for the glass ionomer cement. This is due to the cement maturation process.

is chemically bound to the matrix, this is insufficient to hold the particles in place. Figure 9.17 shows wear on a glass ionomer after 3 years. There are occasions where erosion may occur in a mouth when the pH remains low for long periods of time.

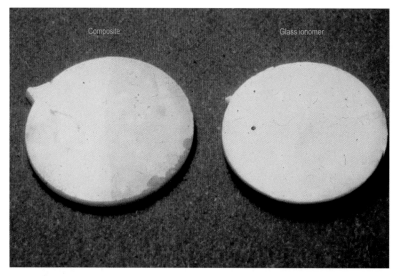

Fig. 9.16 Two discs of material: resin-based composite on the left and glass ionomer cement on the right. Half of each disc was protected by foil and the other half exposed to sunlight for 3 months. Note the marked change in colour on the composite disc, not observed with the glass ionomer sample.

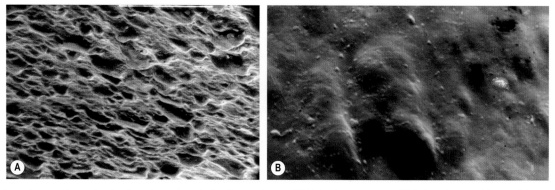

Fig. 9.17 Replicas of the surface of a glass ionomer cement after 3 years in use. (A) Note the craters in which the glass particles are lying. (B) A non-load-bearing area of the same restoration after the same time interval.

ADVANTAGES AND DISADVANTAGES

Table 9.3 shows the advantages and disadvantages of glass ionomer cements.

Table 9.3 Advantages and contraindications of glass ionomer cements	
Advantages	**Disadvantages**
Dynamic bond which can regenerate so useful for the restoration of abfraction lesions	Poorer aesthetics compared to resin composites
Chemical adhesion to tooth so can be used in non-retentive cavities	Weaker so not recommended for cores/large cavities
Cariostatic due to fluoride release	Susceptible to washout
Does not require hardware, for example curing lights	Can be damaged by early finishing
Can be used for domiciliary visits and in non 'ideal' situations	Long time to set
Does not need to be used with rubber dam	Needs protection to prevent desiccation
Requires only limited cavity preparation	Early low mechanical strength

INDICATIONS AND CONTRAINDICATIONS

Glass ionomer cements are versatile materials and are indicated in many different situations in restorative dentistry:

- Atraumatic restorative technique (ART)
- Restoration of deciduous teeth
- Restoration of permanent teeth:
  - Tunnel preparations
  - Class III cavities
  - Class V (especially non-carious tooth surface loss) cavities

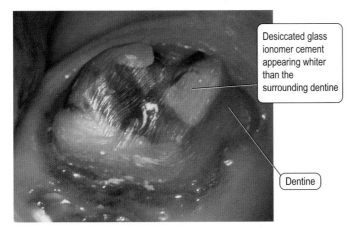

Fig. 9.18 A completed crown preparation where glass ionomer cement has been used as the core material. In order to differentiate between the tooth-coloured core material and the dentine, the dentist has air dried the preparation. This has had the effect of desiccating the glass ionomer cement so rendering it whiter than the surrounding tooth tissue and it can be identified more easily, especially when preparing margins (see Chapter 6).

Desiccated glass ionomer cement appearing whiter than the surrounding dentine

Dentine

- Inter-visit endodontic access cavity restorations (especially with respect to resin-based composite (see below))
- Long-term intermediate restoration
- Core construction (provided sufficient tooth tissue remains to support the material)
- Preventive resin restorations
- As a base or liner
- Dressings
  - Non-retentive cavities
  - When it is envisaged that resin composite will be used as the definitive restorative material (instead of the use of a zinc oxide eugenol cement whose eugenol constituent may inhibit the setting reaction of the resin composite)
- Fissure sealants
- Luting of crown and bridge retainers
- Orthodontic cements.

Atraumatic restorative technique (ART): a technique which uses non-mechanical cavity preparation with minimal removal of softened dental caries from a tooth prior to restoration.
Tunnel preparation: a means of accessing approximal caries from the occlusal surface with minimal tooth destruction.
Base: a dentine replacement material used to decrease the bulk of restorative material or block out any undercuts in indirect restorations.
Liner: a material placed with minimal thickness, usually less than 0.5 mm acting as a cavity sealer. It may release fluoride, adhere to tooth structure and may have an antibacterial action that promotes the health of the pulp.

There are certain situations where the use of glass ionomer cements is contraindicated:

- Where high load is anticipated, e.g., Class I or Class II cavities
- In large cavities in the posterior region of the mouth
- Cores where little or no tooth is remaining to support the material
- Where aesthetics are of primary concern.

CLINICAL MANIPULATION

Cavity preparation

As the material is brittle, the cavity shape should have a rounded internal form with no sharp edges. Any sharp edges where stress concentrations can occur may lead to premature failure of the material due to fracture. As the material bonds to tooth tissue, there is no need to prepare extensive retentive features in the cavity.

When removing tooth-coloured restorative materials from a cavity, it is often difficult to differentiate the material from the surrounding tooth tissue. If this is the case, the cavity should be dried thoroughly. Any material remaining will dehydrate thus appearing whiter. The material can be more easily identified and removed without inadvertent sacrifice of sound tooth tissue. This is particularly true with glass ionomer cements (Figure 9.18).

Conditioning the cavity

The 25% polyacrylic acid supplied by the manufacturer should be used to condition the dentine (Table 9.4) by applying to the tooth surface for 15–30 seconds using a brush or cotton pledget. It should then be rinsed off using water from a three-in-one syringe and the tooth surface gently dried.

Table 9.4 Some dentine conditioning solutions currently available on the market

Product	Manufacturer	Active ingredient
Ketac Conditioner	3M ESPE	20–30% poly(acrylic acid)
ChemFil Tooth Cleanser	Dentsply	25% poly(acrylic acid)
Fuji Dentine Conditioner	GC	10% poly(acrylic acid)
Fuji Cavity Conditioner	GC	20% poly(acrylic acid)
Hi-Tooth Cleanser	Shofu	25% poly(acrylic acid)
Voco Conditioner	Voco	25% poly(acrylic acid)

Commercially available products

As mentioned above, glass ionomer cements are very versatile materials that can be used in many different clinical situations. See Table 9.5 for details. Dentsply has recently produced a glass ionomer (ChemFil Rock) in which the reactive glass filler had been modified by the addition of zinc. This is claimed to increase the fracture resistance and the wear. As yet there is no clinical evidence to confirm this, although laboratory tests suggest that the fracture resistance is better than some other glass ionomer cements.

Always check the expiry date! Although this is true for all dental materials, it is particularly important for glass ionomer cements. In many (anhydrous) products, a desiccant is present in the bottle containing the powder (Figure 9.19) and with exposure to moisture in the air and with time, this loses its efficiency with premature setting of the material in the bottle.

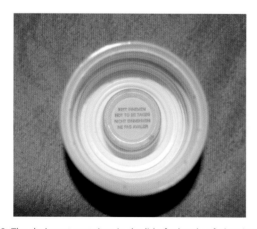

Fig. 9.19 The desiccant container in the lid of a bottle of glass ionomer powder.

Mixing glass ionomer cements: mixing by hand

Hand mixing will produce the optimum results provided that the instructions are adhered to precisely. Failure to observe the correct proportioning, dispensing and mixing instructions will result in a cement with inferior properties (Figure 9.20), although there is scope to vary the material's consistency to suit the clinical application. For example, it may be that a thicker mix using more powder is required if a crown is not fitting as well as it once did yet is otherwise acceptable in the short term. The consistency of this mix would lie between that required of a restorative and that needed to lute a cast restoration. The former more viscous mix may prevent complete seating of the crown, yet the extra powder would impart increased mechanical properties to the cement. This may aid in the retention of the crown until such times as the patient and clinician are able to plan for a definitive replacement. When the manufacturer's recommendations for the powder/liquid ratio are not adhered to, it is essential that the clinician is aware of the consequences and that the intended procedure is a short-term measure.

- *Higher powder/liquid ratio*: When the powder/liquid ratio is increased (i.e. there is addition of more powder), the compressive strength of the final cement will increase and its setting time will be decreased. The material will be much more viscous with limited polyacrylic acid available for bonding. The cement's ability to form chemical bonds will also decrease. The cement must wet the tooth surface adequately and failure to achieve this will result in the decreased retention as bonding is less satisfactory. The rapid decline in mechanical properties is a result of the solid particles of glass not being wetted sufficiently by the acid to start the setting reaction.

- *Lower powder/liquid ratio*: When the powder/liquid ratio is reduced (less powder is added), the properties of the cement decline rapidly and this can have deleterious effects on any restoration. A reduction in mechanical properties of nearly 60% can occur when the powder/liquid ratio is reduced by 25% (Figure 9.20).

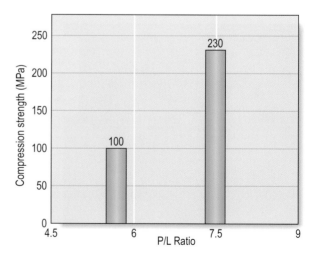

Fig. 9.20 The compressive strengths of a glass ionomer cement mixed at different powder/liquid (P/L) ratios: 6.8:1 (manufacturer's recommendation) and 5:1 (dentist's preference). The latter powder/liquid ratio results in a material with compressive strength which is well below the minimum ISO requirement.

Table 9.5 Some glass ionomer cements currently available on the market

Product	Manufacturer	Indications								
		Base	Dressing	Fissure sealant	Inter-visit temporization in endodontics	Luting	Orthodontic cement	Preventive resin restoration	Restoration of deciduous teeth	Restoration of permanent teeth
AquaCem	Dentsply	X	X	X	X	√	√	X	X	X
ChemFil Molar	Dentsply	X	√	X	√	X	X	X	√	√
ChemFil Superior	Dentsply	√	√	√	√	√*	√	√	√	√
ChemFlex	Dentsply	√	√	√	√	√*	X	√	√	√
CX-Plus	Shofu	X	X	X	X	√	X	X	X	X
Diamond Carve	Kemdent	√	√	√	√	X	X	√	√	√
Diamond Core	Kemdent	X	√	X	√	X	X	X	X	√
Diamond Snappy	Kemdent	X	√	X	X	X	X	X	√	X
Fuji I	GC	√	√	X	√	X	X	X	√	X
Fuji IX (also GP, Extra and Fast)	GC	√	√	X	√	X	X	√	√	√
Fuji Plus (also EWT)	GC	X	X	X	X	√	X	X	X	X
Fuji Triage (formerly Fuji VII)	GC	X	√	√	X	X	X	X	X	√
Glasionomer Type II	Shofu	√	√	√	√	√*	√	√	√	√

Table 9.5 (Continued)

Product	Manufacturer	Indications								
		Base	Dressing	Fissure sealant	Inter-visit temporization in endodontics	Luting	Orthodontic cement	Preventive resin restoration	Restoration of deciduous teeth	Restoration of permanent teeth
Hi-Fi	Shofu	√	√	×	×	×	×	√	√	√
Ionofil Molar AC (also Quick and Plus)	Voco	√	√	×	√	×	×	√	√	√
Ketac Cem (also Aplicap, Maxicap, Radiopaque)	3M ESPE	×	×	×	×	√	√	×	×	×
Ketac Cem μ	3M ESPE	×	×	×	×	√	√	×	×	×
Ketac Fil Plus	3M ESPE	√	√	√	√	√*	√	√	√	√
Ketac Molar (also Aplicap, Quick, Easymix)	3M ESPE	√	√	×	√	×	×	√	√	√
Ketac-Bond (also Aplicap)	3M ESPE	√	×	×	×	√	√	×	×	√
Legend luting	SS White	√	×	×	×	√	√	×	×	×
Legend restorative	SS White	×	√	×	√	×	×	√	√	√
Riva Luting	SDI	√	×	×	×	√	√	×	×	×
Riva Protect	SDI	×	√	√	√	×	√	√	×	×
Riva self cure	SDI	×	√	×	√	×	×	√	√	√

*As a non-definitive measure when cast is not fitting well.

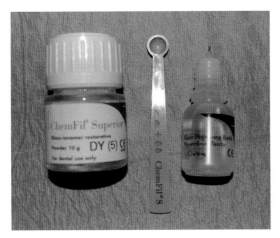

Fig. 9.21 The most common presentation of a hand mixed glass ionomer cement. The bottle on the left contains the powder (and scoop) and the other the liquid.

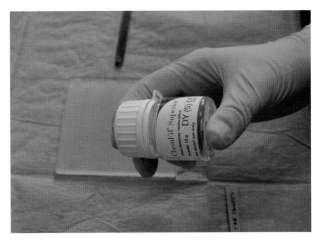

Fig. 9.22 Shaking the powder prior to dispensation on the glass slab.

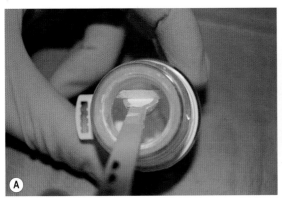
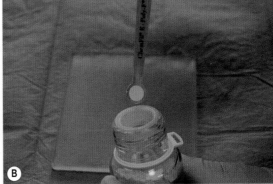

Fig. 9.23A,B Dispensation of correct quantity of powder for a glass ionomer cement.

Most presentations of hand mixed materials come as two components: the powder with a scoop and a dropper bottle with the liquid (Figure 9.21).

 Always shake the bottle! This is particularly true if the cement is one where the polyacid is vacuum dried and incorporated into the glass powder. Shaking the bottle will ensure that the two components are evenly distributed within the powder. This also fluffs the powder. Failure to do so will also alter the powder/liquid ratio and adversely affect the cement (Figure 9.22).

Proportioning

It is important to dispense the correct amount of both the powder and liquid.

Powder

After shaking the bottle, collect the powder in the measuring scoop. Any excess above the top of the scoop is removed by pulling the scoop against the flattener on the inside of the bottle. This ensures that the correct amount of powder required for the mix is dispensed (Figure 9.23).

Liquid

The dropper bottle is designed to dispense a fixed volume of liquid. This is achieved by holding the bottle vertically above the mixing slab before dispensing (Figure 9.24). To compensate for variation between drop volumes manufacturers recommend that two drops of liquid should be dispensed. This reduces the variation in liquid volume dispensed. An analogy is the situation in the kitchen when the enthusiastic amateur chef divides and multiplies up the number of portions required from a recipe. When volumes and ratios are changed, the dish may not turn out as anticipated if the original recipe had been used!

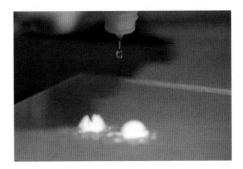

Fig. 9.24 Two drops of liquid being dispensed on to the slab separate from the powder. Note that the bottle is held vertically and that two scoops of powder have already been dispensed.

Spatulation

Vigorous spatulation is necessary and the use of an agate spatula (Figure 9.25) will reduce the risk of metal contamination of the restorative as glass can abrade a stainless steel spatula, turning the material grey. The use of a plastic spatula is inappropriate as plastic will also abrade and the small diameter does not permit easy incorporation of the powder into the water.

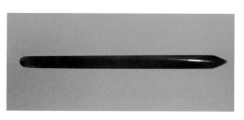

Fig. 9.25 An agate spatula should be used when hand mixing glass ionomer cements.

 Agate: this is a microcrystalline variety of quartz (silica).

The two components should be mixed on a glass slab as this allows the powder to be spread over the surface and quickly wetted by the acid.

✓ **Should dental cements be mixed on a glass slab or paper pad?**

While this may well be a matter of personal preference, there are advantages and disadvantages of each (Table 9.6). Mixing pads made of silicone are also available but the aqueous materials do not wet the surface well and it is more difficult to achieve a satisfactory mix.

Hand mixing protocol

Box 9.1 shows how to mix glass ionomer cement to restore a cavity using ChemFil Superior (Dentsply). While the principles of mixing this material hold true for all glass ionomer cements, it is essential to read the manufacturer's instructions and follow these carefully when using other materials.

Immediately after dispensation, the slab and mixing instrument should be placed in water to facilitate the cement's removal.

Table 9.6 Glass slab versus paper pad for mixing cements

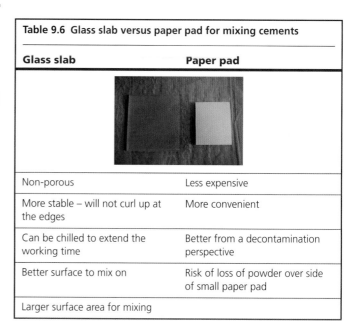

Glass slab	Paper pad
Non-porous	Less expensive
More stable – will not curl up at the edges	More convenient
Can be chilled to extend the working time	Better from a decontamination perspective
Better surface to mix on	Risk of loss of powder over side of small paper pad
Larger surface area for mixing	

Mixing encapsulated glass ionomer cements

The encapsulated presentation reduces the problems associated with hand mixing but is not foolproof. The liquid component is usually stored in an aluminium pillow and incorporated in the capsule,

Box 9.1 Clinical mixing protocol for use of glass ionomer cement as a restorative material

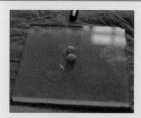 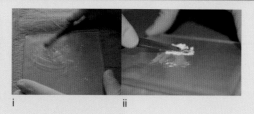 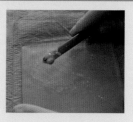 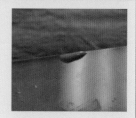

Dispense powder and liquid on slab prior to mixing. Note the short distance from the powder so that the two components are not in contact

All of the powder should be combined into the liquid at one time and the mass is vigorously spatulated together to ensure complete mixing

Mixing is almost complete and the glass ionomer is being collected on the spatula. Note all powder has been incorporated into mix

The final mixed material is placed on the edge of the slab and presented to the clinician for use

which has a means to rupture the pillow to deliver the liquid to the powder (Figure 9.26).

Care must also be taken when expelling the liquid into the capsule by maintaining pressure on the pillow for at least 2 seconds to expel the viscous liquid (see Chapter 1). Insufficient liquid incorporated into the mix will also make it difficult to expel the material from the capsule via the nozzle. The diameter of the nozzle also determines the viscosity of the mixed cement to be dispensed (Figure 9.27). In general the powder to liquid ratio of encapsulated materials is less that the recommended powder to liquid ratio for their hand mixed counterparts.

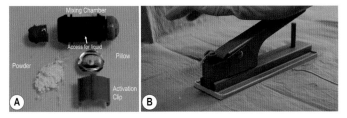

Fig. 9.26A,B The constituents of a glass ionomer cement capsule and the activation device. The aluminium pillow containing the liquid lies over the access hole in the mixing chamber. When pressure is applied to the activation clip by the activator, the pillow ruptures and liquid is forced into the mixing chamber.

Moisture control

As with all restorative materials, the area to be restored should be clean and dry. Failure to achieve good moisture control will result in the material becoming contaminated with saliva during placement and decrease in its properties and ability to adhere to the tooth. Glass ionomer cements are one of the few generic groups of modern materials where the use of rubber dam is not essential in achieving the optimum results. However, it is necessary to ensure that the cement is not allowed to give up water during the setting reaction and the water balance within the material should be maintained throughout the life of the restoration.

Placement

Glass ionomer cements are generally placed using instruments routinely used in restorative dentistry such as a **flat plastic** (Figure 9.28). In some cases, the viscosity of the material makes clinical manipulation difficult as its consistency is slightly sticky. If an instrument becomes coated with the material during placement, it is likely that the already placed material will be pulled from the cavity. Water may be used sparingly as a separating medium. Alcohol or petroleum jelly are not suitable as separating media as they become incorporated within the cement leading to damage to the material.

Incremental packing helps push the material under pressure into the undercuts. The use of matrix strips and other matrices (Figure 9.29) has been advocated to aid placement by applying pressure to the material until it has set. Furthermore, the surface smoothness of the material placed in this way is much improved.

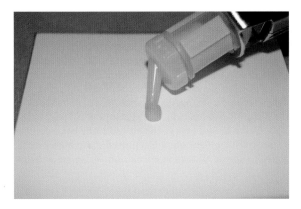

Fig. 9.27 Mixed glass ionomer cement being expressed from a capsule (Chemfil Superior, Dentsply). Note the wide bore of the nozzle.

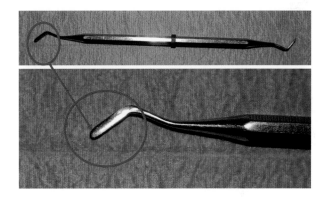

Fig. 9.28 A flat plastic instrument may be used to place glass ionomer cements.

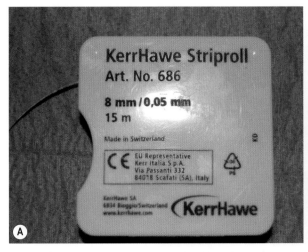

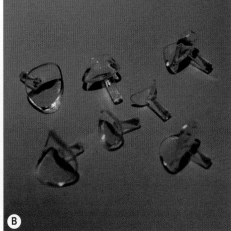

Fig. 9.29 (A) Matrix strips and (B) cervical matrices used to place glass ionomer cements.

When placing a Class V restoration a cervical matrix should be used. A matrix of the appropriate size and shape is selected and held using a pair of locking tweezers (Figure 9.30). The matrix is placed on the bracket table so that when the cement is ready to be placed into the cavity, the cervical matrix can be easily applied to it. The clinician must then hold the tweezers undisturbed against the tooth surface and cement until the material has fully set.

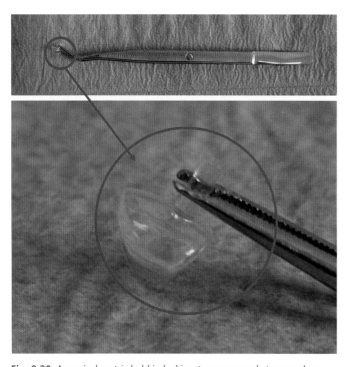

Fig. 9.30 A cervical matrix held in locking tweezers ready to use when placing a Class V glass ionomer cement restoration.

Gross excess should be removed initially with a flat plastic or an explorer (dental probe) before the setting has commenced. Any further excess should be left until the material has set, which can be confirmed by leaving a small increment of the mixed material on the mixing slab. Once this material has set, the material within the oral cavity will also have set as the intraoral temperature is higher. (The rate of reaction is faster at higher temperatures.) At this time any excess material may be fractured away using a sharp instrument (e.g. Ward's carver or a scalpel blade).

> **!**
>
> Always wait until the glass ionomer luting cement will break cleanly before removing the excess at the margins of a crown. If removed in its rubbery state, fragments of the cement under the cast can be lost causing leakage because the seal is broken between tooth tissue and cement. This is also true for a glass ionomer restoration so ensure that the material has set before tampering with it.

Finishing

A further consequence of the slow maturation phase of glass ionomer cements is that premature finishing can cause considerable damage to the forming cement matrix. Under no circumstances should finishing commence before the manufacturer's recommended time. This can be up to 6 minutes after placement of the restoration. Most of the currently available cements require at least a 3-minute wait before finishing. Failure to follow these recommendations will lead to damage to the surface of the restoration (Figure 9.31).

In fact, many regard the finishing of glass ionomer cements as a damage limitation exercise as whatever method of finishing is used, the surface produced is inferior to that achieved against a matrix strip. It is also possible to desiccate the restoration during the finishing process. Studies investigating the most effective method of finishing have shown the use of a finishing instrument under a fine water spray will do the least damage. Use of lubricants such as petroleum jelly on the finishing instrument has proved to be highly detrimental as the petroleum jelly allows the restoration to heat up and desiccate.

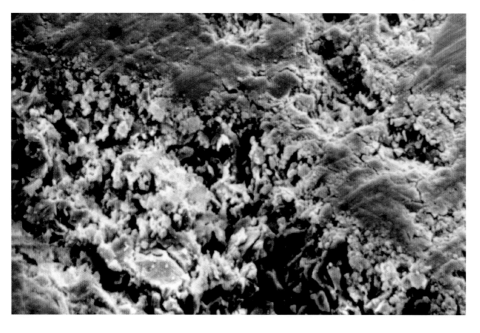

Fig. 9.31 The surface of a glass ionomer cement that was damaged during setting. The finishing has been carried out prematurely with a white abrasive stone and the rotation of the instrument has dragged the surface of the cement and created the fissure.

Ideally finish glass ionomer cements at least 24 hours after placement. Consider scheduling placing these restorations earlier in the treatment plan so they can be polished at a subsequent visit. This is not only more convenient for the patient but also more time efficient rather than making a dedicated appointment for this purpose.

Protection from water contamination

During the initial phases of the setting reaction the cement is susceptible to changes in moisture concentration. Any contamination with saliva at an early stage can disrupt the matrix and damage the surface of the restoration and so protection from water contamination is essential for at least an hour after placement. An additional disadvantage of early contamination with water is that the ultimate mechanical properties may be substantially reduced. The effect of this contamination may be minimized by protecting the outer surface of the restoration with some form of water barrier. A range of products (Table 9.7 and Figure 9.32) can be used to protect the restoration for periods of up to 24 hours after placement. This period is usually sufficient to achieve the optimum performance for these materials. Light-cured fissure sealant may be used but usually residual uncured resin remains on the surface due to oxygen inhibition of the curing process. Figure 9.33 illustrates the effect of flexural strength on glass ionomer cements after being protected using various proprietary varnishes.

Table 9.7 Materials used to protect a glass ionomer cement's surface during setting

Petroleum jelly	Vaseline (Lever Faberge)
Copal ether varnish	Copalite varnish (Cooley and Cooley)
Acetate varnish	Fuji varnish (GC)
Resins	Easy Glaze (Voco), Final varnish LC (Voco), Fuji Coat LC (GC), G Coat Plus (GC), Hi Glaze (Shofu), Ketac Glaze (3M ESPE), Riva Coat (SDI)

It is strongly advised to protect the setting surface of glass ionomer cement, and also crown margins when a glass ionomer luting cement has been employed, by using a material for such a purpose.

Protection against desiccation

A further consideration relating to the later protection of these types of materials is that they should not be allowed to **desiccate**. Under normal conditions in the mouth this will not occur but on occasions where the area is isolated for further work on other teeth, the restoration can become desiccated, causing cracking and crazing which can be extensive. This occurs rapidly and although rehydration occurs, the cracks never 'heal' and often pass down into the bulk of the material. The effect of this crack propagation is potential bulk fracture of the material leading to failure (Figure 9.34).

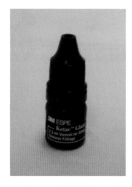

Fig. 9.32 A varnish (Ketac Glaze, 3M ESPE) used to protect glass ionomer cement post placement.

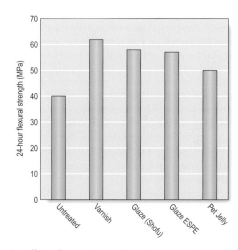

Fig. 9.33 The effect of protection with various proprietary varnishes on the 24-hour flexural strength (MPa) of glass ionomer cements.

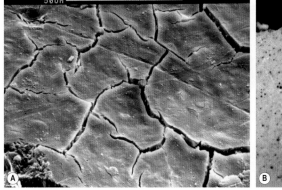
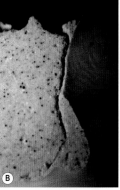

Fig. 9.34 Photomicrographs showing (A) cracking of the surface of a glass ionomer cement after being allowed to desiccate and (B) a crack generated within a restoration after desiccation. Note that the fracture is within the material while the bond to the tooth tissue remains intact.

> ⚠
>
> When carrying out restorative treatment on a tooth adjacent to one restored with glass ionomer cement, the restoration should be protected with either a varnish or petroleum jelly to prevent desiccation.

CERMETS, ADMIXES AND RECENT ADVANCES

One type of glass ionomer cements are those in which metals have been incorporated or alloys have been added to the glass powder. These fall into two groups:

- **Cermets**: here **silver** particles are sintered onto the surface of the glass. Other metals such as **gold** have been used, but these variants have never become commercially available
- **Admixes**: here amalgam alloy is added as an additional filler to the powder.

The theoretical benefits of these modifications are considered to be enhancement of the mechanical properties and improvement in the finishing of these materials as the use of metal would allow burnishing of the restoration. However, these materials have never been used with great frequency as they are not tooth coloured but rather silver or grey in appearance. Furthermore, mechanically they are generally no stronger than the conventional glass ionomer cements. One group of admixed materials has shown some promise: addition of 18–20% alloy to the glass powder led to an increase in the mechanical properties of about 30%.

There is some variation in the other properties depending on material type. The cermets show reduced fluoride release, primarily because there are fewer sites for release as the silver particles are attached to the glass. In the admixed materials, some interaction with the oxide layer on the alloy particles and the polyacid takes place and there is some binding of the alloy into the cement. Interestingly, these materials release slighter greater amounts of fluoride than conventional glass ionomer cements (Figure 9.35).

Microscopic examination of the surface shows that the admixed materials have three phases where as the cermets have only two (Figure 9.36).

More recently other manufacturers have modified the fillers either by the addition of inert materials or already-set glass ionomer cement which has been reground to size. Other modifications have included ceramics and polysiloxane fillers. To date none of these materials has shown any significant advantage over the conventional materials.

Indications

Due to their grey colour, the primary application of these materials is core build-up in the posterior part of the mouth. Other indications are:

- Class V cavities
- Core construction
- Dressings
- Open sandwich (laminate)
- Repairs to restorations
- Restoration of deciduous teeth
- Semi-permanent restorations.

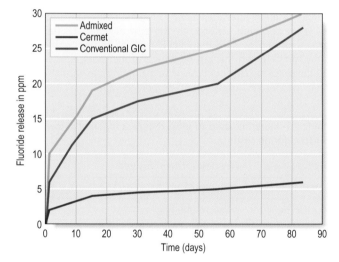

Fig. 9.35 The fluoride release with respect to time shows that the greatest release comes from the admixed material, which exceeds the conventional materials during the initial stage of release. The cermet shows a much smaller release at a much slower rate.

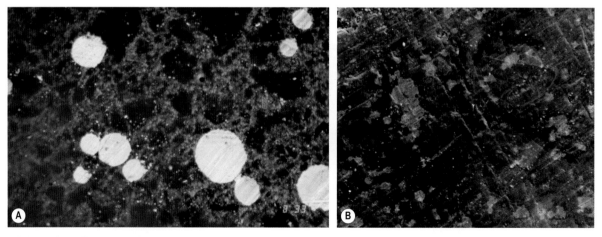

Fig. 9.36 (A) The surface of an admixed glass ionomer cement. Note the three phases: black = glass; white alloy; green = matrix. (B) The surface of a cermet: light grey = silver-coated glass; dark grey = matrix.

Commercially available products

Cermet and admixed materials have failed to live up clinically to the theoretical benefits. While some products are available on the market (Table 9.8) these materials are now used relatively infrequently.

Table 9.8 Some modified glass ionomer cements currently available on the market

Product	Manufacturer	Class
Amalgomer	Advanced Healthcare	Admix
Hi-Dense	Shofu	Admix
Ketac-Silver	3M ESPE	Cermet
Legend Silver	SS White	Admix
Miracle Mix	GC	Admix
Riva Silver	SDI	Admix
Voco Silver	Voco	Admix

SUMMARY

- Glass ionomer cements contain glass and acid and set by an acid–base reaction to a salt plus water.
- Their mechanical properties are inferior to resin composite but they release fluoride ions and bond to tooth tissue without the use of an intervening resin.
- Glass ionomer cements require protection from both moisture contamination and desiccation after placement.
- Addition of metals or alloys has provided increased mechanical properties but at the expense of aesthetics.

FURTHER READING

Frencken, J., van Amerongen, E., Phantumvanit, P., Songpaisan, Y., Pilot, T., Manual for the Atraumatic Restorative Treatment Approach to Control Dental Caries. Available at: <http://www.dentaid.org/data/dentaid/downloads/ART_Manual_English.pdf>

van Noort, R., 2007. Introduction to Dental Materials, third ed. Mosby Elsevier, Edinburgh. (See Chapter 2.3)

Wilson, A.D., McLean, J.W., 1988. Glass-ionomer cements. ART manual. Quintessence, Chicago. Available at: <www.art.com>

SELF-ASSESSMENT QUESTIONS

1. What are the advantages and disadvantages of a glass ionomer cement?
2. Why is it deleterious to finish glass ionomer cement restorations at the placement visit?
3. Summarize the indications for use of glass ionomer cements.
4. What is the difference between the adhesion of glass ionomer cement to tooth tissue and that of a resin-based composite?
5. What are the similarities and differences between encapsulated and powder/liquid presentations of glass ionomer cements with respect to mixing?
6. What are the similarities and differences between glass ionomer cements and compomers?

Chapter 10

The tooth-coloured restorative materials IV: Resin-modified glass ionomer cements

INTRODUCTION AND HISTORY OF DEVELOPMENT

Resin-modified glass ionomer cements (RMGICs) were developed in an attempt to address the perceived limitations of the conventional glass ionomer cements and to utilize the advantages of resin composite materials (Table 10.1). In other words, RMGICs aim to maintain the benefits of fluoride ion release and adhesion of glass ionomer cements while overcoming their disadvantages with the more favourable attributes of resin-based composites.

COMPONENTS OF A RESIN-MODIFIED GLASS IONOMER

Essentially RMGICs are conventional glass ionomer cements containing glass, polyacid, tartaric acid and water, with the addition of a water-soluble resin and modified poly(acrylic acids) (Figure 10.1). These modified polyacrylic acids have **pendant methacrylate groups** or **methacryloxy groups** grafted onto the polyacid chain and are called **copolymers**. Chemicals that allow light activation are also incorporated. These materials may therefore be regarded as **hybrid glass ionomers**. They behave

Table 10.1 Advantages of resin-based composites and disadvantages of glass ionomer cements in relation to the development of resin-modified glass ionomers

Advantages of resin-based composites	Disadvantages of glass ionomer cements
Command set by visible light	Low early strength
Better wear resistance	Susceptibility to erosion
Lower solubility	Slow setting phase
Early high compressive and flexural strength	Risk of desiccation
Good polishability	
Ability to retain its polish	

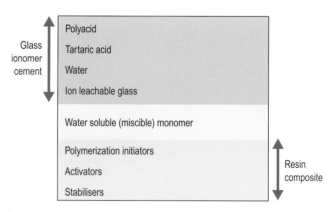

Fig. 10.1 Generic composition of RMGICs. The upper (mauve) constituents are found in a conventional glass ionomer cement while the lower (blue) components are from conventional resin composites. The middle constituent (yellow) is the resin that will bind all these together.

primarily as glass ionomer cements as only a small amount of resin has been added, which is usually **hydroxyethylmethacrylate (HEMA)**.

What is HEMA?

HEMA is the monomer that is used to make the polymer **polyhydroxyethylmethacrylate (polyHEMA)**. In the monomeric form HEMA is a small, highly reactive molecule. The polymer is **hydrophilic** and so once it is exposed to water it will swell. Depending on the physical and chemical structure of the polymer, it will absorb between 10% and 600% of its own dry weight of water. This property has been utilized successfully in the manufacture of flexible contact lenses. HEMA's hydrophilic properties mean that it has become a common constituent in a range of dental materials including RMGICs and adhesive resin systems. It is one of the few resins which is miscible with water.

Biocompatibility of HEMA

The HEMA monomer is **cytotoxic** and so care should be taken in the application of the unset material to any soft tissue. The

cytotoxicity is minimal after polymerization, however, if the level of conversion is low then unconverted monomer can leach out as polyHEMA, which will absorb water very quickly. HEMA is known to cause chemical dermatitis (Figure 10.2) if it comes into contact with skin or mucous membrane.

Any dental materials containing HEMA should be handled with extreme care because of its potentially adverse dermatological effects. Unfortunately, surgical gloves are porous and HEMA is known to penetrate through the glove to reach the skin. For this reason, the dental team should avoid touching any HEMA-containing products when mixing and placing these materials.

Furthermore if the polymer degrades, the resulting release of freed monomer into the surrounding dental hard and surrounding tissues may potentially have toxicological effects on the dental pulp and osteoblasts (see Chapter 3).

Even in its polymerized form bound in the RMGIC, if HEMA is placed directly onto vital dental pulpal tissue it may cause the death of the pulpal tissue. For this reason the use of RMGICs in direct contact with the pulp is contraindicated. In a very deep cavity, microexposures may be present and not obvious to the dentist. If there is any doubt, consider the use of another lining material such as a setting calcium hydroxide cement placed on the pulpal floor as a **sublining**. A layer of RMGIC may then be placed over the set calcium hydroxide cement and the surrounding dentine. This will seal the dentinal tubules opened during cavity preparation and decrease the risk of microleakage (Figure 10.3).

There should always be an adequate thickness of dentine present (at least 0.2–0.5 mm) between the base of the cavity and the pulp when placing an RMGIC lining. This is due to:
- HEMA's cytotoxicity to vital pulp tissue
- The excessive heat released during curing, which may be detrimental to the pulp especially if the material is used in bulk.

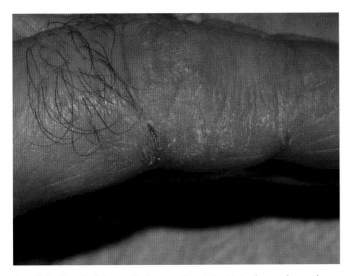

Fig. 10.2 Chemical dermatitis in an active state. Note the cracks on the skin and the erythema (redness).

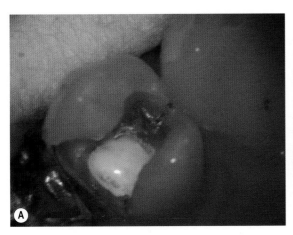
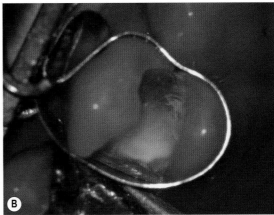

Fig. 10.3 (A) Sublining of setting calcium hydroxide cement (Life, Kerr Hawe) placed over the pulpal floor of a deep cavity in tooth 24. (B) A RMGIC (Vitrebond Plus, 3M ESPE) has then been applied to cover the sublining and the rest of the pulpal floor to seal the dentinal tubules on the cavity floor.

Chemical constituents of RMGICs

The chemical constituents of RMGICs are shown in Table 10.2.

Table 10.2 Chemical components of a resin-modified glass ionomer cement		
Powder	**Liquid**	**Purpose for their inclusion**
Barium, strontium or aluminosilicate glass		Improved strength Imparts radiopacity
Vacuum-dried polyacrylic acid	Polyacrylic acid	Reacts with the glass to form the poly salt matrix
Potassium persulphate Ascorbic acid		Redox catalyst system to provide the methacrylate (dark) cure
Pigments		Varies shade
	HEMA	Water miscible resin
	Polyacrylic acid with pendant methacrylates (copolymer)	Ability to undergo both acid–base and polymerization reactions Helps form interpenetrating network
	Tartaric acid	Sharpens the acid–base reaction set
	Water	Permits reaction between the polyacid and the glass
	Photo-initiators	Achieves light curing

Effect of particle size

As with all cements, the particle size of the glass is related to the application. The finer glasses are used in the cements intended for luting. Particle size also affects the setting reaction. The smaller the particle, the faster the setting reaction as its surface area available for reaction is greater with respect to its volume. The size of the particles is therefore often a compromise to achieve set in a clinically acceptable time while leaving an adequate surface finish. Generally speaking, in RMGICs intended for use as restorative materials there is a progressive loss in translucency as the particle size is reduced.

SETTING REACTION

The polyacrylic acid reacts with the glass to form the poly salt matrix as for the conventional glass ionomer cement (see Chapter 9). This extended setting reaction means that the salt matrix is liable to damage for some time after placement if exposed to water. The addition of a water-miscible monomer to the material permits a polymerization reaction to take place during the initial stages of the setting of the material, which provides it with early strength as the secondary acid–base reaction between the glass and the polyacrylic acid goes to completion. In other words, the polymerized resin phase is designed to form a scaffolding while the ionomer cement matrix is

being formed. As the resin content is increased so the acid–base reaction is slowed. The effect of the resin addition is primarily seen during the initial stages of set when the glass ionomer cement is at its weakest. It is essential that the resin is soluble in water as the cement remains water based. In the absence of water, no reaction will occur between the polyacid and the glass. This restriction limits the number of resin systems which may be used in these materials as most are **hydrophobic**.

Thus two types of setting reaction take place within the material: an **acid–base** reaction and a **polymerization** reaction. The polymerization reaction is a free-radical methacrylate reaction effected by light activation. Unfortunately, light transmission through these materials is limited and in thicknesses greater than 0.5 mm the base of the material does not polymerize adequately. The methacrylates in the material essentially remain uncured in the absence of light. Therefore in materials designed for restoration or core build-up, it is essential to place the material in increments and light cure each layer in order to obtain a thoroughly cured material. With lining materials this is not a problem as only a thin layer of material is required.

To compensate for the limited light-cure polymerization reaction, a second **dark-cure** initiator system has been incorporated into some RMGIC products. This system aims to achieve adequate free-radical methacrylate polymerization within the deeper parts of the restoration where light cannot penetrate. This gives the dentist confidence that the material will reach a full cure. The disadvantage is that the end product is not as well cross-linked as in the areas where light activation is achieved and the mechanical properties of the material where dark curing has occurred are reduced by approximately 25–30%.

> The dentist should always ensure that light curing is effective over as much of cement surface as possible because the chemical dark cure is less effective and results in a material which has usually about 70% strength of the light-cured component.

Reliance on the redox reaction for the cure leads to a reduction in the level of conversion of the material and reduced mechanical properties. This is illustrated in Figure 10.4, which shows the difference in compressive strength of a RMGIC when light cured and when the redox setting reaction is relied on alone. The magnitude of shrinkage

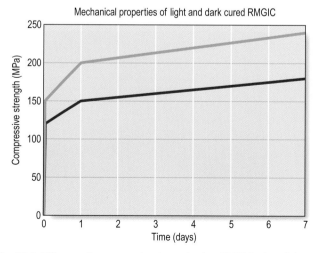

Fig. 10.4 Difference in compressive strength of an RMGIC when light cured (upper line) and when allowed to set by dark cure alone (lower line).

is in excess of the resin-based composites so considerable care must be taken to control the effect of the stresses which are generated. In thin sections, particularly when used as a liner, the margins of the cement layer may curl up away from the surface to be protected. As with the conventional acid–base cements, the acid–base reaction is not involved with the shrinkage. It will only contribute if there is desiccation of the material.

Dual- and tri-cure

The two types of setting reaction seen in RMGICs are referred to as:

- **Dual-cured**: acid-base reaction + light activation
- **Tri-cured**: acid-base reaction + light activation + dark redox.

Redox: stands for *reduction-oxidation* reaction. The term is used to describe all the chemical reactions in which the atoms have their oxidation state changed.

Stages of the RMGIC setting reaction

The setting reaction of RMGICs is complex as two or three chemical reactions are occurring concurrently depending on whether the product is a dual- or tri-cure material (Figure 10.5).

Dual-cured products

- *Acid–base reaction*: This commences at the start of mixing and often continues for a substantial time after all other setting reactions have been completed, which may be up to 6 hours from start of mixing. During this time, the matrix is susceptible to damage by extraneous water.
- *Light activation*: This takes place at the end of placement and is completed within 10 seconds of light activation. Little post curing occurs but the material in the path of the light will have formed a solid resin matrix at this point. Water uptake by the polymer will start from the saliva in the oral cavity at this time.

Stage	Chemical reaction	Clinical stage
1	Polyacrylic acid in one component is mixed with aqueous solution of HEMA in the other starting an acid base reaction	Commences when powder and liquid are mixed together
2	Methacrylate group on HEMA reacts with other HEMA molecules and with pendant methacrylate groups on side of polyacrylic acid chain	Light activation of polymerization reaction
3	Light polymerization reaction completed	Light activation stopped
4	Acid base reaction continues for some hours thereafter	Restoration finished and patient leaves surgery

Fig. 10.5 The sequence of the two setting reactions in a dual-cured resin modified glass ionomer cement. The boxes coloured mauve indicate the glass ionomer cement reaction, while those in blue indicate the resin polymerization reaction initiated by light.

Tri-cured products

Tri-cured products involve **dark-cure** activation at the commencement of mixing, which may be completed within about 4–6 minutes after start of mix (Figures 10.6 and 10.7).

Stage	Chemical reaction	Clinical stage
1a	Polyacrylic acid in one component is mixed with aqueous solution of HEMA in the other starting an acid base reaction	Commences when powder and liquid are mixed together
1b	Redox (dark cure) reaction commences	
2	Methacrylate group on HEMA reacts with other HEMA molecules and with pendant methacrylate groups on side of polyacrylic acid chain	Light activation of polymerization reaction
3	Light polymerization reaction completed	Light activation stopped
4	Redox (dark cure) reaction continues for a maximum of five minutes thereafter	Finish restoration
5	Acid base reaction continues for some hours thereafter	Finish restoration and patient leaves surgery

Fig. 10.6 The sequence of the three setting reactions in a tri-cure resin-modified glass ionomer cement. The boxes coloured mauve indicate the glass ionomer cement reaction, while those in blue indicate the resin polymerization reaction initiated by light. Boxes in grey indicate a redox polymerization reaction initiated chemically.

Setting phase	Dark cure reaction				
	Acid base reaction				
Clinical stage	Working time		Light curing	Maturation	
	Mixing	Clinical placement			
Time	45s	135s	40s	140s	→ 6 hours

Fig. 10.7 A working time-line illustrating the relationship of the various setting reactions to the clinical handling of a tri-cure RMGIC. A dual-cured product is identical but with the omission of the dark-cure reaction.

It is important that both the acid–base and the polymerization setting reactions are initiated at the same time. It would also be beneficial if they proceeded at the same rate as the material would be fully set at the same time. However, this is not normally achieved as the addition of the HEMA adversely affects the acid–base reaction, retarding its setting rate. The reaction, therefore, continues for sometime after the material appears to be hard clinically. The effect of this is that ions from this acid–base reaction can potentially wash out from the restoration. In early variants of the cements, where no modifications were made to the polyacrylic acid, two different cement matrices could be produced with no continuity between them, which could lead to a catastrophic failure of the material. The additional grafting of the **methacryloxy groups** onto the polyacrylic acid chain permits cross-linking between these groups and HEMA, producing what has been described as an **interpenetrating network**. Even with further development of these materials, there is still a difference in the rate of setting of the two phases.

To protect or not to protect from water?

There is a divergence of views as to the need for protection of RMGICs from water after placement as required by the glass ionomer cements. However, to ensure the optimum outcome, they should be protected for some time, until the acid–base reaction is complete. Poly-HEMA, although providing some protection, absorbs water very quickly and this can affect the salt matrix formation that is taking place.

CONSEQUENCES OF SETTING REACTION ON THE MATERIAL'S SHORT TERM PROPERTIES

Polymerization shrinkage

The inclusion of the resin phase immediately brings with it the problem of **polymerization shrinkage**, which is greater than that in resin-based composites. The measured shrinkage is more akin to an unfilled acrylic resin, being in the region of 3–4%. This shrinkage can lead to loss of adhesion as stresses at the interface between the tooth and the restorative are generated with the onset of the light-activated polymerization reaction.

Exothermic setting reaction

When HEMA polymerizes, there is a marked exothermic reaction (Figure 10.8). The temperature rise is dependent on the bulk of material present, but temperature rises of up to 12°C have been recorded. These values are more common in the lining materials, one of the most important uses for this family of materials. This is an obvious disadvantage in very deep cavities where little dentine is available between the material and the pulp so the effects of heat generated will be more significant.

Adhesion: to tooth tissue

The mechanism for bonding to tooth tissue of RMGICs is essentially the same as that for the glass ionomer cements, namely calcium chelation and subsidiary collagen bonding (see Chapter 9). However, various factors limit the success of the adhesive bond:

- There is a limited acid–base reaction as less acid is present. Carboxyl groups are needed for adhesion and they may not be readily available at the tooth–restoration interface.
- Since the shrinkage of the resin phase will stress the interface between the cement and the tooth, there is frequently a risk of pulling away from the tooth surface just at the time any bonding may be taking place.
- There may be some micromechanical interlocking between the tooth and the restorative but this again is likely to be disturbed during the polymerization process.
- With time, the water uptake may allow readaptation of the cement to the tooth but fewer carboxyl groups will be available because by the time the water becomes available, these will be bound within the resin structure. The likelihood of repair to the bond is reduced.

The bond strengths quoted for the materials are similar or slightly better than those for conventional glass ionomer cements in the absence of any additional intervening adhesive system.

Adhesion: to other materials

As illustrated earlier, RMGICs are commonly used over a sublining of calcium hydroxide. There is no interaction or bonding between these two materials. It is therefore important that the RMGIC layer is extended beyond the extent of the calcium hydroxide cement to gain adhesion to the surrounding dentine and to form a seal.

The surface of RMGICs when used as a lining material is rough. Micromechanical retention will therefore be likely between the RMGIC lining material and the material placed over it. Additionally, as RMGICs contain HEMA, bonding can potentially occur chemically with other resin-containing materials. A cross-linking reaction will occur provided that there are reactive groups available at the time of

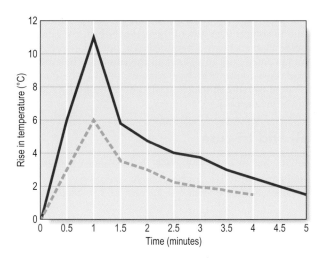

Fig. 10.8 Temperature rise within a resin-modified glass ionomer cement. The continuous line represents the temperature rise associated with the dark-cure exothermic and light-cure reactions combined. The dashed line represents the temperature rise associated with light curing alone.

placement. As such the material can be used as a part of the sandwich technique (see Chapter 9).

When RMGICs are used for luting, they will form chemical bonds with the dental tissue of the tooth preparation but not to the cast restoration being cemented. For this reason, this is another example of grouting.

If the RMGIC lining material is inadvertently etched during cavity preparation prior to the placement of a resin-based composite material, there will be no deleterious effects on the material.

Phase separation

The affinity of polyHEMA for water can have other problems particularly if the material has not been mixed correctly and a higher proportion of monomeric material is included in the mix. Figure 10.9 shows the result of an early RMGIC being incorrectly mixed. The liquid phase had separated and almost all the liquid was HEMA. The

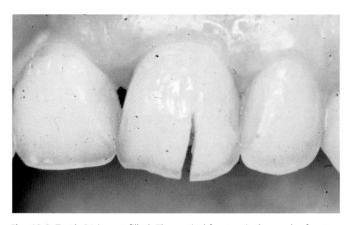

Fig. 10.9 Tooth 21 is root filled. The vertical fracture is the result of water uptake by the restoration containing excess polyHEMA due to failure to shake the liquid bottle.

material was mixed and placed in an access cavity of a root canal. During the subsequent 48-hour period the restoration absorbed a substantial amount of water and expanded. The result was a vertical fracture of the tooth.

LONG-TERM PROPERTIES

Mechanical properties

The addition of the polymerized resin component has an immediate effect on the mechanical properties with the result that these are improved substantially initially. However, as discussed in the previous section, as polyHEMA absorbs water, the mechanical properties begin to fall, the extent of which is related to the HEMA concentration. This means that the restoration is at its strongest immediately after placement and partly why these materials are more popular as lining materials since these do not come in contact with saliva and the amount of water sorption which occurs will therefore be minimized.

Fluoride release

These materials provide a sustained release of fluoride, which occurs in the same way as with conventional glass ionomer cements. The majority of the release occurs in the early life of the cement, usually during the first 10–15 days, which is slightly higher than that observed for conventional glass ionomer cements. Thus longer-term release with RMGICs is slightly greater, which may be due to the slower setting of the glass ionomer phase of the cement. It may also be because the polyHEMA matrix could provide an easier pathway for the ionic species to migrate through the cement. The clinical significance of this is that the initial external fluoride concentration is increased. However, this may be at the expense of the restoration as it starts to degrade. Fluoride release is also much reduced in linings so its benefits may outweigh the risks associated with the slow degradation (Figure 10.10).

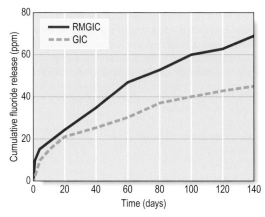

Fig. 10.10 Fluoride release (parts per million) with respect to time from a resin-modified glass ionomer cement and a conventional glass ionomer cement. The former releases more fluoride than the conventional cement.

Staining

There is some evidence of staining of the RMGIC restoration with time. This is almost certainly due to the uptake of oral fluids which occurs during the time the restoration is in the mouth and causes intrinsic staining which cannot be removed by polishing or removing the surface layers of the material. This problem is also seen with compomers. The degree of staining which occurs varies with individual materials but both categories of material can stain significantly.

EFFECT OF INADEQUATE CURING

For the material to reach its optimal properties it must be fully light cured. The dentist should therefore be aware of the depth of cure when placing and curing the material. Where this is not possible, it is essential that a tri-cure system is selected to ensure complete set of the restoration.

Biological considerations

The failure to completely cure RMGICs means that any unconverted monomer can easily leach out from the filling. The adverse reactions reported above with the HEMA monomer means that there is a potential risk of damage to pulpal tissue where material will be in contact. However, the better the polymerization the greater the exothermic reaction so that again the pulp can be at risk if minimal dentine separates the restoration from the pulp. Care should be exercised in the selection of cases for use of these materials.

ADVANTAGES AND DISADVANTAGES OF RMGICS

The advantages and disadvantages of RMGICs are shown in Table 10.3.

Table 10.3 Advantages and disadvantages of resin-modified glass ionomer cements

Advantages	Disadvantages
Fluoride ion release	Exothermic reaction on curing
Early strength	Shrinkage on curing
Adhesion – molecular bonding	Incomplete cure produces weak material
Long working time	Monomer leach
Limited moisture sensitivity	Swelling due to moisture uptake
Low solubility or erosion of cement margins	Phase separation
Simple to use	Moisture-sensitive powder
Command set	Effect of command set in reducing the rate of acid–base reaction
Can be finished immediately after light curing	Release of benzoyl iodides and benzoyl bromides which can be cytotoxic
Seals dentinal tubules	Where redox setting of the resin phase is used, material will be weaker
Release of benzoyl iodides and benzoyl bromides see pp. 131	

INDICATIONS AND CONTRAINDICATIONS

RMGICs are versatile materials that can be used in many different clinical conditions (Table 10.4). The differences in handling between these chemically similar products is due to the amount and type of resin incorporated into them and the curing mechanisms employed.

Table 10.4 Indications and contraindications of resin-modified glass ionomer cements	
Indications	**Contraindications**
Restoration of small Class I cavities	Restoration of anything larger than a small Class I cavity
Restoration of Class III and V cavities	Restoration of Class III and V cavities where aesthetics are of paramount importance
Core build-ups when a substantial amount of tooth tissue remains	Core build-ups when more than 50% tooth tissue is missing
Sandwich (open and closed)	Luting of (unreinforced) all ceramic crowns
Dressings	Direct placement on vital pulp tissue
Definitive cementation (luting) of cast metal restorations, metal bonded to ceramic restorations, strengthened core ceramic restorations, metal posts, orthodontic bands	Direct placement on periradicular tissue
Restoration of deciduous teeth	
Lining of cavities	
Blocking out undercuts for indirect restorations	
Used (in its uncured state) to bond dental amalgam	

Restoration of small Class I, Class III and V cavities

RMGICs may be used as a restorative material. However, the material has only sufficient strength to withstand forces in small-sized Class I cavities. Under no circumstances should the material be used as a replacement for the wall of a tooth. RMGICs have been used with success for restoring non-carious tooth surface loss lesions such as abfraction lesions. This is because their matrix has some flexibility and so the material may be retained in the cavity during function where the tooth surrounding it may be flexing (see Chapter 7,8 and 9).

When the material is intended for use in the aesthetic zone, a few products are available in a number of shades.

Core build-ups

The material can be used effectively when a substantial amount of tooth tissue remains to construct the core prior to the placement of a crown or bridge, in both root-filled and vital teeth. It is important to note that if more than 50% of the tooth tissue has been lost then the use of this material is contraindicated as it is not strong enough to withstand the forces applied to the tooth.

To assist in the identification of the restorative against tooth tissue, one product (Vitremer, 3M ESPE) has a blue colouring agent. This facilitates the placement of a finishing line for any preparation below the core margin and follows the same principles as with amalgam cores (see Figure 6.2, p. 57).

With regards to temporary restorations, any preparation constructed using a RMGIC core material should be kept moist to prevent against bonding of the chemically cured temporary material to the core.

Sandwich (open and closed)

RMGICs have been used in the laminate (sandwich) technique where the resin-modified glass ionomer material lies under another restorative material such as resin-based composite (Chapter 9).

Dressings

These materials work well as short-term dressings to protect the pulp and restore form and function to the tooth. They can be used in cavities which lack suitable retention as they rely on adhesive bonding but the clinician must bear in mind the limitation of this.

RMGICs may be selected particularly if resin-based composite is envisaged to be used as the definitive restorative material, as there is no eugenol in the material to react with the resin-based composite (see Chapters 7 and 12). Many clinicians select them as an alternative to traditional glass ionomer cements because the ability to command set the resin phase is regarded as saving time. Whether this is justified is not clear clinically as there is potential of inadequate seal. Since the RMGICs bond to tooth tissue they may occlude the dentinal tubules and potentially decrease sensitivity.

Definitive cementation (luting)

RMGICs have been used successfully for some years to definitively lute cast metal, metal bonded to ceramic and strengthened core ceramic restorations to tooth tissue as well as metal posts and orthodontic bands. The advantages of this material for this purpose are:

- Adequate strength
- Sustained fluoride release
- Relatively good biocompatibility once set
- Limited susceptibility to dissolution
- Good retention
- Good marginal seal
- Reduced postoperative sensitivity.

Some products are supplied in an extended working time (EWT) version, which has a longer working and setting time. This is indicated when the clinician is luting more than three units at the same time. While the EWT is a benefit, the commensurate extension in setting time may be a problem as the restoration will need to be supported until the cement is fully set.

As mentioned earlier, the continued uptake of water in the mouth can lead to an expansion in the order of 3%, which can have a significant clinical impact. If the RMGIC has been used to lute an all-ceramic crown, when the cement expands pressure will be transmitted to the ceramic with the potential for fracture of the crown. Therefore use of this material to lute (unreinforced) ceramic crowns is contraindicated.

RMGICs should not be used to lute unreinforced all-ceramic crowns as water uptake expands the luting cement that can cause the crown to fracture.

The first products to be marketed were supplied in a powder/liquid formulation. More recently, some manufacturers have moved onto a paste/paste presentation for ease of mixing. Unfortunately for the end user, the latter version is more expensive.

Restoration of deciduous teeth

The RMGICs are used for the restoration of deciduous teeth because:

- The command set reduces the procedure time, which is advantageous for both the child patient and the dentist.
- The material bonds to tooth tissue so minimally invasive, unretentive cavities may be prepared, thus conserving tooth tissue.
- The material leaches fluoride with its attendant anti-caries benefits.

Lining

One of the main uses of RMGICs is as a lining material prior to the placement of the intracoronal restoration. These materials have the following properties:

- They seal the dentinal tubules so decreasing microleakage and reducing postoperative sensitivity.
- During the polymerization reaction, chemical breakdown products, **benzoyl iodides** and **benzoyl bromides** are released from the material. These chemicals are cytotoxic and are effective against residual cavity bacteria.
- Fluoride is released from the material and has antibacterial and anti-caries effects.
- Its radiopacity is comparable with that of dentine (Figure 10.11).

- The powder/liquid ratio can be varied by the dentist to accommodate their preferred handling without detriment to the properties of the material. Of course, as with other cements, increasing the powder will increase the strength of the material and decrease its retention to tooth tissue. Less powder will have the opposite effect.

It should be emphasized that these materials are contraindicated for direct placement on both pulpal and periradicular vital tissue. They should not therefore be used as a direct pulp capping material or to repair a root perforation.

Blocking out undercuts for indirect restorations

These materials are indicated for this application as they:

- Are light cured, permitting the clinician to continue the procedure even before the chemical phase of the setting reaction has gone to completion
- Have favourable handling properties and can be placed precisely where required
- Bond to tooth tissue.

Bonding dental amalgam

RMGICs have been advocated to be used as an intermediate bonding agent to bond dental amalgam into cavities. The potential advantages of the technique are discussed on p. 61. The important difference is that the material must be used in its **uncured state**.

COMMERCIALLY AVAILABLE PRODUCTS

The commercially available products are set out in Table 10.5.

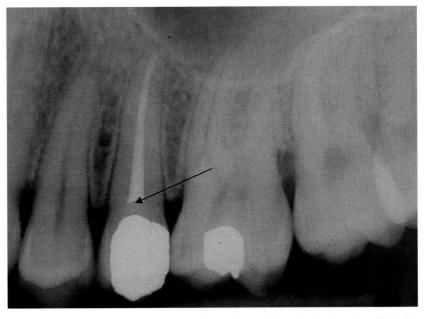

Fig. 10.11 A RMGIC (Vitrebond, 3M ESPE; arrow) covering the gutta percha and floor of the pulp chamber in tooth 25. Note its radiodensity is similar to that of the dentine of the tooth.

Table 10.5 Some resin-modified glass ionomer materials currently available on the market

Product name	Manufacturer	Type of reaction (dual-/tri-cure)	Indications for use										
			Small Class I	Class III	Class V	Core Build ups	Sandwich technique	Dressings	Luting	Restoration of deciduous teeth	Lining	Blocking out undercuts for indirect restorations	As a bonding agent for dental amalgam
Fuji II LC	GC	Tri	×	×	×	×	×	√	×	×	√	√	√
Fuji II LC Improved	GC	Tri	×	×	×	×	×	√	×	×	√	√	√
Fuji Ortho LC	GC	Tri	×	×	×	×	×	×	√	×	×	×	×
Fuji Plus	GC	Tri	×	×	×	×	×	×	√	×	×	×	×
Fuji Plus EWT	GC	Tri	×	×	×	×	×	×	√	×	×	×	×
FujiCEM	GC	Dual	×	×	×	×	×	×	√	×	×	×	×
Ketac Cem Plus	3M ESPE	Dual	×	×	×	×	×	×	√	×	×	×	×
Ketac N100	3M ESPE	Dual	√	√	√	√	√	√	×	√	×	×	×
Photac-Fil Quick	3M ESPE	Tri	√	√	√	√	√	√	×	√	×	√	×
Multi-Cure Glass Ionomer Orthodontic Band Cement	3M Unitek	Tri	×	×	×	×	×	×	√	×	×	×	×
Vitrebond Plus	3M ESPE	Dual	×	×	×	×	×	×	×	×	√	√	√
Vitremer	3M ESPE	Tri	×	√	√	√	√	√	×	√	×	√	×

PRESENTATIONS OF RESIN-MODIFIED GLASS IONOMER CEMENTS

RMGICs are marketed in three forms:

- Powder/liquid
- Encapsulated
- Paste/paste systems.

The powder and liquid presentation is initially mixed by the dental nurse. The mixed mass is then loaded into the delivery system which is supplied with the product (Figure 10.12). This facilitates the placement of the material directly into the cavity as its consistency can be difficult to manipulate. It also minimizes the inclusion of air bubbles and voids. However, the delivery system has been criticized for being fiddly and cumbersome as it can be difficult to load the material into the syringe.

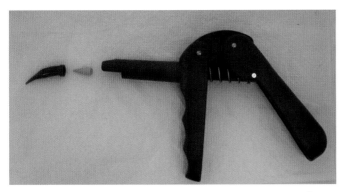

Fig. 10.12 The delivery system used with a resin-modified glass ionomer cement. The two component parts are dispensed onto the mixing pad and mixed. The mixed mass is then loaded into the syringe and the plunger placed. The loaded compule is then placed into a compule gun and the material is placed directly into the cavity.

The phases in the paste/paste presentations may become separated during storage leading to a non-uniform mix. They should be used at room temperature.

Other RMGICs are supplied in the encapsulated form (Figure 10.13) and the material can be syringed directly into the cavity on completion of mixing in the mixing machine. More recently, paste/paste presentations have become available (Figure 10.14) for the advantages discussed in Chapter 1. Nanotechnology has been utilized and is claimed to enhance the polishability of the material together with its wear resistance. This product also uses the clicker delivery system previously mentioned.

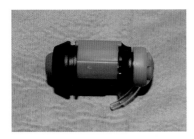

Fig. 10.13 An encapsulated resin-modified glass ionomer cement (Photac-Fil Quick, 3M EPSE).

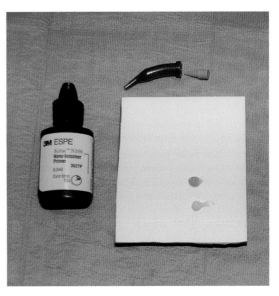

Fig. 10.14 A paste/paste resin-modified glass ionomer cement (Ketac N100, 3M ESPE).

Primers

Some products are supplied with primers. These are visible light-cured liquids which are composed of HEMA, ethanol, photo-initiators and a modified polyacrylic acid. These primers are acidic in nature and act by modifying the smear layer and wetting the tooth surface to allow adhesion of the RMGIC. They tend to be tinted yellow to facilitate visibility during placement and removal. The disadvantage of these materials is that they usually infiltrate the dentine and make alternative adhesive restorations less successful.

The primer supplied with this product should always be used to permit bonding to tooth tissue. The primer may also be used sparingly as a separator to prevent the material sticking to the instruments used to manipulate the product in the same way an unfilled resin may be used when manipulating resin-based composites.

Commercially available primers include:

- Fuji Dentine Conditioner (GC)
- Vitremer primer (3M ESPE)
- Nano-Ionomer primer (3M ESPE).

For more details about primers and bonding, see Chapter 11.

CLINICAL MANIPULATION

Cavity preparation

Cavity design should resemble that of glass ionomer cement. Prior to the placement of the material, the dentine should not be dehydrated.

The recommended technique for using the accompanying primer depends on the product so always consult the specific manufacturer's directions for use. Generally, primers are applied for 20–30 s using a brush and lightly air dried. This is critical as the ethanol must evaporate. The primer is then light cured for 20 seconds.

Moisture control

As with all dental restorative materials, good moisture control is very important to ensure maximal clinical performance. Moisture contamination prior to final curing will have deleterious effects on bonding, material properties and clinical longevity.

Mixing

Hand mixing requires care as some powder/liquid RMGIC presentations use **microcapsular technology**. The fine walls of the microcapsules need to be broken during mixing to allow their contents to escape and react with the liquid. This is the dark-cure redox catalyst system. The technology is similar to the 'scratch and sniff' advertisements in lifestyle magazines which allow readers to sample a perfume or aftershave. When a reader scratches the panel with their fingernail, it breaks open the microcapsules thus releasing the aroma (see Chapter 1).

When mixing materials based on microcapsular technology, spatulation must be carried out vigorously on the surface of the mixing slab so that the microcapsules are effectively broken down and all of their contents are released to react. The material often appears to be rather gravelly on mixing initially. Using a large-bladed spatula will assist in breaking down of the microcapsules as the flat blade can be pressed down onto the mixed material so crushing the capsules.

Initially this form of the material presented difficulties in encapsulated presentations as the shear stresses during machine mixing were insufficient to break down the glass microspheres. This problem appears to have now been minimized. However, care must be taken to ensure that the correct mixing time is used. Undermixing will result in the microspheres not being ruptured in total. Extension of the mixing time will substantially increase temperature as the mixing procedure generates heat. This in turn accelerates the chemical reaction and reduces the working time.

- With RMGICs it is essential that both the powder and liquid bottles are shaken prior to dispensation. The liquid is usually a combination of the polyacrylic acid and HEMA, and as the two liquids have different densities, separation can occur (see Fig. 10.9). Similarly the bottle containing the powder should be shaken to fluff up the powder which will ensure that the volume of powder dispensed is similar on each occasion, as previously discussed in relation to other cements.
- The powder or liquid should not be dispensed until immediately before mixing. They should be stored in their light-proof bottles as the material will react with visible light (including the operating light) so leading to premature curing.

Placement

The placement of this family of materials is similar to the placement of glass ionomer cements. The operator may choose to use the delivery system provided as previously discussed or to place the material into the cavity using a flat plastic.

Finishing

One of the advantages of a command set is that the material is set clinically and therefore after light curing initial finishing may be carried out. This is in contrast to conventional glass ionomer cements, where minimal finishing is carried out immediately after placement. Finishing of the RMGICs may be carried out by removing excess material (**flash**) using a sharp instrument. Alternatively, rotary instruments with water spray and either diamond or tungsten carbide finishing burs may be used. Final polishing can be done using aluminium oxide polishing discs or silicone polishers. However, it should be remembered that the acid–base setting phase is likely to be still in progress and so excessive finishing and polishing at the initial appointment should be avoided.

Finishing glosses are available with some products. These are light-cured, resin-based solutions that contain bis-GMA and tri(ethylene glycol) dimethacrylate (TEGDMA). Their use is optional but they provide a smoother surface by filling any surface irregularities. Their use is not recommended when the product is being used as a core build-up material as the oxygen inhibited surface may react with some of the currently available impression materials.

SUMMARY

- RMGICs have limited advantages over conventional glass ionomer cements.
- They can have adverse biological effects for the dental staff.
- They have improved fluoride release.
- Their initial mechanical properties are better than those of the glass ionomer cements.
- They may be used particularly for luting restorations.

FURTHER READING

McCabe, J.F., Walls, A.W.G., 2008. Applied Dental Materials, ninth ed. Blackwell, Munksgaard. (See Chapter 25)

Mount, G.J., Hume, W.R., 2005. Preservation and Restoration of Tooth Structure. Mosby, London. (See Chapter 8)

Powers, J.M., Sakaguchi, R.L. (Eds.), 2006. Craig's Restorative Dental Materials, twelfth ed. Mosby Elsevier, St Louis (p. 632).

van Noort, R., 2007. Introduction to Dental Materials, third ed. Mosby Elsevier, Edinburgh. (See Chapter 2.3)

SELF-ASSESSMENT QUESTIONS

1. Describe the importance of spatulating RMGICs well in terms of their setting reaction.
2. List the indications of RMGICs and the advantages and disadvantages for each application.
3. What are the similarities and differences between RMGICs and compomers?
4. What are the benefits of RMGICs compared with conventional glass ionomer cements?
5. Root caries is present distally in a lower permanent canine. There is an acrylic denture abutting the tooth and the lesion has cavitated. What materials could you use to restore this? What are the pros and cons of each material?
6. What materials could be used to definitively restore a non-carious tooth surface loss cervical lesion in an upper first premolar? What are the pros and cons of each material?
7. What problems occur with the inclusion of HEMA in compomers?

Chapter | **11** |

Bonding systems

LEARNING OBJECTIVES

From this chapter, the reader will:

- Understand the purpose of the bonding systems and the principles behind their use
- Understand the chemistry behind bonding systems
- Understand the properties of these materials and the significance of these on clinical manipulation and performance
- Understand their indications, contraindications and limitations
- Have an increased appreciation of how to use these materials to their best effect
- Know the names of currently available commercial products.

INTRODUCTION

Probably one of the most significant aspects of dental materials advancement in the past 50 years is the development of adhesives for dental applications. This has greatly increased the options open to the restorative dentist. The advantages of an adhesive approach are:

- Tooth tissue is preserved as restorations which may be bonded to the underlying tooth structure do not require the preparation of any mechanical retentive features
- The bonding process will enhance the retention of the restoration to tooth tissue
- The bonding process may seal the margins of the restoration with the tooth so reducing or eliminating bacterial penetration into the dentinal tubules (microleakage). This in turn decreases postoperative pulpal sensitivity and the potential for recurrent caries.
- Polymerization shrinkage (which occurs when using resin composite) may be reduced. This shrinkage leaves a marginal gap which may be accentuated during thermal cycling and may allow bacterial ingress.
- Bonding to tooth tissue may have a reinforcing effect on the weakened tooth structure.
- Many restorative materials which are bonded are tooth coloured so offering a more aesthetic option.

The obvious potential of dental bonding has led to the production of innumerable bonding agents and systems. This chapter explains the principles behind the bonding of restorative materials to dental hard tissue and attempts to simplify the confusion and complexities behind many of these systems.

PRINCIPLES OF ADHESION, BONDING AND SEALING IN DENTISTRY

What is meant by adhesion, bonding and sealing? In order to understand the processes, a clear understanding of what these terms mean is essential and a good knowledge of the structure of the substrate i.e. enamel and dentine, is also required. The reader is therefore advised to consult a dental anatomy textbook to review the structure of the dental hard tissues if required.

- **Adhesion:** is the force which binds two differing materials together when they are in intimate contact with one another.
- **Dental bonding:** is the process of attaching a resin composite-based material to the underlying tooth tissue using some form of intermediate material.
- **Sealing:** is the achievement of an impermeable barrier between the cavity wall and the restorative material to prevent the passage of bacteria.

The difference between bonding and sealing

The terms bonding and sealing are commonly used synonymously but they have distinct meanings. Although a material may appear to be 'stuck' to another material, every part of the two surfaces may not be in intimate contact with each other. This may be illustrated by considering a piece of sticky tape stuck to a bench (Figure 11.1). Although the tape is stuck to the table surface, small air bubbles and voids are present between the tape and the bench. The tape has therefore not sealed.

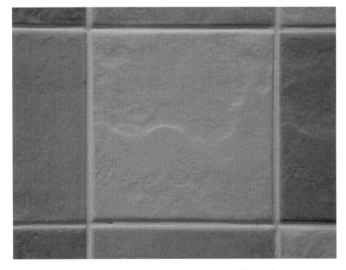

Fig. 11.1 A piece of sticky tape stuck to a bench. Although it has bonded to the table surface, there is no seal as demonstrated by the numerous air bubbles present between the tape and bench.

Bonding and luting

Further confusion arises when dentists discuss bonding and luting.

- **Luting:** is the filling up of the potential gap between a cast restoration and tooth, which is essentially a **grouting** effect. An everyday example is that of kitchen or bathroom tiles, where the grout (cement) is used to fill in the gaps between the tiles but not necessarily to bond them together (Figure 11.2).

There is therefore an important difference between luting and bonding. Luting materials may be divided into **conventional cements** and **luting composites**. The latter are more wear resistant, aesthetic and insoluble in oral fluids. However, it is a paradox that although they fill up the microgap between the tooth and cast restoration, they are usually bonded to the underlying tooth surface by means of an intermediate agent.

When luting a cast restoration, the cement should be applied sparingly to the axial surfaces of the restoration. Filling the retainer with cement may prevent its full seating, however. The aim is to fill up the potential gaps between the cast and tooth but not have much excess (Figure 11.3).

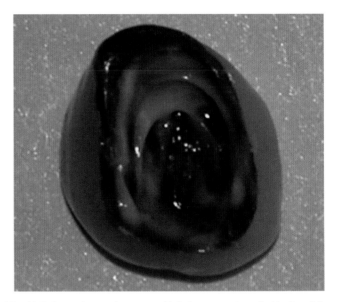

Fig. 11.3 A metal ceramic crown with luting cement applied to its axial walls just prior to placement on the prepared tooth.

Characteristics of dental bonding

In dentistry, two phenomena can occur in bonding. Firstly, it is a solid–liquid interface that is commonly encountered when bonding a dental material to tooth tissue. The intervening layer (adhesive) is generally applied as a liquid. The advantage of using a liquid is that the liquid will more readily **wet** the surfaces to be bonded to each other. This will achieve the intimate microscopic contact with the solid surfaces much more effectively than could be achieved with a solid on solid. Increased wetting results in better bonding. However, even with a liquid interface, there may be some limitations, as the **viscosity** of the liquid will limit the degree to which it wets the surface. This is the effect of surface tension (Figure 11.4).

Secondly, solid surfaces that need to be joined often have microscopic irregularities, giving the surface a rough texture. If both surfaces are uncontaminated, the irregularities on them may connect with one another. Depending on their respective roughness, the two surfaces will become intimately related. This means that any attempt to slide one against the other will be resisted by friction.

The aim with dental bonding is to use a combination of these two phenomena. The first surface, the tooth surface, is usually rough and an intervening layer of resin fills these micro- and macroscopic irregularities. The second surface is the restoration, which will be either a cast that may have a relatively rough fitting surface (perhaps achieved by sandblasting or etching) or a direct filling material. This material contains a filler that will provide microscopic irregularities on its surface (Figure 11.5).

Fig. 11.2 Kitchen ceramic tiles with grout between them. The grout serves no adhesive function for the tiles, it merely fills the gap between them. This analogy represents the intimate contact between a cast restoration and the tooth with the gap between them being filled by a cement.

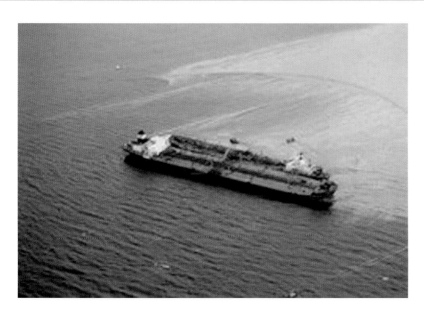

Surface tension: is the property of the surface of a liquid that allows the liquid to resist an external force. The higher the surface tension, the lower is the ability of bonding to it. Oil has high surface tension although the oil is heavier than the water (Figure 11.4). Conversely from a bonding perspective, the low surface tension of the intervening layer of water between two sheets of clean glass will hold them together with the glasses only being easily separated by sliding one away from the other. If the water was absent, the glasses would not stay together unless supported.

Adhesion in dentistry

Three types of adhesion are possible at the interface:

- Mechanical
- Physical
- Chemical.

Mechanical

Mechanical adhesion involves the interlocking of the roughened surface of two substrates, which leads to mechanical bonding. This is clearly illustrated in the bonding of resin to etched enamel. A liquid resin (bonding agent) will flow into the irregularities produced by the surface modification of the enamel. On polymerization, the resin solidifies and the two materials become mechanically bound together.

Physical

There can be a physical attraction between two surfaces that need to be bonded. This is usually achieved using molecules with different charges at ends of the molecule. These molecules are referred to as **dipolar**. This means that if there is an opposing charge on the other substrate, the molecule will be attracted to it. The substrates will orientate themselves so that the oppositely charged ends of the molecules are adjacent to each other. This type of bond is relatively weak and readily breaks down.

In dentistry, the bonding agent normally infiltrates the substrate. In most cases it does not dissolve into the substrate but will infiltrate any irregularities in the surface. This is how the majority of the dentine adhesives function. It is, however, essential that the surface of the substrate is wetted effectively to achieve this.

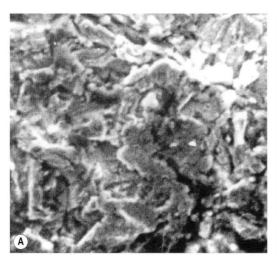 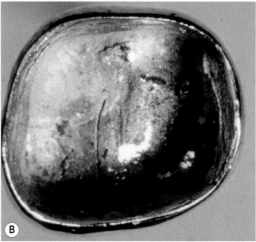

Fig. 11.5A,B (A) Micrograph of the internal surface of a metal casting which has been sandblasted and (B) the macroscopic view of the fit surface of a full gold crown. Both show micro- and macroscopic irregularities into which the bonding agent will flow, providing mechanical retention.

Chemical

It is possible that the structure of one of the substrates will result in its dissociation after application on to the surface of the other. This may result in different components bonding to the substrate. Glass ionomer cement attaches to enamel and dentine in this way. Failure of this type of adhesion occurs within one or the other of the substrates rather than at the interface.

Molecular entanglement

Adhesion is a complex phenomenon and one which is difficult to achieve. The bonding of materials to one another is more successfully achieved when an intervening adhesive layer is used. This is possible mainly when there is a large surface area of tooth or restoration to which to bond. However, it is doubtful whether there is complete attachment over all the surfaces being bonded, which reinforces the difference between bonding and sealing. Whether dental adhesives can achieve a complete seal is a topic of great debate among dental clinicians.

BONDING TO ENAMEL

The acid etch technique

Attempts to bond to tooth tissue date back to the 1920s but it was Buonocore in the 1950s who first reported the bonding of restorative materials to enamel using the **acid etch technique**. This technique has proved to be one of the most durable techniques in dentistry and defined one of the critical requirements of any bonding process: the need to prepare the substrate.

Substrate

The structure of the substrate plays a considerable part in the success of any adhesive process. Any adhesive system demands that:

- The surface should be clean, that is:
  - Free from debris and organic material
  - Dry
- The surface must have low surface energy
- It must have good wetting properties.

Any fluid with a low surface tension when applied will flow readily across the surface and adapt to its irregularities. In addition, when the fluid contains a chemical which will interact with the substrate surface then the bonding process will be enhanced.

Enamel as a substrate

Preparing enamel presents far fewer problems than preparing dentine due to its microscopic structure. Enamel is acellular, which means it is almost totally inorganic in nature (Figure 11.6). Enamel is generally prepared by using an acid to partly demineralize the crystalline structure. This part demineralization process results in preferential and differential removal of the crystallites so that the surface produced has micromechanical irregularities. These irregularities extend into the enamel structure, forming clefts and greatly increasing the surface area for contact by the bonding agent. The microscopic structure produced by etching enamel is shown in Figure 11.8 later in the chapter. The clefts usually penetrate between 20 and 30 μm and are found in the areas where the interprismatic material is present. The crystallites are partly removed. This effect is accentuated in freshly cut enamel and hence it

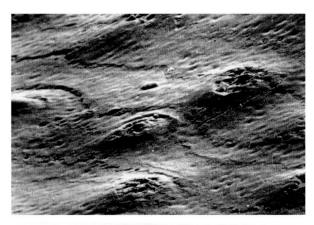

Fig. 11.6 Surface of human enamel showing its amorphous structure, which provides very limited means of retention for a restoration.

is frequently recommended that enamel is roughened using a bur prior to bonding. The bond formed by acid etching is **micromechanical** in nature. Etching enamel with an acid will therefore:

- Increase the surface area for bonding
- Increase the surface roughness
- Decrease the surface tension
- Increase wettability
- Increase the surface energy so the surface is more reactive so more receptive to bonding.

When etching enamel, the dentist needs to look out for a loss of sheen on the etched area, which takes on a frosted appearance (Figure 11.7).

The outer 5 μm of the enamel surface is amorphous and is less susceptible to etching, so the surface preparation of the enamel will ensure that the surface is clean. Pretreatment with a non-organic-based abrasive paste will remove organic smear. Furthermore, the effect of the acid will make the surface more receptive to the placement of a low-viscosity fluid. The nature of the structure of enamel means that it may also be dried sufficiently, so that its surface may be wetted by an intermediate resin without the risk of water forming a barrier between the adhesive fluid and substrate. In order to achieve

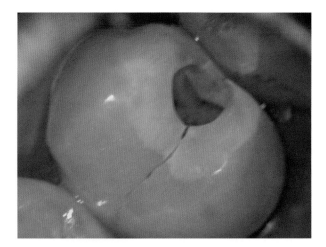

Fig. 11.7 The well-recognized frosted appearance of enamel after acid etching.

a successful etch on unprepared enamel, the exposure time should be extended. This is also recommended with older enamel particularly if it has been exposed to fluoride for a significant period of time. The solubility of the enamel will be decreased due to the effect of the fluoride ion. Effective etching still forms a major part of any adhesive system available for dental use.

- The surface of the tooth should be thoroughly cleaning with a pumice slurry (prophylaxis) (Figure 19.49) prior to etching to remove pellicle and plaque.
- Proprietary pastes should be avoided as they contain oils, which can contaminate the surface to be bonded so reducing its wettability and ability to bond effectively.

> **Pellicle:** a protein film that forms on enamel by selective binding of the glycoproteins from saliva. It forms in seconds after the tooth surface has been cleaned.

Etching considerations for deciduous enamel

Primary enamel contains more prismless enamel at the surface but it is also less calcified than permanent enamel. It takes longer for the acid to penetrate the prismless layer to create the etch pattern on the underlying prismatic enamel. This means that the clinician should increase the etching time. Bond strengths to deciduous enamel are generally lower as a result.

Deciduous enamel may require a longer exposure to etching agents to produce the ideal etching pattern.

Problems with etching

Over-etching

It is possible to over-etch enamel. Note the difference between a 30- and 60-second etch in Figure 11.8. There is a substantially greater removal of the enamel prism sheath after 60 seconds and the porosities produced are not so numerous. This will decalcify the substrate to too great a depth, that is, the etch pattern will be lost, thus decreasing ability of the resin to form tags which may penetrate the etched pattern. The result will be lower bond strength. It is impossible to determine clinically when the enamel has been over-etched, so attention must be paid to the length of time of application of the acid.

Re-etching

Etching can only be done once on the same surface. Repeating the etching process will result in over-etching (see Figure 11.8B). If the tooth surface becomes contaminated by blood or saliva during the bonding process then etching may require to be repeated. This is a common clinical problem when the dentist is working on teeth not isolated by rubber dam. If contamination does occur, then the dentist should re-prepare the tooth and re-etch, removing approximately 50 µm of enamel.

Bevelling enamel

The quality of the etching pattern may also be improved by bevelling the enamel. Bevelling removes the outer amorphous enamel, so exposing fresh enamel for bonding and roughening its surface. In addition, this takes account of the angulations of the enamel prisms and ensures that no unsupported prisms remain. Hence bevelling aids in the production of a better etch pattern so that higher bond strengths may be achieved.

> **Bevelling:** when the dentist prepares the enamel margins at an angle of approximately 120°, using a diamond bur.

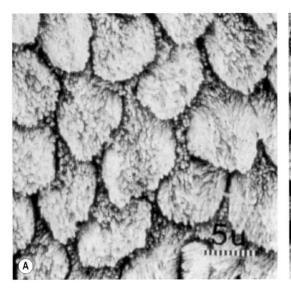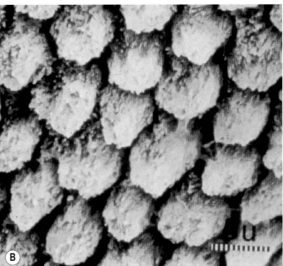

Fig. 11.8 Microscopic patterns in enamel produced by etching for (A) 30 seconds and (B) 60 seconds. Note the difference in the depth of the clefts.

Acids used

A number of acids have been proposed over the years to etch enamel. The most commonly used chemical is **phosphoric acid** (ortho-phosphoric acid), and the optimum concentration is between 30% and 50%. The acid must be strong enough to effect an etch pattern but not too concentrated so that the small amount of water present does not get saturated with reaction by-products quickly, as this would slow the dissolution rate. The most commonly used concentration is 35–37% and this is applied for a period of 15–30 seconds.

When the technique was first used clinically the recommended etching times were longer, but this increased the risk of over-etching the surface. Other acids have been introduced to market in an attempt to decrease the etch time, for example maleic acid was introduced by 3M some years ago. Unfortunately few dentists read the directions-for-use (DFU) accompanying the material, which recommended a shorter application time. The result was that the enamel surface was over-etched so bond failures resulted. As a result this product was withdrawn.

> **Ortho-phosphoric acid:** term synonymous with phosphoric acid, signifying a stereo-chemical difference.

Liquid	Gel
Tends to run over the enamel surface and could chemically traumatize the oral soft tissues	Stays in situ more readily so easier for the dentist to control its application
Easier to remove	Must be removed thoroughly by rinsing otherwise the residual colloidal silica may decrease bond strength gained
Applied by a brush	Applied by a fine needled syringe
More effective as no additives	May not penetrate to the same depth as solution

Fig. 11.9 Advantages and disadvantages of a liquid versus gel presentation of acid for etching enamel.

Presentation of etching agents

Modern etching materials are available as **liquids** or **gels** (Figure 11.9). Liquids are difficult to control as they may run off the tooth surface, causing undesirable etching of enamel that will not be bonded. There is also the potential for causing chemical burns to the gingival tissues. The viscosity of the acid liquid may be increased with the addition of fine particles of **colloidal** or **amorphous silica**, which is used in many industries as a thickening agent. This aids localization of the acid solution, which then may be applied precisely to the areas to be etched (Figure 11.10).

When a thickening agent is added to the aqueous 37% phosphoric acid solution in quantities less than 2%, a transparent paste is produced, which may be extruded from a syringe. A colouring agent is frequently added to make gel identification easier against the white of the tooth surface. When using an etching gel, great care must be taken to ensure that the gel is washed away completely by thoroughly washing with air and water from the three-in-one syringe before the application of the bonding system. Otherwise the fine particles of colloidal silica will remain within the retentive features of the clefts within the enamel. This will prevent the bonding material adapting to the surface of the tooth tissue and will reduce the performance of the bond.

- A balance must be reached with regard to the viscosity of the gel.
- It should be viscous enough to be able to be placed precisely and for it to remain there.
- It should not be so viscous that it cannot penetrate into the smallest fissures.
- It must be easy to remove completely.

> The surface of the enamel should not be scrubbed during etching as the newly etched surface and exposed crystallites are friable and may break down. However, the acid should be gently agitated during its application as this will remove etch solution at the surface of the tooth which has been contaminated with products of dissolution. The movement of the fluid will introduce fresh acid to the surface so enhancing the efficacy and effectiveness of the etch process.

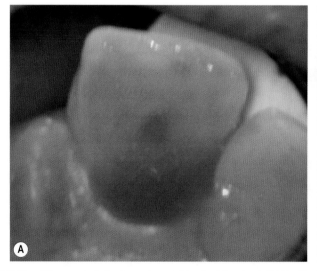
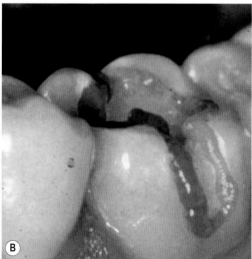

Fig. 11.10A,B The difference in behaviour of an etching liquid and gel. (A) The liquid has run off the area being etched. It is now in contact with enamel that does not need to be etched and, worse still, the soft tissues, which may result in a chemical burn if not removed. (B) The etching gel retaining its position on the periphery of a cavity.

> - It is essential to wash the tooth thoroughly after etching to remove all the acid, the products of etching and the gel thickening agent. Failure to do this may mean that the silica carrier is retained in the enamel clefts, so reducing the bond strength.
> - When etching (high acidic) products are being used, the patient and dental team should wear protective equipment such as protective clothing and eye wear. The application of rubber dam is also advisable.

Normally the bonding material is a dilute dimethacrylate resin system with a low viscosity. The most commonly used material is bis-GMA diluted with TEGDMA. Urethane dimethacrylates are rarely used. These materials are applied to the enamel surface after etching and flow into the crevices formed during the etching process. The resin monomer is then polymerized to form a solid polymer. The resin tags impregnate the enamel surface to a depth of about 30 μm (Figure 11.11).

During the polymerization process, oxygen inhibition of the curing process means that the surface of the resin layer is only partly polymerized. This part-polymerized resin should be wiped away with a cotton pellet before the patient is discharged. Alternatively, the addition of a restorative or another methacrylate-based material to the resin followed by polymerization results in union of the overlying material with the bonding resin and indirectly with the enamel.

One of the difficulties with this type of procedure is that during the polymerization process the resin tags shrink and have a tendency to **neck**. This means that just beneath the enamel surface the resin tag is narrower than the aperture it is occluding. During thermocycling, this thin neck of resin is likely to be stressed and fail, resulting in separation of the tag from the overlying surface resin.

In addition the resin may not penetrate to the full depth of the fissure that has been created by the etching process as air becomes entrapped during the resin application. This may lead to microleakage. The newer self-etch bonding systems have attempted to overcome this.

Commercially available products

Commercially available materials are shown in Table 11.1.

Table 11.1 Some acid etching products

Product name	Manufacturer	Active ingredient (phosphoric acid in %)	Liquid or gel
Ana Etch Gel Maxi	Nordiska	37	Gel
DeTrey Conditioner 36	Dentsply	36	Gel
Email Preparator Blu	Ivoclar Vivadent	37	Liquid
Etch 37	Bisco	37	Semi-gel
Etchant 15	Coltène Whaledent	15	Gel
Etchant Gel S	Coltène Whaledent	35	Gel
Etching Gel	DMG	37	Gel
Etching Gel MiniTip	3M ESPE	32	Gel
Gluma Etch 20 Gel	Heraeus	20	Gel
Gluma Etch 35 Fluid	Heraeus	35	Liquid
Gluma Etch 35 Gel	Heraeus	35	Gel
iBond Etch 20 Gel	Heraeus	20	Gel
iBond Etch 35 Gel	Heraeus	35	Gel
Kerr Gel Etchant	Kerr Hawe	37.5	Gel
K-Etchant Etchant Agent	Kuraray	40	Liquid
Sci-Pharm Etchant Gel	Sci-Pharm	33	Gel
Scotchbond Etchant	3M ESPE	35	Gel
SS White Etch Gel	SS White	40	Gel
Super Etch	SDI	37	Gel
Total Etch	Ivoclar Vivadent	37	Gel
Ultra-Etch	Ultradent	35	Gel
Uni-Etch	Bisco	32	Semi-gel
Unitek Etching Gel	3M Unitek	35	Gel
Voco Etch Gel	Voco	35	Gel

Enamel surface
Etched surface
Resin

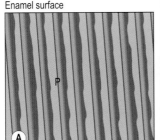
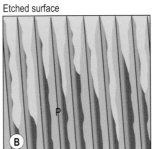
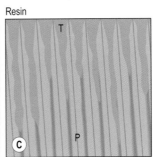

Fig. 11.11 (A) Cross-section of enamel showing the orientation of the enamel rod structure. (B) After acid etching there is preferential etching of the enamel rods to a depth of between 10 and 30 μm. (C) After resin application and polymerization, formation of tag within the enamel. P, prism sheath; T, resin tag.

BONDING TO DENTINE

Dentine unlike enamel is a 'living' tissue. This causes problems for bonding, as:

- It is always wet.
- Its surface is difficult to clean
- It is frequently contaminated with debris from the cutting process (**smear**).

The smear layer has to be removed but when this has been done fluid starts to flow out from the dentinal tubules. This will continually contaminate the surface. Any material that is designed to bond onto dentine must therefore be miscible with water. Unfortunately most of the materials used as bonding agents are hydrophobic, which presents a problem as these are not compatible with the bonding agent.

The process for bonding to dentine consists of three chemical processes:

1. The removal of the smear layer and the etching of the dentine.
2. The impregnation of the dentine by a water-miscible fluid or one which will substitute for the water.
3. The application of a fluid which will bond to both the impregnated material and the overlying restorative or cast restoration.

The above processes occur whatever bonding system is used. Each of these stages should be completed without any antagonistic processes intervening to ensure that the resulting bond is as good as possible. Ideally, each stage should be carried out alone, but to be more time efficient, most dental adhesives are designed to do at least two of these stages together. This means that frequently there are two chemical reactions taking place at the same time. For example, the demineralization of the dentine occurs at the same time as the impregnation of the dentine.

Since smear layer removal opens the dentinal tubules, the dentinal fluid outflow that follows will always cover the surface of dentine with a thin fluid film. The clinician, therefore, may need to make a choice between (Figure 11.12):

- Maintaining the smear and reducing the amount of fluid (which may interfere with the wetting of the dentine by the bonding agent)
  and
- Removing the smear and allowing fluid outflow from the dentinal tubules (which must be displaced for successful bonding).

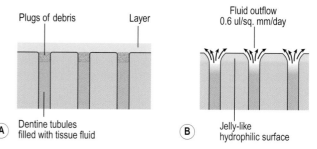

Fig. 11.12 Cross-section of dentine. (A) The smear layer is intact and the dentinal tubule openings are plugged with debris. When the smear layer is removed, fluid may flow out from the now opened dentinal tubules (B).

Removal of the smear layer and dentine etching

This is the initial stage of any dentine bonding process and a range of chemicals have been developed for it. These are normally known as dentine conditioners and include:

- Phosphoric acid
- Nitric acid
- Maleic acid
- Citric acid
- Ethylene diamine tetra-acetic acid (EDTA).

Dentine conditioning agents are generally acids which are designed to remove the smear layer produced by cavity preparation and modify the surface of the underlying dentine. Depending on both their concentration and the time period of application, these materials modify or remove the dentine smear layer and preferentially partly demineralize the intertubular dentine and the periphery of the dentinal tubules. This normally extends to a depth of approximately 10 μm, leaving the collagen matrix intact and uncollapsed. The partly demineralized collagen matrix acts as a scaffolding which may be impregnated with the primer (Figure 11.13). Sclerosed dentine requires a longer exposure time for the same effect to be produced. Some conditioning agents also incorporate glutaraldehyde, which acts on the collagen fibres by fixing them by a process of cross-linking. This is supposed to strengthen the fibres and prevent their collapse.

The conditioning process is fraught with problems as the smear layer is of variable thickness at different points on the surface. The time available to treat the underlying dentine is dependent on how quickly the

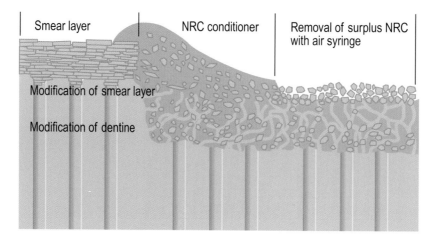

Fig. 11.13 The conditioning process: application of the conditioner demineralizes the smear layer and removes the inorganic phase of the dentine; after drying of the surface the excess conditioner infiltrates the collagen and interlocks when the resin is polymerized. (NRC: no rinse conditioner)

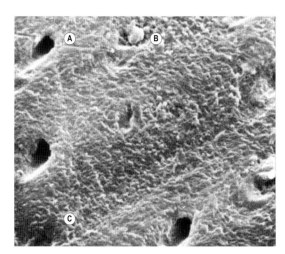

Fig. 11.14 Dentine surface after treatment with conditioner: as a result of the very thick smear present the conditioner has only been partly effective. Note the open dentinal tubule (A), a dentinal tubule still completely occluded with debris (B) and a dentinal tubule partially cleared (C).

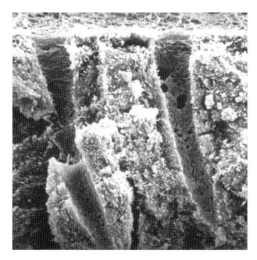

Fig. 11.15 Aggressive etching of the dentine exposing the underlying collagen matrix. The risk with this extensive etch is that unless care is exercised the structure may collapse.

smear layer is removed, making the process less predictable. Figure 11.14 shows the variable results achieved with application of a conditioning agent on a smear layer. The varying thickness of the smear layer has led to differential opening of the dentinal tubules. Figure 11.15 shows a much more aggressive etching process. Here the demineralization has been much more extensive and extends more deeply into the dentine. This may cause an inflammatory response in the pulp if the cavity is deep.

If the dentine is over-treated and the dentine is excessively demineralized, the residual collagen will not act as a scaffold but will collapse. Excessive drying may also have this effect, making infiltration of the primer very difficult as no inter-penetration of the dentine structure is achieved. The selection of the conditioner and its concentration is therefore critical.

Use of too strong an acid will lead to the various stages of the process being completed too quickly in some areas of the preparation, leading to over-etching. If the acid is too weak then the dentine preparation will only be partially complete and less inter-penetration of conditioner with tooth will occur. In either case the bonding process will be sub-optimal.

Priming the dentine surface

The next stage in the bonding process is priming of the prepared dentine surface with a material that can bond the hydrophobic material (such as resin composite or compomer) to the hydrophilic dentine. A **primer** is a solution which is applied to the conditioned surface of the dentine. It infiltrates the collagen network to stabilize it and provides a link between the dentine and the sealer, i.e. between the hydrophilic dentine and the hydrophobic **sealer**. The composition of the primer is generally a bifunctional monomer (**coupling agent**) in a solvent (**carrier**). The bifunctional monomer has the role of ionically linking to the (hydrophobic) methacrylate groups in the sealer to the collagen and hydroxyapatite in the (hydrophilic) dentine. These molecules are referred to as amphiphilic and the linking is achieved by having a molecule with a methacrylate group at one end. This is connected to an inert backbone and on the opposing end is a reactive group that carries a charge which will be attracted to the hydroxyapatite in the tooth. Whether there is any chemical interaction with this reactive group varies with each manufacturer's adhesive. The molecule should not be too rigid, however, as strains may be set up in the bond or sites for bonding may be reduced due to the decreased ability of the reactive groups to line up. All dentine bonding agents therefore have similar basic structure:

$$M–R–X$$

where M is the methacrylate molecule bonding to composite, R is the linking molecule on the backbone and X is the molecule interacting with dentine or smear.

Amphiphilic: a term used to describe a molecule that has a polar, water-soluble group attached to a non-polar, water-insoluble hydrocarbon chain.

! | **Confusing terms!**

- Unfortunately there are a number of terms which are frequently defined in different ways by different authors and manufacturers. This can be very confusing to the student and qualified clinician alike! For simplicity the following guide may be helpful:
- **Primers** are often referred to as dentine conditioners, which are acids used to alter the appearance and characteristics of the dentine surface.
- **Coupling agents** do the chemical linking but are often described as primers.
- **Sealers** flow into the dentinal tubules and seal the dentine with a surface layer rich in methacrylates and bond to the resin composite. They are sometimes referred to as the bond, resin or adhesive.

    In the research literature the latter terms, i.e. dentine conditioner, primer and sealer, are used respectively and the reader should be mindful of this.

The coupling agent within the primer varies from manufacturer to manufacturer since no one molecule appears to be have universal acceptance. The most commonly used ones are:

- Hydroxyethylmethacrylate (HEMA)
- N-phenylglycine-glycidyl methacrylate (NPG-GMA)
- 4-methacryloyloxyethyl phenyl phosphoric acid/ methylmethacrylate-tri-*n*-butyl borane (4-META/MMA-TBB) or 4-methacryloyloxyethyltrimellitate (4-META)
- Dimethacryloyloxyethyl phenol phosphate (MEP-P)

All of these contain a methacrylate reactive group and some form of ionic charge at the opposite end. Probably the most popular primer at the present time is HEMA (see Chapter 10). This very small molecule is water soluble and therefore is attractive to manufacturers as the dentine is itself rich in water. When carried by a solvent, it can penetrate into the demineralized collagen and saturate it. This creates a entangled network of polyHEMA molecules with collagen.

The potential of sensitization with HEMA has been stressed throughout this text. A no-touch technique should be employed to avoid contact of the chemical with gloves. See Chapter 10 (p.125) for more details.

Primer carriers

All the primers have some form of solvent into which the coupling agent is dissolved. These are generally hydrophilic chemicals which will rapidly pass through the conditioned dentine carrying the coupling agent with them. The primer may infiltrate the partly demineralized layers as well as passing into the dentinal tubules. Solvents commonly used are **alcohol** (such as ethanol or butanol) and **acetone** (Table 11.2). Both these solvents have the ability to displace the water in the dentine and may be removed after they have served their function by evaporation. Not all alcohols may be used, as the higher-molecular-weight alcohols (such as tertiary butanol) do not work effectively with the methacrylate resins due to their molecular structure. **Water** is also sometimes used as this will rapidly pass into the dentine tubules as the pulpal outflow pressure is low and water is readily miscible with any fluid outflow.

The caps of bottles containing bonding chemicals should always be kept on as failure to do so will result in the solvent being lost by evaporation. The solutions usually thicken. Both the loss of the solvent and the thickening will reduce the ability of the primer and sealer to wet and get into the surface of the dentine, with a decrease in bond strength.

If the primer contains a higher concentration of solvent, then better penetration of the dentine surface is possible but since each layer is very thin, more layers will need to be placed. A low-solvent-containing primer usually requires only one layer as it forms a better film. Solvents which contain a filler tend to separate.

In order to achieve complete saturation of the demineralized dentine, several coats of the bonding agent may be required. It may also take

Table 11.2 Advantages and disadvantages of the various bonding system carriers

Alcohol-based	Acetone-based	Water-based
Evaporate less quickly	Evaporation may be too fast, limits penetration of the solute into the dentine	Hydrophilic, so better for substrate
Less sensitive to dentinal moisture	More sensitive to dentinal moisture so more technique sensitive if the dentist over-dries the tooth	Does not need to evaporate but has a long drying time
Not as good at water chasing as acetone	Seeks out moisture from dentinal tubules more aggressively (water chasing)	Rehydrates demineralized collagen after drying of the primer
Decreased postoperative sensitivity	More volatile than alcohol so easier to evaporate once monomers have been carried into dentine	Not sensitive to dentinal moisture
May increase shelf-life (*cf.* acetone-containing products)	Bad odour	Water may interfere with adhesion
	Multiple coats may be required	Difficult to remove

some time to penetrate and get absorbed. Multiple layers make the layer more flexible, which may allow stresses on the bond to be dissipated. A thick layer of bond will cover all of the dentinal surface, which may not occur with a thin layer. Some products that are designed to yield a thicker bonding layer tend to be more syrupy in presentation.

Hybridization

The primary objective of the priming stage is to ensure that the dentine is fully infiltrated and that the partly unsupported scaffold of collagen does not collapse. The infiltration of the partly demineralized dentine with the conditioning agent is known as hybridization and the area affected is known as the **hybrid layer**. Failure to achieve hybridization results in the primer floating on the surface of the demineralized dentine with voids underneath. This will lead to microleakage in the long term (Figure 11.16).

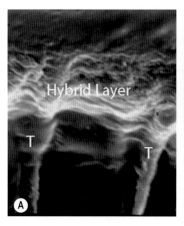
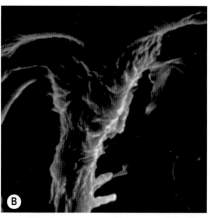

Fig. 11.16 (A) A well-formed hybrid layer. However, in (B) there is no hybrid layer as the collagen network has collapsed prior to application of the conditioner. Note that the only conditioner present is that which has passed down the open dentinal tubules. To show this, the dentine has been dissolved post preparation using ethylene diamine tetra-acetic acid (EDTA).

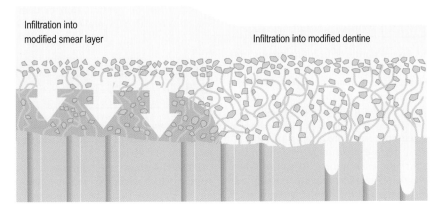

Infiltration into modified smear layer

Infiltration into modified dentine

Fig. 11.17 Following application of the conditioner to the etched dentine, the figure illustrates the penetration of the conditioner into the collagen scaffold.

Wet bonding

The solvents used to carry the primers are very good at displacing the water in the conditioned dentine. However, great care must be taken not to then dry the dentine or the collagen will become desiccated and the scaffold of collagen will collapse (Figure 11.17). This has led to the term **wet bonding** being used and the dentine should be kept moist.

When the dentine has been conditioned the collagen fibres are hydrated and stand up. This is advantageous as the bonding agent may attach to these fibres. However, if the dentine is desiccated then these collagen fibres collapse making bonding to them much less effective. The behaviour of the collagen is illustrated using spaghetti to represent the collagen fibres in Figure 11.18.

The dentine should never be over-dried (desiccated) prior to wet bonding as this will cause the collagen network to collapse so significantly compromising the bond strengths gained. However, if the dentine is inadvertently over-dried, then remoistening with water will rehydrate the collagen, causing the fibrils to stiffen slightly and stand up again, but the collagen does not revert to normal.

✓ After lightly air drying, the surface of the dentine should be left moist with a glassy appearance when wet bonding.

Sealing

Once the priming process has been completed, the sealer is applied to the surface. This material is invariably a methacrylate-based material which will cross-link with the methacrylate chain in the coupling agent. A range of methacrylates have been used but the most commonly available today are bis-GMA and HEMA. This combination is effective in wetting the surface of the primer and ensuring good adaptation of the sealer to the primer. The viscosity of the sealer will affect the penetration into the surface. Lower viscosity resins will achieve greater penetration than those of higher viscosity. Some sealers may have had fillers added to them. This will increase their viscosity and may prevent complete bonding to the tooth surface. Furthermore, air may become entrapped leading to a zone of oxygen inhibition and consequent bond failure.

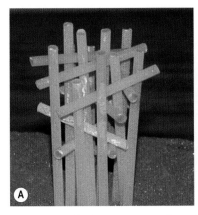
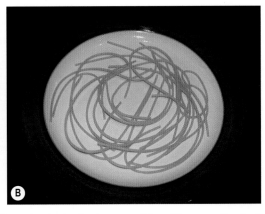

Fig. 11.18A,B (A) Illustration using spaghetti to represent collagen fibres: the dentine has been conditioned in preparation for the bond to be applied. Note the spaghetti (collagen fibres) standing up so permitting the bonding agent to readily attach. (B) If the dentine is desiccated then the collagen network will collapse, so creating a less favourable environment for bonding.

MOISTURE CONTROL

As mentioned elsewhere the vast majority of bonding agents and the materials to which they are attaching are hydrophobic in nature. To maximize bond strengths and therefore success excellent moisture control should be maintained by the dentist. Moisture contamination may come from intraoral fluids such as saliva or from exhaled air.

Rubber dam is the most effective and predictable method of achieving moisture control and its use is strongly recommended. Some dentists would argue that the environment so gained when teeth are isolated is too dry and therefore not conducive to wet bonding. This, however, is a facile argument as the dentist is much more in control of the environment when working under rubber dam. They are therefore in a better position to achieve the correct surface condition of the dentine. Rubber dam will also prevent corrosive solutions reaching the oral soft tissues. See page 140.

COMMON CHEMICAL CONSTITUENTS OF BONDING SYSTEMS

There are many chemicals contained in the bonding agents used in modern dentistry (Table 11.3). The table also gives the reasons for inclusion of each agent.

Table 11.4 shows the representative composition of a resin luting cement, which would be used in conjunction with the bonding agent. As can be seen from the composition there are several similarities between the two. The luting cement, however, contains a substantially higher amount of filler and is unlikely to have bifunctional monomers.

Table 11.3 Commonly used chemicals in dental bonding agents

Chemical name/abbreviation	Type of chemical	Reason for its inclusion
PENTA	Acidic monomer	Adhesive promoter Wetting aid Cross-linker
Polyalkenoate methacrylates including TCB	Acidic methacrylate resin	Difunctional monomer with both carboxylate and methacrylate groups
Urethane dimethacrylate (UDMA) Tri(ethylene glycol) dimethacrylate (TEGDMA)	Methacrylate resins	Regulates strength Viscosity regulator
Hydroxyethylmethacrylate (HEMA)	Water-miscible methacrylate resin	Wetting agent Cross-linking monomer
Barium glass Silicon dioxide	Nanofillers	Increase strength Marginal integrity Ensure adequate film thickness
Acetone t-butanol Ethanol Water	Solvents	Carrier for resin, may varies with adhesive type
Bifunctional acrylic amides	Acidic acrylic amides	Etchant and wetting agent Cross-linker, more stable than acrylic esters
Phosphoric esters	Acidic polymer	Etchant Adhesion promoter Wetting aid used in some products as more hydrolytically stable
Acrylic acid	Carboxylic acid	Dentine conditioner and chelating agent with calcium Wetting aid
Glycerol methacrylate Glycerol dimethacrylate	Hydrophilic swellable monomer	Wetting agent
Maleic acid	Dicarboxylic acid	Dentine conditioner Chelating agent with calcium
Camphorquinone	α-diketone	Photo-initiator
Benzoyl peroxide	Organic peroxide	Part of dual-cure system
Butylated benzenediol	–	Extends shelf-life Stabilizes monomer during storage
Glutaraldehyde	Hydrated dialdehyde	Collagen fixation
Potassium fluoride Ytterbium trifluoride	Inorganic fluoride salt	Fluoride release
Antibacterial agents	–	Control of bacterial contamination

Table 11.4 Typical composition of a resin luting cement (Rely X ARC, 3M ESPE)

Base paste	Catalyst paste
Bis-GMA	Bis-GMA
Tri(ethylene glycol) dimethacrylate (TEGDMA)	TEGDMA
Zirconia/silica filler	Zirconia/silica filler
Dimethacrylate polymer	Dimethacrylate polymer
Amine	Peroxide
Photo-initiator	Inhibitor
Pigments	

Some chemicals (such as eugenol, hydrogen peroxide or alkalis) interact with the camphorquinone light initiator in the resin composite-based adhesive. This retards the setting of the polymerizable material and plasticizes the polymeric components of the bonding agent. Decreased bond strengths will therefore result. These chemicals should therefore have no direct or indirect contact with bonding agents based on resin composites.

TOTAL ETCH TECHNIQUE

Most modern bonding materials provide for preparation for both enamel and dentine in one application. This means that the etching process is the same for both enamel and dentine. There was some concern originally about the use of an acid on the dentine particularly with respect to pulpal trauma. However, more recent investigations have shown that the acid penetrates less than 15 µm before it is neutralized. As such, the risks to the pulp are minimal. As a result, most modern bonding systems use an acid such as phosphoric acid which will etch both tissues. This avoids the rather more time-consuming approach of having two differing etching agents that are applied in turn (see also Table 11.5).

Table 11.5 Advantages and disadvantages of the total etch technique

Advantages	Disadvantages
Higher bond strengths	Over-drying causes collapse of collagen network
Quicker	Time consuming
Easy to do as etching solely one substrate is difficult	Highly technique-sensitive
	More potential for failure with more steps
	Nanoleakage as demineralized layer is too thick to be penetrated within a given time by the adhesive

BOND STRENGTHS

All published bond strengths are based on that achievable to acid-etched enamel, which is quoted as being 20 MPa. The bond strengths gained on freshly cut enamel using the techniques above are similar to this. Modern products now approach or exceed it in dentine using wet bonding techniques. That said, whether there is a need for bond strengths above a certain level is debatable. The self-etch systems while having a lower bond strength appear fit for purpose. As indicated in Chapter 4 there is a trade-off between number of steps in a procedure and reliability. Similarly, materials that exhibit both very low and very high bond strengths are less suitable than materials which have an average, consistently achievable bond strength.

To evaluate bond strengths in the laboratory, manufacturers can measure bond strengths either in tension or shear. Tension testing is carried out by pulling away a block of cured composite material bonded to the surface of the dentine. Shear testing is carried out by applying a knife edge tip to the interface and driving this down the interface. Neither gives a true indication of the bond strength as many additional factors influence the bond. Microtensile testing has become very popular as the test area is very small. This probably gives the closest guide to the bond strength but is misleading in judging clinical performance as minor failures at any point over the areas of bonding in a cavity will immediately affect the performance of the adhesive.

In the selection of an adhesive system for bonding material to tooth, the clinician should prioritize ease of use, a minimal number of stages of the operation and reliability of bond, before considering the ultimate bond strength desired.

Factors affecting bond strength

While bond strength is important it is not the sole factor in successful bonding. It is essential that the bond achieved initially is durable to withstand the stresses which are placed on it. There are two immediate problems.

- The cross-linking of the primer will apply the first stress to the system
- The next stress applied almost immediately after the setting has occurred is when overlying resin restorative itself undergoes polymerization shrinkage.

There are then a series of longer-term and cyclical stresses to which the bonding system will be subjected. These include:

- The effect of the regular thermocycling of the restorative in the mouth
- The loading applied to the restoration in function
- The slow and insidious long-term chemical degradation of the restorative and the bonding system.

It should be remembered that the bond strength obtained increases in the short term after placement and that the initial bond strength, when the polymerization stresses occur, will be substantially below that finally achieved after 24 hours to 1 week, depending on the system used.

Table 11.6 'Generation' classification of bonding agents

Generation	Description	Explanation
1st	Supposed chemical adhesion to smear using chelating chemicals	Calcium chelation with co-monomers, no removal of smear layer
2nd	Conditioning and priming with no etchant used	Bonding of calcium ions in tooth tissue and smear layer, polymerizable phosphates added to bis-GMA
3rd	Separate etchant for each tissue followed by conditioning, followed by primer applications, followed by adhesive application	Modification or removal of smear layer, separate conditioning stage
4th	Etchant (conditioner) + primer + adhesive	Total etch: removal of dentine smear and hybridization
5th	Etchant + (primer and adhesive)	Total etch: removal of dentine smear, attempt to achieve hybrid layer in dentine, wet bonding
6th	(a) Primer and adhesive	Self-etching multi-component primers, light- and dual-cured options, dissolving smear later
	(b) One-step 'all in one' and mixing products	
7th	Etch and bond in one	Self-etching single component primers
8th	One-step, dual-cure, self-etch, nano-particles reinforced	Mixed in blister pack before applying

Patients should be advised to avoid putting stresses on a newly bonded resin composite restoration for up to 24 hours. This is because initial bond strengths are lower due to polymerization shrinkage (causing the bond to be stressed before it is fully matured). As time goes on the bond matures and the full bond strength develops. Further information on the effects of polymerization shrinkage of resin composites on bonding is given in Chapter 7.

PRESENTATION OF THE BONDING AGENT

It has become a habit in the development of bonding agents to refer to each new bonding agent as being of a new 'generation'. This is a facile use of the term that has no meaning. However, the reader will undoubtedly encounter discussion of these products in terms of their 'generation' in other texts and in manufacturers' promotional literature. The 'generation' classification in Table 11.6 is given only for completeness.

It is far better to refer to the bonding agents by the number of stages involved. There are currently three types: three-, two- and one-stage presentations.

Three-stage bonding agents

In the original presentation, the three components of the system (conditioner, primer and sealer) were applied in turn as separate stages (Figure 11.19). While these multiple stages optimize the performance, the clinician is confronted a number of bottles of chemicals. Each of these has to be applied in a specific way and for a fixed time to produce the desired result. The benefit of this process was that each reaction at the tooth surface was carried out alone and not inhibited by the next process, nor were there competitive reactions proceeding at the same time.

Two-stage bonding agents

The original three stage bonding agents are now not commonly used, as clinicians have been presented with simplified systems that reduce the number of components by combining stages of the procedure. This has also reduced the number of chemicals used separately.

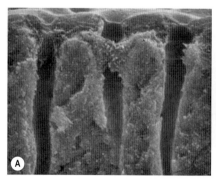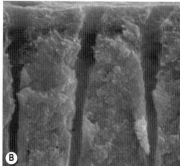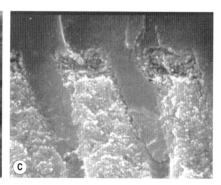

Fig. 11.19 Using a three-stage bonding system, the smear layer present in (A) has been removed and the upper layers of the dentine have been partially etched (B). In (C) the resin tags in the dentinal tubules are clearly seen as is the partial infiltration of the demineralized dentine near the surface. This is not complete and polymerization shrinkage is evident as the resin tags are not adapted closely to the tubule wall in some areas.

When combining number of steps, the manufacturer has three options (Figure 11.20):

- Providing a conditioner (etchant) and mixing the primer and sealant together. These are known as **one bottle bond** or **etch and bond** systems.
- Mixing the primer and conditioner (etchant) and presenting the sealer separately. These are known as **self-etch primers**
- Mixing etchant primer and bond into one system applied as one solution.

Of the systems shown in Figure 11.20, those using a separate primer and bonding agent (three-step and two-step self-etch primers) tend to result in a complete sealing of the cavity by the subsequent application of the adhesive bond. These products have higher bond strengths and are more effective than the 'all in one' materials with the primer and bond blended together.

Bonding system	Presentation		
Three-step	Etch	Primer	Bond
Two-step etch and bond	Etch	Primer	Bond
Two-step self-etch primer	Etch	Primer	Bond
One-step self-etch adhesive	Etch	Primer	Bond

Fig. 11.20 Summary of currently available bonding systems.

It is essential that the dentist is aware of the type of adhesive that they are using and understands what each of the stages is attempting to achieve as different systems combine different stages.

Etch and bond systems

Composition

The etchants in these systems are often not provided by the manufacturer and the recommendation is that conventional phosphoric acid solution or gel is used. The priming and bonding agent is generally based on water-soluble resins, as the dentine structure remains wet, or a combination of water-displacing agents.

Example of a clinical technique for an etch and bond system (Box 11.1)

The principles of using the etch and bond system are similar for all etch and bond products.

The clock in the surgery should have a second hand (Figure 11.21) so that the dentist can accurately time the length of each stage of the bonding procedure.

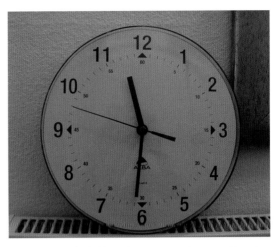

Fig. 11.21 A surgery clock. Note the presence of a second hand.

Clinicians should be aware that manufacturers may prescribe a different regimes for the preparation of the tooth surface prior to the application of the resin composite restorative material or adhesive. It cannot be stressed enough that the dentist must read and follow the manufacturer's instructions meticulously to maximize performance of the system. However, manufacturers are aware that dentists are often remiss at this and their timings may not be precise. They therefore design materials to have some tolerances and their instructions do take account of this.

It is not possible to provide a comprehensive standard operative procedure for every dental adhesive product available, including their idiosyncrasies; there is no universal technique as they all have different requirements. It is therefore essential that the instructions are read and followed precisely, otherwise inferior results will result.

When a bonding agent is air thinned (and to evaporate the residual solvent), the three-in-one syringe should be held some distance away from the tooth surface and a small steady flow of air directed in the direction of the tooth. If a strong blast of air is applied, the bond is not air thinned but blown off the surface of the tooth. This results in the incomplete covering of the cavity, formation of voids and may lead to bond failure and postoperative sensitivity. It is important that any residual water in the nozzle of the syringe is expelled before starting to air thin the agent.

Air lines should be regularly checked that they are free from oil and moisture as these will have a detrimental effect on bonding efficiency. Draining the compressor daily (at the end of the day) will help to reduce oil and moisture build up in air lines. Some dentists prefer to use oil-free handpieces for adhesive dentistry to minimize potential oil contamination.

Box 11.1 Clinical protocol for an etch and bond system using Adper Scotchbond 1 XT (3M ESPE)

Step 1	Step 2	Step 3	Step 4	Step 5	Step 6	Step 7
Apply etch for 15 seconds	Rinse with water for 10 seconds	Lightly air dry or blot dry with a cotton wool pledget to achieve a dentine surface that appears moist and shiny. Note the appearance of the dentine required for optimal bonding	Apply two coats of bond and gently massage into surface of tooth	Lightly air dry	Light cure for 20 seconds	Apply resin composite
Reason	Reason	Reason	Reason	Reason	Reason	Reason
Forms an etch pattern in enamel and removes smear layer in dentine ('total etch')	Removes all of the etch, particularly any thickening agent used in gel presentations	Removes excess moisture. Care is required at this stage not to desiccate the dentine surface	Bond wets substrate and penetrates collagen network and dentinal tubules	Thins bonding layer and evaporates the carrier	Cures the bond	The restoration

Commercially available products

Commercially available materials are shown in Table 11.7.

Self-etch systems

The self-conditioning (etch) adhesive systems attempt to combine conditioning, priming and bonding in a single step. This reduces working time and is possibly less technique-sensitive. The penetration/depth of the etch and the penetration of the monomer (primer) into the tooth should be similar. However, it is likely that the depth of penetration is less than the other systems. There may be reduced leakage as these materials are thought to be better at sealing. It is claimed that the smear layer adhering to dentine is dissolved and becomes part of the hybrid layer, as a result of which there is reduced postoperative sensitivity. A good analogy of a self-etch system is that of a train going into a tunnel (Figure 11.22).

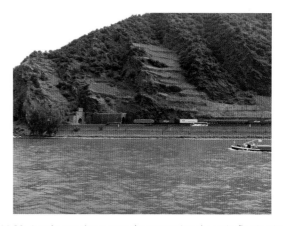

Fig. 11.22 A train entering a tunnel representing the resin flowing into a dentinal tubule as seen with a self-etch bonding system.

Table 11.7 Some bonding agents used after etching to bond direct restorative materials to tooth tissue currently available on the market

Product name	Manufacturer	Notes
A.R.T. Bond	Coltène Whaledent	
Adper Scotchbond 1 XT	3M ESPE	
Adper Scotchbond Dual Cure	3M ESPE	
Adper Scotchbond Multi-Purpose Adhesive	3M ESPE	
Adper Scotchbond Multi-Purpose Plus	3M ESPE	Activator available to allow a dual cure
All Bond 2	Bisco	
All Bond 3	Bisco	
ExciTE	Ivoclar Vivadent	
Excite DSC	Ivoclar Vivadent	Dual-cured
ExciTE F	Ivoclar Vivadent	Fluoride release
Gluma Comfort Bond	Heraeus	Single component
Gluma Solid Bond	Heraeus	
Heliobond	Ivoclar Vivadent	Use with Syntac
iBond Total Etch	Heraeus	
Mirage Bond	Chameleon Dental Products	
One Coat Bond	Coltène Whaledent	
One-Step	Bisco	
One-Step Plus	Bisco	Filler particles incorporated
Optibond FL	Kerr Hawe	Also acts as a liner
Optibond Solo Plus	Kerr Hawe	Fluoride release
PQ1	Ultradent	Ethyl alcohol carrier, releases fluoride
Prime & Bond NT	Dentsply	Fluoride release, when used in conjunction with Self-Cure Activator product becomes dual cure
Solobond M (Mono)	Voco	One component
Solobond Plus	Voco	
Stae	SDI	Fluoride release
Syntac	Ivoclar Vivadent	Use with Heliobond
Tenure Multi-Purpose	Den-Mat	
Tenure Quik with Fluoride	Den-Mat	Fluoride release
Transbond XT Primer	3M Unitek	Orthodontic bonding, contains fluoride
XP Bond	Dentsply	When used in conjunction with Self-Cure Activator product becomes dual cure

The train locomotive (the etching part of the molecule) enters the tunnel (dentinal tubule) pulling its carriages behind it (bonding component). When the train gets some way into the tunnel it may stop (etching depth) but the carriages are still attached. The penetration depth of the acid and the bonding agent are the same with no intervening gap (void) where leakage or incomplete curing may result.

Constituents

Self-etch systems consist of a mixture of an acidic etchant to demineralize the tooth surface, a linking molecule or primer and the bonding agent. A solvent is also present to carry the mixture to its site of action.

The demineralization component is often a **methacrylated phosphoric acid ester**. This is a long-chain methacrylate with a phosphoric acid group and dissolves calcium from hydroxyapatite. A satisfactory etch pattern is achieved when these products are applied to freshly cut enamel, however, the result is not as good if the enamel has not been freshly prepared. In order to achieve as good a bond as an etch and bond system, a separate etching step is required which tends to defeat the objective of having an all-in-one system!

The solvent is water based. This promotes dissociation of the acid groups and allows hydrogen ions to be released for etching. After etching has been completed, the excess solvent needs to be removed by evaporation. This is potentially problematic as any water left behind may be trapped within the bonding material, which may lead to failure at the adhesive layer.

Manufacturers have a problem with the presentation of this type of adhesive as one bottle. In order to incorporate all the necessary chemicals into the one solution, high concentrations of solvent are necessary. Attempts to evaporate the solvent by air drying may not be successful. This has a direct effect on the bond strengths achieved. Polymerization may be reduced by water and HEMA retention within the hybrid layer. Long-term storage is difficult to achieve with the mix of acids and hydrophilic and hydrophobic monomers in a single bottle. To overcome this, manufacturers often supply self-etching systems in two bottles for mixing by the dental team at the chairside just prior to application.

These self-etch systems provide a means of demineralizing the dentine at the same time as the infiltration process is carried out. This can present problems as two reactions which are distinctly different are taking place at the same time. That is, the presence of the sealer may well reduce the passage of the primer component within the already etched dentine. This is less of a problem with the one bottle bond.

Example of a clinical technique for a self-etch system

The principles of using the self-etch system (Box 11.2) are similar for all self-etch products. Unfortunately, manufacturers do not define what they mean by a thin film and it is a very arbitrary decision which the clinician must make, leaving the system open to misuse and failure.

Self-etch bonding systems should be rubbed on the surface being treated to ensure adequate etching action. This also prevents the neutralization processes on the tooth surfaces taking place too quickly.

Use with dual-cured or chemically cured resin composites

Self-etch bonding systems should not be used with either dual-cured or chemically cured resin composites as they are chemically incompatible. The acidic monomers required for the etching process react with the amine initiator that is needed for the chemical curing mechanism in self- or dual-curing systems.

Self-etch bonding systems are contraindicated with both dual-cured or chemically cured resin composites as they are chemically incompatible.

Commercially available products

Commercially available materials are shown in Table 11.8.

Table 11.8 Some self-etch bonding systems

Examples on the market	Manufacturer	Notes
AdheSE	Ivoclar Vivadent	Contraindicated for zirconium oxide ceramic or pulp caps. Activator available for dual cure
AdheSE One F	Ivoclar Vivadent	Fluoride releasing
Adper Easy Bond	3M ESPE	
Adper Prompt L-Pop	3M ESPE	
Adper Scotchbond SE	3M ESPE	Changes colour
All-Bond SE	Bisco	
Clearfil DC	Kuraray	Dual-cured
Clearfil S3 Bond	Kuraray	One bottle
Clearfil SE Bond	Kuraray	
Contax	DMG	
ED Primer 2.0	Kuraray	Dual-cured
Filtek Silorane SE Adhesive	3M ESPE	Should not be used with methacrylate-based composites
Futurabond M	Voco	
Futurabond NR	Voco	Fluoride release
G-Bond	GC	
Go! Bond	SDI	Fluoride release
iBond Self Etch	Heraeus	
One Coat 7.0	Coltène Whaledent	
One Coat SE Bond	Coltène Whaledent	
ParaPost Adhesive Conditioner	Coltène Whaledent	
Optibond All in One Adhesive	Kerr Hawe	
Optibond Solo Plus Self Etch Adhesive	Kerr Hawe	
ParaBond	Coltène Whaledent	
Peak SE Primer	Ultradent	
SEA2	3M ESPE	
Tenure Uni-Bond	Den-Mat	
Transbond Plus Self-etching Primer	3M Unitek	For bonding in orthodontics, contains fluoride
Xeno III	Dentsply	Fluoride releasing
Xeno V	Dentsply	

Box 11.2 Clinical protocol for a self-etch bonding system using Adper Prompt L-Pop (3M ESPE)

Step 1	Step 2	Step 3	Step 4	Step 5	Step 6	Step 7
Activate the product as directed and mix components together	Apply the product by brushing over the cavity surface. Work fluid into the surface for 15 seconds, applying pressure. Larger cavities require a longer application time	Thoroughly air dry the adhesive, leaving a thin film	Apply a second coat	Thoroughly air dry the adhesive leaving a thin film	Light cure for 10 seconds	Apply resin composite
Reason	Reason	Reason	Reason	Reason	Reason	Reason
Activates the product for clinical use	Cavity surface etched, conditioned and covered with bonding agent	Thins bonding layer and evaporates the carrier	Ensures complete saturation of the demineralized dentine	Thins bonding layer and evaporates the carrier	Cures the bond	The restoration

One-stage bonding agents

These are generally two components which are mixed and then applied to the enamel and dentine without any prior treatment to the tooth tissue. While these are simple they are not suitable for use in stress-bearing areas and rely on polar bonding rather than micro-mechanical entanglement, which appears to be more consistent.

Comparison of etch and bond versus self-etch bonding techniques

The advantages of the etch and bond and self-etch techniques are compared in Table 11.9.

Table 11.9 Comparison of the etch and bond and self-etch bonding techniques

Etch and bond	Self etch
Higher bond strengths gained	Quicker
Greater consistency	Better sealing of dentine
	Less postoperative sensitivity
	Cannot be used with dual-cured or chemically cured resin composites
	Less good etch pattern produced

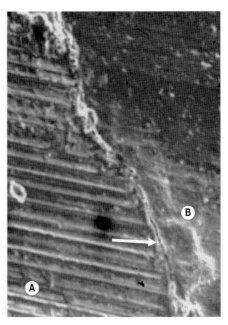

Fig. 11.23 Photomicrograph of a cross-section though a resin composite restoration bonded to tooth showing partial failure of the adhesive interface (arrow). (A) dentine, (B) resin composite.

BOND FAILURES

It is important to ascertain the reason for failure if this occurs. Failure occurs at the weakest link and may be:

- **Adhesive:** This is failure at the interface between two differing materials.
- **Cohesive:** This is failure within the substrate or adhesive.
- **Mixed:** This occurs partly at the interface and partly (cohesively) within the substrate or adhesive.

Failure may also be **partial** or **total**, when the bond may break down due to the effects of:

- Polymerization shrinkage
- Thermal cycling
- Internal stresses caused by occlusal forces on the tooth
- Chemical attack such as hydrolysis

Partial bond failure (Figure 11.23) may manifest clinically as:

- Loss of the restoration
- Sensitivity due to bacterial ingress (microleakage)
- Recurrent caries
- Staining of the cavity/restoration margins.

Ultimately the success of the bonding procedure and the marginal seal gained depends on wetting properties of the resin composite, its shrinkage during polymerization and the stresses caused by this shrinkage and its level of adhesion. For successful use, the correct combination is required (Figure 11.24).

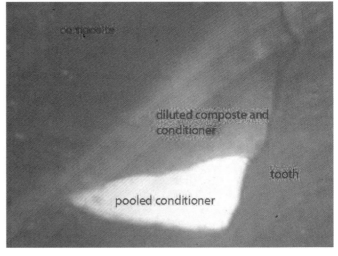

Fig. 11.24 A bonding system that has been applied incorrectly: use of excess conditioner and adhesive has resulted in pooling of these materials at the angle of the cavity. In addition, the adhesive has not been polymerized adequately and this is affecting the overlying composite as the adhesive has blended with the composite.

CONSISTENCY OF BONDING AND SUBSEQUENT PRODUCTS

Due to differing chemical constituents used by different manufacturers it is strongly advised that the dentist is consistent in their selection of the bonding product and subsequent products, be it a restorative material or an adhesive. For example it the dentist is using a 3M ESPE resin composite then they should use a 3M ESPE bonding system. Chemically these will be compatible and the combination will work well clinically if carried out as directed. Furthermore, should there be any problems such a premature debond, the manufacturer will be in more of a position to help resolve the issue than if another, perhaps incompatible, product had been selected.

The process of dental bonding is a technique-sensitive one and operator error is a significant factor in bonding failure. The clinical team must therefore pay close attention to all parts of the process and execute them fastidiously in order to maximize success.

RESIN ADHESIVE SYSTEMS FOR BONDING INDIRECT RESTORATIONS

Resin luting composites are widely used for the definitive cementation of indirect restorations to tooth tissue. They usually require to be used in combination with bonding agents as they have no natural affinity to bond to tooth tissue. Usually the etch and bond systems are used, as self-etch and dual-cured luting composites should not be used together (see p. 152). This bonding agent also forms a bond with the luting material. Some of the newer resin adhesive products are self-etching and may be used directly on the prepared tooth.

Light-cured, dual-cured or self-etch?

The dentist has three types of resin luting composite agents to choose from;

- **Light-cured:** These tend to be used where the light from the curing lamp may predictably access the cement to ensure it will be fully cured, for example, ceramic veneers. Light-cured products do not contain tertiary amines, which may result in a shade shift that is significant in the aesthetic zone.

- **Dual-cured:** These products are useful as the dentist need not worry about light penetration into inaccessible areas. They are therefore indicated for crowns, bridges, inlays/onlays (ceramic, metal or resin composite) and non-metallic posts.

- **Self-etch:** These save time and are easier to use as no intermediate bonding procedure is required prior to their application.

For further information on light- and dual-cured resin composite cements, see Chapter 7.

Commercially available products and clinical technique

There are too many products on the market (Table 11.10), and it is beyond the scope of this chapter to describe clinical protocols for them all. The prior use of an intermediate dentine bonding system is usually required but not with the self-etch products. The reader is advised to consult the DFU prior to using any product.

> The dentist is advised to maintain a constant seating pressure on the indirect restoration until the cement has set. This not only ensures that the restoration is correctly seated onto the preparation but it also suppresses any diffusion of water from the dentine. If water is allowed to diffuse, it can form globules in the setting cement which will reduce bond strength. Resin cements are relatively permeable.

The products designed to bond feldspar-based ceramics (see Chapter 22) such as veneers or resin-bonded crowns often come in a range of shades (Figure 11.25). This allows the dentist to slightly vary the colour of the cement and therefore the restoration to facilitate more exact shade match to the adjacent teeth as the ceramic is thin and the colour of the cement shines through it. The final

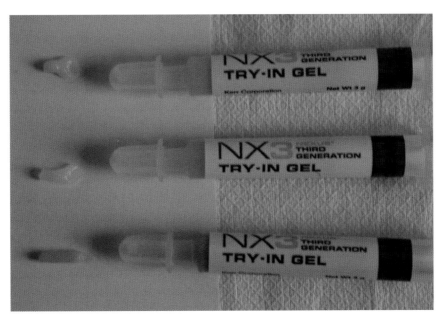

Fig. 11.25 Try-in pastes are supplied in a range of shades in a resin composite bonding kit, which allows the clinician to refine the shade of the final restoration such as a ceramic veneer.

Table 11.10 Some luting composites to bond indirect restorative restorations to tooth tissue, usually in conjunction with a dentine bonding agent, currently available on the market

Product name	Manufacturer	Notes
Adherence	Septodont	Dual-cured
BisCem	Bisco	Dual-cured
C & B Cement	Bisco	Chemically cured
Calibra	Dentsply	Light/dual-cured, fluoride release
Choice 2 Veneer Cement	Bisco	Light-cured
Clearfil Esthetic Cement	Kuraray	Dual-cured
Clearfil Liner Bond	Kuraray	Light/dual-cured and chemically cured, direct and indirect restorations
Clearfil SA Cement	Kuraray	Self-etching, fluoride release
Dual Cement	Ivoclar Vivadent	Dual-cured
Duo Cement Plus	Coltène Whaledent	Light/dual-cured and chemically cured
DuoLink	Bisco	Dual-cured
Futurabond DC	Voco	Self-etching, dual-cured
G-Cem	GC	Self-etching, dual-cured, fluoride release
Heliosit Orthodontic	Ivoclar Vivadent	Light-cured for orthodontic brackets
iCem Self Adhesive	Heraeus	
MaxCem Elite	Kerr Hawe	Self-etching
Multilink	Ivoclar Vivadent	Self-etching, dark-cured
Multilink Implant	Ivoclar Vivadent	Dual-cured
NX3	Kerr Hawe	Light/dual-cured
ParaCem Universal DC	Coltène Whaledent	Light/dual-cured
Rely X ARC	3M ESPE	Dual-cured
Rely X Unicem	3M ESPE	Self-etching, dual-cured
Rely X Unicem 2 Automix	3M ESPE	Self-etching, dual-cured
Rely X Veneer	3M ESPE	Light-cured
Resinomer	Bisco	Dual-cured
seT	SDI	Self-etching, dual-cured
seT PP	SDI	Self-etching, dual-cured, paste/paste
Smart Cem2	Dentsply	Self-etching, dual-cured, fluoride release
SpeedCEM	Ivoclar Vivadent	Self-etching, dual-cured
Tansbond XT Light Cure Adhesive	3M Unitek	Light-cured for orthodontic use
Transbond LR Adhesive for lingual retainers	3M Unitek	For orthodontic use, increased working time
Transbond Plus Color Change Adhesive	3M Unitek	For orthodontic use, contains fluoride, light cure
Transbond Supreme LV Low Viscosity Light Cure Adhesive	3M Unitek	For orthodontic use, flowable presentation for indirect bonding or direct light cure, increased strength
Twinlook	Heraeus	Light/dual-cured
Unite Orthodontic Adhesive	3M Unitek	For orthodontic use, chemical cure
Variolink II	Ivoclar Vivadent	Light/dual-cured
Variolink Ultra	Ivoclar Vivadent	Dual-cured, high viscosity
Variolink Veneer	Ivoclar Vivadent	Light-cured
Vitique	DMG	Light/dual-cured

shade may be ascertained prior to fitting by using the try-in pastes supplied with the kit. The shade of the try-in paste matches the set cement and not the unset cement, which may undergo a colour shift when cured. It is very important to thoroughly remove these prior to attempting to bond the restoration otherwise the bond achieved will be reduced.

- Some products are supplied with glycerine-based try-in pastes with varying pigmentations. This should be thoroughly washed off as failure to do so will result in an inferior bond.
- Many manufacturers refer to some products as **self-cure**. This means either chemical or dual cure. It should not be confused with self-etch.
- Products containing non-acid-resistant monomers should be stored in a refrigerator to slow down their degradation. Newer materials contain hydrolytically stable monomers and so this advice is less pertinent.

ANAEROBIC SET RESIN COMPOSITE LUTING CEMENTS

These cements are based on **phosphonated esters** such as MDP (10-methacryloyloxydecyldihydrogenphosphate). They originally gained popularity for cementation of resin-retained bridges. Today, they are mainly used to bond metal to tooth tissue such as the nickel chrome alloy of resin-retained bridges or adhesive gold restorations (see later).

In order to achieve an anaerobic environment to allow the setting phase to commence, the dentist must apply a glycerine gel to the margins of the restoration. This is supplied as Oxyguard II with the Panavia products (Kuraray) and is also available as Liquid Strip (Ivoclar Vivadent). The material cures from the interface towards the centre of the cement and its setting time is 4 minutes. In the case of the light-curing variety (Panavia F, Kuraray), when the cement at the margins of the restorations is exposed to the curing light the cement sets. An anaerobic environment is therefore created so allowing the rest of the cement not reached by the light to set. Alternatively, Oxyguard II could still be used if desired.

Commercially available products

Commercially available product are shown in Table 11.11.

Table 11.11 Phosphonated ester-containing resin bonding cements currently available on the market

Product name	Manufacturer	Notes
Panavia 21	Kuraray	
Panavia Ex	Kuraray	Chemical cured
Panavia F 2.0	Kuraray	Dual-cured
		Fluoride release due to the inclusion of sodium fluoride
		Available in six shades

The setting and therefore working time of anaerobic cements may be lengthened by spreading them out thinly on the mixing pad (Figure 11.26). This large surface area is exposed to oxygen in the atmosphere, which will inhibit its set and is particularly useful when a hybrid restoration is being fitted. The dental nurse mixes the phosphonated ester-containing product and spreads it thinly as described. Then they mix the conventional luting cement and, lastly, load both their respective bridge retainers for placement in the mouth.

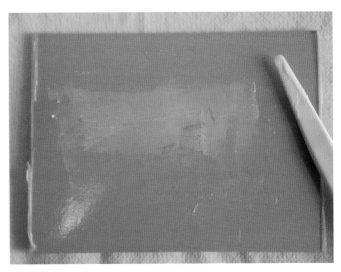

Fig. 11.26 A phosphonated ester-containing resin bonding system (Panavia Ex, Kuraray) spread thinly on the mixing pad to increase its working time.

BONDING TO METALS

Micromechanical bonding

Adhesive bonding to metal alloys such as nickel chrome and gold alloys is frequently employed in dentistry. Bridgework has been revolutionized by the advent of resin-retained bridges which are chemically bonded into place with resin composites. This has been made possible by the treatment of the fitting metal surface to enhance the bond of the resin adhesive to it by either sandblasting or acid etching. These processes both increase the surface energy, surface roughness, surface area for bonding and wettability, and decrease the surface tension, so improving the ability of the resin adhesive to contact and 'hold' the surface.

Chemical adhesion

The other method is to alter the surface chemically. As the resin bonds to metal oxides, the surface is treated to optimize this. In the case of nickel chrome, a thick oxide layer is produced by the nonprecious metals and this must be thinned, otherwise cohesive failure may occur within this oxide later. Gold alloys in contrast do not oxidize well and therefore other metals must be added to the gold, which will more readily oxidize. Copper and iridium are examples. If the metal surface is heat treated prior to fitting, a thin oxide layer is formed at the surface to facilitate bonding to the resin adhesive.

This heat treatment involves heating the gold restoration at 400°C in air for 9 minutes. This generates a copper oxide layer on the alloy surface (see Chapter 21). The restoration may now bond to the tooth tissue by a combination of chemical and micromechanical bonding. When the luting composite is applied to the gold alloy restoration, adhesion to gold is via disulphide methacrylate, which forms a methacrylate gold compound that bonds via the sulphur atom.

Another method in which gold may be bonded to a luting composite is by **tin plating**. The tin-plated surface immediately oxidizes to create an oxide layer of stannous oxide. This technique, however, is much less frequently used.

Restorations based on zirconium oxide, aluminium oxide and base metals should not be cleaned with phosphoric acid.

Zirconium oxide, aluminium oxide and base metals react with phosphoric acid forming a stable phosphate layer. This renders them inert and unreactive. Instead, the fitting surface should first be sandblasted, and then alcohol should be used to clean the fitting surface prior to cementation. A similar effect is observed with zirconium oxide as a layer of zirconium phosphate is created which inhibits the adhesion of the metal/zirconia primer, rendering it ineffective. Methacrylated phosphoric acid esters are used, creating a stable chemical bond to the oxide layers produced.

Metal, alumina and zirconia cores should be sandblasted to enhance micromechanical bonding with resin composites.

As MDP (e.g. Panavia Ex, (Kuraray)) and 4-META are chemically active and can form chemical bonds to base metals, they create stronger bonds to nickel chrome alloys than those cements based on bis-GMA.

Commercially available products

Commercially available products are shown in Table 11.12. These are frequently alloy specific. Alloys used in dentistry are discussed in Chapter 21.

Table 11.12 Some metal conditioning agents (used when bonding metal to tooth tissue via a luting resin composite cement) currently available on the market

Product	Manufacturer
Clearfil Alloy Primer	Kuraray
GC Metal Primer II	GC
Metal/Zirconia Primer	Ivoclar Vivadent
Monobond Plus	Ivoclar Vivadent
Signum Metal Bond	Heraeus

BONDING AGENTS AND ORTHODONTICS

Fixed orthodontic appliances often comprise **bands**, which are fitted around the molars, and **brackets**, which are bonded to other teeth (Figure 11.27). Increasingly brackets are used on the molars in preference to bands.

Bands are constructed from stainless steel and are usually **luted** in situ using a glass ionomer or resin-modified glass ionomer cement. Stainless steel is chosen as it is hard enough to function satisfactorily yet is malleable enough to be burnished so that its shape may be adapted more closely to the tooth surface. The inner surface is commonly roughened by micro-etching to facilitate luting.

Brackets are bonded onto the enamel surface with resin composite. These brackets may be made from stainless steel, gold or ceramic. Many manufacturers provide a mesh to bond mechanically to the resin (Figure 11.28). In some systems, the brackets are supplied precoated with adhesive. Other fixed orthodontic systems such as Incognito (3M Unitek) are constructed of gold alloy. These are bonded as previously described.

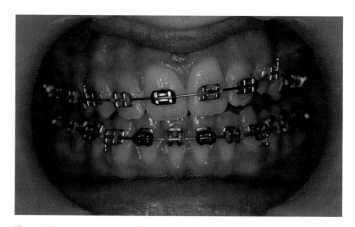

Fig. 11.27 Upper and lower fixed orthodontic appliances in situ with brackets bonded to the enamel surfaces of the teeth.
(Photograph courtesy of Mr Richard Buckle.)

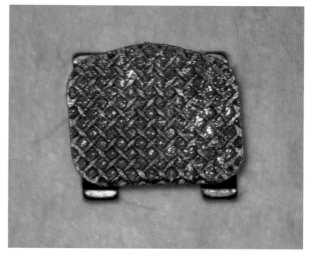

Fig. 11.28 Stainless steel orthodontic bracket that will be bonded onto the tooth surface using resin composite. Note the mesh, which will aid the micromechanical retention with the resin composite.

Ceramic brackets are also available to the orthodontist should the patient prefer a more aesthetic solution. These brackets are also bonded using resin composite cement and a silane coupler will be required to chemically bond the resin composite to the ceramic. To simplify the clinical procedure, many ceramic brackets are supplied presilanated.

The bonding procedure is essentially similar to the placement of a direct resin composite restoration. The enamel surface is etched as usual prior to the application of a bonding resin and placement of the bracket coated with resin composite cement.

Certain ceramics used to construct crowns (such as Techceram) are less amenable to bonding (see next section). This may present a problem for the orthodontist should a tooth which has been restored using a ceramic crown be required to be included in the orthodontic treatment.

Commercially available products

Commercially available orthodontic bonding products are shown in Table 11.13.

Table 11.13 Some luting resin composite cements used especially for orthodontic use currently available on the market

Product name	Manufacturer	Notes
3M APC II Adhesive Coated Appliance System	3M ESPE	Used with a light-cured adhesive, fluoride release (fluoride releasing glass)
3M PLUS Adhesive Coated Appliance System	3M ESPE	Pink, which fades when cured, used with a light-cured adhesive, fluoride release (fluoride releasing glass)
3M Concise Orthodontic Bonding System	3M Unitek	Suitable for metal, ceramic and plastic brackets (plastic prier must be used); two-paste composite system

BONDING TO CERAMICS

Etching ceramics

A 9.5% solution of hydrofluoric acid may be used to etch the glass phase of feldspathic ceramic both in the dental laboratory and in the clinic (Table 11.14). This creates a micro-retentive etching pattern in the same way as enamel will etch when an acid is applied to it, roughening it microscopically to enhance bonding. Hydrofluoric acid is a very noxious, toxic and caustic chemical and must be used with extreme caution. When used intraorally, the use of rubber dam is **mandatory** with all soft tissues covered. The face of the patient also has to be covered using paper towels for the 10 minutes it takes to create a sufficient etch pattern.

As a result of the shortcomings of the clinical use of hydrofluoric acid its usage has declined in recent years in favour of safer methods such as Cojet (3M ESPE) (see Chapter 19 for further details). However even Cojet may have its limitations, as an alkali is used which will impair the effects of the acidic part of the self-etch adhesive if this is being used.

Unfortunately, high-density polycrystalline ceramics especially those with more than 95% alumina or zirconia do not etch as easily due to their decreased glass content. This may present a problem if the dentist needs to repair a defect in the ceramic or wishes to bond an orthodontic bracket to it.

Table 11.14 Some ceramic etching agents currently available on the market

Product name	Manufacturer	Notes
Porcelain Etchant	Bisco	9.5% hydrogen fluoride Also available in 4%
Porcelain Etch	Ultradent	Usually 9.6% hydrogen fluoride

- Silane degrades quickly with time so it is advisable to apply silane coupling agents at the chairside just prior to use to maximize its effectiveness. They should be stored in the refrigerator to slow their degradation.
- After trying in a ceramic restoration, its fit surface should be thoroughly cleaned with phosphoric acid using a scrubbing motion.

Silanation

After etching the ceramic surface or treating it with Cojet, a **silane coupling agent** is applied to the surface of the ceramic. This is because resin composite is unable to bond chemically to ceramic without the application of an intermediate chemical y-methacryloxy-propyltrimethoxysilane, a **silane**. This is supplied in a volatile solvent such as acetone and links the resin adhesive to the ceramic to achieve high bond strengths. Bonding is achieved via the trialkoxy silane groups on methacrylic monomers (silane methacrylate) reacting with the silicate surface to form a methacrylate silicate compound. The reaction is hydrolysis of the trimethoxy silane and the intermediate product reacts with the silicate surface via a condensation reaction. Silane is inherently unstable and quickly degrades by hydrolysis. In order to maximize its effect it should be placed on the etched ceramic just prior to bonding.

Commercially available products

Commercially available products are shown in Table 11.15.

Table 11.15 Some silane coupling agents currently available on the market

Product	Manufacturer
3M ESPE SIL	3M ESPE
3M RelyX Ceramic Primer	3M ESPE
Bis-Silane	Bisco
Choice 2	Bisco
Clearfil Porcelain Bond Activator	Kuraray
GC Ceramic Primer	GC
Monobond 2	Ivoclar Vivadent
Monobond Plus	Ivoclar Vivadent
Porcelain Primer	Bisco
Silane 2	DMG
Ultradent Silane	Ultradent

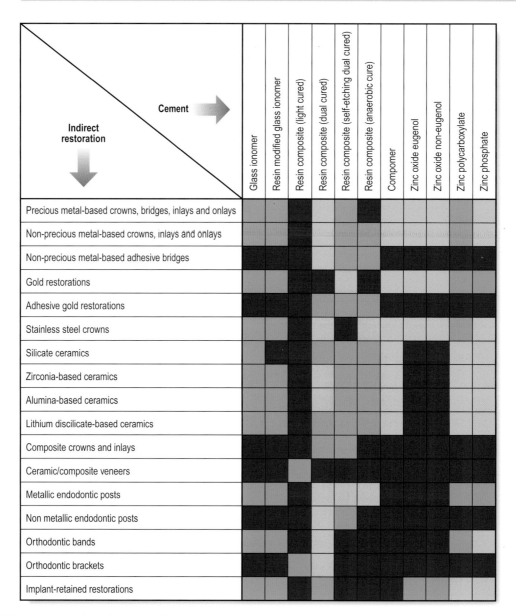

Fig. 11.29 A traffic light system guide to the luting or bonding material of choice with respect to the indirect restoration. The preferred combinations are in green, those which would work but are not first choice are in amber and those combinations contra-indicated are in red. *(Table courtesy of* Dental Update.*)*

As with resin composite and bonding systems, the chemical structure of the silane coupling agents varies between manufacturers. It is strongly advisable to keep systems consistent by matching the silane coupling agent with the luting resin composite of the same manufacturer otherwise a reduction in bond strength may be seen.

ADHESIVE SYSTEMS FOR EPOXY RESIN-BASED RESTORATIVES

The change in the base resin in the newer epoxy resin composite (such as Filtek Silorane, 3M ESPE) means that the composition of the adhesive has also been modified. It consists of two components, a self-etch primer and an adhesive sealer.

The self-etch primer contains acid methacrylate groups and also acid carboxylate groups which will demineralize the dentine. In addition, resin including HEMA and bis-GMA are included to infiltrate the dentine. This is then suspended in a solvent system that includes water and ethanol, a combination that aids the penetration of the resin. Silane-coated colloidal silica (of about 7 nm in size) is included to enhance the strength of the system as well as acting as a viscosity regulator. The presence of the ethanol means that the bottle should be refrigerated otherwise the alcohol will evaporate and the primer will thicken.

The sealer has to bond both to the primer and to the silorane molecule. This is rather more demanding than the normal adhesive as siloranes are more hydrophobic. While the sealer contains methacrylate resins it also has a hydrophobic bifunctional monomer which will bond with the silorane base resin. In addition, the sealer contains acidic monomers that initiate the ring-opening process which leads to the curing of the silorane.

The sealer also contains colloidal silica, which increases the mechanical properties and also is said to assist in a process known as shear thinning. The sealant is initially quite viscous but once it is applied to the surface and either air thinned or spread with a brush, the viscosity drops substantially allowing a more uniform thickness to be formed on the dentine surface.

> **Shear thinning:** this occurs when the viscosity of a material decreases as the shear stress applied to it is increased. An example is tomato ketchup. When the bottle is squeezed the force causes the ketchup to go from being thick like honey to flowing like water. It is also a common property of polymers. Materials that exhibit shear thinning are described as **pseudoplastic**.

SO WHAT TO USE?

In short, what should the clinician faced with a plethora of restorative and adhesive products use? Generally speaking, resin composite-based cements have higher strength and low solubility and will provide better and stronger bonding to tooth tissue. However, this may be undesirable for the clinical situation and so each case should be assessed on its merits. Figure 11.29 gives an indication of the adhesive product that should be used to fit each type of indirect restoration or appliance.

SUMMARY

- Bonding to tooth tissue requires careful preparation of the surface of the tooth to achieve success.
- Bonding is generally micromechanical although some chemical interactions occur.
- Bonding to tooth tissue requires three distinct stages. Modern adhesives attempt to combine these stages.

- Surface preparation of both metal alloys and ceramics is necessary to achieve adequate bonding.
- Bonding systems vary greatly and the DFU should be consulted prior to their use.
- Bonding is a very technique-sensitive procedure and should be carried out meticulously.

FURTHER READING

Powers, J.M., Sakaguchi, R.L. (Eds.), 2006. Craig's Restorative Dental Materials (twelfth ed.). Mosby Elsevier, St Louis. (See Chapter 10)

van Noort, R., 2007. Introduction to Dental Materials, third ed.. Mosby Elsevier, Edinburgh. (See Chapter 2.5)

SELF-ASSESSMENT QUESTIONS

1. What is the difference between luting and bonding?
2. Compare and contrast etch and bonding with self-etching when attaching resin-based composite to tooth tissue.
3. A Class IV resin composite that is out of the occlusion in all excursions of the mandible keeps debonding. What could be the possible causes for this problem?
4. What cements may be used to cement a resin-retained bridge? What are the pros and cons of each?
5. The dentist has just etched the enamel surface of a tooth and thoroughly rinsed off the etching gel. The procedure is being done without the use of rubber dam and the patient inadvertently swallows, so contaminating the newly etched surface. What should the dentist do now?
6. There is a cohesive fracture of the ceramic on one of the retainers of an eight-unit bridge. How may the dentist retrieve the situation?

Chapter | **12** |

Other dental cements

From this chapter, the reader will:

- Be aware of the range of other dental cements currently available
- Understand the setting mechanisms and the ways they may be manipulated
- Understand their indications, contraindications and limitations
- Have an increased appreciation of how to use these materials more effectively and to their best advantage.

INTRODUCTION

This chapter deals with the other, more traditional, cements that dentists have used for many years. While their use has diminished to some extent in recent years as a result of the development of new materials, traditional cements are still available and widely used. It is therefore important that their composition, uses and handling characteristics are still understood by the dental team.

Essentially, these cements are varying permutations of a combination of an **acidic liquid** and a **basic powder** (Table 12.1), which,

Table 12.1 Acids and bases participating in the formation of traditional dental cements

Acids	Bases
Phosphoric acid	Zinc oxide
Poly(acrylic acid)	Magnesium oxide
Maleic acid	Copper oxide
Eugenol	Fluoro-alumino-silicate glass
Mellitic acid	

when mixed together, form a **salt** plus **water**. The acids and bases react to form different materials. The permutations of these interactions are illustrated in Figure 12.1. Glass ionomer cement has already been discussed in detail in Chapter 9. **Silicate cement** is no longer used in modern dentistry and therefore there is no need to consider it further. The other cement permutations are:

- Zinc phosphate
- Zinc polycarboxylate
- Zinc oxide eugenol.

As they are derived from similar building blocks, these products have common principles of use and share many properties as might be expected.

Zinc oxide eugenol cement has further been modified with the addition of other active ingredients, marketed as a steroid/antibiotic cement. This modified cement and other materials such as setting calcium hydroxide cements and cavity varnishes are also discussed in this chapter.

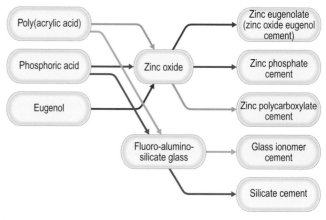

Fig. 12.1 The relationship between the various acids and bases that are used to synthesize traditional dental cements.

GENERAL STRUCTURE

Zinc phosphate, zinc polycarboxylate and zinc oxide eugenol cements have the same structure (Figure 12.2). This is because these products have the same base (zinc oxide) and the different cements are produced by the reaction of this base with different acids. In each case, only the surface of the zinc oxide particles will react with the acid when mixed. The set cement is therefore composed of unreacted cores of zinc oxide powder surrounded by the matrix of the reaction product, namely zinc phosphate, zinc polycarboxylate or zinc eugenolate, respectively.

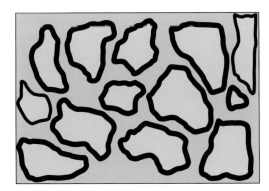

Fig. 12.2 Diagrammatic representation of the structure of zinc oxide-based cements. The centre core of zinc oxide (light blue) remains unchanged. The matrix (light green) is the acid salt. The dark blue band around each particle is the reacted part of the zinc oxide.

ZINC PHOSPHATE CEMENTS

Chemical constituents

Zinc phosphate cements have been used in dentistry for many decades. The material is generally supplied as **zinc oxide** powder and **phosphoric acid** liquid. Other chemicals are added to both the powder and liquid to modify the properties of the product (see Table 12.2).

Difference between stannous and stannic fluoride

These chemicals derive from the tin ion, stannum (Sn). When this ion reacts with the fluoride ion, stannous fluoride (SnF_2) and stannic fluoride (SnF_4) are produced. The difference between the two is that tin exists in two valent states. These compounds are often added to dental cements to convey caries resistance to the tooth in which they are placed as they leach fluoride. Stannous fluoride is more commonly used. Occasionally, there is a reference to 'tannin fluoride'. This refers to a mixture of tannic acid and a fluoride salt, which used to be known commercially as the HY agent. It purports to cause remineralization of dentine, but has not been mentioned in the literature for the past decade. Addition of any of these materials to zinc phosphate cement is at the expense of the cement matrix formation and so will weaken the cement. Their inclusion does, however, impart some cariostatic properties to the cements.

Setting reaction and structure

The setting reaction of zinc phosphate cements is a two-stage process. In the first part of the reaction, the zinc oxide in the powder reacts with the phosphoric acid in the liquid to form zinc phosphate and water. This newly formed zinc phosphate reacts with more zinc oxide, forming **hopeite**. This compound is **hydrated zinc phosphate**. Aluminium when present prevents crystallization and permits the formation of an amorphous cement, which is very similar in structure to the glass ionomer cement (see Chapter 9).

This matrix is almost insoluble but the set cement is porous, making it highly permeable as water which was not consumed in the reaction forms globules within the material. The water produced during the setting reaction is in both free and bound form within the cement. While the water exists in its free form the cement is weaker and more soluble. As the cement matures (the **maturation phase**), water is bound more strongly into the cement, leading to a stronger and less soluble cement.

Properties

Exothermic reaction and factors affecting the speed of set

The chemical reaction of zinc phosphate cement is the most exothermic of all the dental cements and so there is a potential risk that the heat produced during the setting reaction could cause pulpal

Table 12.2 Typical chemical constituents of zinc phosphate cement

Constituent	Reason for inclusion	Amount (%)
Powder		
Zinc oxide	Main reactive ingredient	89–92
Magnesium oxide	Maintains white colour Increases compressive strength	3–10
Aluminium oxide	Improves mechanical properties	0–6.8
Silicon dioxide	Affects colour Aids the calcination process	0–2.1
Stannous or tannin fluoride	Leaching of fluoride	<2
Liquid		
Phosphoric acid	Main reactive ingredient	38
Water	Aqueous solution with the phosphoric acid	30–40
Phosphoric acid combined with aluminium	Buffer, essential to form the cement	1–3
Phosphoric acid combined with zinc	Buffer, stabilizes the pH and reduces the reactivity so increasing working time, which in turn facilitates the mixing of the cement	0–10

inflammation. There are two methods by which manufacturers attempt to reduce this:

- By including buffers in the liquid component
- Treating the powder by heating it to above 1000°C. The higher this temperature, the less reactive is the powder.

Heat treatment of the powder causes **granulation** which, as the name suggests, converts the product into granules. The product is then sintered with other less reactive oxides (Figure 12.3) before being ground to a fine powder. The smaller the particles are ground, the greater is their reactivity.

> **Sintering:** a heating process to densify and purify a mixture of components. Heating is carried out below the temperature of the lowest melting component.
> **Densify:** to heat a product so that its particles coalesce but no ingredients are lost in the process. This can be compared to melting an Aero bar (Nestlé). None of the chocolate is lost, but as its constituents come closer together as a result of the heating, its volume decreases.

As well as varying the particle size, the reactivity of the powder also depends on the degree of calcination and its composition.

> **Calcination:** process of heating a raw material or ore to thermally decompose it with the loss of volatiles in gaseous form.

Mixing on a cooled glass slab permits the heat produced in the reaction to dissipate more easily and slows the chemical reaction, providing the dentist with a longer time for manipulation of the cement. Care must be taken not to cool the slab below the dew point or water condensation will form and affect the properties of the cement (Figure 12.4). Further regulation of the rate of setting is possible by varying the rate of incorporation of the powder to the liquid. The slower the incorporation of the powder fraction, the more slowly the cement will set. This is partly due to the fact that there is a reduction in temperature rise observed as each increment of cement powder starts to react at a different time. All of these factors may be used in the clinic to control the setting time of the cement.

Dimensional stability

The cement shrinks slightly during the setting reaction. This is probably not significant with respect to its clinical behaviour.

Lute thickness

Depending on the size of the particles of zinc oxide, the cement lute gained with this material is the thinnest of all the currently available luting agents. Generally quoted figures state that the cement lute is approximately 25 μm (range 15–40 μm).

Mode of retention

Zinc phosphate cements do not adhere to either tooth tissue or restorative materials. They function by grouting the potential space between the cast and tooth preparation. The cement forms tags between the micro-irregularities on the two surfaces being luted. For this reason these surfaces should not be polished. In fact, sandblasting the fitting surface of the cast restoration prior to luting will increase retention.

Solubility

This material has a low solubility. However, any change in the water content of the liquid component can adversely affect the set cement. That is, there is crystallization of the matrix, which leads to a weakening of the cement structure.

Erosion

While the solubility of the cement is low, it further reduces with age as the cement matures and the water becomes bound into the matrix. The set cement starts to erode in an acid medium when the pH drops below 4.5, and the erosion becomes more marked with increasing

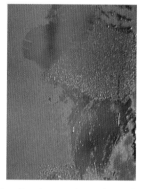

Fig. 12.4 Water droplets forming on the surface of glass slab after it has been cooled too much.

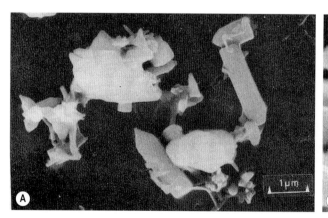
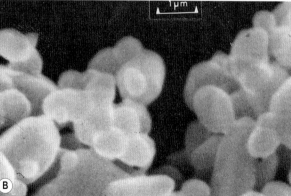

Fig. 12.3 (A) Zinc oxide powder produced from zinc oxalate as a result of sintering. (B) Note the reduction in size and the alteration in shape achieved by raising the temperature to below the melting point of the solid.
(From Prosser and Wilson 1982, J of Biomedical Materials Research 16, 585–98).

acidity. In the clinical scenario, the set cement exposed to the oral environment will be subjected to cyclical changes in pH, which frequently falls below 4.5 (see Chapter 1).

Viscosity

The material's viscosity increases as setting starts. To enable full seating of the cast restoration and to achieve the optimal film thickness, the dentist must either maintain the seating pressure on the cast restoration or vent the restoration, especially if it is a full crown.

The cementation process should therefore be completed with minimum delay.

Cariostatic properties

Inclusion of fluoride into the cement may impart some cariostatic properties. This is borne out clinically as little caries is seen under inlays when the cement has washed out over time. The addition of the fluoride salt does, however weaken the cement because it is present as inclusions which disrupt the matrix.

Mechanical properties

The mechanical properties of the final cement are dependent on the powder/liquid ratio used. The mechanical properties increase with increased powder content until a point is reached where the material will not mix to a homogeneous mass. The more powder that is incorporated, the thicker the cement lute that is produced. The consistency of the mixed cement produced will depend on the clinical indication. Table 12.3 sets out the effects of some handling variables on the properties of the final cement.

Zinc phosphate, zinc polycarboxylate and zinc oxide eugenol cements have a common base, zinc oxide. However, the powder supplied by the manufacturer usually has a different chemical composition depending on the material. In other words, the powder is not composed solely of zinc oxide. These powders should therefore not be used interchangeably as mixing and matching them will produce a substandard product.

Effect of the acid

Phosphoric acid is highly acidic and for this reason there has been concern that its acidity may have detrimental effects on the pulp, such as pulpal inflammation and possibly pulpal death. Clinically this would manifest as postoperative sensitivity or pain. The more liquid that is used, the greater is the initial acidity of the cement. In very runny mixes

the pH could be as low as 2. Stiffer mixes produce an initial pH of about 3. It is known that the pH approaches neutrality with time. However, the more liquid used, the longer it takes for the pH to rise. Generally the pH is higher than 4 at 60 minutes after mixing and returns to neutral after 24 hours. The moisture in dentine can have a buffering effect.

There is still no evidence to confirm whether the incidence of pulpal death or postoperative pain is higher with these cements when compared with other cements. This is not particularly surprising in that the acidic nature of the cement is not very different from that of the etching gels used currently as part of the adhesive process with resin-based filling materials. The pulpal reactions which have been reported are more likely to be attributable to the porosity of the cement and consequential bacterial leakage. However, if the clinician is concerned, they may choose to apply a cavity varnish (see p. 181) as a barrier in an attempt to reduce or eliminate postoperative sensitivity. Alternatively, another material could be selected as a base.

Advantages and disadvantages

The advantages and disadvantages of zinc phosphate cement are set out in Table 12.4.

> **Sharp set:** a short time interval between the end of working time and the completion of set.

The set material is opaque and thus it may shine through all ceramic restorations, which can compromise the aesthetic result. Another luting material may therefore be more appropriate for use in this situation if this is a potential concern.

Table 12.4 Advantages and disadvantages of zinc phosphate cements

Advantages	Disadvantages
Easy to mix	Possibly irritant to the pulp
Sharp set	Does not bond to tooth tissue or restorative materials
Acceptable properties for purpose	Brittle
Cheap	No antibacterial effects
Long successful track record	Soluble in the mouth
	Opaque

Table 12.3 Handling variables influencing the properties of zinc phosphate cement

Handling variables	Property				
	Compressive strength	Film thickness	Solubility	Acidity	Setting time
Reduced powder/liquid ratio	Reduced	Reduced	Increased	Increased	Increased
Increased rate of powder incorporation	Reduced	Increased	Increased	Increased	Reduced
Increased mixing temperature	Reduced	Increased	Increased	Increased	Reduced
Water contamination	Reduced	Increased	Increased	Increased	Reduced

Indications and contraindications

Indications and contraindication are set out in Table 12.5.

Table 12.5 Indications and contraindications of zinc phosphate cement

Indications	Contraindications
Definitive cementation of inlays, metal-based crowns, metal-based bridges and orthodontic bands	Definitive cementation of all ceramic crowns and bridges
As a base	When in very close proximity to the pulp without another intermediate material such as calcium hydroxide
Temporary restorations where adequate retention is present	

When using zinc phosphate to lute orthodontic bands, the cement should be at a consistency between that used to lute castings and that used for bases or temporary restorations.

Commercially available products

Commercially available products are shown in Table 12.6.

Table 12.6 Some zinc phosphate cements currently available on the market

Product name	Manufacturer
De Trey Zinc	Dentsply
Hy-Bond Zinc Phosphate Cement	Shofu
Zinc Cement	SS White
Zinc Phosphate Cement	Heraeus

Mixing

It is very important that the cement is mixed correctly as the properties of the cement will be determined by the reaction between the powder and liquid. The recommended method of mixing zinc phosphate cement to lute a cast restoration is illustrated in Box 12.1 and should be followed precisely.

The bottle containing the liquid should only be open to the atmosphere for the shortest possible time necessary to dispense the liquid. If the stopper is left off for any extended period of time, water will either be lost or gained depending on the humidity and temperature of the surrounding environment. This will adversely affect the setting reaction and the final physical properties of the cement. If the liquid is cloudy or crystals are present in the bottle, the material should be discarded, as the concentration of the acid will have changed and will no longer be optimal.

The dental nurse should not continue to mix the cement after its viscosity has started to increase. This is because it means that the zinc phosphate matrix is starting to form (i.e. the material is beginning to set). Further mixing at this stage will significantly weaken the cement by disrupting the salt matrix formation.

Moisture control

Good moisture control is important when placing these materials as water contamination will adversely affect the setting reaction and cement's final physical properties.

Summary

Some (more traditional) operators still use this material routinely but zinc phosphate cement is less frequently used in current practice mainly as developments of other cements which have superseded it.

ZINC POLYCARBOXYLATE (POLYALKENOATE/POLYACRYLATE) CEMENTS

Chemical constituents

When **zinc oxide** powder is mixed with **poly(acrylic acid)** liquid, **zinc polycarboxylate** cement is produced, this being the primary chemical reaction. The cement is also referred to as **zinc polyacrylate** or strictly speaking, in modern chemical terminology, **zinc polyalkenoate**.

Most products are presented as a powder, which is primarily zinc oxide (Table 12.7). The powder is mixed with the liquid, a viscous

Table 12.7 Typical chemical constituents of zinc polycarboxylate cement

Constituent	Reason for inclusion	Amount (%)
Powder		
Zinc oxide	Main reactive ingredient	85–96
Stannous fluoride	Improves the set Leaches fluoride – anti-cariogenic Improves mixing qualities Enhances strength by about 50%	4
Magnesium oxide	Acts as a densifier Preserves white colouration	4–10
Silica	Improves sintering process	0–2
Alumina	Can form complexes with acid	<5
Liquid		
Poly(acrylic acid) 32–42% aqueous solution (copolymer)	Main reactive ingredient	32–43
Itaconic acid	Stabilizes liquid to prevent gelation Substitutes for some of poly(acrylic acid)	trace
Maleic acid	Substitutes for some of poly(acrylic acid) as it is more reactive due to its two carboxylate groups	32–43

Box 12.1 Protocol for mixing zinc phosphate cement to lute a cast restoration

Step 1	Step 2	Step 3	Step 4	Step 5	Step 6	Step 7
Shake both bottles prior to dispensation	Cool glass slab but not too much! (Figure 12.4)	The proportion of powder and liquid is not measured precisely	Incorporate the powder into the liquid in small increments (4–6)	Mix the material over a wide area of the slab	Luting consistency strings 2.5 cm above the slab	Apply the cement to the restoration and not the preparation. Complete the procedure within 60–90 seconds
Reason	Reason	Reason	Reason	Reason	Reason	Reason
Ensures all the constituents are mixed together	Decreasing the slab temperature will increase the working time (see p. 164)	The consistency of the cement required will be gained by experience	This delays the onset of setting so increasing working time. Also allows the heat to dissipate	This keeps the temperature of the mix lower, increasing working time	The cement is correctly mixed and ready for use	The intraoral temperature is higher than the cast. Placing the cement onto the cast will increase working time

solution of poly(acrylic acid). Some manufacturers, however, vacuum dry the poly(acrylic acid) and add it to the zinc oxide powder. In these products the setting reaction is initiated by the addition of water to the powder.

The advantage of blending the poly(acrylic acid) and zinc oxide together in one composition is that the component will be in optimized proportions for use. The disadvantage is that the powder must be kept completely dry or the setting reaction will commence prematurely. In climates where the humidity is high this can be a major problem even with a desiccant being incorporated into the storage bottle cap (see Figure 9.19, p. 114).

In those presentations where the poly(acrylic acid) is in an aqueous form there is a risk that loss of water from the solution will cause thickening of the mixture making mixing more difficult. It also adversely affects the concentration of the acid solution. It is essential that the liquid container is kept sealed at all times except during dispensation.

Powder manufacturing process

The most common method of preparing the powder is to heat the two main ingredients for 9 hours to sinter the constituents. This is similar to the manufacture of zinc oxide powder for the zinc phosphate cements. The sintered mass is ground to reduce particle size and then reheated for a further 8–12 hours. Pigments are added to control shades.

Other chemicals (such a stannous or strontium fluoride) have been added to some products in an attempt to confer the benefits of fluoride leaching. The fluoride release is transitory and usually stops within 30 days. Stannous fluoride also enhances the mixing and mechanical properties and the set of the cement.

Setting reaction and structure

When the zinc oxide and poly(acrylic acid) come into contact, a salt (zinc polyacrylate) matrix is formed only on the surface of the zinc oxide particles. Poly(acrylic acid) chains cross-link through the zinc ions of the zinc oxide. The set material has cores of zinc oxide within the zinc polyacrylate matrix binding the unreacted zinc oxide cores together as previously described.

The mixed cement goes through a rubbery phase as it is setting and it should not be disturbed during this phase. This is because the adhesive bond of the cement will be ruptured. There is a risk that microleakage will then occur if the cement has been pulled away from the tooth surface. The cement should be left undisturbed until it can be fractured away cleanly from the margin of a cemented restoration.

Properties

Mechanical properties

The compressive strength of zinc polycarboxylate is less than that of zinc phosphate cement. Once set, the cement has a lower modulus and is therefore slightly more elastic and less likely to fracture under heavy load. While it appears thick after mixing, the cement is more fluid and it exhibits shear thinning under load allowing restorations to be seated completely under pressure.

Biocompatibility

Poly(acrylic acid) is a weak acid with a relatively high molecular weight. As such it will not diffuse readily along the dentinal tubules and is rapidly immobilized in them. The cement's pH returns to neutral within a short period of time after mixing and the cement is less acidic than zinc phosphate. The biological compatibility of the cement with the pulp is regarded as being excellent. There is some release of zinc fluoride and poly(acrylic acid) but these do not appear to affect the tissues in clinical use.

Viscosity

Mixing these cements has proved to be difficult as the viscous nature of the poly(acrylic acid) when in liquid form often results in less powder being incorporated into the mix than is recommended by the manufacturer. This in turn results in inferior properties. One reason that the materials which contain vacuum-dried poly(acrylic acid) were produced was to improve the mixing properties of the cements. This has enhanced the mixing properties to some extent but these cements are still notoriously difficult to mix. The material's viscosity increases as setting starts and the material stretches if disturbed with a probe before setting is complete. It returns to its original position but the seal between restoration and tooth will be compromised. This effect is termed **rebound**.

Lute thickness

Film thickness has been reported to vary from 20 to 100 µm but this is dependent on the plasticity of the cement at the time of placement. The longer the material has been mixed, the lower the plasticity and hence the thicker the cement lute. The minimum cement lute thickness is governed by the particle size of the cement powder.

Solubility

Solubility of the cement is relatively low, ranging from 0.1% to 0.6% after 24 hours. One of the disadvantages of the addition of stannous fluoride is that it tends to increase the dissolution. This process appears to start at the site of the zinc oxide particles and the solubility increases with increasing concentrations of magnesium oxide in the powder.

Erosion

The cement is prone to erosion as the pH of the mouth becomes more acidic. In fact, this type of material exhibits less resistant to erosion than the zinc phosphate cements.

Aesthetics

The presence of a substantial volume of zinc oxide in the set cement results in a rather opaque cement which necessitates using a tinted cement in cementation of ceramic restorations. Opacity may be a problem for all ceramic restorations especially at the margins, thus as with zinc phosphate cement this property may preclude its use.

Adhesion

Glass ionomer cement and zinc polycarboxylate cement are based on the same liquid, poly(acrylic acid) so they adhere to tooth tissue in the same way (a chelation reaction with the calcium ions in enamel and dentine). The bond to enamel is better than dentine due to the increased amount of calcium ions available. It is also believed some subsidiary collagen bonding also contributes to the adhesion. Clinically this means that zinc polycarboxylate cements can be used in non-retentive cavities and for luting crowns. Good moisture control is important when these cements are placed as the presence of saliva reduces bond strength to enamel considerably. Those cements containing fluoride appear to bond better.

The cements will also bond to metals. However, the bond strength is reduced where there is little or no oxide formation on the metal. More effective bonding to precious metal may be achieved by **tin plating** the surface to be bonded. Alternatively the fitting surface may be **sand blasted** to surface-activate it and increase the bond strength. Zinc polycarboxylate cements are particularly effective when used with stainless steel bands. The bond is durable and frequently failure of the bond is cohesive rather than at the junction between the cement and restoration substructure. It has no chemical reaction with ceramic materials and retention is by micromechanical interlocking.

> **Cohesive failure:** failure within a material rather than at the interface between it and another material.
> **Adhesive failure:** failure at the interface between two different materials.

Zinc polycarboxylate materials bond effectively to stainless steel. Care should therefore be taken to totally remove any set material from instruments prior to sterilization. If instruments with cement on them are subjected to high temperatures in the autoclave, the cement will bake onto the instruments, making its removal all but impossible thereafter. Placing the glass slab and stainless steel instruments in water immediately after use will facilitate cleaning (Figure 12.5). Alternatively, an alcohol wipe can be used to remove the unset cement from the instruments although is more difficult as the cement is itself sticky.

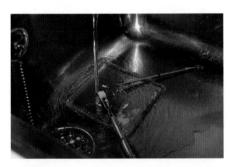

Fig. 12.5 The glass mixing slab and the instruments used to mix zinc polycarboxylate cement are placed under running water immediately after use to facilitate cleaning.

Powder/liquid ratio

The more zinc oxide powder added to the liquid, the stronger will be the cement but its ability to bond is reduced as there is less poly(acrylic acid) freely available to bond with the calcium in the dentine. The amount of powder added to the liquid will also depend on the application. A mix required to lute a crown has to be much thinner (less viscous) than one required for a temporary restoration that may be subjected to higher forces being placed on the material during function.

Advantages and disadvantages

Advantages and disadvantages of zinc polycarboxlylate cement are set out in Table 12.8.

Table 12.8 Advantages and disadvantages of zinc polycarboxylate cements

Advantages	Disadvantages
Bonds to tooth tissue or restorative materials	Difficult to mix
Long-term durability	Opaque
Acceptable mechanical properties	Soluble in the mouth particularly where stannous fluoride is incorporated in the powder
Relatively inexpensive	Difficult to manipulate
Long and successful track record	Ill-defined set

Indications

Zinc polycarboxylate cement has a variety of uses:

- Temporary restorations (see Box 12.2):
  - Non-retentive cavities: as chemical bonding occurs between the cement and the tooth tissue, zinc polycarboxylates are particularly useful to temporarily restore non-retentive cavities so avoiding needless tooth tissue removal to create mechanical retention

Box 12.2 Correct procedure for mixing a zinc polycarboxylate cement as a temporary restoration, using Poly F Plus (Dentsply)

Step 1	Step 2	Step 3	Step 4	Step 5
		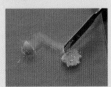	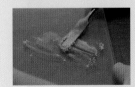	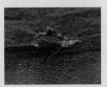
Shake the bottles. Dispense the correct amount of powder by using the scoop (two scoops) provided	Place two drops of liquid adjacent to the powder on a (cooled) glass slab. Divide each scoop into two increments	Work one increment initially into the liquid and mix	Combine the other increments into the mix quickly and continue to spatulate mix until all the powder is incorporated into the mix. Takes 30–40 seconds	Collect the final mixed mass and gather on the edge of the slab for presentation to the dentist

- Inflamed pulp: due to its low flow characteristics this cement is unable to enter the dentinal tubules; it is sedative and can be used in cases where the patient has been experiencing pulpal pain
- Where resin-based composite is envisaged to be used subsequently: this is because there is no eugenol present in the material (eugenol use is contraindicated with resin-based composites – see p. 82)

- Bases: the adhesive properties of these cements fulfil the role of a base as they will seal the dentine, but their manipulation presents difficulties. Due to the difficult handling characteristics of the material, i.e. it sticks to instruments often displacing the cement already placed, its usage for this indication has decreased in favour of other cements such as a resin-modified glass ionomer cement
- Definitive luting of metal/metal ceramic crowns/core-reinforced ceramic crowns
- Cementation of orthodontic bands.

Commercially available products

Commercially available products are shown in Table 12.9 and Figure 12.6.

Table 12.9 Some zinc polycarboxylate cements currently available on the market and their potential uses

Product name	Manufacturer	Potential uses		
		Temporary restorations	Base	Luting
Durelon (inc Maxicap)	3M ESPE	√	√	√
Hy Bond Polycarboxylate Cement	Shofu	√	√	√
Poly F Plus	Dentsply	√	√	√
Polycarboxylate Cement	Heraeus	√	√	√

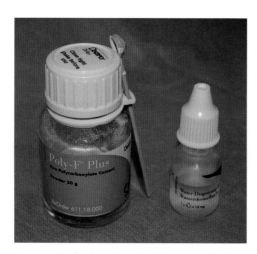

Fig. 12.6 An example of a zinc polycarboxylate cement (Poly F Plus, Dentsply).

Mixing

As previously mentioned, the consistency of the mixed cement will depend on the application for which the cement is used. The powder to liquid ratio is changed to achieve this. It is advisable that a glass mixing slab is used. The viscosity of the liquid and the mixed material means that a large stable surface area facilitates the mixing, which may be difficult to achieve on a paper pad.

 Accurate proportioning of components of a cement

After shaking the bottle, collect the powder in the measuring scoop. Any excess above the top of the scoop should be removed by drawing the scoop against the flat bar across the top of the inside of the bottle. This ensures that the correct amount of powder required for the mix is dispensed (Figures 12.7 and 12.8).

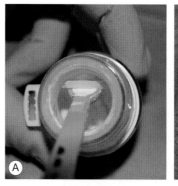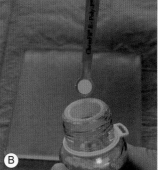

Fig. 12.7A,B Dispensation of the correct volume of powder for the cement.

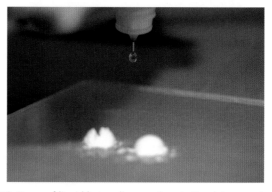

Fig. 12.8 Drops of liquid being dispensed on to the slab separate from the powder. The bottle is held vertically to ensure that the correct volume of liquid is dispensed. The powder has already been dispensed as this obviates any risk of powder contaminating the liquid before mixing commences. This is similar to mixing a glass ionomer cement.

A dappens dish of isopropyl alcohol should be available to act as a separator when placing zinc polycarboxylate cements. Applying alcohol to the surface of the setting cement will render it smooth using either an instrument or a gloved finger! The alcohol can also be used to remove excess unset material from instruments.

Box 12.3 Correct procedure for mixing a zinc polycarboxylate cement to lute a cast restoration, using Poly F Plus (Dentsply)

Step 1

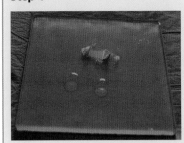

Shake the bottles. Consider cooling the glass slab to increase working time. Place one scoop of powder and two drops of liquid close together on the slab

Step 2

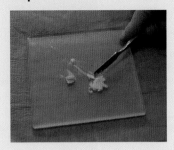

Incorporate all the powder into the liquid as rapidly as possible. Mix for 30–40 seconds. Use a small area of the slab

Step 3

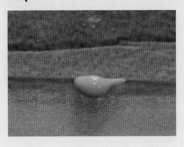

End of mix. Note the creamy final consistency

Luting

See Box 12.3. The mixing of this cement has been termed pseudo-plastic: that is, as spatulation increases so does the force placed on the cement and as a consequence its flow increases.

- The liquid should never be refrigerated as the poly(acrylic acid) may develop a jelly-like (gel) consistency due to hydrogen bonding and then cannot be used.
- It is not a problem if the cement appears too thick as it will flow under pressure. A runnier consistency should *never* be prepared as this will seriously compromise the properties of the final cement.
- The cement is no longer useable when its lustre is lost and it becomes stringy. This is termed as becoming '**cobwebbed**' (Figure 12.9).

- Zinc polycarboxylate cement flows under (intermittent) pressure. When seating a crown the dentist should allow the long poly(acrylic acid) molecule to unravel so that stress is not created in the cement lute. This is done by seating the crown axially then removing the force on the cast before reapplying it. This may be done twice or thrice. Failure to do this may result in a white cement luting line being seen at the margin.
- Zinc polycarboxylate cements have a short working time. This may pose a problem when multiple units must be cemented at the same time, for example a bridge with many retainers. Cooling a glass slab will slightly reduce the setting time and therefore increase the working time. Good team work between the dentist and dental nurse in this case is critical to ensure efficient mixing, placement into the retainers and then seating of the multiple unit restoration without delay.

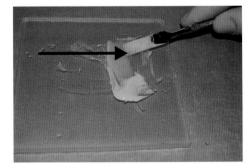

Fig. 12.9 A zinc polycarboxylate cement beyond the point of being used clinically. Note the stringy consistency with a strand linking the spatula and the glass slab.

ZINC OXIDE EUGENOL CEMENT

Chemical constituents

Zinc oxide eugenol cements have also been used in restorative dentistry for many years as they were believed to have a sedative effect on the pulp. The familiar smell of **oil of clove (eugenol)** is synonymous with the atmosphere of the dental surgery. Their usage has decreased in the past few years but they are still widely used in contemporary practice. The principal reaction is that of **zinc oxide** with **eugenol** but manufacturers have added various other chemicals in an attempt to improve the cement's physical properties.

Depending on the intended usage, zinc oxide eugenol products are available in two forms: **powder and liquid** (Figure 12.10 and Table 12.10) or a **two-paste** (Figure 12.11 and Table 12.11) cements. The two-paste presentation is mainly used as an endodontic sealer or temporary luting cement and these indications are discussed further below as well as in Chapters 13 and 14, respectively.

A small quantity of zinc acetate is added to accelerate the set of the material as it creates a more reactive medium in which the setting reaction can occur. The zinc oxide used in these cements differs from

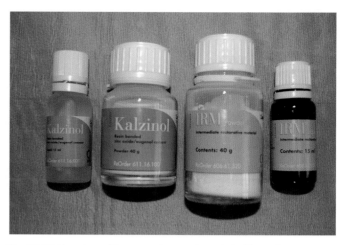

Fig. 12.10 Two zinc oxide eugenol cements made by Dentsply.

Table 12.10 Typical chemical constituents of a zinc oxide eugenol cement

Constituent	Reason for inclusion	Amount (%)
Powder		
Zinc oxide	Main reactive chemical	69
Rosin	Reduces brittleness	29
Zinc acetate or other salts	Accelerator	0.1–8
Zinc stearate	Plasticizer	1
Liquid		
Eugenol	Main reactive chemical	85–95
Olive or cotton seed oil	Modifies viscosity Masks taste of eugenol	5–15
Acetic acid	Accelerator	0.1–2

Table 12.11 Typical chemical constituents of a two-paste zinc oxide eugenol cement

Constituent	Reason for inclusion	Amount (%)
Base		
Zinc oxide	Main reactive salt former	69
Rosin	Reduces brittleness	29
Zinc acetate or other salts	accelerator	1
Accelerator		
Eugenol	Main reactive salt former	85–95
Other oils	Modify viscosity Mask taste of eugenol	5–15

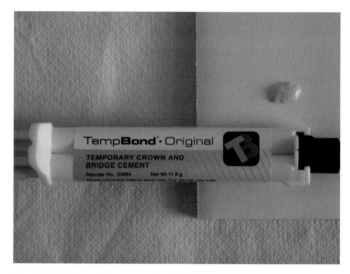

Fig. 12.11 A zinc oxide eugenol-containing temporary cement (TempBond, Kerr Hawe).

that in the zinc phosphate cements in that it is an active form and is prepared by thermal decomposition of zinc salts at 350–400°C. This underlines that the zinc oxide powders of different cements should not be mixed or interchanged.

Reinforced materials

The plain zinc oxide eugenol cement is weak and mainly used as temporary cement. Different chemicals have been added in an attempt to improve the strength and the material's inherent poor long-term stability in water by reducing the solubility. The composition of individual materials within this category is quite varied (see Table 12.12).

EBA-reinforced zinc oxide eugenol cements

Ortho-ethoxybenzoic acid (**EBA**) is added to zinc oxide eugenol cements to increase their mechanical properties. EBA forms a crystalline form of zinc eugenolate which is stronger and less soluble. A higher powder to liquid ratio can be used (up to 7:1) and will enhance the strength of the cement.

The liquid in this type of cement is a mixture of 62.5% EBA and 37.5% eugenol. The powder has also been modified as **hydrogenated rosins** are commonly added (6%) to reduce brittleness and film thickness, facilitating mixing.

The setting characteristics of the EBA-reinforced cement are more or less the same as zinc oxide eugenol cements. The material is also affected by moisture in the same way as other zinc oxide eugenol products. Depending on the mixture produced when the cement is mixed, its film thickness may vary and is generally between 25 and 35 μm. EBA-containing cements should be mixed on a glass slab. The powder should be incorporated as quickly as possible in large increments or at once into the liquid. These products are not used so much in the UK these days but are still widely available in the USA.

Setting reaction and structure

EBA-reinforced cements are usually presented as a powder and liquid and when they are mixed together a set cement of amorphous zinc eugenolate is formed by a chelation reaction. The eugenol is not an aqueous solution but forms a salt with zinc oxide. Additionally, another salt is formed, zinc 2-ethoxybenzoate. As with zinc phosphate cements, the set material has cores of zinc oxide set in the zinc eugenolate/zinc 2-ethoxybenzoate matrix, which binds to the surface layer of the zinc oxide particles (Figure 12.12). A small amount of water is required to act both as an initiator and a catalyst for the setting reaction.

The rate of setting of the cement depends on:

- The powder particle size
- The amount of accelerator added to the liquid

The setting reaction of eugenol-containing cements is catalysed by water. Exposure to water or heat will make the cement set more rapidly.

- The powder/liquid ratio: increasing the powder/liquid ratio accelerates the set.

Properties

Mechanical properties

Zinc oxide eugenol cements have poorer mechanical properties than other dental cements. They may break down during amalgam condensation or under occlusal load. When this cement is used as a cavity base, it should be used in a thickness of more than 2 mm for it to have sufficient strength to function effectively. Additionally, the cement mass may contain air voids causing it to collapse under load and leave the restoration unsupported, leading to failure. However, they do appear to perform satisfactorily in clinical use.

Biocompatibility

Traditionally, zinc oxide eugenol cements have been used as a temporary restoration. The set cement is neutral in pH and for this reason is regarded as a bland (sedative) material to the dental tissues. It is bactericidal as it inhibits bacterial metabolism. This reduces bacterial leakage and hence reduces pulpal inflammation. However, if eugenol-containing cement is placed directly onto vital pulp tissue, an acute inflammatory reaction will result and the patient will complain of pain. The presence of an intervening dentine layer appears to modify the pulpal response.

The high level of filler makes the material a good insulator with low thermal and electrical diffusivity. For this reason it was used

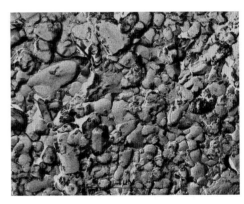

Fig. 12.12 Scanning electron micrograph showing a set zinc oxide eugenol cement. The zinc oxide particles are covered by the zinc eugenolate matrix, which holds the cement together.
(From Wilson Clinton and Miller 1973 J Dent Res 52, 253–60).

Table 12.12 Composition of reinforced zinc oxide and eugenol cements

Zinc oxide (%)	Reinforcing chemical (%)		Chemical present in	Reason for inclusion	Generic name	Product examples (manufacturer)
80	Polymethylmethacrylate	20	Either as an inclusion on its own or as coating to the powder	Increases strength	Polymer reinforced	IRM (Dentsply)
90	Polystyrene	10	Liquid	Increases strength	Polystyrene bonded	Kalzinol (Dentsply)
60–75	Alumina/fused quartz	20–35	Powder	Reinforcing agent	EBA cements	SuperEBA (Bosworth)
90	Hydrogenated rosin	10	Powder	Reinforcing agent	EBA cements	SuperEBA (Bosworth)

extensively, especially under metallic restorations. Unfortunately, this meant that more tooth tissue often needed to be sacrificed to accommodate both layers of material. The use of this type of cement has decreased because modern thinking entails:

- Removing only the minimal amount of tooth tissue possible and adapting the restorative material to the clinical conditions
- Microleakage prevention (and therefore pulpal inflammation) by dentinal tubule occlusion and not by thickness of lining material or thermal insulation.

Eugenol is cytotoxic to pulpal tissue leading to pulpal necrosis. Direct placement on an exposed pulp is therefore contraindicated. A thin layer of setting calcium hydroxide cement should be placed on the pulpal floor prior to the placement of a eugenol-containing cement if micro-exposure is suspected.

Mode of retention

Zinc oxide eugenol cement does not have any chemical adhesion to tooth tissue or other dental materials. Thus a cavity into which such a cement will be placed must therefore be mechanically retentive and this fact may limit its use. Rather than remove more (sound) tooth to create a retentive cavity, another material which does adhere to the tooth or restoration (such as zinc polycarboxylate or glass ionomer cement) may be selected instead. The cement's retention may, however, be enhanced by micromechanical means.

If a eugenol-containing material has not been used for some time, the liquid has a tendency to thicken as some of its volatile solvent is lost by evaporation. This makes the material difficult to mix as it may be very stiff to handle. The cap should be kept on the bottle at all times other than during liquid dispensation. The expiry date should also be checked.

Solubility

One of the drawbacks of this family of materials is high solubility in water. Eugenol is constantly released from the cement, which consequently gradually breaks down. The cement hydrolyses to leave soft zinc hydroxide, which will slowly wash away. For this reason it is not generally recommended for use as a definitive luting cement.

Eugenol is known to adversely affect the polymerization setting reaction of resin composites and those materials containing polymerizable monomers. The eugenol will react with the resin composite causing it to plasticize. This will have a detrimental effect on the mechanical properties of the restorative. Therefore the cement should not be used as a base under such materials.

Any tooth tissue which has been in contact with a eugenol-containing cement may be contaminated. It is therefore inadvisable to place eugenol-containing products onto prepared enamel and dentine where the definitive restoration is likely to contain resin composite or where a resin composite system is being used as an intermediate layer, for example in bonding.

Similarly eugenol reacts with addition silicone impression materials, and these should not be selected where eugenol has been used previously.

Advantages and disadvantages

The advantages and disadvantages of zinc eugenol cements are set out in Table 12.13.

Table 12.13 Advantages and disadvantages of zinc oxide eugenol cements

Advantages	Disadvantages
Sedative	Difficult to mix
Bactericidal	Opaque
Adequate mechanical properties	Does not bond to tooth tissue or restorative materials
Inexpensive	Interacts with resin composite
Good and long track record	Soluble in the mouth

Indications and contraindications

As well as being mainly used as a dental cement, zinc oxide eugenol-containing products are used for many other purposes: see Table 12.14.

Table 12.14 Indications and contraindications of zinc oxide eugenol materials

Indications	Contraindications
Temporary restorations	Temporary restorations in non-retentive cavities
As a base	Direct placement on an exposed pulp
(Temporary) luting of cast restorations	Under a resin composite-containing material
Long-term temporary restorations	Definitive luting of cast restorations
Root end fillings	Where a resin composite-containing material may be used in future
Endodontic sealer	Where resin-based materials are being used as an intermediate layer between restoration and tooth
Impression material (working cast/rebase/reline of dentures)	Where the cement will be exposed to oral and tissue fluids as it will slowly dissolve

Temporary luting cements

Zinc oxide eugenol cements can also be used to lute temporary crowns and bridges and be used for trial cementation of definitive indirect restorations to assess the aesthetics and occlusion.

They are usually presented as a bespoke two paste system. Many of the powder and liquid presentations are also indicated for temporary luting. Their film thickness is 25 µm. The cements are also unreinforced and therefore soft, which facilitates the easy removal of the temporary restoration. The set material is quite rigid in nature and this is advantageous as, if left to set, it can be easily and cleanly chipped away from the margins of the crown using a probe.

- The dentist should wait until the excess material is fully set before removing it. It may seem a longer wait but the clean-up will be much quicker and less messy.
- Zinc oxide eugenol-containing products stick to hard and soft tissues. This can be avoided by coating the soft tissues with petroleum jelly prior to their use or using oil of orange (Orange solvent) on a cotton wool roll or gauze to remove any smeared, set temporary cements.
- Additionally, a third tube is presented with this product called a '**modifier**'. The modifier acts to retard the final set and produces a softer set cement (see Chapter 14). This aids the removal of the temporary restoration particularly when the preparation is very retentive. Alternatively petroleum jelly may be mixed with the cement to have the same effect.

Non-hardening materials which are also based on zinc oxide eugenol are also available for short-term trial cementation such as Opotow Trial Cement (Teledyne Water Pik). For more information on this, see Chapter 14.

Long-term temporization

Due to it superior strength, IRM (Intermediate Restorative Material) (Dentsply) is indicated for longer-term temporization. It also has high wear resistance and so temporized teeth can be maintained in the correct occlusal relationship. The use of this material is indicated in patients with high caries rates and with many teeth requiring stabilization prior to definitive restoration. It can also be used to build up badly destroyed teeth and in particular when an extensively restored tooth has been investigated prior to the commencement of endodontic therapy.

The need for a temporary restoration which is dependable, strong and is capable of maintaining a good coronal seal is particularly desirable while an endodontic procedure is being performed. Reinforced zinc oxide eugenol materials among others have a significant role to play in this situation. The materials used for inter-visit restorations in a patient undergoing an endodontic procedure are discussed in more detail in Chapter 13.

Other uses for zinc oxide eugenol-containing materials

As mentioned earlier, zinc oxide eugenol-containing materials have other uses apart from dental cements:

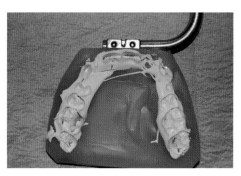

Fig. 12.13 Zinc oxide eugenol temporary cement being used on the wax wafer of a facebow registration to improve the definition of the tooth indentations.

- Improved definition: the rigid nature of these cements combined with their good surface detail is ideal to improve the definition on a facebow wax wafer (Figure 12.13). This is particularly so when the study casts have been constructed with an elastomer impression material as its accuracy is much greater than that of alginate.
- Endodontic sealers: the use of zinc oxide eugenol **endodontic sealers** is discussed in more detail in Chapter 13.
- Denture impression material: **impression paste** used to record edentulous ridges either as a second (working) impression or as a reline (rebase) is chemically zinc oxide eugenol (see Chapter 15).

Facebow: a device used by the dentist to record the relationship of the temporomandibular joint to the maxillary arch in three dimensions outwith the mouth so allowing the casts to be mounted onto an articulator.
Articulator: a device which holds the upper and lower study casts in the relationship to each other and may permit various movements that the mandible may make during function.

Commercially available products

There is a plethora of zinc oxide eugenol-containing materials on the market (Table 12.15). They vary in their exact chemical formulation determined by their indication.

Mixing

Box 12.4 shows the correct technique which should be employed when mixing zinc oxide eugenol cements.

Box 12.4 Protocol for mixing a zinc oxide eugenol cement

Step 1	Step 2	Step 3	Step 4	Step 5*	Step 6
	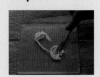				
Shake the bottle containing the powder. Dispense the powder and liquid in a ratio of approx 3:1. Ensure that the liquid is kept separate from the powder until mixing commences	Incorporate bulk of the powder into the liquid at one time. A glass slab and a stainless steel spatula are used	Add further small increments until desired consistency is achieved	Increments are incorporated over a 30-second period until the desired consistency of mix is achieved	For EBA cements, mix for a further 60 seconds to ensure that all the powder is wetted by the liquid	Present to dentist in a sausage shape with a little powder to use as a separating medium

*Note the additional time in Step 5 that is required if an EBA cement is used.

Table 12.15 Some zinc oxide eugenol-containing materials currently available on the market

Product name	Manufacturer	Additional chemical	Uses						
			Temporary restoration	Long-term temporary	Base	Temporary luting of crowns	Root end filling	Endodontic sealer	Denture impression material
Cavity Lining	SS White	Acetic Acid	X	X	√	X	X	X	X
Hy Bond Zinc oxide Temporary Cement	Shofu	–	X	X	X	√	X	X	X
Impression paste	SS White	–	X	X	X	X	X	X	√
IRM	Dentsply	Acrylic	√	√	√	√	√	X	X
Kalsogen Plus	Dentsply	Polymer	√	X	√	√	X	X	X
Kalzinol	Dentsply	Polystyrene	√	X	√	√	X	X	X
Optotow Trial Cement	Teledyne Water Pik	–	X	X	X	√	X	X	X
Rely X Temp E	3M ESPE	–	X	X	X	√	X	X	X
Sedanol	Dentsply	–	√	X	√	√	X	X	X
SuperEBA	Bosworth	EBA	√	√	√	√	√	X	X
Temp Bond	Kerr Hawe	–	X	X	X	√	X	X	X
TubliSeal	Sybron Endo	–	X	X	X	X	X	√	X
TubliSeal EWT	Sybron Endo	4-allyl-2-metoxyphenacid resin and mineral oil	X	X	X	X	X	√	X

The mix has reached the correct consistency when it does not stick to gloves or instruments. It can then be picked up and rolled into a cylinder and packed into the cavity using a plugger or a flat plastic instrument. A little of the cement powder acts as a good separating medium on the instruments during this phase of the placement. The spatula and slab should then be wiped clean before the cement sets.

The EBA cements require to be mixed for a further 60 seconds after the initial 30 seconds taken for incorporation of the powder into the liquid. This ensures that the powder particles are sufficiently wetted by the liquid to achieve a good working consistency and form a cement that will set satisfactorily.

SETTING STEROID/ANTIBIOTIC CEMENT

Another product commercially available is based on zinc oxide eugenol cement but has been modified by the addition of a **steroid** and an **antibiotic** (Table 12.16). The cement is hard setting and is placed as a cavity base with the intention of the active ingredients having a therapeutic effect on the pulp.

Table 12.16 Chemical constituents of a steroid/antibiotic setting cement

Chemical	Reason for inclusion
Powder	
Demeclocycline hydrochloride	To kill microorganisms locally
Triamcinolone acetonide	To reduce pulpal inflammation
Zinc oxide	filler
Calcium hydroxide	pH controller
Barium sulphate	imparts radiopacity
Hardener F*	
Eugenol in rectified turpentine oil	Reacts with zinc oxide to form cement matrix
Hardener S*	
Eugenol	Reacts with zinc oxide to form cement matrix
Polyethylene glycol in rectified turpentine oil	Plasticizer

*Depending on the clinician's preference, the choice of hardener will determine rate of set of the materials. F, fast set; S, slow set.

Chemical constituents

Steroid component

The steroid contained in this cement is **triamcinolone**. It is believed to reduce pulpal inflammation by suppressing the inflammatory process and therefore the patient's symptoms of pain. Unfortunately, use of this chemical in this situation has been reported to cause pulpal necrosis. No reparative dentine is laid down as the odontoblasts are destroyed.

Antibiotic component

The cement also contains **demeclocycline**, which is a derivative of tetracycline, a broad-spectrum antibiotic. This medicament is included to kill any susceptible microorganisms present in the proximity of the cement as it only acts as a topical antibiotic. If the infection is more extensive, bacteria will proliferate away from the directly affected site but with a suppressed pulpal response, leading to pulpal necrosis in the long term.

> **Rectified:** a chemical process whereby a solvent has been purified by means of repeated distillation with the result that it is highly concentrated.

Advantages and disadvantages

The advantages and disadvantages of medicated zinc oxide/eugenol cement are set out in Table 12.17.

Table 12.17 Advantages and disadvantages of steroid/antibiotic cements

Advantages	Disadvantages
Sedative	Causes necrosis of dental pulp
Bactericidal	Opaque
Adequate mechanical properties	Does not bond to tooth tissue or restorative materials
Good and long track record	Interacts with resin composite Soluble in the mouth Corticosteroid suppresses any reparative processes

Indications and contraindications

This cement has been advocated for use in cases of irreversible pulpitis or periradicular periodontitis. The ideal treatment in these scenarios is the complete removal of microorganisms and necrotic tissue by preparing and disinfecting the root canal system. The cement's main indication is therefore as a palliative temporary restoration prior to root canal therapy, particularly when there is an exposed pulp due to caries. It should not be used when the pulpal inflammation is considered reversible nor should it be used as a definitive base.

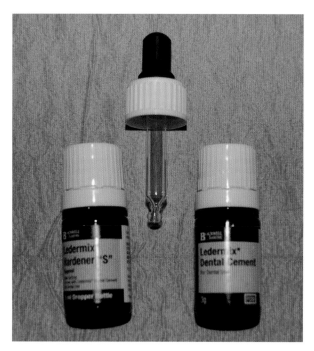

Fig. 12.14 An example of the steroid/antibiotic cement, Ledermix (Lederle).

Commercially available product

There is only one product available on the market. Ledermix (Lederle) is presented as a cement (Figure 12.14) and in paste form, the latter being used in endodontics. The indications for the paste presentation is dealt with in Chapter 13.

Mixing

The dentist should select the hardener to use depending on how quickly they wish the cement to set. Manufacturers report that the slow set catalyst retards the set by three to four times, although as with other products setting time is influenced by ambient temperature and humidity.

One drop of the selected hardener (depending on the speed of set required) should be placed on a glass slab with a small quantity of the powder. The two are combined together by mixing until a homogeneous mix is obtained. The mix is then collected and handed to the dentist for application to the cavity floor. The mixing sequence for this type of cement is the same as that for zinc oxide eugenol (see Box 12.4 above).

SETTING CALCIUM HYDROXIDE CEMENTS

Another group of traditional dental cements comprises the setting calcium hydroxide materials. In contrast to other cements discussed in this chapter, these materials are employed solely as lining materials. They should not be used as structural bases as they are relatively weak.

Chemical constituents

These cements are based on the reaction between **calcium hydroxide** and **salicylate esters** forming a **calcium disalicylate complex**.

They are presented as a two-paste system and the contents of a typical product are shown in Table 12.18.

A less satisfactory means of incorporating calcium hydroxide into a sublining for pulpal protection is by mixing calcium hydroxide with either distilled water or methylcellulose to form a non-setting paste. This is due to difficulties with the proportioning and mixing. Some light-curing calcium hydroxide cements are available but the chemistry means that the calcium hydroxide is not available for any reaction with the tooth as it is bound up in the resin.

Table 12.18 Typical formulation of calcium hydroxide chelating cements

Constituent	Reason for inclusion	Composition (%)
Base*		
Calcium hydroxide	Main reactive ingredient	51
Zinc hydroxide	Filler Imparts radiopacity	9–10
Zinc stearate	Filler	0.3
All of the above are suspended in a plasticizer, *N*-ethyl toluene sulphonamide (38%)		
Catalyst		
Titanium dioxide	Filler	13–14
Calcium sulphate	Filler	32
Calcium tungstate	Filler Imparts radiopacity	15.2
All of the above are suspended in 1-methyl trimethylene disalicylate butane-1-3-diol ester (39%)		
*Zinc oxide may be added as an additional filler and barium sulphate may be added as a radiopacifying agent.		

Setting reaction of the chelating calcium hydroxide cements and structure

The setting reaction is a **chelation** reaction between the **calcium** and **butylene glycol disalicylate**. It requires the presence of water to proceed and in the absence of water there is only a very slow reaction or no reaction at all. This explains why although calcium ions are available in the catalyst paste no reaction occurs. The reaction is slightly exothermic in nature but this is of negligible significance. The final structure is that of calcium disalicylate complexes surrounding the unchanged calcium hydroxide, similar to a zinc oxide eugenol cement.

Properties

Mechanical properties

The mechanical properties of this cement are poor. It is the weakest of all the setting dental cements and even after 24 hours it remains weak. It shows plastic deformation once set upon loading. This may well be the reason why it does not fracture (but probably deforms) when amalgam is condensed on the surface. The cement should be used in thin section, preferably air-thinned prior to setting.

Solubility

Calcium hydroxide cements are unstable and soluble. In the presence of water they start to degrade. A hydrophilic **sulphonamide** plasticizer is included to control the viscosity of the cement but this chemical permits rapid water permeation which facilitates the breakdown of the cement and determines the rate of the degradation. Some manufacturers use hydrophobic **hydrocarbon** plasticizers and these resist water ingress.

If leakage should occur at the margin of the restoration, the cement will continue to degrade and will slowly be lost. Studies have shown setting calcium hydroxide material linings to disappear under restorations due to the presence of moisture from dentine and via microleakage.

Biocompatibility and mode of action

As previously mentioned, degradation of these cements is not particularly desirable but this property does have a biological benefit, in that calcium hydroxide is available for release. There is a rapid increase in the alkalinity of the surroundings (pH 12 has been recorded), which has either a bactericidal or a bacteriostatic effect on microorganisms beneath the lining. The extent of this effect depends on the pH of the surrounding in which the bacteria thrive. Cariogenic bacteria survive in an acid environment and a change to an alkaline habitat will mean that the bacteria either become dormant or die. The degree of hydrophobicity of the plasticizer will determine the release of calcium hydroxide. A more hydrophobic plasticizer will release calcium hydroxide more slowly and so the cement will have decreased antibacterial properties.

> **Cariogenic:** causing or inducing dental caries.

The cement's reparative property is based on its high alkalinity having an irritating effect on the odontoblasts in the pulp chamber. Necrosis initially occurs when the cement in placed in direct contact with pulpal tissue. The odontoblasts are stimulated to lay down reparative (tertiary) dentine and a calcified layer eventually develops. This forms a bridge of dentine so walling off the pulp from the base of the cavity. Radioactive isotope research studies have proved that the calcium in this new reparative dentine is derived from the cells in the pulp and not the calcium in the cement. Figure 12.15 shows radiographs of reparative dentine being laid down after the application of a setting calcium hydroxide cement.

There is evidence that calcification of the carious dentine occurs. Whether this is assisted by the presence of the calcium hydroxide or whether it is an extension of the normal reparative process is not entirely clear.

Mode of retention and light-curing varieties

The material does not adhere to dentine either chemically or micromechanically. To overcome this and to allow a command set of the cement, light-activated varieties have been produced by adding various resins such as urethane dimethacrylate (UDMA), bis-GMA and hydroxylethylmethacrylate (HEMA). In these formulations, the calcium hydroxide plays no part in the setting reaction and any effects are dependent on diffusion from a resin matrix. The HEMA permits water ingress so there will be some diffusion of fluid within the cement similar to the resin-modified glass ionomer cements. Methacrylated glycerol salicylates may also be used. These appear to improve the cement's effects as observed with the conventional materials. The methacrylated glycerol salicylates work in a similar manner as the hydrophilic sulphonamide plasticizer.

The materials containing these resin additions show a much higher exothermic reaction during the polymerization process and thus, when placed close to the pulp, may present some risk. The strength of the resin-modified cements is slightly enhanced but they are less brittle. With the inclusion of the resin also comes polymerization shrinkage, often noted as the lifting away of the periphery of the cement from the cavity floor.

There is a limited degree of thermal protection afforded by both types of cement although the thermal conductivity and diffusivity is similar to other cements, since they are only used in thin section. However, they are effective at sealing dentinal tubules which is generally regarded of much greater importance.

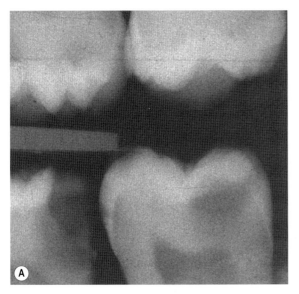
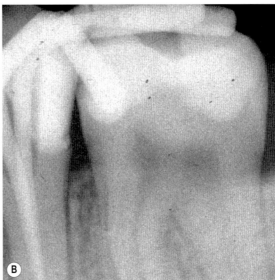

Fig. 12.15A,B Radiographs showing how reparative dentine has been laid down in tooth 37 over a period of 12 months after the application of a setting calcium hydroxide cement. Note the difference in the shape of the distal pulp horn.

Advantages and disadvantages

Advantages and disadvantages of calcium hydroxide cements are set out in Table 12.19.

Table 12.19 Advantages and disadvantages of setting calcium hydroxide cements

Advantages	Disadvantages
Stimulates the formation of reparative dentine	Low compressive strength
Forms a physical barrier over exposed pulp, allowing a dental material to seal the tubules	Soluble so tends to break down during use
	Non-adherent to dentine
	High pH on setting, which may cause local irritation
	Exothermic reaction
	Light-polymerized material – shrinks during setting

Indications

The indications of setting calcium hydroxide cements are:
- Deep cavity over the pulpal wall
- Indirect pulp capping
- Direct pulp capping.

The use of setting calcium hydroxide cements has decreased in recent years, mainly due to increased understanding of the prevention of microleakage, and manufacturers have seen sales of this family of materials decrease. Many dentists still place this material but are more selective in its usage. Current thinking indicates that retention of some softened dentine over the pulp at the base of the cavity is permissible, particularly if exposure of the pulp is likely. The margins should be cleared of softened dentine to allow a seal to be created with the restorative material thus depriving the residual bacteria of their substrate. The risk of iatrogenic exposure of the pulp is therefore reduced and may even be eliminated.

The clinician may elect to use this type of material in the deepest part of the cavity (without a pulpal exposure or potential exposure) in an attempt to stimulate dentine deposition. However, the perceived view that sealing of dentinal tubules is more important in preventing passage of bacteria (microleakage) means that other materials which have this ability are now preferred, such as the variants of glass ionomer cements.

Pulp capping

It is a contraindication of many base materials, for example zinc oxide eugenol and resin-containing materials, to be directly placed on exposed pulp as they are cytotoxic. If the clinician is concerned that a micro-exposure may be present in a deep cavity or if indirect or direct pulp capping is indicated, a setting calcium hydroxide cement may be used to form a physical barrier between the (exposed) pulpal tissue and the other material(s) used to restore the cavity. More recently, **MTA** is a likely alternative as an indirect or direct pulp capping material instead of a setting calcium hydroxide cement because of its ability to form a seal and its excellent biocompatibility. This material is described in full in Chapter 13.

Commercially available products

Commercially available calcium hydroxide products are shown in Table 12.20.

Table 12.20 Some setting calcium hydroxide cements currently available on the market

Product name	Manufacturer	Comments
Calcimol LC	Voco	Light-cured
Dycal	Dentsply	
Dycal VLC	Dentsply	Light-cured
Fluoroseal LC Liner	SciPharm	Light-cured
Life	Kerr Hawe	
Renew 2	SS White	
Septocalcine Ultra	Septodont	

Mixing

The mixing of the conventionally setting cements is simple as the two pastes used are of similar consistency and the amount of each component required is usually the same (Box 12.5). The two pastes should be blended together within 30 seconds. The uniformity of the mix can be confirmed in that the two pastes are slightly different

Box 12.5 Correct procedure for mixing a setting calcium hydroxide cement, using Life (Kerr Hawe)

Step 1	Step 2	Step 3
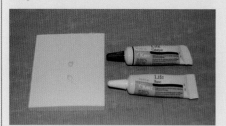	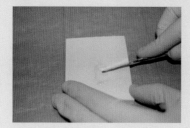	
Dispense equal amounts of base and catalyst onto a mixing pad	Mix the two pastes together until a uniform colour is achieved (30 seconds)	Collect the mixed mass together and hand to the dentist for application

colours. Once a streak-free mix has been obtained the cement may be applied to the cavity floor. Setting is rapid, particularly in the presence of water, and is usually complete within 2–3 minutes.

Clinical placement protocol

Calcium hydroxide cement should be placed in a small thin layer on the base of the cavity, which is then covered with variant of glass ionomer cement. The clinical procedure for placing this material is illustrated in Box 12.6.

NOVEL BULK DENTINE REPLACEMENTS

Recently, further development in the cement arena has led to the production of a tricalcium silicate cement claimed to be both bioactive and biocompatible (for an example see Figure 12.16). It is related to **MTA** (see Chapter 13). The material primarily contains tricalcium silicate, calcium carbonate and zirconium oxide and water with a superplasticizing agent, which reduces the water content of the mixture while helping to retain the workability of the material. It has a setting time of 10 minutes and a pH in the region of 8.2. It is designed to be placed both on dentine and vital pulp tissue and is reported to encourage the formation of reparative dentine. Plugs of the material have been observed in the dentinal tubules and there appears to be good adaptation to the cavity. This material has been described as a dentine substitute. It is too early to say whether the initial encouraging results will be confirmed in the longer term.

> **Superplasticizer:** a dispersing agent used to reduce water content.

Commercially available products

One tricalcium silicate cements currently available on the market is Biodentine (Septodont).

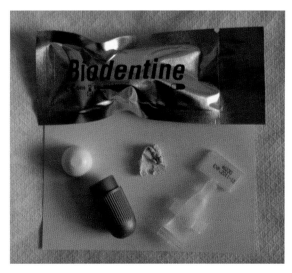

Fig. 12.16 An example of a currently available tricalcium silicate cement product (Biodentine, Septodont).

CAVITY VARNISHES

Cavity varnishes are natural **rosins** (such as copal, colophony or sandarac resin obtained from pine trees) or synthetic **resins** (polystyrene) dissolved in a **solvent** (alcohol, ether, chloroform or acetone).

Once applied on the walls and floor of the cavity using a brush, the solvent evaporates leaving a thin (4 μm) thick film on the cavity walls. The rationale behind this material's use is that it will fill the potential gap between the dentine and the restorative material. This decreases postoperative sensitivity and retards the progress of microorganisms into the potential space.

The evaporation of the solvent usually means that the thin film is not totally intact as shrinkage occurs and often there are voids where the dentine is left unprotected. This material is generally used with amalgam and gold. It is soluble and has a tendency to wash out with

---

Box 12.6 Correct procedure for placing a setting calcium hydroxide cement into a cavity, using Life (Kerr Hawe)

Step 1

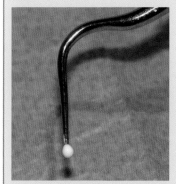

Pick up a small amount of mixed paste on a base (Thymozin) applicator

Step 2

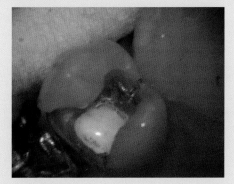

Apply to the base of the cavity. Gently air dry the material to thin it before it sets. If a light activated calcium hydroxide material is being used, it should be light cured

Step 3

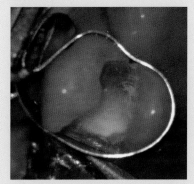

Place a resin-modified glass ionomer cement over the set calcium hydroxide to cover it and the surrounding dentine. Light cure the resin-modified glass ionomer cement and restore the cavity

time in the mouth with the result that its use has decreased in recent years in favour of other materials that can bond to tooth tissue and occlude dentinal tubules. There are consequently few such products on the market (Table 12.21).

Table 12.21 Some cavity varnishes currently available on the market

Product name	Manufacturer
Copal Varnish	SciPharm Inc
Copal Varnish	PD
Copaliner	Bosworth, Cooley USA

SUMMARY

- Acid–base cements have similar chemical structures and setting reactions.
- Zinc phosphate cement was one of the first cements and provides a basis for all cements but it is now primarily used for luting restorations.
- Zinc polycarboxylate cement has similar properties to zinc phosphate cement but adheres to tooth tissue and is bland with regard to the pulp.
- Zinc oxide eugenol cements have multiple applications and may be used in a wide range of temporary and provisional applications.
- Calcium hydroxide-based cements interact with the tooth tissue but are weak and are generally used as pulp protection materials.

FURTHER READING

Ford, P., 2004. Harty's Endodontics in Clinical Practice, fifth ed. Wright Elsevier, Edinburgh (See Chapter 4).

McCabe, J.F., Walls, A.W.G., 2008. Applied Dental Materials, nineth ed.. Blackwell Munksgaard, Oxford (See Chapters 28–30).

Mount, G.J., Hume, W.R., 2005. Preservation and Restoration of Tooth Structure, second ed. Knowledge Books, Brisbane (See Chapters 11–13).

Powers, J.M., Sakaguchi, R.L. (Eds.), 2006. Craig's Restorative Dental Materials (twelfth ed.). Mosby Elsevier, St Louis (See Chapter 20).

van Noort, R., 2007. Introduction to Dental Materials, third ed.. Mosby Elsevier, Edinburgh (See Chapter 3.8).

Wilson, A.D., Nicholson, J.W., 2005. Acid Base Cements: Their Biomedical and Industrial Applications. Cambridge University Press, Cambridge.

SELF-ASSESSMENT QUESTIONS

1. What are the factors governing the rate of set of zinc phosphate cement?
2. What are the similarities and differences between the properties of zinc phosphate and zinc polycarboxylate cements?
3. What are the advantages and disadvantages of zinc oxide eugenol cements?
4. What materials may be used for an iatrogenic pulpal exposure?
5. What are the similarities and differences between glass ionomer and zinc polycarboxylate cements?
6. Describe the procedure from start of mix to the final seating of a full gold crown when using a zinc polycarboxylate cement.

Chapter | 13 |

Materials used in endodontics

LEARNING OBJECTIVES

From this chapter, the reader will:

- Appreciate the basic principles underpinning endodontics
- Be aware of the types of rubber dam and the necessity for its use during conventional endodontic therapy
- Be aware of the various types of endodontic file and how these should be used during root canal instrumentation
- Understand the importance of thorough disinfection of the root canal system by chemical irrigation and other more novel means
- Be aware of the materials used to temporize a tooth undergoing root canal therapy
- Be aware of the materials used to fill the root canal system and restore the tooth postoperatively
- Know the names of currently available commercial products.

INTRODUCTION

Endodontology is the branch of dental science concerned with the form, function, health, trauma and disease of the dental pulp. **Endodontics** is the practice of endodontology. Many patients will report that they have had **root treatment**, which is a misleading term. The correct technical term is **root canal therapy (RCT)**, which more accurately describes the process, i.e. of cleaning and filling all of the root canals in the tooth. The term **root filling** is often used synonymously with root canal therapy but this only refers to the material that is used to fill the root canal system.

> ✓
>
> It must be emphasized at the outset that the dental team's primary objective should be to preserve the vitality of the tooth. Endodontic procedures should only become necessary if, despite best efforts, the pulp has become irreversibly compromised and requires partial or full removal.

The objective of successful root canal therapy is to **access** the entire root canal system, and thoroughly remove any necrotic (dead) tissue and microorganisms by **canal preparation**. This preparation involves **cleaning** and **shaping** the canals to facilitate the subsequent **obturation** (filling) of the dead space. It is critical that a **coronal seal** is then gained and maintained to prevent subsequent reinfection of the root canal system by oral microorganisms. Should this seal become compromised, the treatment is likely to fail, so underlining the importance of this final stage.

This chapter discusses the materials and the instrumentation used during endodontic procedures.

RUBBER DAM

Reasons for use

The battle in endodontics is against the bacterial infection. To achieve a sterile root canal system the tooth should be isolated to prevent contamination with oral bacteria. The only predictable and effective method is the use of **rubber dam**, which is also referred to as **dental dam** (see Figures 13.1B, 13.2 and 13.4 below). The benefits of using rubber dam in relation to endodontics include:

- Protection of the oropharynx and prevention of inhalation or ingestion of instruments or medicaments
- Isolation of the operating field, rendering it aseptic
- Prevents ingress of saliva, and reinfection of the root canal system, by oral bacteria
- Improved access and vision
- Containing irrigants extraorally
- Improved patient comfort
- Improved treatment efficiency.

As well as being used in endodontics, rubber dam also has many applications in general operative dentistry, particularly when the dentist is using hydrophobic materials, hence the many references to it in this text.

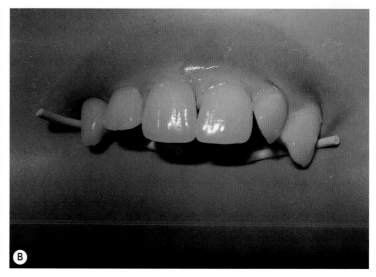

Fig. 13.1 (A) Rubber dam stabilizing cord, Wedjets (Hygienic). The orange cord is thicker than the yellow. (B) Cord retaining the dental dam during isolation of the upper anterior teeth.

The rubber dam system

The rubber dam system consists of a sheet of an **elastic material** held taut over a **frame**. Some products have a frame incorporated in them, e.g. OptraDam (Ivoclar Vivadent). A hole or holes are punched into the sheet corresponding to the teeth that need to be isolated. The dam is retained by the use of a **clamp** or clamps or **stabilizing cord** such as Wedjets (Hygienic) (Figure 13.1).

Types and presentation of rubber dam

Rubber dam is available in **latex** and non-latex (**elastic plastomer** or **polyolefin**) presentations (Figure 13.2 and Table 13.1). It should be noted that the words 'rubber' and 'dental' in relation to dam are used synonymously although the elastic plastomers and polyolefins are polymers.

Table 13.1 Commercially available dental dam types

Dam type	Properties	Notes	Example commercial product
Latex	Good handling properties	Contraindicated in patients with a latex allergy. Take care with solvents like chloroform.	Dental Dam (Hygenic)
Elastic silicone plastomer	Better tear resistance than latex. Very elastic, stretching 1000% prior to tearing.	Should be stretched before use. Use a smaller hole than the latex product otherwise dam will slide off the clamp/teeth.	Flexi Dam Non Latex (Roeko)
Polyolefin	Similar properties to latex	Avoid direct contact with: bis-GMA, chloroform, copal varnish, eugenol, formocresol, methylmethacrylate monomer	Non-Latex Dental Dam (Hygenic)

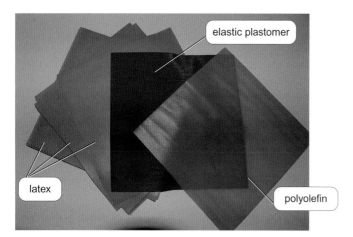

Fig. 13.2 Three types of dental dam in common usage: latex (Hygenic), elastic plastomer (Roeko) and polyolefin (Hygenic).

Rubber dam is either presented in precut squares of material (Figure 13.2) or in rolls where the dentist cuts off the desired amount. Different sheet thicknesses are available, the thicker sheets may be more difficult to place but they have a greater tear resistance and will retract the tissues more. Products are also available in different colours. Darker colours contrast with the operative site better so decreasing eye strain. Lighter shades, however, can naturally illuminate the area due to their greater translucency. Some products are supplied flavoured or scented in an attempt to improve the patient's experience.

Rubber dam sealers

When rubber dam is placed for endodontics, it is advisable to create a seal around the dam using a **caulk** material. This prevents irrigants reaching the mouth and equally prevents saliva from leaking back into the operating field. The caulk material used is **hectorite clay**, which belongs to a group of materials called **smectitec clays**. In these materials platelets of a metal oxide are sandwiched between plates of silicon dioxide. This layered structure allows the clays to swell in contact with water. The metallic oxide in hectorite clay is magnesium (Figure 13.3). On taking up water the clay will expand to up to 35 times its original size effectively sealing any gaps adjacent to the dam.

An example of such a product on the market is OraSeal (Ultradent). The rubber dam is applied and the sealer is syringed around the now isolated tooth (Figure 13.4).

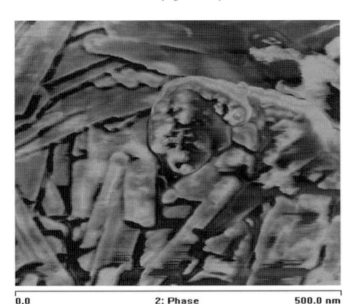

Fig. 13.3 Photomicrograph from atomic force microscopy showing the platelet-type layered structure of hectorite.
(Photo courtesy of Elementist.*)*

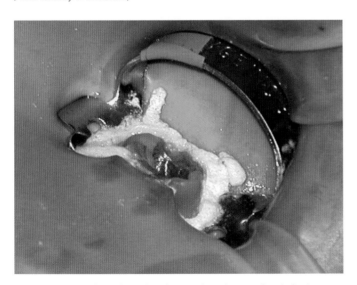

Fig. 13.4 Latex rubber dam placed around tooth 17 and sealed using OraSeal (Ultradent).

ENDODONTIC FILES

The aim of root canal preparation is to remove as many of the microorganisms as possible and to shape the root canal to facilitate its subsequent **obturation** (filling) with an inert material. Effective cleaning of the complex root canal system requires using both mechanical and chemical means. Metal **files** are used to remove necrotic material from the lumen of the canals and also to remove hard tissue from the canal walls. It also removes the microorganisms that have penetrated the dentinal tubules in the canal walls. This process also facilitates the penetration of disinfecting agents so they can reach the bacteria in the root canal system.

Additionally files shape the root canals to provide a uniform-sized dead space, which may be filled using standard-sized cones of plastic material. This is not easy as the root canal system is complex (unlike a chimney!) and the internal anatomy is more akin to a three-dimensional spider's web of major and minor canals within a network. It is therefore impossible to completely prepare the whole root canal system and the obturating material must be able to be adapted to the root canal walls to achieve a seal.

File preparation of root canals is done either by **hand** or using **rotary files** in a speed-reducing, torque-controlled handpiece (Figure 13.5). Rotary systems are much more efficient than those used by hand; however, hand files may be preferred to negotiate very curved root canals as rotary instruments may not be able to get round the curve due to lack of sufficient flexibility. The file may also break (**separate**) during use. The sharper the curve of the canal, the greater the incidence of fracture of the file due to **cyclic fatigue**.

Fracture may also occur due to **flexural fatigue** (i.e. overuse) or **torsional fatigue**, that is, forces placed on the instrument in rotation while the instrument is prevented from moving. The use of a **torque controller** is important so that the rotation of the file is stopped prior to receiving excessive torque, which may cause fracture. For further information on speed-reducing handpieces and torque, see Chapter 19. From this brief description, it can be seen that the selection of the material of which the file is made and its method of construction is critical in determining the performance of the instrument.

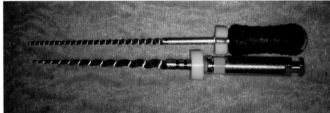

Fig. 13.5 Hand (top) and rotary (bottom) endodontic files.

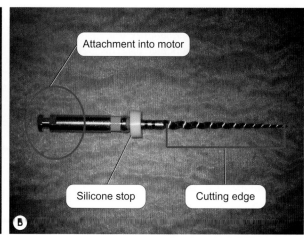

Fig. 13.6 The parts of (A) hand and (B) rotary files. The silicone stop is used as a measuring device: the required canal length is measured and the silicone stop is placed at this same distance measured from the tip of the file.

Anatomy of endodontic files

Hand and rotary files both have a cutting edge along the length of the file and at the other end is either a handle or an attachment that fits into the handpiece, respectively (Figure 13.6). The instrument cuts when its **radial lands** are in contact with the canal wall, the lead angle determining its cutting efficiency. Radial land areas are required for conventional helically fluted files because they prevent the file from over-engagement in the canal (Figure 13.7). Lack of radial land areas reduces friction. If a file becomes suddenly engaged or self-threaded, it may fracture. Radial lands are especially important for files that have positive rake angles. That is, the angle of action of the cutting blade is similar to a snow plough which is forced downward towards the surface of the road. Many files are designed so that the radial lands cannot screw themselves into the canal wall. Thus, the dentinal debris is directed towards the coronal part of the canal so that it is not compacted apically.

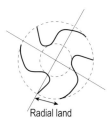

Radial land

Fig. 13.7 Diagrammatic representation of the microscopic structure of an endodontic file in cross-section showing the radial lands.

There are many different types of file available. For the clinician's convenience and from a quality-control perspective, files are standardized according to their physical properties and dimensions (i.e. diameter and taper). To indicate the increase from one instrument size to the next, these are often numbered and colour coded. Files are available in a range of different shapes, tapers, lengths, cutting or non-cutting tips, safe edged (only cutting on one side). The material of which they are constructed is either **stainless steel** or **nickel-titanium**.

Stainless steel files

The traditional material used in the construction of endodontic files is **stainless steel**. This is an alloy of **iron**, **carbon** and **chromium**. **Nickel** may also be present. Originally steel was made by forming an alloy of carbon and iron. This was known as **carbon steel**. This alloy was prone to rusting in the presence of water, but the addition of a percentage of chromium was seen to prevent this rusting. Normally between 13% and 26% of a stainless steel alloy is chromium. The chromium forms a passivation layer of chromium oxide on the surface when exposed to air. This thin layer is not visible but preserves the steel from rust. If scratched, the oxide layer will rapidly re-form, preventing degradation.

> **Passivation layer:** the non-reactive surface film (usually an oxide) that prevents further corrosion.

Endodontic instruments are manufactured by machining stainless steel wire into a blank of the desired shape (for example either square or triangular in cross-section). This is then twisted into a spiral. During the twisting the material becomes work hardened. The greater the number of twists, the greater the work hardening. The other means of producing the instruments is by directly machining of the shape from a stainless steel rod into the final shape. This machining process also work hardens the material.

> **Work hardening:** is the strengthening of a metal by plastic deformation. This strengthening occurs because the crystal structure of the material is dislocated by the movement. Any material with a fairly high melting point such as metals and alloys can be strengthened using this technique. Alloys such as low-carbon steel and stainless steel which are not amenable to heat treatment are often work hardened.

Particularly with larger sizes, stainless steel files do not bend easily and in order to maintain the canal shape which is invariably a curve, the clinician should bend or **precurve** the file prior to its introduction to the canal. It should be remembered that bending the instrument will further work harden the metal and make it more brittle. This can lead to fracture.

Stressing

The mechanical properties of the file will depend on the composition of the material, the geometry of the file and the way in which it is loaded. Anticlockwise twisting of a file is inadvisable as this increasing the twisting of the file, which may result in brittle fracture.

Files should therefore not be stressed in this way and definitely not when they are bound in the canal. Some irrigants such as sodium hypochlorite and ethylene diamine tetra-acetic acid (EDTA) can reduce the cutting ability of stainless steel files and so they should be rinsed immediately after use. The risk of this occurring has been substantially reduced as the current recommendation is that files should only be used once and discarded. However, if canal preparation is extended over a long period of time at one appointment, prolonged immersion of these instruments in these solutions in the canal will start the process of degradation.

All files should be regularly inspected for damage after their removal from a root canal. If any damage is seen then the file should be discarded and a new file used. Continued use of a stressed instrument (Figure 13.8) has a high risk of instrument separation with the fractured fragment being retained in the root canal system. If the file cannot be removed, or the canal negotiated beyond it, the success of the treatment will be compromised. Unfortunately, fracture of files can also occur without any visible signs of previous permanent deformation. In order to minimize file breakage, files should only be used in a wet canal and in accordance with the manufacturer's instructions.

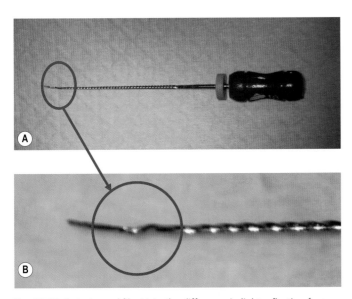

Fig. 13.8A,B A stressed file. Note the difference in light reflection from the instrument, with a matt appearance. This file should now be discarded and not reused.

Debris retained on an endodontic file after use is called **swarf**. It may contain neural tissue with **prions**, which are theoretically associated with **new-variant Creutzfeldt–Jakob disease** (**nvCJD**). Prions are proteins that cannot be destroyed by the usual methods of surgical disinfection. Endodontic files should therefore be considered as single use (to be used only on the same patient) and then discarded. The other advantage of the single use policy is that instrument separation fracture is decreased as the file is used less. Furthermore, autoclaving can decrease the cutting ability of some files and may result in metal fatigue.

Types of stainless steel file

As previously mentioned, there are many different types of file made of stainless steel, for example, Hedströem and K-Flex (Figure 13.9).

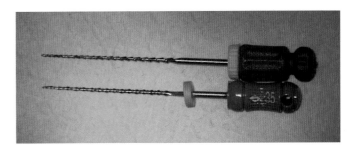

Fig. 13.9 Two examples of stainless steel endodontic files: the upper file is a Hedström file and the lower file a K-Flex file, both size 35 02. Note the difference in the shape of their cutting parts.

Nickel-titanium files

An alloy which has been more recently used to produce endodontic files is **nickel-titanium** (**NiTi**). This material is extremely flexible (Figure 13.10), some 500% more than stainless steel and has been termed **super-elastic**. This means that it is more likely to maintain the canal shape during preparation as it can memorize its original shape. It is also less likely to straighten curved canals as occurs with stainless steel. With nickel-titanium instruments, after a finite number of rotations cyclic fatigue leads to failure. However, they are three times stronger and have a superior resistance to torsional fracture compared with the equivalent stainless steel file. They are also corrosion resistant. It is the alloy of choice for rotary systems although hand files are also available (Figure 13.6).

When the alloy is stressed during use, its structure changes from an **austenitic crystalline structure** to a **martensitic crystalline structure**. This happens progressively and as a result the stress on the file reduces even though the strain may be increased. The modulus of elasticity is much higher for an austenitic structure than for the martensitic form, meaning that the latter state is more brittle than the

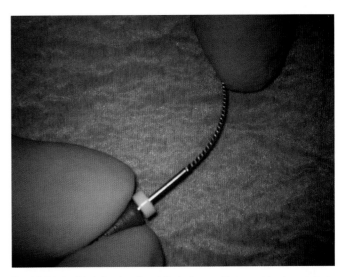

Fig. 13.10 A nickel-titanium hand file being gently curved to demonstrate its flexibility.

former. When the stress on the alloy decreases, spring back occurs without permanent deformation and the alloy returns to the austenitic phase. This allows an 8% strain deformation with complete recovery compared with less than 1% with stainless steel.

The nature of this alloy dictates that to make a file, the desired shape must be machined out of the blank rather than just twisting a blank before grinding the cutting pattern into it. The production costs are thus increased as this process is more complicated than merely twisting the blank as with stainless steel instruments.

Commercially available products

There are so many files and file systems available to the endodontist these days that to list even a small selection would be prohibitive from a space perspective! Many systems have various nuances which may appeal to various operators. Practitioners are therefore advised to select the file system which they find most effective and are comfortable using. They should use the instruments within the principles of their recommended usage and should consult the manufacturer's instructions prior to clinical use. Comprehensive lists of files and file systems are available from companies manufacturing or distributing them.

ROOT CANAL DISINFECTION

Successful outcome of the treatment is dependent on the removal of microorganisms from the root canal system. Studies have shown that root canals free of infection at the time of obturation have a higher success rate, whereas residual bacteria retained in the canal at the time of obturation leads to a higher risk of failure. The dentist has a number of medicaments available to achieve this objective. **Irrigants** are used during root canal preparation. Other novel antibacterial systems that are now available include **ozone** and **bacterial photo-dynamic therapy**, which may also be used at this stage. Root canals may be dressed with antibacterial **inter-visit intracanal medications** if the procedure is to be carried out over more than one appointment.

Endodontic irrigants

It is imperative that root canals are not prepared dry. Fluids introduced into the root canal system have a number of purposes. They should:

- Lubricate endodontic files so facilitating their passage in the canal
- Wet canal walls and remove debris by flushing
- Contain any dentinal shavings in suspension, so facilitating their removal from the canals. This prevents impaction of debris in the apical portion of the canal which may prove difficult to renegotiate due to the blockage
- Facilitate dissolution of organic matter
- Remove smear layer and soften dentine
- Aid cleaning of areas inaccessible to mechanical cleansing methods
- Disinfect the canal system: mechanical root canal preparation alone is ineffective at microbial removal. It is essential that solutions used during root canal preparation can disinfect the root canal system.

The irrigants available can be divided into two groups based on their mode of action:

- Those used to clean and expose the bacterial contaminants
- Those used to disinfect the root canal system.

Biofilm and smear layer

Bacteria colonize not only on the necrotic material in the lumen of the root canal but also infect its walls. Microorganisms can penetrate

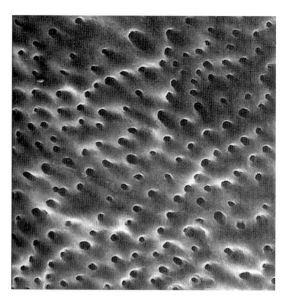

Fig. 13.11 Dentine surface with the smear layer removed.
(From Pathways to the Pulp, *8th edition, Cohen and Burns, p. 306, Mosby.)*

into the dentinal tubules as well as forming complex, highly developed ecologies on the surface of the canal wall. This has been termed a **biofilm**. In order to kill these organisms the biofilm must be disrupted and penetrated. Furthermore, during instrumentation organic material is left behind on the dentinal surface, termed the **smear layer**, which must also be removed to allow the disinfectant to gain access to lateral canals (Figure 13.11). If this is achieved, then the disinfection process will be enhanced.

The removal of the smear layer (and so opening of the dentinal tubules) is achieved primarily by using chelating agents such as **citric acid** or **EDTA**. These also have some benefit in disrupting the biofilm but they are ineffective at killing bacteria. Disruption of the biofilm may be achieved, albeit slowly, by using sodium hypochlorite, which will break up proteinaceous material. The action of a chelating agent also provides a cleaner surface against which the final filling materials will adapt.

Irrigants for cleaning

Citric acid

Citric acid is a chelating agent that removes calcified tissue. It was first used in dentistry as a surface cleaner in conjunction with glass ionomer cements to prepare the tooth surface for bonding to these materials. It has been reported to successfully remove the proteinaceous material on the surface of dentine, allowing an interaction between the cement and the clean dentine surface. It is also effective as a decalcifying agent. It is used in solution at a concentration of 10–12.5%.

Bespoke citric acid-containing endodontic irrigation solution products are available such as d2d Endo citric acid or it can be obtained from a pharmacy on prescription by a registered dentist.

EDTA

EDTA may also be used as a chelating agent as an alterative to citric acid, its action being more aggressive. It is used as either a synthetic amino acid or sodium salt of EDTA and is highly effective at removing the smear layer and emulsifying soft tissue. EDTA demineralizes and softens root canal wall dentine by 20–50 µm. Although it is neither bactericidal nor bacteriostatic, EDTA-containing compounds (Figure 13.12) will eventually kill bacteria by starving them of the metallic ions needed for growth as the chemical chelates the ions. It is non-toxic and non-corrosive to instruments.

preparation easier and faster. The increased viscosity of this presentation is better for holding debris in suspension.

Some products contain **carbamide** or **urea peroxide**, which effervesce during use, resulting in an 'elevator action' that helps to remove debris from the root canal system, so optimizing cleaning. Effervescence is caused by release of oxygen, which occurs when the product comes into contact with sodium hypochlorite solution. The release of oxygen may also kill anaerobic bacteria.

Commercially available products

Commercially available materials are shown in Table 13.2.

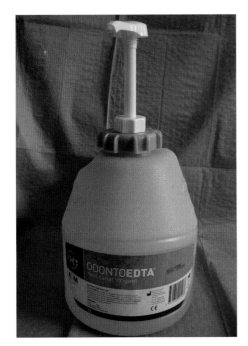

Fig. 13.12 Example of an EDTA-containing endodontic irrigation product (OdontoEDTA, Smart Dental).

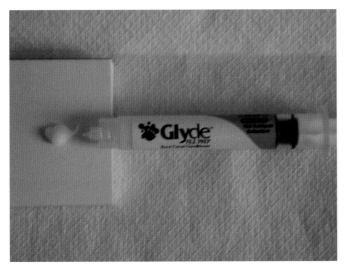

Fig. 13.13 Example of a product containing EDTA in a gel form (Glyde File Prep, Dentsply Maillefer).

Bacteriostatic: the ability of a chemical to inhibit the growth or reproduction of bacteria.
Bactericidal: the ability of a chemical to kill bacteria outright.

EDTA is normally used in solution at a concentration of 15–17%. Products available include Endo-Solution EDTA (Cerkamed Dental-Medical Company). Alternatively, in the UK, a dentist can request a pharmacist to make up the required concentration by writing a prescription.

EDTA gel

EDTA is used in liquid form for endodontic irrigation but is also available in gel form (Figure 13.13). These products are used to coat endodontic files. They act as lubricants as well as helping to remove smear when the file is used within the root canal, making canal

Table 13.2 Some EDTA-containing gels used during root canal preparation currently available on the market

Product	Manufacturer	Active ingredient	Comments
Canal +	Septodont	10–25% EDTA 10–25% carbamide peroxide	
Endo-Prep Cream	Cerkamed Dental-Medical Company	15% EDTA 10% urea peroxide	
FileCare EDTA	VDW	15% EDTA 10% urea peroxide	
File-Eze	Ultradent	19% EDTA	
Glyde File Prep	Dentsply Maillefer	EDTA Carbamide peroxide	
Largal Ultra	Septodont	15% EDTA Cetrimide less than 1%	Cetrimide has a bactericidal action and reduces surface tension
RC Prep	Premier	Propylene glycol Urea peroxide EDTA	Propylene glycol lubricates
Smear Clear	Sybronendo	17% EDTA	

!

- Chelating materials should be thoroughly washed from the root canal system as their retention for any length of time will continue to soften the dentine. This effect is eventually self-limiting as the chelator is used up. For best results, these irrigants should:
  - Always be used in combination with a disinfecting irrigant
  - Not be used as the last irrigant.
- Chelating materials soften the dentine within the tooth and so should not be initially used to negotiate the canals as a false canal may be cut iatrogenically.

Iatrogenic event: inadvertent complications as a result of a clinical intervention.

Irrigants for disinfection

Many disinfecting agents have been used for endodontic irrigation over the years. These include halogenated compounds such as sodium hypochlorite, iodine potassium iodide, chlorhexidine and a number of potent phenolic disinfecting agents. There is a significant problem with many disinfectants where the concentrations producing effective bactericidal activity are close to those concentrations where tissue toxicity has been reported.

Sodium hypochlorite solution

Of the disinfectants now commonly used, sodium hypochlorite (bleach) solution is preferred by the majority of endodontists. It is a potent organic tissue solvent that is proteolytic and dissolves necrotic organic material. It releases free chlorine, a powerful disinfecting agent which has a wide spectrum of bactericidal effects, so disinfecting the area of application. It is the chlorine that breaks down tissue and proteins into amino acids. These amino acids are then degraded by hydrolysis through the production of chloramine molecules. This is an oxidation reaction with the bleach. The bleach pH can be in excess of 11 and it has no effect on the calcium deposits in the smear layer.

Since the disinfecting component is consumed, i.e. it breaks down during use, the solution must be constantly replaced otherwise it will lose its efficacy. Some workers advocate constant washing of the root canal system for at least 30 minutes for the solution to be effective. This substantial **dwell time** is also desirable to ensure that the biofilm structure which the bacteria inhabit is disrupted allowing the disinfectant to effectively reach the bacteria. Current canal preparation techniques especially using rotary instrumentation are very efficient and canals may be prepared in no time at all. It is important that the clinician continues to flush the canal long after canal preparation has ceased for this disinfectant to be effective.

The therapeutic and toxic concentrations of sodium hypochlorite are undesirably close together. There is no difference in the antibacterial effect between 0.5% and 5% solutions but the efficiency of weak solutions decreases rapidly. A solution with concentration greater than 1% is required for pulpal tissue dissolution to occur. However, at higher concentrations, although the disinfecting process is faster, it is more likely that untoward tissue damage will occur as the chemical is more toxic at these concentrations. This is especially the case if the chemical is inadvertently extruded outwith the root canal system.

A further problem with sodium hypochlorite is that it has a higher surface tension than water. It does not wet the root canal walls as well as some other disinfecting solutions. This results in the canal walls being incompletely covered, and consequently the biofilm layer may not be disrupted effectively. This is more likely at higher concentrations as the solution is thicker.

The effects of the solution are increased if the solution is warmed prior to use as more chlorine is released as the temperature increases. Most dentists use a solution of 1% which presents a balance between effective disinfection and toxicity. The solution should be warmed just as it is about to be used.

Sodium hypochlorite is not totally effective at killing all the microorganisms found in the root canal system. Pathogens such as *Enterococcus faecalis* have been isolated from root canals which have been previously treated with this solution.

As its active ingredient is the chloride ion, sodium hypochlorite is a bleaching agent. It will damage clothes if it comes into contact with them so it is advisable that the patient's clothes are adequately protected during treatment. It also has an unpleasant taste and is an irritant to the eyes, skin and oral mucosa. The patient and dental team's eyes should be covered and rubber dam should be placed and sealed during treatment. This bleach effect is of course an advantage when the solution is used in the root canal system as it will lighten any stained tooth tissue. When a tooth loses its vitality, staining happens not infrequently due to the breakdown of blood products (iron from haemoglobin) and these molecules may penetrate into the dentinal tubules.

- Commercial sodium hypochlorite endodontic irrigant products include Parcan Solution (Septodont), which is a 3% solution, or Chlorax (which is available as a 2% or 5.25% sodium hypochlorite solution from Cerkamed Dental-Medical Company). It can also be obtained from a pharmacy. The advantage of using these products is that they do not have to be made up at the chairside and they are buffered. Buffering maintains the solution's properties throughout its shelf-life and extends this time. There are also products containing other chemicals to enhance the effect of the solution. For example, Chlor-Xtra (Vista) is a combination of sodium hypochlorite and Triton-X. This latter chemical is a surfactant that lowers the viscosity of the irrigant so improving its penetration in the dentinal tubules and narrow canals.
- An alternative is household bleach bought from a supermarket. This is usually supplied as a 1% solution in which case should be used neat or it can be diluted with tap water if required. However, the clinician must be satisfied that any material being used on a patient is approved for contact with humans or has been certified with a CE mark for dental or medical applications. This may preclude the use of supermarket-bought household bleaching products.

Care should be taken with all materials used intraorally as the material safety data sheet (MSDS) has instructions on hazards, including those related to swallowing or inhalation. This means that the use in the oral cavity would be regarded as a hazard. In the UK, failure to carry out a risk assessment under COSHH regulations would be a potential problem if anything untoward occurred. This is a particular problem as proprietary solutions specifically for dental use are available.

When the solution is made up, its shelf-life is short. To ensure that it remains effective it is recommended that it is made up daily in the surgery as it is more effective just prior to its use.

Many endodontists use sodium hypochlorite solution in combination with an ultrasonic instrument as they believe that the acoustic streaming that occurs enhances the cleaning effect.

Acoustic streaming: the application of ultrasonic vibrations produces a continuous flow of bubbles in the line of the sound wave.

!

Milton sterilization fluid (Proctor and Gamble) should *not* be used as a source of sodium hypochlorite. Milton solution is a solution of sodium hypochlorite and sodium chloride. The sodium chloride may precipitate out and the salt crystals may block the root canals and corrode instruments.

Extracanal extrusion of endodontic irrigants

It is not uncommon for endodontic irrigating solutions to be extruded outwith the root canal system during use. Depending on the chemical involved the effects can range from insignificant to very serious. There are many documented cases in the literature where sodium hypochlorite solution has been inadvertently extruded outwith the root canal system. When sodium hypochlorite comes into contact with vital tissues it can cause severe inflammation and tissue necrosis. Severe complications such as neurological damage, facial atrophy, anaphylaxis and airway problems have also been reported.

Clinically, the problem manifests as immediate severe pain for the patient (even though local anaesthetic has been administered), rapid swelling and ecchymosis (bruising). Secondary infection and persistent pain may result subsequently. Management of this distressing problem for both patient and clinician involves:

1. Stopping the irrigation, and considering giving additional local anaesthesia
2. Irrigating with sterile water or saline

3. Closure of the root canal with no medication and dressing the tooth
4. Analgesic advice
5. Considering prescription of an antibiotic, a steroid (such as dexamethasone) and an antihistamine.
6. Considering referral to an oral and maxillofacial surgical unit for specialist care and monitoring.

✓

To reduce the risk of extracanal extrusion of endodontic irrigants, the dentist is advised to use a side exiting endodontic irrigating needle. This should not bind tightly in the canal so that irrigating fluid may pass out in a coronal direction. The needle and syringe should be kept moving while performing slow, gentle irrigation.

Chlorhexidine

Chlorhexidine digluconate (Figure 13.14) is used by many endodontists as it has a number of beneficial properties. This chemical is a cationic bis-biguanide that is bacteriostatic at low (0.2%) and bactericidal at higher (2%) concentrations. Its mode of action is to cause cell wall decomposition, leading to the loss of cellular components. It does not, however, dissolve any organic tissue. It is active against a wide spectrum of microorganisms, with its antibacterial properties similar or greater to that of sodium hypochlorite. It is known that the bacterial flora and ecology of endodontic cases which have failed is different. In these cases, chlorhexidine is thus preferred because it may have an effect on microorganisms resistant to sodium hypochlorite. Other clinicians use it in preference to sodium hypochlorite as it is a safer alterative (see below).

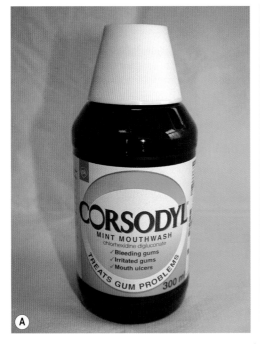
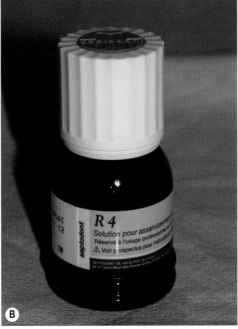

Fig. 13.14 Examples of products containing chlorhexidine that can be used for endodontic irrigation: (A) Corsodyl (GlaxoSmithKline) and (B) R4 (Septodont). The former product is also very effective against periodontal pathogens and is thus widely used in the treatment of periodontal disease (see Chapter 17).

Chlorhexidine binds to hydroxyapatite on the root canal walls and has a good substantivity, that is about 12 hours after application (with some products claiming much longer times than this). It should therefore be the last irrigant to be used in the canal.

Substantivity: the length of time that a medicament remains effective after application.

If chlorhexidine is used in direct combination with sodium hypochlorite solution, an acid–base reaction between the two may occur with formation of an insoluble precipitate that can be difficult to remove. This potential problem may be circumvented by irrigation with sterile water or saline between these two chemicals.

Some chlorhexidine products have been specifically designed for endodontic irrigation. They commonly have a higher concentration of chlorhexidine (2%) and also contain a wetting agent to lower surface tension to improve its penetration into dentinal tubules and small canals. Examples include R4 (Septodont), which is 20% chlorhexidine digluconate in denatured alcohol and commonly used as a final soak, and Gluco-Chex 2.0% (Cerkamed Dental-Medical Company). Concentrations lower than this are likely to be ineffective.

Some products are supplied as a gel that can be coated onto endodontic files prior to their insertion in the root canal to lubricate their passage. Two examples are Hibiscrub (Regent Medical), which contains 4% chlorhexidine, and Gluco-Chex gel 2% (Cerkamed Dental-Medical Company) which is 2%.

Iodine potassium iodide

Iodine potassium iodide is an organic compound that releases iodine. Iodine is a potent antibacterial agent with a broad spectrum of action: it is bactericidal, fungicidal, tuberculocidal, virucidal and sporicidal. It is effective for a limited period of time, about 2 days. Its mode of action involves attacking proteins, nucleotides and fatty acids leading to cell death. It has a low toxicity but some patients are allergic to iodine so its use in these individuals is contraindicated. It is supplied as an irrigating solution containing 2% solution of iodine in 4% aqueous potassium iodide. In the UK, Videne (Adams), which is povidone iodine, can be sourced from the pharmacy.

Iodine is know to discolour teeth as it stains dentine but use of sodium hypochlorite solution early in the procedure will help negate this side effect. It can also stain clothing so care should be taken during its use to avoid contact with the patient's or dental team's clothing.

Hydrogen peroxide

Hydrogen peroxide degrades to form water and oxygen, produces hydroxyl free radicals, which are effective against bacteria, yeasts and viruses as they attack proteins and DNA. Unfortunately it has not been shown to reduce bacterial load in root canals significantly. Furthermore due to effervescence of the chemical, oxygen may penetrate into the periradicular tissues causing surgical emphysema. In contemporary endodontics, it is considered to be a product of the past and should not be used. It is still available as Acqua ossigenata 12 V (Septodont), which is a 3.6% hydrogen-stabilized peroxide solution.

Other irrigants

Hypochlorous acid

This has some support, as it is less toxic than sodium hypochlorite although its mode of action is similar. In solution, it dissociates into hypochlorite ions but the reduced level of dissociation compared with sodium hypochlorite means that any adverse effects are also reduced. Similarly, with solutions of the same concentration of hypochlorous acid and sodium hypochlorite, the efficiency of sodium hypochlorite is greater as there is more chlorine available.

Electronically activated water

This is a spin off from the medical industry in which a device electrochemically generates, through the process of electrolysis, a solution of hypochlorous acid from the raw materials water and common salt, sodium chloride. The solution is regarded to be safer than other disinfectants as is less irritant if extruded into the periradicular tissues but it is still strongly bactericidal. The acid produced has a pH of near neutral (5–7). It is marketed to the dental profession as Sterilox.

MTAD

MTAD is a mixture of tetracycline isomer (doxycycline), an acid (citric acid) and a detergent (Tween 80). It is usually used in conjunction with sodium hypochlorite. The solution will disrupt pulp tissue and dentine to the same extent as EDTA. The doxycycline present in MTAD binds to the dentine and has also been reported to be effective against *Enterococcus faecalis*.

With every new product there is always concern about the cytotoxicity to the underlying tissue and the effect it may have on the strength of dentine. MTAD has been compared with commonly used irrigants and medications, and its level of cytotoxicity appears to be less than eugenol but greater than a 1% sodium hypochlorite solution.

Isomer: a compound with the same chemical formula but a different mode of arrangement of atoms.

Some dentists have advocated using **sterile water** or **local anaesthetic** solution to irrigant the root canal systems. While these solutions will lubricate the files and carry the swarf in solution, they do not have any disinfectant properties and are therefore not recommended to be used as the sole irrigant.

Combinations of irrigants

A number of techniques have been developed which use co-irrigants, to enhance the bactericidal effect, proteolytic disruption or removal of residual calcified debris on the root canal walls. The co-irrigants usually consist of an acid or chelating agent to dissolve the smear and assist in biofilm destruction, together with sodium hypochlorite, acting primarily as the disinfectant. They also may include alternative or additional disinfectants such as chlorhexidine.

Ozone

Ozone is used in the food and environmental industries for large-scale sterilizing of water supplies. The gas is a very effective sterilizing agent but at levels close to which it has toxicological effects can damage normal tissue. Devices are now available whereby the gas can be produced and delivered down a handpiece to the operating site in

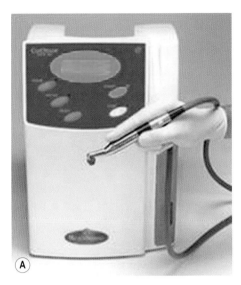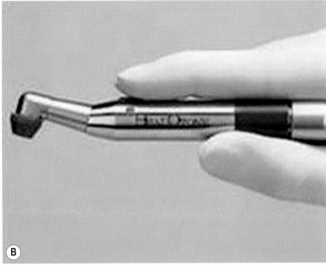

Fig. 13.15 (A) Healozone (CurOzone) device for using ozone and (B) handpiece delivery.

the mouth (Figure 13.15). In one device the area is sealed from the surroundings. The residual gas is then drawn back to the generator and neutralized using a platinum filter. More recent devices deliver the ozone down a fine tip directly into the canal for very short exposure times. This system does not require a seal around the tooth.

Commercially available products

Commercially available products are shown in Table 13.3.

Table 13.3 Some ozone-producing devices currently available on the market

Device name	Manufacturer
Healozone	CurOzone
Prozone	W & H

Bacterial photo-dynamic therapy (bacterial PDT)

Despite major advances in instrumentation and techniques, it is still not possible to consistently disinfect the root canal system. Accessing parts of the complex internal root canal system anatomy where bacteria are harboured can be challenging with conventional instruments and irrigants. This possibly explains why the success rate of endodontics even under ideal conditions is no better than 87%. Another reason is that currently available disinfectants such as sodium hypochlorite, chlorhexidine and calcium hydroxide are ineffective against some organisms, such as *E. faecalis* and *Streptococcus faecalis*.

It has been known for a number of years that the combination of a **photo-sensitizer** and a specific **wavelength of light** is effective against all microorganisms found in the mouth. This system is called **Bacterial photo-dynamic therapy (bacterial PDT)**. Some clinicians are using such a system to disinfect the root canal system during root canal therapy in an attempt to eradicate all microorganisms prior to obturation.

Photo-sensitizer

Depending on the system, there are a number of photo-sensitizers available with differing excitation wavelengths. The most commonly used photo-sensitizer is pharmaceutical grade **tolonium chloride**, a member of the phenothiazine family of compounds and a close relative of toluidine blue O, a vital stain. It is supplied as a solution at a concentration between 13–80 µg/ml.

Tolonium chloride has a lower surface tension and so it has better wetting properties than sodium hypochlorite solution, which means that it can penetrate into the dentinal tubules. It is also more biocompatible and does not pose a problem if it is inadvertently extruded outwith the root canal system.

Light

The light source is generally a laser diode or LED, which produces a red light at 635 nm ± 2 nm. The light acts as a means of exciting the photo-sensitizer molecules and minimal heat is produced. The light is delivered through an endodontic tip which is tapered in shape, allowing it to be placed into the root canal to be treated (Figure 13.16).

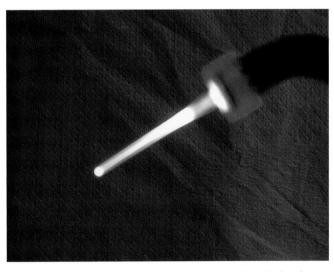

Fig. 13.16 Red light emitting from the endodontic light guide (Denfotex Research).

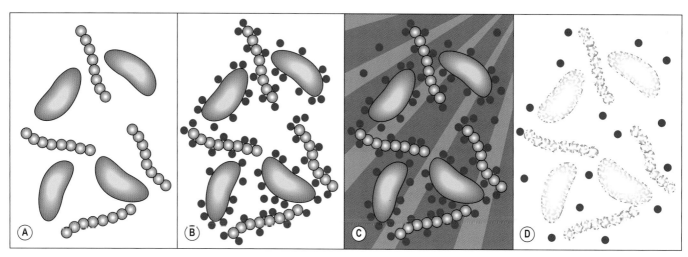

Fig. 13.17 A pictorial sequence demonstrating how bacterial PDT works. (A) Mixture of lactobacilli and streptococci in an infected area. (B) Photo-sensitizer solution (in blue) attached to the bacteria. (C) Photo-sensitizer activated by red light. (D) Bacteria destroyed by bacterial PDT.

Mechanism of action

The photo-sensitizer is preferentially taken up by rapidly dividing cells, of which microorganisms are examples. If the chemical is in contact or in very close proximity to the bacteria, the photo-sensitizer will be taken up by the liposomes on their cell walls. When the light energy is applied, the photo-sensitizer molecule becomes excited and free oxygen radicals are produced. The singlet oxygen species is a protoplasmic poison which causes oxidative injury to the bacterial cell wall, leading to death of the microorganism. This is very similar to the effect of inserting a pin into a balloon (Figure 13.17).

When the light is switched off, the photo-sensitizer returns to its unexcited state and causes no further effect. There is no collateral damage to any of the surrounding tissues. Unlike conventional antimicrobial therapy, resistant strains do not build up. It is important to note that it is the combination of the laser and photo-sensitizer which will result in the death of the microorganisms. Both the light and the photo-sensitizer are ineffective when used separately. The system is also effective against other microorganisms such as viruses and fungi, and thus may have other potential applications in dentistry and medicine in the future.

Commercially available products

Some of the commercially available products are set out in Table 13.4.

Table 13.4 Some bacterial PDT disinfection systems currently available on the market

Product	Manufacturer	Type of light source
CumdentPACT	Cumdente Dental concepts	Laser diode
FotO₂San	CMS Dental ApS	LED
PAD Plus	Denfotex Research	LED
Theralite laser	Helbo photo-dynamic systems	Laser diode

INTER-VISIT TEMPORIZATION

Inter-visit canal medicaments

Some clinicians prefer to carry out endodontic treatments over a number of appointments. This may be due to time constraints, as rarely is there sufficient time to fully clean and prepare the root canal system and then obturate it at the same appointment. The clinician and patient may both become fatigued!

Multiple-visit treatment also affords another opportunity to disinfect the root canal system by filling the prepared root canals with a medicament with antimicrobial properties. This is particularly so when concerns exist that conventional irrigants would not have totally disinfected the root canal system. Additionally, necrotic tissue is difficult to eradicate in one clinical session and the dentist will want any infection to resolve completely prior to obturation. Alternatively the tooth may still be tender to percussion and therefore contraindicate obturation at that time.

> **Apexification:** the procedure aimed at inducing apical closure with a hard tissue barrier across the open apex in a non-vital immature tooth.

In other cases such as trauma, the dentist may wish to encourage root formation to complete by apexification, which necessitates numerous appointments to change the inter-visit medication. In all of these cases the dentist restores the tooth temporarily prior to completing the procedure at a subsequent visit. The inter-visit (**intracanal**) medicaments available are:

- Steroid/antibiotic combination
- Non-setting calcium hydroxide
- Chlorhexidine
- Phenol or phenol derivatives
- Halogens
- Formaldehyde.

These are discussed in turn below. Once the selected medicament has been placed in the root canal system, the crown of the tooth is restored so establishing a coronal seal to prevent ingress of microorganisms.

Steroid/antibiotic combination

This paste is advocated in endodontics for the treatment of irreversible pulpitis and as an intracanal dressing between endodontic appointments. It is a mixture of a steroid **triamcinolone** and an antibiotic, **demeclocycline**. It is also available as a hard setting cement (see Chapter 12). The only product on the market is Ledermix (Lederle; Figure 13.18).

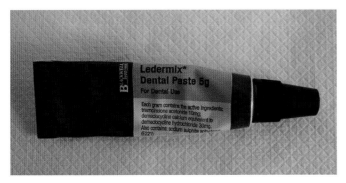

Fig. 13.18 Ledermix (Lederle), a steroid/antibiotic paste for the inter-visit dressing of endodontic canals.

The paste used in endodontics contains one-third more steroid than the cement. However, there is not more than 10% of either of the active ingredients in the paste. It is useful therefore in cases of irreversible pulpitis, particularly when sufficient analgesia cannot be gained to fully extirpate the canals. It is also recommended in cases when the pulp has been exposed. The antibiotic acts topically, only killing the bacteria adjacent to the dressing, while the steroid suppresses any inflammatory response, permitting bacteria at a distance from the surface of the lesion to proliferate, so leading to death of the pulp.

Some clinicians prefer to use the paste as an intracanal dressing between endodontic appointments. Since the paste is water soluble it can be easily rinsed from canals. The rationale of the paste use as an inter-visit dressing is not clear as the material is only effective when it is in contact with vital tissue. In a necrotic canal there is no vital tissue so it is unable to be used to its full potential.

There is a synergistic effect with non-setting calcium hydroxide paste when used in root canals in combination with a steroid/antibiotic paste. However the two materials should be placed separately into the root canal as the resultant mixture is too viscous to be placed easily, particularly into a narrow canal. Ledermix should be placed on a paper point to carry it into the canal followed by the non-setting calcium hydroxide being syringed into the canal.

Non-setting calcium hydroxide

The non-setting calcium hydroxide products are probably the most popular and commonly used intracanal medicaments. The active chemical (calcium hydroxide) is provided as a slurry in a water base. Some products are methylcellulose based, which is intended to facilitate removal of the products from the canal. They are also radiopaque,

which is advantageous. The pH is normally in the order of 12. Refrigerating these chemicals does not prolong their shelf-life.

Non-setting calcium hydroxide:

- Is **bactericidal**. It is a slow-acting antimicrobial agent which has a therapeutic effect after being in situ for at least a day. Effective disinfection in most cases of infected necrotic cases is seen in about a week
- Neutralizes the acidic endotoxins secreted by bacteria
- Inhibits the activity of osteoclasts due to its high pH. This is useful in cases of inflammatory root resorption as this process is arrested
- Is able to hydrolyse the lipid component of bacterial lipopolysaccharides. This renders the bacteria biologically inactive and reduces the toxic effects sometimes produced by the cell wall debris
- Denatures proteins found in root canals
- May activate the calcium-dependent adenosine triphosphatase reaction associated with hard tissue formation, so stimulating periradicular healing

Indications

Non-setting calcium hydroxide products have been advocated for use in the following clinical situations:

- As an **inter-visit intra-canal medicament**. Due to its antimicrobial properties, it may assist in the disinfection of the root canal system.
- The **control of exudation**. Non-setting calcium hydroxide has been used in cases of persistent infection, the exudate being a product of the inflammatory process for the same reasons.
- In a **Cvek (partial) pulpotomy**. This is done most commonly in trauma cases. Calcium hydroxide is used to create a calcific barrier with the intention of maintaining the vitality of the tooth.
- **Apexogenesis**.
- **Apexification**. Calcium hydroxide has been used traditionally to induce apical closure in non-vital immature teeth. The root canal is dressed with non-setting calcium hydroxide, and which is replaced every 6 weeks until a hard tissue barrier is formed across the open apex.
- **Resorption**. Calcium hydroxide is effective at inhibiting the activity of osteoclasts due to its high pH. Thus it can arrest the inflammatory process seen in cases of root resorption.

There are no contraindications to its use.

Pulpotomy: procedure in which only the most inflamed pulpal tissue is amputated, leaving the vital tissue in place.
Apexogenesis: process by which the apex of the root is closed in a vital tooth.

Use of non-setting material may cause calcification of the canal if left in situ for prolonged periods of time in excess of 6 months. The long term use of calcium hydroxide is also associated with an increased risk of root fracture as it has a denaturing effect on the collagen.

Mode of delivery

The material is presented as a paste supplied in a tube. Very often a fine endodontic needle may be attached to the Luer lock syringe

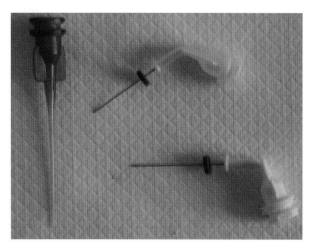

Fig. 13.19 Three Luer lock endodontic tips that may be used to place calcium hydroxide paste into a root canal. The purple tip is called a Capillary Tip whilst the two (blunt) needles on the right are NaviTips. Both products are made by Ultradent. Note the silicone stops on the NaviTips that allow the dentist to control the depth to which the needle is inserted into the root canal, thus preventing inadvertent extrusion of material outwith the root canal system.

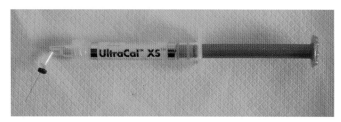

Fig. 13.20 A non-setting calcium hydroxide paste with a fine endodontic needle used to place the material in the canal (UltraCal, Ultradent).

attachment to deliver the paste into the canal. A range of needles are available (Figures 13.19 and 13.20).

The consistency of the calcium hydroxide should be as thick as possible to completely fill the root canal system. Some dentists advocate the use of a spiral filler to introduce the material into the canal which then can be compacted.

Non-setting calcium hydroxide can be difficult to remove completely from the root canal system once introduced. As both citric acid and EDTA are acidic in nature they will react with the calcium hydroxide, removing it more readily. One of these chelating irrigants should therefore be used to remove the calcium hydroxide prior to using sodium hypochlorite solution.

Another method of delivery of the calcium hydroxide as an inter-visit dressing is in a gutta percha matrix, marketed as Calcium hydroxide PLUS points (Roeko) which are 58% calcium hydroxide. This presentation is claimed to have a number of advantages over calcium hydroxide paste such as:

- Greater release of calcium hydroxide, which is more effective over a longer period
- The points are ready to use and do not require mixing
- They are easy to apply and remove and therefore save time
- There is no smearing around the access cavity during insertion.

Commercially available products

Table 13.5 shows some of the commercially available non setting calcium hydroxide cements.

Table 13.5 Some non-setting calcium hydroxide-containing products for inter-visit endodontic placement currently available on the market

Product	Manufacturer	Notes
ApexCal	Ivoclar Vivadent	
Calasept	JS Dental	Mixed with water or saline
Calcium hydroxide with iodoform	TG Pex	With iodoform
Endocal	Septodont	52% calcium hydroxide
Hydrocal	Cerkamed Dental-Medical Company	
HypoCal	Ellman	
UltraCal	Ultradent	
Vista-Cal	Vista Dental Products	
Vitapex	Neo Dental	With iodoform

Chlorhexidine

In the similar manner that calcium hydroxide has been incorporated into gutta percha and used as an inter-visit dressing so has chlorhexidine. Activ point (Roeko) is 5% chlorhexidine diacetate on a gutta percha matrix, which is usually placed in the canal for 1–3 weeks. They conform to the ISO specification (see The regulation of dental materials and the International Standards Organization' on the inside back cover of this book) for GP points for size and diameter (see p. 199), which matches their shape to that of the prepared root canal. A drop of sterile water can be used to accelerate the release of the chlorhexidine. The effects are similar to those described for the same material as an irrigant.

Phenol and phenol derivatives

The phenols and their derivatives (such as **para-monochlorphenol**, **thymol** and **cresol**) are quite effective antimicrobials. The derivatives of phenol are stronger antiseptics than phenol itself. However, their effect is only of a short duration. Phenol is a protoplasmic poison and works at an optimal concentration of 1–2%. Unfortunately many dental preparations containing phenol have too high a concentration (30%), which has a less than optimal effect. One study has demonstrated that phenols were unable to fully disinfect the root canal system after 2 weeks. This may be due to insufficient vapour being released for effective antimicrobial action when the product is placed on a cotton pellet in the pulp chamber. It may also be that their potency was exhausted.

An example of one such product on the market is Cresophene (Septodont). This product contains para-chlorphenol and dexamethasone (an anti-inflammatory agent) together with thymol and camphor, two antiseptic agents. However, due to these materials' high toxicity and concerns that they may be carcinogenic, their use is no longer be considered appropriate in contemporary endodontic practice.

Halogens

Halogen-containing products have been used as antimicrobial intracanal medicaments. Chlorine-containing products (**chloramines**) are available but iodine is more popular. Available as iodine potassium iodide, this chemical releases vapours that are an effective antimicrobial. A 2% iodine preparation is quicker at reducing bacterial load than an inter-visit dressing of calcium hydroxide. It may also prevent growth of *E. faecalis* within 1–2 hours.

- Some patients may be hypersensitive to iodine so products containing iodine are contraindicated in these individuals.
- Iodine-containing products may also stain clothing and care should therefore be taken when using to avoid contact except in the operating area.

Commercially available products

Table 13.6 lists some of the commercially available halogen-based products.

Table 13.6 Some halogen-based products currently available on the market

Product	Manufacturer
Cresophene	Septodont
Tempophore	Septodont

Formaldehyde

Inter-visit materials containing formaldehyde include Caustinerf Forte (Septodont). Various concerns have been raised with respect to the toxicity of formaldehyde-containing medicaments and as a result their use cannot be justified these days. More detail on formaldehyde and formaldehyde-containing dental materials can be found later in the chapter.

Inter-visit temporary dressings

When a multiple-visit procedure is planned the endodontist needs to temporarily restore the tooth until the next appointment. It is essential that this restoration is able to prevent any bacterial ingress into the root canal system by forming and maintaining a good coronal seal. It should also be strong enough to withstand occlusal loads, have sufficiently low solubility and high wear resistance, so that it will function satisfactorily for the length of time of treatment, which

may be over a potentially longer period. Materials used for this purpose are discussed in Chapters 9, 12 and 14 and include:

- Glass ionomer cement
- Zinc polycarboxylate cement
- Reinforced zinc oxide eugenol cement
- Zinc oxide-containing putties.

Thought should be given to the final restorative material when the dentist is selecting the temporary material. When a resin composite core or restoration is envisaged after the endodontic treatment has been completed, a eugenol-containing cement is contraindicated, and a material compatible with resin composite such as glass ionomer or zinc polycarboxylate cement should therefore be considered. This is also applicable to anterior teeth, where resin composite is likely to be the restorative material of choice.

The prudent clinician will also take some measures to prevent tooth fracture. Endodontically treated teeth are more susceptible to fracture as a substantial amount of tooth will have been removed to access the pulp chamber, so weakening the tooth. The placement of a tightly fitting copper or orthodontic band (Figures 13.21 and 13.22) has been advocated to hold the tooth together. This helps the tooth resist any splitting forces on it during mastication and also facilitates the placement of the rubber dam clamp. That said, copper rings are now becoming more difficult to source and in future orthodontic bands may be the only alternative.

Some clinicians may construct a core in a semi-permanent material after investigating the tooth for restorability by forming a core using a resin-modified glass ionomer cement or amalgam.

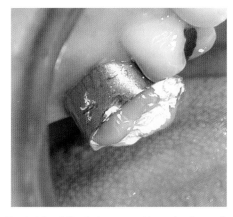

Fig. 13.22 Tooth 16 stabilized after coronal investigation and removal of caries with a copper ring and cored using IRM (Dentsply). Endodontic treatment can now be performed.

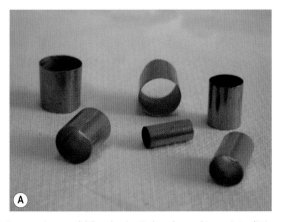

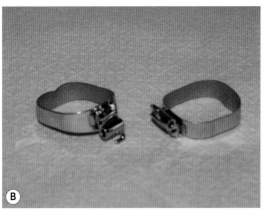

Fig. 13.21 (A) Copper rings and (B) orthodontic bands used to resist splitting forces on teeth which are undergoing endodontic treatment. If orthodontic bands are chosen then the component into which the archwire is placed can be removed prior to fitting as it is superfluous for this purpose.

OBTURATING MATERIALS

Once the root canal system has been fully cleaned, disinfected and shaped, it must be **obturated** (filled). This is to prevent any subsequent ingress of microorganisms by creating a seal at both the coronal and apical ends, not forgetting any lateral canals and the dentinal tubules. The material also completely fills the dead space, i.e. the whole root canal system, so removing air which may expand or contract if the patient is in a pressurized environment, such as in an aeroplane or when diving. Failure to do this may result in breakage of the tooth or pain (**aerodontalgia**) due to the difference in pressure. The most commonly used technique is when the root canal is filled using a semi-solid material (such as **gutta percha**) in combination with a **root canal sealer**. In modern endodontics, many clinicians use a **hybrid technique** in an attempt to utilize the best features of both techniques. An alternative technique involves the injection of a paste into the prepared root canal so obturating it; however, there are a number of problems associated with this technique and the material used for the purpose.

Gutta percha

Gutta percha (GP) primarily consists of the rubber **polyisoprene**, which comes from the rubber tree. Polyisoprene exists in two isomeric forms. The *cis* form is natural rubber and the *trans* form is gutta percha. The *trans* form further has two phases. The α phase is heated and used in the molten form. The commercially available gutta percha **points** or **cones** are consist of the β form. These are used at room temperature and are semi-solid. These two different crystalline forms are manufactured by heating the gutta percha to a high temperature. If the gutta percha is cooled quickly, the crystalline β phase is formed whereas if the material is cooled slowly the α phase is formed. The α form is denser and has better thermoplastic characteristics. It is therefore used in obturation techniques which require higher temperatures.

Polyisoprene in gutta percha is mixed with other chemicals to facilitate clinical handling. Table 13.7 lists the constituents of commercially available gutta percha together with their approximate proportions and the reasons for their inclusion.

Table 13.7 Chemical constituents of gutta percha

Constituent	Percentage range	Reason for inclusion
Gutta percha	19–22	Rubber
Zinc oxide	59–79	Filler
		Antimicrobial properties
Resins	1–4	Plasticizer
Waxes		Plasticizer
Metal sulphates	1–17	Confers radiopacity

Properties

Gutta percha is:

- A highly biocompatible material that causes minimal tissue changes even if it is inadvertently placed in the periradicular tissues

- Inert, with minimal toxicity and tissue irritability
- One of the least allergic materials available
- Dimensionally stable and packable
- Thermoplastic, softening at 60–65°C and melting at 100°C
- Stretchable, which means it is easily deformed and therefore may not fit the canal as intended.

Gutta percha also has some antibacterial properties. Due to the addition of metal sulphates, the form used clinically is radiopaque.

As such, gutta percha may not be heat sterilized. Acetone or alcohol should also not be used to disinfect gutta percha as these chemicals may be absorbed by it, so causing the material to swell. Therefore, if disinfection is necessary prior to placement, sodium hypochlorite should be used. Modern gutta percha tips are often presented in individual packets, having been sterilized by the manufacturer.

> **!**
>
> On exposure to light, gutta percha oxidizes and so will degrade and become brittle. Therefore gutta percha containing materials should be stored in a dark place.

Gutta percha lacks rigidity which may mean that smaller gutta percha points may be more difficult to fully seat into the canal. In its cold form, it displays poor adaptation to the tooth walls and does not adhere to dentine. Thus it offers poor resistance to bacterial ingression if the coronal seal is compromised. Some endodontists would advocate complete revision of the case if the coronal seal has been lost for more than 24 hours. Gutta percha can be softened with organic solvents, which is advantageous. Some dentists advocate dipping the gutta percha point in solvent prior to fitting so that its adaptation to the irregularities in the root canal can be improved. However, a minimum shrinkage in the order of 2% is seen with this technique.

Removal of gutta percha

Removing gutta percha from root canals is usually a difficult procedure. It does not cut cleanly and does not completely dissolve in solvents. However it can be softened by the action of solvents and this facilitates its removal from the root canal, for example should the case require to be re-treated. That said, the process is much easier these days as bespoke re-treat (root canal material removal) files are available on the market that are very efficient at removing gutta percha (Figure 13.23). These, in combination with an organic solvent,

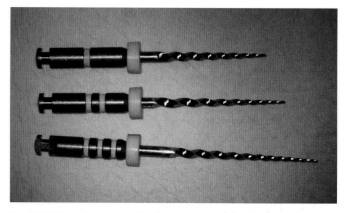

Fig. 13.23 Bespoke re-treat files (Protaper Universal Retreatment, Dentsply Maillefer) used to remove gutta percha from root canals.

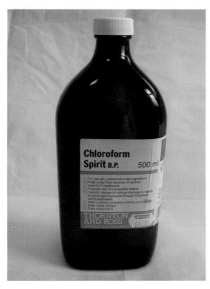

Fig. 13.24 Chloroform spirit used to soften gutta percha and facilitate its removal from root canals.

- Solvents used to dissolve gutta percha should be used with care as inadvertent spillage on rubber dam may cause it to break down, so compromising the aseptic environment.
- These solvents, particularly chloroform and halothane, require a well-ventilated clinical environment.

Solvents used to dissolve gutta percha should be used sparingly, that is, they should be used with an endodontic syringe and needle to precisely place the liquid onto the gutta percha, one drop at a time.

should with time and patience allow the endodontist to re-establish a patent root canal. The most effective and efficient solvent is chloroform (Figure 13.24). This can be sourced from a pharmacy; in the UK it is available to registered dentists on prescription.

Other solvents that also soften root canal filling materials are also available (Table 13.8) but are less effective and efficient. Many of the chemicals used for this purpose, including chloroform, are also toxic and therefore should be used with care. For this reason, inexperienced dentists may be advised not to use chloroform but to select a less potent and less toxic alternative.

Presentation

In the cold form, gutta percha is supplied as points or cones (Figure 13.25) and the dentist selects the appropriate size to fill the root canal to be obturated. The taper of the cones may vary and should match the taper of the last file used in the canal.

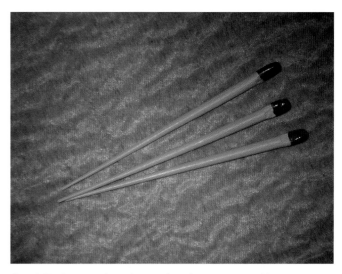

Fig. 13.25 Gutta percha points used to obturate root canals.

Manufacturing tolerances

Gutta percha cones are subject to ISO standards, however, there are some variations with respect to size tolerances and proportion of chemical ingredients. Cones are made to a tolerance of ±0.05 mm, which is less than that for files. This may therefore cause a mismatch that would only become apparent on fitting the cone. Furthermore, different products are composed of different proportions of chemicals and so variations in properties such as brittleness and stiffness may be encountered.

Cold obturation

Cold obturation techniques essentially use gutta percha cones with an endodontic sealer to fill the root canal. An example of one such

Table 13.8 Some products currently available on the market for the removal of root canal filling materials

Product	Manufacturer	Active chemical	Used to soften
Chloroform	Thornton and Ross	Chloroform	Gutta percha
DMS IV Solvent	Dentsply Maillefer	Ethyl acetate	Eugenol-based cements
Endosolv E	Septodont	Tetrachloroethylene	Zinc oxide eugenol
Endosolv R	Septodont	Formamid	Phenolic resin
Eucalyptus oil	Cerkamed Dental-Medical Company	Cyclic ether and a monoterpenoid often known as **cineole**	Gutta percha
Halothane/ fluothane	Wyeth-Ayerst Labs	Halothane	Gutta percha
Oil of Wintergreen	Available on prescription from a pharmacist	Methyl salicylate	Gutta percha
Turpentine oil		Turpentine	Gutta percha
xylol		Xylol	Gutta percha

technique, **cold lateral condensation**, has been considered to be the gold standard for many years. In this technique, a gutta percha cone that corresponds in size to the canal preparation (**master cone**) is coated with a root canal sealer and introduced into the root canal. It is pushed laterally using an instrument called a spreader. This creates a space so that the next cone (**accessory cone**) can be placed. Other accessory cones coated with sealer are then introduced into the canal one at a time. This process is continued until the root canal is fully obturated. Accessory cones tend to be thinner and more tapered than master cones.

If a gutta percha cone needs to be trimmed to gain a closer apical fit, this should be done using a scalpel blade. Scissors should not be used as they will distort the cone during cutting (Figure 13.26).

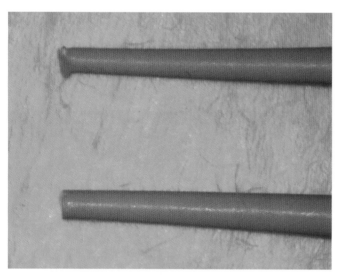

Fig. 13.26 Two gutta percha cones, one trimmed using scissors (top) and the other trimmed with a scalpel blade (bottom). Note that the point cut with the scissors has been deformed, which will compromise the quality of the apical seal achieved.

Cold lateral condensation is time consuming and due to the potential shortcomings of using cold gutta percha, many clinicians have moved onto using a technique that uses a more liquid presentation of gutta percha. The more fluid material may flow into the irregularities of the root canal system so improving the quality of the obturation achieved. This may be achieved by either using a gutta percha product which is in a semi-liquid form at room temperature (e.g. GuttaFlow, Roeko) or by use of a warm technique that involves additional hardware.

GuttaFlow combines gutta percha and an addition cross-linking poly(dimethyl siloxane). Other chemicals in the product are listed in Table 13.9. As no heat is required to use this product, no shrinkage is seen. In fact, there is a slight expansion of the material in the order of 0.2%, which is claimed to improve the seal obtained. The particle size is $30\,\mu m$ and this facilitates its flow. It has virtually zero solubility.

Table 13.9 Chemical constituents of GuttaFlow (Roeko)

Constituent	Reason for inclusion
Gutta percha powder	Main obturating component
Zinc oxide	Filler and radio-opacifier
Zirconium dioxide	Filler and radio-opacifier
Silicone oil	Binder and consistency modifier
Paraffin oil	Binder and consistency modifier
Colloidal silver	Inhibits reinfection
Hexachloroplatinic acid	Catalyst
Colouring agent	Optimizes colour

GuttaFlow is used effectively as a sealer (it is a modification of RoekoSeal (Roeko), mentioned later) in combination with a master gutta percha cone. While heat is not required for this technique the application of heat will reduce the working time. It is presented in a capsule which is mixed for 30 seconds. A faster setting product is now available (GuttaFlow FAST, Roeko) (Figure 13.27).

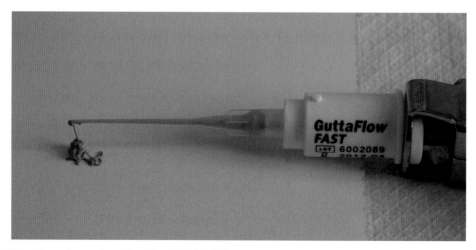

Fig. 13.27 A cold flowable gutta percha product, GuttaFlow FAST (Roeko).

Warm gutta percha

Gutta percha used at a higher temperature is supplied as little pellets. These are placed in a gun with a small oven to warm the gutta percha (Figures 13.28 and 13.29). The recommended temperature depends on the product. It is usually 150–200°C with the selection of the product being determined by the gauge of needle used to express the gutta percha into the canal. The narrower (smaller) the gauge, the lower temperature material should be used. The product is chemically similar but there is a difference in the manufacturing process whereby the lower temperature material is heat treated. Once it has come to the correct temperature the molten material can be expressed out of the needle of the gun directly into the root canal to be obturated.

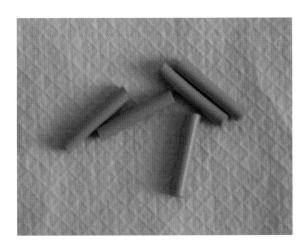

Fig. 13.28 Gutta percha pellets used into conjunction with Obtura II (Obtura Spartan) (see Figure 13.29).

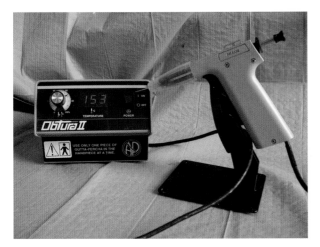

Fig. 13.29 Obtura II gun (Obtura Spartan).

Many clinicians prefer to have secured an apical stop prior to using molten gutta percha to prevent extrusion of the molten material outwith the root canal system and into the periradicular tissues. The molten gutta percha by its nature can obturate anatomical irregularities within the root canal system such as fins, isthmuses and irregularities caused by pathological changes (Figure 13.30).

Due to its thermoplastic nature, gutta percha may be cut using heat. Traditional methods involved heating an instrument in a Bunsen burner and searing the gutta percha. This is not desirable due to the presence of the naked flame, the potential for burning other objects between the Bunsen and the tooth, and the effect of

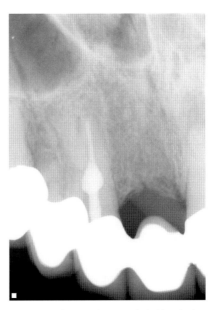

Fig. 13.30 Tooth 13 was obturated using a hybrid technique of a gutta percha cone heated with System B (SybronEndo) and then backfilled using Obtura II (Obtura Spartan). Note that the warm gutta percha has completely obturated the defect caused by internal resorption.

heating tempering the steel of the instrument, so damaging it. The modern instruments used to sear gutta percha such as System B (SybronEndo) have a wire inside a probe which when current is initiated heats up very quickly and then cools likewise when the current is switched off. This is much easier and safer.

Another popular system on the market consists of a metal or plastic point coated in gutta percha. These cones are heated in an oven to the recommended temperature and then inserted into the root canal. An example of this system is Thermafil (Dentsply Maillefer). Root canals can be obturated very quickly using this method and the softened gutta percha will flow. The disadvantage is the central carriers may be difficult to remove and this may be significant if a post space preparation requires to be done subsequently or if the endodontic treatment needs to be repeated. Another similar product in design is Real Seal 1 (SybronEndo) but this product is resin based (see later).

Latex-sensitive patients

As gutta percha is a rubber-based product, there is the theoretical possibility of allergy in those patients sensitive to latex. In these cases, it may be prudent to avoid the use of gutta percha and the root canals could either be obturated using a paste which has sufficient volume stability to maintain a seal such as AH Plus (Dentsply) or Ketac-Endo (3M ESPE). Care would have to be taken by the dentist as the use of a paste on its own may result in extrusion of the material into the periradicular tissues as there is nothing to contain the material within the root canal system. Achievement of a good apical seal is also likely to be compromised.

Another (and better) alterative is to use a product such as RealSeal 1 (SybronEndo). This is made from polymers of polyester and so does not contain rubber or rubber-based materials.

Commercially available products

As with root canal files, there are too many gutta percha products available on the market to list here. The dentist should select a product with which he or she is comfortable and considers compatible with the root canal preparation technique they have used.

Resin points

A recently introduced product to the market consists of endodontic obturation points composed of a hydrophilic polymer. These have the ability to swell when water is absorbed from the tooth tissue. The point swells only laterally, preventing extrusion apically or coronally. It also has a controlling hoop system, which prevents excess swelling that could cause root fracture, and is flexible for placement into curved canals and can be removed easily should the need arise. The points are radiopaque and come in two taper sizes.

The system is marketed as Smartseal (Smartseal DRFP Ltd) and consists of the points (Smartpoint) and a sealer (Smartpaste) to be used in combination. This sealer contains an active polymer that also swells to fill any voids in the root canal system. The amount of swelling is controlled by the quantity of active polymer used. The problem is exactly controlling the expansion to fit every case.

Another resin-based product is EndoREZ (Ultradent) (Figure 13.31). This is a hydrophilic, primarily dual-cured resin obturation system based on urethane dimethacrylate (UDMA) and triethylene glycol dimethacrylate. The chemical polymerization is achieved using a system similar to chemically activated resin composites. The material is presented as a base and catalyst in a cartridge for self-mixing. The dark-cure reaction takes 20 minutes but this reaction time may be speeded up by using the accelerator provided. The set can also be accelerated by mixing with an additional accelerator paste. Filler is added for radiopacity. In a similar technique to cold lateral condensation, a master cone is inserted, followed by accessory cones that are then light cured for 40 seconds.

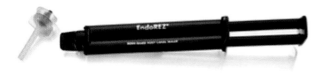

Fig. 13.31 A resin-based endodontic sealing product EndoREZ (Ultradent).

Products containing UDMA, such as EndoREZ (Ultradent), should not be used following preparation with products containing peroxide or iodine (for example Glyde File Prep or RC Prep) as this may affect the polymerization process.

A resin system that resembles Thermafil (Dentsply Maillefer) in concept as it requires an oven to heat the obturation point is RealSeal 1 (SybronEndo). Formerly known as Resilon, it is a thermoplastic synthetic resin material based on the polymers of polyester. The glasses provide radiopacity. This material is presented as a primer and sealer, which are based on dimethacrylate technology. The points are made of polyester with barium sulphate and silicate as the radiopaque filler.

The core is resin based with a Resilon outer coating. It is non-toxic, non-mutagenic and bonds to dentine. As RealSeal 1 is constructed from polymers of polyester and not gutta percha, it does not contain rubber or rubber-based materials. Thus it is indicated for patients who are sensitive to latex. It is soluble in chloroform and may be removed in a similar manner to gutta percha.

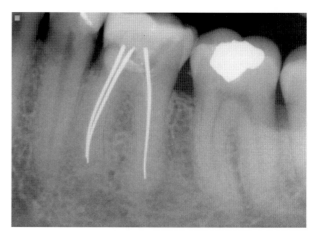

Fig. 13.32 Tooth 36 obturated with a silver point in each canal.

Silver points

Silver points were used for many years to obturate root canals. Due to their rigidity these cones were easy to place and to identify on radiographs (Figure 13.32). Silver is also a known bactericide. However, use of silver points did present some shortcomings:

- They do not fully obturate the canal as they are not shaped to match the final shape of the canal. There is a reliance on the root canal sealer to do this, which is not ideal as explained later.
- They are prone to corrosion, which is exacerbated by the very small amounts (1–2%) of copper and nickel present. The corrosion products are highly toxic and may leak out from the root canal system causing tissue injury. Corrosion may also result from galvanism.
- They are difficult to remove as they tend to fracture. This can be particularly troublesome if a post space preparation is indicated or if the case requires to be re-treated.
- They are rigid in nature and so cannot adapt to the canal walls.
- The products of corrosion may permeate the dentinal tubules so causing unsightly staining of the tooth tissue.

Silver points have fallen into disuse for the above reasons and are considered to be obsolete in contemporary endodontic practice.

Other endodontic obturation materials

Acrylic and titanium points are also available to obturate root canals. They are produced by Produits Dentaires. They are rarely used as they do not provide good adaptation to the apical third of the root canal.

ENDODONTIC SEALERS

An endodontic sealer is a paste, usually presented as a base and catalyst. After mixing together, the paste is coated onto the endodontic point prior to its insertion into the root canal. The sealer subsequently hardens by a chemical reaction. The purpose of a sealer is to:

- Lubricate and facilitate the full placement of the endodontic master point and accessory cones in a technique such as cold lateral condensation
- Fill any voids between the obturation points due to their physical limitations
- Fill and seal lateral canals and pass through the lateral canals to the root surface. This may been seen radiographically as a 'puff' on the side of the root.
- Provide a disinfectant action if they contain an active component.

Clearly, endodontic sealers must be non-toxic. However, transient adverse biological activity may occur during the setting phase. Provided that this does not continue after setting, the material may be acceptable. Various products have different setting times, so thought should be given as to the selection of the product to be used. For example, extended working time (EWT) products are available and the dentist may select these products in cases with multiple canals or in difficult cases that may require more time to obturate.

Likewise, other physical properties which should be considered are: flow, film thickness, solubility and radiodensity. The ability of the sealer to flow will determine how effectively voids between the master cone and accessory cones and any accessory canals may be obturated. It is desirable that the film thickness is minimal as the sealer is by far the most likely material to degrade. As most sealers are soluble and are absorbed to some extent when exposed to tissue fluid, the amount of sealer should be kept to a minimum. The material should also be radiopaque.

Several chemically different categories of endodontic sealer are available:

- Zinc oxide eugenol
- Calcium hydroxide
- Epoxy resin
- Glass ionomer cement
- Poly(dimethyl siloxanes).

Zinc oxide eugenol

Zinc oxide eugenol-containing endodontic sealers are probably the most commonly used and give good results, especially with cold techniques.

They are essentially similar to the traditional dental zinc oxide eugenol cements and their setting reaction is the same. The difference lies in their particle size, which is finer to enhance flow compared with restorative zinc oxide eugenol cements. They are weak and porous and thus susceptible to decomposition in tissue fluids. They do with time lose some volume, as eugenol and zinc oxide are released. In an attempt to decrease this dissolution and render the product more insoluble, some manufacturers have added resins or rosins such as colophony. This may increase the potential of the sealer to act as an sensitizing agent (see Chapter 3).

Some patients are sensitive to colophony and this should be determined when the patient's medical history is taken. Colophony is also present in other dental materials such as topical fluoride varnish (e.g. Duraphat (Colgate), see Chapter 17).

Zinc oxide and zinc eugenolate are antimicrobial and so these cements have potent antibacterial potential. They are cytotoxic and in high doses mutagenic. However, this does not appear to be an issue clinically. Some products have other chemicals added for various reasons. Germicides have an antiseptic action, rosin or Canada balsam increase the adhesion of the sealer to dentine, corticosteroids suppress inflammatory reactions and paraformaldehyde has a mummifying and antimicrobial effects. Products containing paraformaldehyde are contraindicated as is explained later in the chapter.

There are numerous chemical ingredients contained in zinc oxide eugenol endodontic sealers; Table 13.10 lists the ingredients of three

Table 13.10 Typical ingredients of three zinc oxide eugenol endodontic sealers

Ingredient	Reason for inclusion	Proportion in Kerr's sealer (~%)	Proportion in Grossman's sealer (~%)	Proportion in Tubli-Seal (~%)
Powder				
Zinc oxide	Filler	34–41	42	57–59
Silver	Radio-opacifier (may cause discolouration)	25–30	–	–
Oleoresins	Viscosity regulator	16–30	–	18–21
Staybelite resin	Binder	–	27	–
Dithymoliodide	Antiseptic	11–13	–	–
Bismuth subcarbonate	Radio-opacifier	–	15	–
Bismuth subiodide	Radio-opacifier	–	–	–
Bismuth trioxide	Radio-opacifier	–	–	7.5
Barium sulphate	Radio-opacifier	–	15	–
Sodium borate	Filler	–	1	–
Thymol iodide	Antiseptic	–	–	3–5
Oils and waxes	Binder and viscosity regulator	–	–	10
Liquid				
Oil of cloves	Cement former	78–80	–	–
Eugenol	Cement former	–	100	*
Canada balsam	Viscosity regulator	20–22	–	–
Polymerized resin	Reinforcing agent	–	–	*
Annidalin		–	–	*

All three materials are available from SybronEndo.
*Constituent present but proportion unavailable.

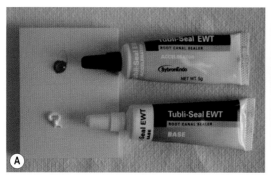
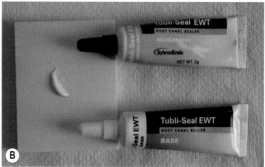

Fig. 13.33 A zinc oxide eugenol endodontic sealer (Tubli-Seal EWT, SybronEndo): (A) note the higher viscosity of both pastes and (B) the final mixed material.

zinc oxide eugenol endodontic sealers. For a comprehensive list of ingredients in a particular product, the manufacturer should be contacted for full details.

Presentation and mixing

These sealers are presented as a two-paste system (See Box 12.5, p. 180). The viscosity of both pastes is higher than other dental materials presented in this form. However, the principles behind their mixing are the same as other paste/paste systems (Figure 13.33). See Box 12.5 for a pictorial illustration of the sequence of mixing of a paste/paste presentation.

Calcium hydroxide

These sealers became popular when they were first introduced, as they claimed to offer therapeutic effects due to the calcium hydroxide. When the calcium hydroxide dissociates into an ionic form, these ions may confer an antimicrobial effect and may promote healing. Unfortunately, for this to happen, the sealer must dissolve, so leaving voids in the obturated material, thus negating one of the principal functions of a sealer and weakening the remaining cement. This sealer is therefore more soluble. It has a poor cohesive strength but its sealing ability is similar to zinc oxide eugenol-containing endodontic sealers. There is no evidence that calcium hydroxide sealers provide any advantage for obturation or desirable biological effects.

As with zinc oxide eugenol endodontic sealers, there are numerous chemical ingredients in calcium hydroxide-based endodontic sealers. Table 13.11 lists the ingredients of two calcium hydroxide endodontic sealers as an illustration.

Table 13.11 Typical ingredients of two commonly available calcium hydroxide endodontic sealers

Ingredient	Reason for inclusion	Proportion in Sealapex (SybronEndo) (~%)	Proportion in Apexit Plus (Ivoclar Vivadent) (~%)
Base			
Calcium hydroxide	Cement former	25	32
Zinc oxide	Cement former	6.5	5.5
Calcium oxide	Cement former	–	5.6
Silicon dioxide	Viscosity regulator	–	8
Zinc stearate	Binder	–	2.3
Hydrogenized colophony	Binder	–	31.5
Tricalcium phosphate	Antiseptic filler	–	4.1
Polydimethyl siloxane	Viscosity regulator	–	2.5
Activator			
Barium sulphate	Radio-opacifier	18.6	–
Titanium dioxide	Filler/colouring agent	5.1	–
Zinc stearate	Binder	1.0	1.4
Trimethyl hexanedioldisalicylate	Cement former	–	25
Bismuth carbonate	Radio-opacifier	–	18.2
Bismuth oxide	Radio-opacifier	–	18.0
Silicon dioxide	Filler and viscosity moderator	–	15
1,3-butanedioldisalicylate	Cement former	–	11.5
Hydrogenized colophony	Binder	–	5.4
Tricalcium phosphate	Antiseptic filler	–	5

Epoxy resin

Epoxy resin endodontic sealers are **polymers** composed of an **epoxy amine**. They have gained in popularity in the recent past, particularly with the heated obturation techniques. The resins demonstrate many of the attributes of an ideal sealer, such as good flow and sealing ability, high dimensional stability, low shrinkage, sufficient working time, adhesion to other materials and dentine, and antibacterial properties. These sealers are less porous and have greater hardness than zinc oxide eugenol sealers and the same radiodensity as gutta percha. However, their lower solubility and greater film thickness may prove problematic if the material needs to be removed. They are soluble in chloroform, which facilitates removal.

When first mixed they are toxic, however, this decreases during setting and after 24 hours they are the least toxic of all the endodontic sealers. Some patients, however, may be sensitive to the epoxy resin contained in the material so the dentist should check for allergy prior to selecting the material.

Ingredients

These sealers are presented as a paste/paste system, a base and catalyst (Table 13.12), which are mixed by hand on a pad. One product, AH Plus (Dentsply), is also now available in a cartridge mixing presentation.

Setting reaction

AH Plus (Dentsply) is a two-paste system (Figure 13.34) that sets by an addition polymerization reaction. It is an exothermic reaction in which the epoxides and the amine react to form long chains. Since this is an addition reaction, there is no residual monomer remaining and no by-products. The diamines present in the cement are reported to provide high dimensional stability.

The poly(addition) reaction is temperature dependent and takes a substantial amount of time. This does provide an extended working time in the region of 4 hours. Interestingly, the setting process is dependent on the two reactive components being put together and by addition of small amount of heat.

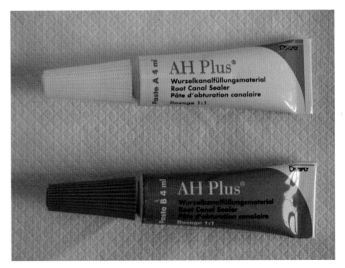

Fig. 13.34 An epoxy resin endodontic sealer (AH Plus, Dentsply) supplied as two pastes.

Table 13.12 Typical ingredients of two commonly available epoxy resin-based endodontic sealers

Ingredient	Reason for inclusion	Proportion in AH Plus (Dentsply) (~%)	Proportion in Diaket (3M ESPE) (~%)
Base			
Silver powder	Radio-opacifier	10	–
Zinc oxide	Filler	–	98
Bismuth oxide	Radio-opacifier	60	–
Bismuth phosphate	Radio-opacifier	–	2
Hexamethylenetetramine	Hardening agent	25	–
Titanium oxide	Colouring agent/filler	5	–
Catalyst			
Bisphenoldiglycidyl ether	Cement former	100	–
2,2 dihydroxy 5,5 dichlorodiphenylmethane	Cement former	–	*
Propionylacetophenone	Setting agents	–	*
Triethanolamine	Setting agents	–	*
Caproic acid	Setting agents	–	*
Copolymers of vinyl acetate, vinyl chloride and vinyl isobutylether	Cement former	–	*

*Constituent present but proportion unavailable

Glass ionomer cement

Glass ionomer cements have been modified to be used as endodontic sealers. They have a low toxicity and induce little tissue irritation. They are cytotoxic but this and any inflammatory responses decrease with time.

These cements adhere to dentine but may be less good at sealing. Their physical properties are better than zinc oxide eugenol, with less coronal leakage. Like restorative glass ionomer cements, they leach fluoride, which is taken up by dentine. They are more susceptible to dissolution if exposed to liquids before maturation is complete. The composition and setting reaction are similar to those of a luting glass ionomer (see Chapter 9 for further details).

Polydimethyl siloxanes

These sealers are chemically the extension of the addition cured polyvinyl siloxane impression materials. Their chemical constituents are shown in Table 13.13. The material is insoluble, which may be a problem as it is not resorbed so should not be used in deciduous teeth. It is dimensionally stable, although there is an initial slight expansion on setting. Its small film thickness and good flow characteristics allows the material to flow into tubules and fins. It has an excellent biocompatibility but cannot bond to dentine and has no antibacterial properties.

Table 13.13 Chemical constituents of a polydimethyl siloxane endodontic sealer

Constituent	Reason for inclusion
Polydimethyl siloxane	Active component
Silicon oil	Binder
Paraffin base oil	Binder
Platinum catalyst	Catalyst
Zirconium dioxide	Filler

RoekoSeal (Roeko) is an example of one such product and it is supplied as an auto-mix or single-dose presentation (Figure 13.35) that provides a homogeneous mix, free of air bubbles. The material should be applied onto a gutta percha point prior to insertion of the cone into the canal. It can also be used on its own but the clinician must take care that it does not extrude outwith the root canal system. It may be difficult to use with heated techniques as the heat will decrease the working time, and the dentist should be aware of this.

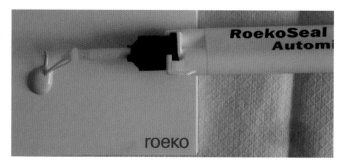

Fig. 13.35 A polydimethyl siloxane endodontic sealer (RoekoSeal, Roeko).

Polydimethyl siloxane-containing materials should be not used in deciduous teeth as they are not resorbable.

Chloropercha

Chloropercha was a root canal obturation material consisting of the combination of chloroform and gutta percha. It has fallen out of favour and is no longer used as it is prone to shrinking.

- Most paste/paste presentations are used sparingly in combination with gutta percha cones to prevent extracanal extrusion and decrease amount of sealer needed.
- Endodontic sealers should also be used sparingly, with the point being only thinly coated with sealer (Figure 13.36). This will prevent extrusion of the sealer into the periradicular tissues and loss of the more soluble sealer over time.

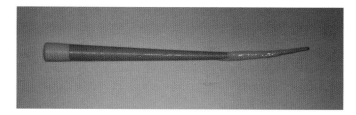

Fig. 13.36 A gutta percha cone with endodontic sealer thinly buttered on the apical portion of the point prior to insertion into the root canal.

Root canal obturating pastes

Some root canal obturating materials are available as pastes. This may prove problematic as the material may extrude outwith the root canal system into the periradicular tissues due to the product's flow properties.

The **formaldehyde**-containing products are supplied in this form. As well as the shortcomings of their physical properties, these materials are chemically toxic. They are usually supplied as **paraformaldehyde**, which is the polymer form of formaldehyde. Paraformaldehyde decomposes to give its monomer, which is a water soluble, protein-denaturing agent. These chemicals are highly toxic, allergenic, genotoxic, mutagenic and carcinogenic. They are known to cause severe inflammatory reactions and necrosis if they come into direct contact with the tissues as they are tissue destructive. This may cause permanent injury if applied to neural tissue on extrusion outwith root canal space. This problem is further compounded as they are not resorbable after setting. There have also been concerns that formaldehyde may be transported to other parts of the body. As an allergen, it can cause contact dermatitis, a delayed-type hypersensitivity, and also has on rare occasions caused type 1 anaphylaxis. Leaching occurs for a long time and results in chronic inflammation. They may prevent or delay healing and mask the inflammatory process.

Traditionally these products were used as a devitalizing agent or to reduce postoperative flare-ups. They were applied to a cotton wool pellet and placed in pulp chamber and due to their volatile nature, they released antimicrobial vapours.

Endomethasone N (Septodont) and N2 (Indrag Agsa) are examples of paraformaldehyde-containing products. These are basically a zinc oxide eugenol sealer with 6–8% paraformaldehyde. A well-known historical product is SPAD (Quetigny), which is now no longer available. The use of paraformaldehyde-containing products should now be considered to be contraindicated and they are now obsolete in contemporary endodontics.

Commercially available products

Table 13.14 show examples of commercially available root canal sealer products.

Table 13.14 Some root canal sealer products currently available on the market, categorized by material type

Product	Manufacturer	Material type
Acroseal	Septodont	Epoxy resin and calcium hydroxide based
AH Plus	Dentsply	Epoxamine resin
Mtwo 2 Seal	VDW	Epoxyamine resin
Apexit Plus	Ivoclar Vivadent	Calcium hydroxide
Diaket	3M ESPE	Polyvinyl resin, polyketone
GuttaFlow	Roeko	Silicon
Ketac Endo	3M ESPE	Glass ionomer
RoekoSeal	Roeko	Polydimethyl siloxane
Sealapex	SybronEndo	Polymeric calcium hydroxide
Endomet Plain	Septodont	Zinc oxide eugenol
Pulp Canal Sealer EWT	SybronEndo	Zinc oxide eugenol
Rickert's sealer	SybronEndo	Zinc oxide eugenol
Tubli Seal EWT	SybronEndo	Zinc oxide eugenol
TubliSeal	SybronEndo	Zinc oxide eugenol
Endomethasone N	Septodont	Zinc oxide eugenol/ paraformaldehyde paste
N2	Indrag Agsa	Zinc oxide eugenol/ paraformaldehyde paste
EndoRez	Ultradent	UDMA resin
RealSeal 1	SybronEndo	UDMA resin

MINERAL TRIOXIDE AGGREGATE

Mineral trioxide aggregate (MTA) has revolutionized endodontics since its invention and availability on the market. It is essentially Portland cement, an α-hemihydrate calcium sulphate plus bismuth oxide, which is included to impart radiopacity to the material. MTA stimulates hard tissue deposition, forms an excellent seal and permits regeneration of the periodontal membrane, so achieving complete repair of the periradicular tissues.

Composition

MTA consists of fine hydrophilic particles that contain a number of mineral oxides:

- Tricalcium silicate
- Dicalcium silicate
- Tricalcium aluminate
- Tetracalcium aluminoferrite
- Calcium sulphate dehydrate (gypsum)
- Bismuth oxide (forms about 20% of the material)
- Other constituents included in trace amounts are:
  - Calcium oxide
  - Magnesium oxide
  - Potassium sulphate
  - Sodium sulphate
  - Crystalline silica.

Setting reaction

The powder is mixed with sterile water and a colloidal gel is formed. It takes about four hours to set and requires moisture to effect this. The most common method of achieving this is to seal a moist cotton wool pledget adjacent to the MTA until the next appointment. The material may then be covered with a resin modified glass ionomer cement and the definitive coronal restoration provided. The setting reaction is similar to that of Portland cement which is a hydration reaction (see Chapter 20).

The material is not adversely affected by blood contamination.

Low pH environments inhibit the setting of MTA. Areas of infection may be acidic and so the material should not be used in areas of acute infection.

Properties

MTA is alkaline in nature with a pH of about 12.5. Its compressive strength is the same as a reinforced zinc oxide eugenol cement– approximately 50 MPa when the powder and liquid are mixed in its recommended ratio of 3:1. The compressive strength develops over a period of approximately 28 days. However, it has been show that MTA discolours with time. In addition it increases the brittleness of the dentine due to denaturing of the collagen.

Biocompatibility

MTA is non-toxic and is biocompatible with the periradicular tissues similar to calcium hydroxide cement. Little or no host inflammatory response is seen when the material is in contact with vital tissues. It is less cytotoxic than zinc oxide eugenol cements.

Its unique property is the new cementum formation and regeneration of the periodontal membrane which occurs over the surface of MTA when it is used as a root end filling material. Collagen fibres may integrate with the material. This is unlike other dental materials used for the same purpose where a fibrous capsule usually forms over them.

MTA is believed to attract growth cells and promotes a favourable environment for formation of cement. The stimulation of osteoblasts increases the production of osteocalcin and other interleukins so inducing bone deposition. Likewise, the stimulation of odontoblasts forms hard (tertiary dentine) tissue following direct pulp capping. Cell adhesion and proliferation has also been shown to be stimulated by MTA.

Sealing ability

MTA has an excellent ability to seal with little or no marginal leakage seen in dye leakage studies. It expands in a moist environment, which is advantageous in adapting the material to the walls of the tooth whether in perforation sites or at the root end. The material is non-resorbable and thus does not break down over time, maintaining the seal.

Advantages and disadvantages

The disadvantages and advantages of MTA are listed in Table 13.15.

Table 13.15 Advantages and disadvantages of MTA

Advantages	Disadvantages
Excellent biological compatibility	Difficult to manipulate
Regeneration of the periodontal membrane	Takes time to set so another appointment required to definitively restore
Encourage hard tissue deposition	Can be washed out when rinsed
Excellent ability to seal	Expensive
Can be used in many situations	

The amount of material presented in a sachet of MTA is too much for one case. As the material is expensive, it is prudent to minimize wastage. The contents of each sachet may be divided into six equal amounts and placed into air tight (MTA degrades in moisture) Epidorph tubes (Figure 13.37). One tube should provide enough MTA for one application.

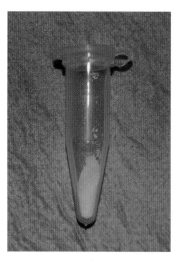

Fig. 13.37 One-sixth of a sachet of ProRoot MTA (Dentsply Maillefer) in an Epidorph tube.

Indications

MTA has a number of indications:

- As a **pulp capping** material: after the removal of caries and rendering the cavity sterile, MTA may be placed over an exposed pulp instead of calcium hydroxide. With MTA the likelihood and rate of tertiary dentine deposition is greater than with calcium hydroxide. Furthermore this occurs without pulpal inflammation.
- **Internal** and **external root resorption**: MTA has been used successfully to not only gain a hermetic barrier between the inside of the tooth and the periradicular tissues but it may also increase the strength of the root.
- **Perforation repair**: in a similar manner as above, MTA can achieve and maintain a hermetic barrier between the inside and the periradicular tissues. Perforation repair may be carried out as an **internal** (i.e. from inside the root canal) or as an open procedure **external**ly (Figure 13.38).
- **Root-end filling** material: this is a common use for MTA due to its excellent biocompatibility and promotion of complete periradicular healing, which is superior to that obtained with other materials indicated for this procedure, such as IRM, SuperEBA and amalgam (Figure 13.39).
- **Apexification**: the traditional method of managing a non-vital immature tooth by regularly changing the non-setting calcium hydroxide dressing to achieve closure of the apex of the root has been superseded by the use of MTA, which can instead be placed as a 3–4 mm sized apical plug to seal the apex of the root. Very commonly, the root will be restored with a non-metallic post by bonding it in situ with a resin-based composite material in an attempt to strengthen the thin, weakened root.
- **Apexogenesis**.

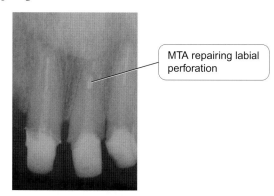

MTA repairing labial perforation

Fig. 13.38 Repair of a labial perforation in tooth 21 using MTA.

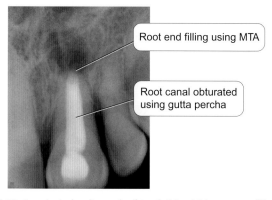

Root end filling using MTA

Root canal obturated using gutta percha

Fig. 13.39 A periapical radiograph of tooth 21, which was root filled with gutta percha. The tooth subsequently underwent periradicular surgery and a root end filling was placed using MTA.

Commercially available products

There are only two commercially available MTA products: ProRoot MTA (Dentsply Maillefer) (Figure 13.40) and MTA Angelus (Angelus). The latter product is not sold in the USA due to patent licences. This product forms a gel when mixed and sets in 10–15 minutes.

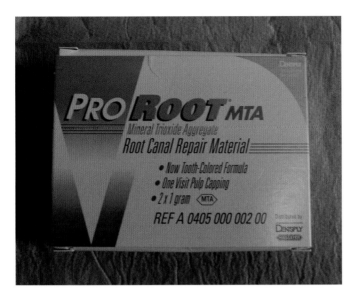

Fig. 13.40 A commercially available product of MTA (ProRoot MTA, Dentsply Maillefer).

The original material was supplied as a grey cement but tooth-coloured presentations are also now available.

Mixing

Box 13.1 shows the recommended technique for mixing MTA.

Placement

The mixed consistency of MTA being like wet sand makes its handling and accurate placement difficult. The dentist may find that using an absorbent material to control the moisture content makes the material easier to manipulate and pack into its desired place. Cotton wool pledgets or paper points are useful in this regard. Equally, if the material is deemed to be in the wrong place, it may be washed out using sterile water prior to another attempt at placement.

The material should be placed with a minimum thickness of 2 mm. This may not always be possible to achieve, for example, when a perforation in the furcation area of a molar requires repair. In this case, a resin-modified glass ionomer cement could be used to form a wall around the defect (a doughnut shape) and set by light curing. The MTA could then be placed into the 'well' so formed. Many dentists use a Buchanan plugger to insert MTA into the operation site (Figure 13.41).

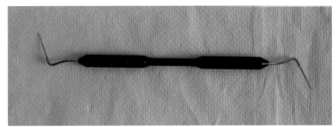

Fig. 13.41 A Buchanan plugger is used to introduce MTA to the site of use.

Some clinicians prefer to use a matrix when placing MTA to contain the material and prevent its extrusion outwith the root. A barrier will provide a more rigid surface to condense the material against. Barriers will also aid in achieving haemostasis and a dry field. Barriers may be either **resorbable** or **non-resorbable**. The choice is often dependent on the material being subsequently used to repair the defect. Although there is a variety of resorbable barriers, most dentists use either **collagen** or **calcium sulphate**. These are pushed non-surgically outwith the root canal into the periradicular tissues.

Box 13.1 Recommended procedure for mixing MTA

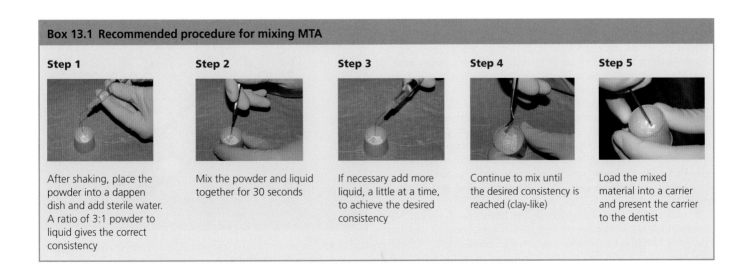

Step 1 After shaking, place the powder into a dappen dish and add sterile water. A ratio of 3:1 powder to liquid gives the correct consistency

Step 2 Mix the powder and liquid together for 30 seconds

Step 3 If necessary add more liquid, a little at a time, to achieve the desired consistency

Step 4 Continue to mix until the desired consistency is reached (clay-like)

Step 5 Load the mixed material into a carrier and present the carrier to the dentist

Collagen barrier materials are easy to manipulate and achieve good haemostasis. They are biocompatible, support the growth of new tissue and resorb in 10–14 days. The material is cut to size and packing incrementally until the desired matrix is achieved. The material absorbs moisture so its use is contraindicated if use of a bonding technique is envisaged in the subsequent definitive restoration as moisture control will be compromised. An example of such a product is Collacote (Sulger Dental), a type 1 bovine collagen.

Calcium sulphate is another barrier and it works by plugging the vascular channels, providing haemostasis. It is biocompatible, resorbs in 2–4 weeks and is syringed into the operation site before setting. Its shape can therefore be smoothed to the desired shape. A commercially available product is Capset (Lifecore Biomedical).

MTA is frequently used as a non-resorbable barrier as well as a restorative material. It is indicated when moisture control is a problem, where access may be problematic or another material requires to be packed against a rigid barrier.

ENDODONTIC MEDICAMENTS FOR DECIDUOUS TEETH

Deciduous (primary) teeth differ morphologically from permanent teeth in size and shape. Their fine roots resorb as the permanent successor tooth moves towards the oral cavity. Traditional root canal therapy is therefore not performed on deciduous teeth. Instead, if the pulp requires to be treated, a pulpotomy may be carried out.

> **Pulpotomy:** surgical amputation of the entire coronal pulp and placement of a dressing over the exposed healthy pulp stumps.

Carious cavities in deciduous teeth may be restored and their pulps protected by the application of a base material to seal the dentinal tubules from microorganisms. This will decrease postoperative sensitivity and future microleakage. Setting calcium hydroxide cements are not generally used for this purpose these days, rather, materials which bond to tooth tissue and seal dentinal tubules are favoured.

If the caries process is approaching the pulp and indirect pulp capping is indicated, setting calcium hydroxide should be placed over the pulpal floor leaving the softened dentine. This base disinfects dentine and walls off the zinc oxide cement from the pulp. In the primary dentition, the placement of a direct pulp cap is inadvisable as calcium hydroxide paste has been implicated in internal resorption due to the high cellular contact of the pulp tissue of primary teeth. Pulpotomy is a better option for primary teeth with carious or traumatic exposures, and has a better outcome.

Materials used in a pulpotomy should ideally be bactericidal and promote healing of the radicular pulp. Thus they should be biocompatible and not interfere with the physiological process of root resorption. Unfortunately, there are few materials if any which conform to these requirements. Pure calcium hydroxide mixed with sterile water is not used anymore as success rates are poor because it induces chronic pulp inflammation and internal resorption.

The other material used traditionally was **formocresol**, the product of **formaldehyde** and **cresol**. Formocresol is very cytotoxic and has mutagenic effects as has been discussed earlier in the chapter. It denatures and fixes protein and bonds with nucleic acid; the latter may

explain its cytotoxic effects. It can also deactivate bacterial toxins. Formaldehyde precludes the healing potential of the pulp by modifying the immune response. One such product is Caustinerf Deciduous (Septodont). This preparation contains paraformaldehyde to enable rapid mummification of the pulp. It also contains camphor and parachlorophenol for their antiseptic properties and lidocaine as an analgesic agent.

To reduce the exposure to formaldehyde, it has been suggested that Buckley's formocresol may be diluted. Other medicaments such as glutaraldehyde or ferric sulphate may be used. The former chemical is an aliphatic dialdehyde and is a mild fixative and less toxic than formaldehyde. Surgical techniques such as the use of lasers or electrosurgery have also been advocated.

Formocresol is no longer recommended by the American Association of Endodontists and the American Academy of Pediatric Dentistry, given the body of evidence and concerns over formaldehyde's toxicity. MTA has shown promise in studies involving deciduous teeth and so this should be used instead due to its biocompatibility.

Other materials that may be used to obturate the root canals in primary teeth include Tempophore (Septodont), which contains zinc oxide, thymol, creosote and iodoform. This radiopaque material is resorbable and thus allows the eruption of the underlying permanent tooth. It has an antiseptic action that helps provide an infection-free canal until the tooth exfoliates.

The indications and procedures for using these techniques are beyond the scope of this text and the reader is referred to a text on paediatric operative dentistry.

ENDODONTIC CUTTING INSTRUMENTS

When preparing endodontic access cavities, there is always a need for a balance between facilitation of access to the root canals and removal of excess tooth tissue, which would weaken the remaining tooth structure. In contemporary practice, endodontists prefer to remove as little tissue as possible and as precisely as possible. This is done using a cutting tip in an ultrasonic handpiece. It is important to use these instruments at a low power setting as they are liable to fracture when used at higher powers. The cutting tip is usually made of **zirconium nitride-coated** or **titanium alloy** (Figure 13.42).

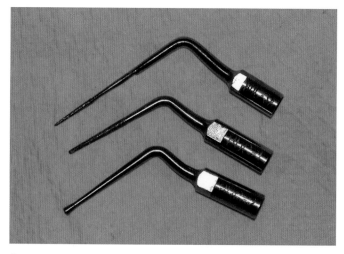

Fig. 13.42 A selection of zirconium nitride coated endodontic cutting tips used in an ultrasonic handpiece.

ENDODONTIC POSTS

Significant amounts of tooth tissue are removed during endodontic therapy to achieve adequate access to the pulp chamber and the canals. Frequently little tooth tissue remains so weakening the remaining tooth structure. Often the dentist has to resort to using the root canal to support the definitive cast restoration required to restore the coronal portion of the tooth. A **post** is therefore placed in the enlarged root canal (**post space**) and the **core** forms the foundation for the crown. The core may be cast onto the post (**post and core**) or may be constructed using a direct restorative material such as resin composite or glass ionomer. The final crown is then placed onto the core. The restoration is therefore known as a **post crown**.

Posts are either **prefabricated** or **cast**. Prefabricated posts may be constructed of either **non-metallic** materials or **metals**. The core is then built up onto the prefabricated post with a direct restorative dental material. This procedure has the following advantages:

- The post space preparation may be carried out and the definitive post fitted at the same appointment as the root canal obturation, under aseptic conditions, so ensuring that the coronal seal is maintained.
- The tooth does not require temporization. Temporary post crowns have a high incidence of non-retention, so compromising the coronal seal.
- No laboratory procedures are required so the definitive crown may be provided more quickly, especially if the post and core and the crown are constructed in two stages.
- It may be a cheaper option, depending on the post system selected.

Cast post and cores are constructed from either a prefabricated plastic blank or a metal blank. The core is constructed on to the post either directly or indirectly using wax or a burnout resin. The final pattern is invested in the dental laboratory and heated to such a temperature that the wax or resin is burnt out. Molten metal is then forced into the void left by the wax to form the core, which is returned to the surgery and cemented into place. This process is known as the **lost wax technique** (see Chapter 20). It is desirable that all materials used to construct posts are radiopaque for ease of identification on a radiograph.

Non-metallic posts

It is desirable that the material of which the post is constructed has a similar modulus of elasticity as dentine. This means that during function there will be a more even distribution of mechanical stresses and the root and post should flex by approximately the same amount. If this was not the case, the weakest structure would fracture. Root fracture is particularly undesirable as it condemns the tooth to extraction. With non-metallic posts a lower incidence of root fracture is seen. These posts have a sufficient strength to withstand high stress without permanent deformation and without breaking. However, there is a risk that the overlaying crown may be disturbed if the post flexes.

The more even distribution of mechanical stresses is dependent on the bonding between the post and the dentinal walls of the post space, which can absorb the stresses and strains of function. Less stress is seen at the post–cement interface. The greater the amount of tooth structure removed, the weaker it becomes. A post space preparation further weakens the root. However, if a post is bonded to the radicular dentine, the strength of the restored tooth should increase as it forms an integral unit with the tooth. Contemporary techniques use non-metallic posts and resin composite to strengthen weaken roots, especially in traumatized immature teeth.

It is essential that teeth into which non-metallic posts are placed have at least 1.5 mm of sound tooth circumferentially further apical to the core. This is required so that the final crown may have a bracing effect, called the **ferrule effect**. Failure to achieve the ferrule effect may result in the post fracturing at the post–core interface. This is evident clinically as the crown moving on the root and must be treated without delay as recurrent caries may occur fairly quickly, destroying the little supporting tooth tissue is present.

The use of a non-metallic post is contraindicated if there is insufficient sound tooth tissue (1.5 mm circumferentially) further apical to the core.

It is considered desirable that the post and core have the same optical properties as natural tooth. A metal post may shine through thin labial gingival tissues, with a blueing or greying effect. The optical properties of the majority of non-metallic posts are much closer to tooth tissue (except for carbon fibre which tend to be dark in colour) and so result in a more pleasing aesthetic result. Furthermore, it is desirable that the material of the post can transmit light. This is particularly so for those posts whose fibres are unidirectional in the long axis of the post as the light may be transmitted down the post so facilitating the curing of light-sensitive bonding adhesives.

Non-metallic posts may be constructed of:

- Zirconia
- Ceramic
- Fibre-reinforced resins
  - Carbon fibre
  - Glass fibre
  - Woven polyethylene ribbon reinforced composite.

Zirconia

Zirconia is being used much more in dentistry these days due to its high strength, and posts have been constructed out of this material. The material is brittle, having a high modulus, and potentially may cause root fracture. The material is hard to cut and remove should this be necessary.

Ceramic

Posts have been constructed using ceramic. This material is brittle and this may lead to failure. The material may be too strong for use as a post as the root may fracture and not the post. Retrievability may be problematic, with the post being difficult if not impossible to remove.

Fibre-reinforced resins

All of these materials are the products of a resin reinforced by some form of fibre strands, mesh or mat.

Carbon fibre

Carbon fibre is essentially a polymer reinforced with carbon. It has many applications in modern life – in aerospace and civil engineering, the military and motor sports. An example is that of a golf club. The carbon fibre shaft of the club is strong but it may flex so imparting more energy to the golf ball. Carbon fibre shows minimum deformation, maximum use range, and absorbs and transfers forces in a similar way to dentine. As previously mentioned, carbon fibre posts tend to be dark in colour and so they cannot transmit light and may shine through, leaving an unaesthetic result.

Glass fibre

Glass fibre (or **fibreglass**) is a polymer reinforced with glass fibres. Fibreglass is less brittle than ceramic posts (e.g. zirconium oxide). One such product is composed of 60% glass fibre and 40% resin (Figure 13.43). Posts with unidirectional fibres are the strongest. It is difficult to produce this material as the twisted fibre bundles need to be infiltrated and wetted with the resin. This is difficult to achieve and often voids are present on the surface of the fibres which weakens the structure.

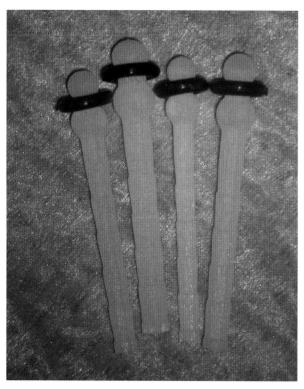

Fig. 13.43 Examples of glass fibre endodontic posts of varying diameters (FibreLux, Coltène Whaledent).

Woven polyethylene ribbon-reinforced composite

These products have already been mentioned in Chapter 7. As well as being used as periodontal splints and bridge substructures, they may also be used to construct post and cores (Ribbond Bondable Reinforcement Ribbon, Ribbond Inc.).

Many non-metallic posts have their heads designed to retain the core. This is often achieved by the use of undercuts. It is important that, wherever possible, a rounded design is used to prevent stress concentrations being formed between the material of the post and the core material. It is also desirable that the post incorporates an antirotation device to prevent rotation forces placing undue stress on the post–dentine interface.

In order to achieve a strong chemical bond between the non-metallic post and the resin composite material used to bond the post into the post hole, the surface of the post is often chemically treated. This is usually by the application of silane but some manufactures use other chemicals. It will also enhance the bond between the head of the post and the core material, which is commonly resin composite (see Chapter 7).

After trying in the non-metallic post and carrying out any adjustment to it, the post may be cleaned with an alcohol wipe. The alcohol should be allowed to evaporate before cementation is carried out.

Non-metallic posts may either be used directly, which is the most common way in which they are used, or indirectly, by being built up in the laboratory by the dental technician.

Retrievability

It is important that any dental restoration must be reasonably easy to remove should the need arise. For example, in the case of posts, endodontic failure or damage to the post itself (such as fracture). Metal posts are difficult to remove as the dentist must cut around the post to loosen it and unscrew it. This often requires much tooth tissue to be removed and may transmit destructive forces to the root which, by definition of having a post placed in it is already compromised. Another advantage of non-metallic posts is that they can be removed from the tooth more easily than those made of metal.

A bespoke drill may be used to initially get between the fibres of the post such as a Tenax starter, Tenax or Kodex drill (Coltène Whaledent) (Figure 13.44). Post space drills are then used, moving from small to the final size to remove the rest of post. This procedure should be done under magnification so that the dentist only removes the post and stays along the axial plane of the root.

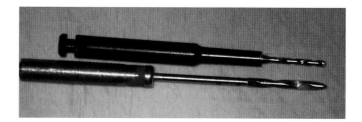

Fig. 13.44 The Tenax drill system designed to remove fibre endodontic posts.

If adjustment of non-metallic posts is required, then this should be done under water spray using a carborundum disc or diamond bur. The post should be rotated during cutting to ensure even removal.

Non-metallic posts should not be bent by the dentist prior to fitting because fatigue will occur during function.

Some systems, such as Luminex (Dentatus), use the post to transmit light by fibreoptic means to set the light-cured resin composite placed in the post space. After etching and bonding, rein composite is placed into the post space and the post is pushed into place. The light is then shone on top of the post so setting the resin composite. The post is then removed and a quartz fibre post subsequently recemented using a resin composite-based bonding system. The resin composite core can then be constructed and prepared to receive the crown.

Commercially available products

The use of non-metallic posts has become more commonplace in the recent past and many different posts are available on the market; see Table 13.16.

Table 13.16 Some non-metallic post products currently available on the market

Product	Manufacturer	Type of post	Comments
Aestheti-Plus	RTD	Quartz fibre	
Carbon fibre Post	Svenska	Carbon fibre	
CosmoPost	Ivoclar Vivadent	Zirconia	
DT Light Post	RTD	Quartz fibre	
DT Light SL	VDW	Quartz fibre	
Ellipson Post	RTD	Quartz fibre	Oval in shape
FRC Postec Plus	Ivoclar Vivadent	Glass fibre	
Light-Post	RTD	Quartz fibre	
Luminex	Dentatus	Quartz fibre	
LuxaPost	DMG	Glass fibre	
Macro-Lock Post	RTD	Quartz fibre	
ParaPost Fiber Lux	Coltène Whaledent	Glass fibre	
ParaPost Fiber White	Coltène Whaledent	Glass fibre	
ParaPost Taper Lux	Coltène Whaledent	Glass fibre	
Peerless Post Kit	Sybron Endo	Fibre reinforced	
Radix Fiber Post	Denstply Maillefer	Glass fibre	
Rebilda Post	Voco	Fibre reinforced	
Rely X Fiber Post	3M ESPE	Glass fibre	
Snowpost	Carbotech SARL	Glass fibre	Epoxy resin
Tenax Fiber White	Coltène Whaledent	Glass fibre	
Twin Luscent Anchors	Dentatus	Glass fibre	

Metal posts

Metal is the traditional material for post construction due to its good corrosion resistance and high yield strength. Metal posts may be **smooth sided**, have a **roughened** surface or may have serrations incorporated into their surface, termed a **serrated** post. Metal posts are passively cemented into the canal with a luting cement. The difference in their surface will give more retention. The smooth sided post has least retention compared with the serrated, with the roughened surface post in between. Some posts incorporate a venting channel to allow excess cement to escape coronally, thus ensuring that the post may be fully seated.

Other metal posts are referred to as **active**. This means that they have threads incorporated into their surface, which engage the dentine on the post space wall to increase retention of the posts. Unfortunately, these cause local stress concentrations as the post is screwed into place, possibly leading to root fracture. This may be exacerbated if the post is tapered, which has a wedge effect on the root (Figure 13.45).

Metal posts may be categorized as **prefabricated** or **cast**. The chemical composition of the metal used will differ with the design.

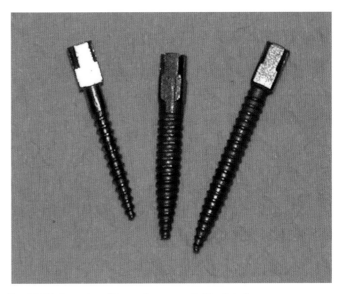

Fig. 13.45 Examples of tapered screw posts (Dentatus).

Prefabricated metal posts

Prefabricated posts are constructed from **stainless steel**, **titanium**, **titanium alloy** or **gold alloy**. Some posts may be a combination of metals such as stainless steel with a gold plate (covering). This may be problematic because if the gold plate is breached, a galvanic cell (see Chapter 6) may be established leading to corrosion of the post. The volume of the post may therefore increase, so causing root fracture, or the corrosion products may not be contained in the tooth, which may be harmful to the patient. These posts may be passive or active in design. Usually the prefabricated post is placed into the post space and the core is constructed with a direct restorative (core) material. However, some products incorporate both the post and the core and so the construction of a core is not required.

Other prefabricated posts are intended to have the core cast onto them. This may be done **directly** (in the mouth) or **indirectly** (in the dental laboratory). These posts tend to be made of type IV gold alloy (containing gold, platinum, palladium and iridium) or platinum, gold and iridium alloys, which are compatible with palladium, and silver-free alloys or platinum, gold, palladium and silver alloy. For more information on these metals, see Chapter 21.

If gold alloys are being used, a non-chloride containing investment material should be used in the laboratory otherwise chemical corrosion will occur.

Many prefabricated posts are examples of **wrought** posts. A wrought post is made from a block of metal that is drawn to form a wire. This results in the stresses within the metal being low, and the post is stronger than a cast post of the same diameter. Wrought posts should therefore be preferred to cast posts if possible.

Stainless stain or Wiptam wire which is a cobalt chromium alloy should not have gold cast on to them as they may corrode. Furthermore, heating alters the characteristics of stainless steel wire and it becomes very ductile.

Ductile: capable of being drawn out.

When a direct technique is being used, the post is placed into the post space and the dentist may build up the core portion using **wax** or a non-residual **burn-out resin**, such as Duralay (Reliance) (see Chapter 15). In the case of the indirect method, the post is placed into the post space on the model and the core built up in the same way. In each case the finished pattern is processed by the lost wax technique as previously mentioned, whereby the wax or resin is converted into metal alloy, usually type IV gold alloy; see Chapter 21.

The Parapost system (Figure 13.46; Coltène Whaledent) is probably the most commonly used post and core construction kit. This is due to its simplicity of use and its versatility, it is used for many techniques.

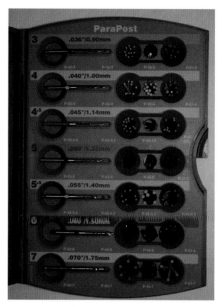

Fig. 13.46 The ParaPost kit (Coltène Whaledent).

Cast metal posts

Cast metal posts are constructed by placing a plastic blank into the post space and the core waxed up in wax or resin onto the post. This is then cast into metal alloy, again usually type IV gold alloy. Unfortunately, when the post and core cools, the metal alloy may **core** (Chapter 21). This means that porosities and irregularities may form within the metal and these represent areas of stress concentrations. The presence of stress concentrations may lead to failure and breakage of the post.

Commercially available products

Examples of commercially available products are show in Table 13.17.

Table 13.17 Some metal posts currently available on the market and their characteristics

Product	Manufacturer	Post material	Shape	Means of retention	Type of post
Filpost	Fil-Hol	Titanium	Tapered	Passive	Prefabricated
Parapost XH	Coltène Whaledent	Titanium alloy	Parallel	Passive	Direct post and core build-up in one appointment
Parapost XP	Coltène Whaledent	Titanium alloy	Parallel	Passive	Prefabricated temporary
Parapost XP	Coltène Whaledent	Stainless steel	Parallel	Passive	Direct post and core build-up in one appointment; prefabricated
Parapost XP G-Alloy	Coltène Whaledent	Wrought gold alloy	Parallel	Passive	Prefabricated
Parapost XT	Coltène Whaledent	Titanium alloy	Parallel	Threaded	Direct post and core build-up in one appointment
Radix Anker	Dentsply Maillefer	Titanium alloy	Parallel	Active	Prefabricated
Surtex	Dentatus	Gold-plated stainless steel	Tapered	Active	Prefabricated
Tenax	Coltène Whaledent	Titanium alloy	Parallel		Nickel free

SUMMARY

- Successful endodontics requires thorough cleaning and disinfection of the root canal system, and this should be maintained with a coronal seal. Root canal treatment is done in an isolated environment (rubber dam), using files and chemicals.
- A range of chemical irrigants and systems are available to clean and disinfect the root canal system.
- The access cavity and root canal system will require to be temporized if the root canal is to be obturated at a subsequent appointment. A number of inter-visit root canal dressings and cements are available for the temporary restoration of the coronal tooth.
- The root canal must be obturated and there are several techniques and materials available for this purpose. A semi-solid material cemented into the canal with a sealer is the most common method of achieving obturation.
- MTA is used to repair or seal the root and is highly biocompatible.
- Endodontically treated teeth often require the provision of a post to retain the definitive crown and a range of posts systems are available for this purpose, both metal and non-metallic.

FURTHER READING

Cohen, S., Burns, R.C. (Eds.), 2002. Pathways of the Pulp (eighth ed.). Mosby Elsevier, St Louis.

Ford, P., 2004. Harty's Endodontics in Clinical Practice, fifth ed. Wright Elsevier, Edinburgh.

Lewis, B., 2009. The obsolescence of formocresol. Br. Dent. J. 207, 525–528.

Ørstavik, D., Ford, T.P. (Eds.), 2008. Essential Endodontology. Blackwell, Oxford.

van Noort, R., 2007. Introduction to Dental Materials, third ed. Mosby Elsevier, Edinburgh. (See Chapter 11)

SELF-ASSESSMENT QUESTIONS

1. What materials may be used to disinfect the root canal system?
2. Which materials could be used to seal the access cavity between visits when doing endodontic treatment in a molar? What are the pros and cons of each material?
3. Why is the clinical manipulation of MTA difficult?
4. What root canal sealers are available? What are the pros and cons of each material?
5. Summarize the types of endodontic post that are available.
6. What inter-visit root canal dressing materials are available to the endodontist?

Section | III |

Materials used with indirect techniques

Chapter | **14** |

Materials used in temporization

LEARNING OBJECTIVES

From this chapter, the reader will:

- Understand why temporary restorations are required prior to the placement of the definitive (indirect) restoration
- Understand how the materials currently used for temporization achieve these aims
- Be aware of the range materials available for temporization
- Understand the indications and contraindications of materials used to temporize
- Have an increased appreciation of how to use the materials more effectively and to their best effect
- Know the names of currently available commercial products.

INTRODUCTION

It is widely acknowledged that good temporization is one of the most important factors in the fabrication of good quality, definitive indirect restorations. While there is some truth in the urban myth that temporary restorations should never be made too good as the patient may not return to have the definitive restorations fitted, it is essential that good-quality temporary cover is provided. Attention to detail during their construction facilitates the subsequent stages of the procedure, so producing a better definitive restoration. Temporary crowns protect the oral tissues and allow the patient to function while maintaining their appearance until the definitive restoration can be fitted. This chapter discusses the various materials used to provide temporary coverage.

> **Temporization:** the construction of a temporary restoration, which restores form and function to the tooth while the definitive restoration is being made.
> **Definitive restoration:** a restoration provided with the intention of being the long-term solution.
> **Indirect restoration:** a dental restoration constructed outwith the mouth.

THE BIOLOGICAL IMPORTANCE OF GOOD TEMPORIZATION

Biologically, it is important to protect the oral tissues following tooth preparation for the following reasons:

- Some 30 000 to 70 000 dentinal tubules are opened per square millimetre during tooth preparation. The passage of oral bacteria into the freshly cut dentine must be minimized as this will cause pulpal inflammation, which manifests as sensitivity if the dentine is exposed to stimuli from the oral environment such as hot, cold and sweet.
- A well-fitting temporary restoration will prevent the gingival tissues from migrating over the preparation margins.
- It also allows the area to be cleaned more effectively and thus maintains a state of gingival health. This decreases the incidence of gingival inflammation and bleeding at the time of fitting the definitive restoration, which is particularly important when the restoration is being bonded using a hydrophobic resin-based composite material.
- A good provisional restoration will maintain occlusal and approximal contacts so preventing over-eruption and tilting of the prepared tooth, or adjacent and opposing teeth. This minimizes the need for occlusal or approximal adjustment of the definitive restoration at the fit appointment.

THE BENEFITS OF QUALITY TEMPORIZATION

Benefits for the dentist

Time and care taken to construct temporary restorations by the dentist is well rewarded as useful supplementary information may be gleaned from these restorations:

- The temporary restoration should be made prior to impression taking for the definitive restoration. When the occlusion has been verified and the temporary deemed satisfactory, the clinician can

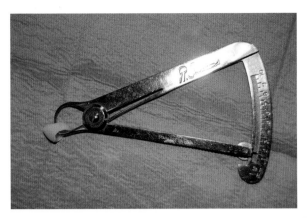

Fig. 14.1 An Iwannson gauge being used to measure the thickness of the occlusal surface of a indirect restoration, in this case a temporary crown.

measure the width of the occlusal part of the restoration using an Iwannson gauge (Figure 14.1). This distance denotes the interocclusal clearance. If this is deemed to be insufficient, the dentist can adjust the preparation to create the required clearance prior to taking the working impression.

- In more complicated cases temporary restorations may provide the clinician with invaluable information for use in diagnosis and treatment planning, such as the construction of a new occlusal scheme or when an aesthetic case is being planned.

Benefits to the patient

It is also important from the patient's perspective that their appearance is maintained and they can continue to function effectively and comfortably. In cases involving a number of teeth, the position and shape of the temporaries will also allow the patient to evaluate their appearance. If this is satisfactory, these features can be incorporated into the definitive restorations.

The purpose of temporization may therefore be summarised as listed in Box 14.1.

Box 14.1 The purpose of temporization

- Maintenance of aesthetics and function
- Protection of prepared dentine from thermal and chemical trauma
- Maintenance of gingival contour and health
- Maintenance of good oral hygiene
- Maintenance of occlusal stability
- Prevention of drifting or tilting of adjacent teeth
- Allows the dentist to check that sufficient interocclusal reduction has been prepared
- Assists the clinician in diagnosis and treatment planning
- Assists the clinician in the construction of a new occlusal scheme
- Allows the aesthetic evaluation of replacements

THE TEMPORIZATION 'BALANCE'

A temporary restoration, be it an inlay, onlay, crown or bridge, must be effectively retained for the period of time between fitting and placement of the definitive restoration. Equally it must be removed easily at the fit appointment without damage to the preparation. A

balance between good retention for this period and ease of removal must be established. Generally speaking, the most satisfactory combination is that of a well-prepared (mechanically retentive) preparation with a well-constructed temporary restoration grouted by a soft luting cement (see Chapter 12).

> **Bridge:** a fixed restoration replacing a missing tooth involving one or more adjacent teeth.
> **Direct restoration:** a restoration made in the mouth by the dentist using materials that set after placement.

TYPES OF TEMPORARY RESTORATION

Most temporary restorations are in clinical use for short periods of time, usually up to 2 weeks. These may be satisfactorily constructed using one of the **directly** placed temporization materials available:

- Acrylate-based materials
- Dimethacrylate composites
- Light-cured temporary materials
- Putties.

Where medium- to longer-term temporization is envisaged (some months or more), consideration should be given to an **indirect** temporary restoration, which is constructed in the dental laboratory. This is particularly true if there is concern that flexion of the material in, for example, a longer span bridge may lead to fracture. Indirect temporary restorations have the following advantages:

- Better fit, particularly at the margins
- Increased strength
- Better wear resistance
- Easier to keep clean
- Better aesthetics and colour stability
- Greater occlusal reliability and stability.

Clearly there is a greater cost implication of an indirect over a direct restoration but failure to provide a satisfactory temporary prosthesis may prove to be a false economy. Laboratory temporary restorations may be constructed of:

- An acrylic, such as heat- or self-cured **polymethylmethacrylate**
- A **bis-GMA**-based material such as resin composite
- **Acrylic or ceramic bonded to metal** – non-precious metal alloys (Chapter 21) are normally chosen on grounds of lower cost.

> **Acrylic**: a generic term for chemical compounds that contain the acryl group derived from acrylic acid
> **Acrylate**: the acrylate ion is the ion of acrylic acid and these are a group of materials that are derived from acrylic acid, that is, they are the salts and esters of acrylic acid. They contain vinyl groups, that is, two carbon atoms double bonded to each other, directly attached to the carbonyl carbon. Acrylates easily form polymers because the double bonds are very reactive. Acrylates and methacrylates (the salts and esters of methacrylic acid) are common monomers in polymer plastics, forming the acrylate polymers
> **Diacrylates** and **dimethacrylates**: have two active groups.

DIRECT TEMPORARY RESTORATIONS

Preformed crown forms

The first method of direct temporization involves the use of a preformed crown, which is trimmed to the margins of the preparation and refined using another material. The crown forms available are made of:

- Polycarbonate
- Cellulose acetate
- Aluminium
- Stainless steel.

Crown forms used to construct tooth-coloured temporaries

Where aesthetics is an issue, i.e. in the anterior and premolar regions of the mouth, the clinician has a choice between a **polycarbonate** or a **cellulose acetate** crown form to use as a template to construct the temporary crown.

Polycarbonate crown forms

These temporary crown forms are made of a polymer with high impact resistance. This means they have sufficient strength to withstand occlusal forces. As the name implies the polycarbonates contain multiple carbonate groups. These may be linked by a variety of chemical groups, with the commonest one being bis-GMA. They are presented in various sizes in a tray (Figure 14.2).

Clinical technique

A crown form of the approximate size is selected by the clinician. It is then adjusted using an acrylic bur to refine its size and shape to closely match that of the preparation. Next, it is refined with another material, which is generally an acrylate (methyl, ethyl or butyl acrylate), although the dimethacrylates and light-cured temporary materials have also been advocated for this purpose. Acrylate-based materials are more suitable than the more elastic materials since it may be necessary to trim through the polycarbonate 'shell' to accommodate the opposing tooth so satisfying the occlusion. The acrylic inside the crown can withstand occlusal forces provided it is at least approximately 1 mm thick. However there is no chemical union between the acrylic resin and the polycarbonate crown form. The interior of the polycarbonate crown should therefore be roughened prior to refining.

One of the limitations of prefabricated polycarbonate crowns is that they are often too broad buccolingually and so they require thinning to achieve a satisfactory contour gingivally.

Cellulose acetate crown forms

These crown forms are transparent (Figure 14.3). They are used in essentially the same manner as polycarbonate crowns: they are trimmed to size using crown shears or scissors and then packed with

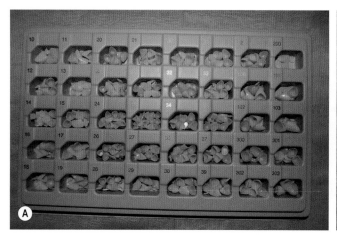
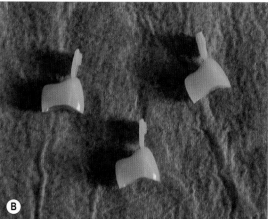

Fig. 14.2 (A) Various sizes of incisors and canine polycarbonate crown forms (Directa, Svenska Dental Instruments AB). (B) Close-up view of some premolar crown forms.

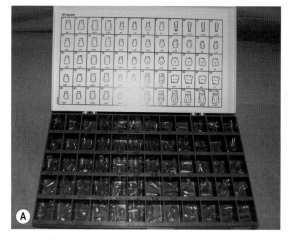
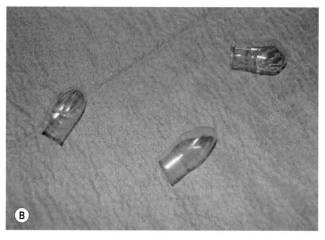

Fig. 14.3A,B Cellulose acetate crown forms (Henry Schein).

another material matching in shade to the surrounding teeth. Some clinicians use resin-based composite for this purpose. These crown forms have the disadvantages that:

- They merely act as a matrix and so must be removed after their refining material has set
- When the cellulose crown form is removed, the thickness of the crown reduces (by about 0.2 mm). This may lead to instability in the occlusion and movement of adjacent teeth
- The refining material (often resin composite or compomer) can lock into undercuts, thus compromising removal of the crown and the patient's ability to keep the (gingival) area clean.

Their main use in operative dentistry is as a matrix to build up teeth (with large defects) using resin-based composite.

Metal crown forms

Due to their appearance, metal crown forms are used in the posterior region of the mouth. Two types of metal crown are available: **aluminium** and **stainless steel**.

Aluminium crown forms

Aluminium crown forms have been used for many years as the material is easy to manipulate, and it is malleable and **ductile**. This makes their handling easy for the dentist as they can be bent and trimmed to shape easily. Aluminium crown forms can corrode with time as

saliva can react with them. There is also a risk that if they are placed adjacent to a freshly packed amalgam or gold restoration, a galvanic cell may be established (see Chapter 6). Figure 14.4 shows some molar aluminium crown forms.

The crown form of the approximate size is selected. It is often expanded using the expander provided to fit over the prepared tooth (Figure 14.5A) and then cut to the approximate size of the preparation using a pair of crown shears (Figure 14.5B). The ability of the aluminium to be worked and shaped lends itself to this process.

> **Malleable:** able to be manipulated into a new shape.

This type of crown form may also be bent to shape before being refined. In exceptional circumstances if the crown form is very close fitting and retentive, it may be possible to only use a temporary cement without refining it. A number of disadvantages are apparent if the crown form is not refined:

- It will not be possible to perforate the metal shell should the occlusion dictate it.
- No other information may be gleaned from it, for example, whether sufficient interocclusal clearance has been prepared, as described earlier.
- If there is any wear on the restoration, the temporary cement will be exposed and the restoration is more likely to fail.

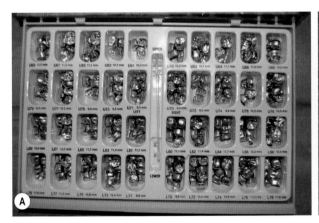
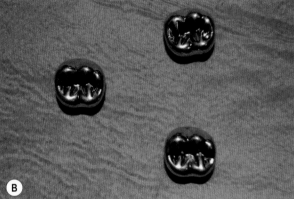

Fig. 14.4A,B The various sizes of molar aluminium crown forms made by 3M ESPE.

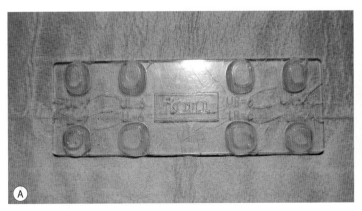
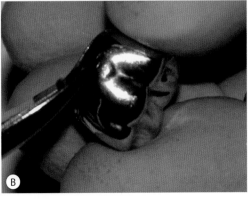

Fig. 14.5 (A) The expander used to manipulate the molar aluminium crown form to the desired shape. (B) The crown is then trimmed using crown shears so that its form approximates the margins of the preparation.

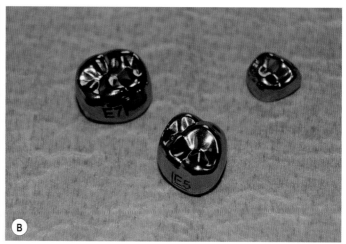

Fig. 14.6A,B The various sizes of paediatric stainless steel crown forms made by 3M ESPE.

Stainless steel crown forms

The other metal crown form available is made of **stainless steel** (Figure 14.6). Its main indication is in paediatric dentistry for the restoration of badly broken down deciduous molars, particularly if pulpal treatment has been performed. These crown forms are much less malleable and ductile than the aluminium crown forms, thus they are harder wearing and are less likely to deform under load. They are usually not refined but trimmed using crown shears until their fit approximates to the prepared tooth. They are placed over the buccolingual bulbosity and snapped into place. They are then luted using a glass ionomer or polycarboxylate cement. The success rate with stainless steel crowns is very high and these crowns are useful to maintain the space that may be lost when a deciduous tooth is lost prematurely.

Acrylic materials used to refine temporary crown forms

All of the aforementioned crown forms except stainless steel crowns are used in conjunction with another material to enhance the fit between their internal surface and the preparation. The closeness of the fit between the inside of the temporary restoration and a retentive preparation will ensure that the restoration is retained

satisfactorily. The original refining materials were chemically cured acrylics formed by mixing **methylmethacrylate** monomer with **polymethylmethacrylate** micro-bead powder. Unfortunately there were some problems associated with these materials (Table 14.1). These shortcomings have made these materials almost obsolete and other materials have evolved in an attempt to eliminate their disadvantages. **Monofunctional acrylate monomers** with a higher molecular weight became available as their properties were an improvement on the original material. This family of materials is called the **higher methacrylates** and these are the most commonly used materials to refine a temporary crown form.

HIGHER METHACRYLATES

Chemically these materials are a combination of **polyethylmethacrylate** beads and the liquid **polybutylmethacrylate** (Table 14.2). The presence of a **tertiary amine** results in these materials tending to turn yellow after setting. This is particularly marked in sunlight as the solar ultraviolet breaks down the amine, causing a colour change.

Table 14.2 Components of a higher methacrylate material and their role in the reaction in the powder and liquid

	Chemical	Role
Powder	Polyethylmethacrylate	Polymer
	Benzoyl peroxide	Initiator
Liquid	Polybutylmethacrylate	Monomer
	Tertiary amine	Activator

Setting reaction

Higher methacrylates set by a **polymerization** reaction, and, as there is no inert filler, they will exhibit significant polymerization shrinkage on curing, which is in the order of 7% linearly. It is important to try to compensate for this large amount of shrinkage clinically (see Box 14.2, p. 223).

When the powder and liquid are combined, a mass is produced which has the consistency of wet sand. At this point the monomer is starting to soften and dissolve the outer surface of the resin polymer beads. The mass then develops a glossy surface. This **dough**

Table 14.1 Disadvantages of methylmethacrylate/polymethylmethacrylate temporary material and their clinical ramifications

Disadvantage	Clinical impact
High polymerization shrinkage	Unsatisfactory fit
Poor mechanical strength	Breakage during function
Highly exothermic setting reaction	Thermal trauma to the pulp
High level of monomer release	Significant pulpal irritation
Poor wear resistance	Undesirable wear during function leading to perforation or fracture of the temporary leading to occlusal instability
Poor aesthetics	Unsightly restoration
Chemical interaction with eugenol	Non-eugenol-containing products should be used

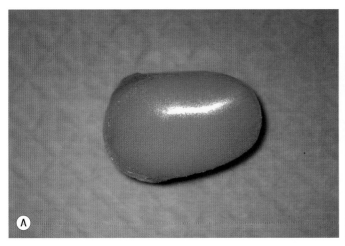 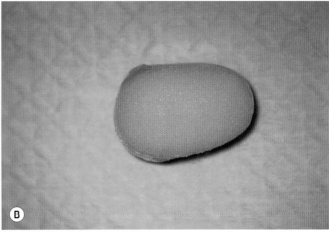

Fig. 14.7 A Directa temporary crown filled with Trim II (Bosworth). (A) The dough stage (note the shiny surface). (B) As the reaction progresses the snap stage is arrived at a minute or so later and the surface losses its glossiness. At this point, the material is now ready to be used.

stage is convenient as it aids clinical handling. As the reaction progresses, the surface of the material loses its gloss and turns to a matt appearance (Figure 14.7). It now corresponds to the **snap stage** and is now ready for use. For more information on acrylics, see Chapter 23. The polymerization reaction is **exothermic** in nature and care must be taken when using this material on a vital preparation to prevent thermal injury to the pulp.

Linear shrinkage: shrinkage in one direction.

Properties

The higher methacrylates have a lower **glass transition temperature** than polymethylmethacrylate. This means that they are more susceptible to temperature change, which will produce softening of the set material. The reason that some materials in this family contain both the ethyl and butyl methacrylates is that the glass transition temperature of the butyl variant is 20°C whereas that of poly(ethylmethacrylate) is 66°C. A temporary restoration made entirely of poly(butylmethacrylate) would distort at mouth temperature. The combined product has an intermediate glass transition temperature and will not be affected by normal mouth temperatures. However, intake of hot foodstuffs and liquids will raise the temperature of the crown to a point where some changes in morphology can occur. The material when compared to poly(methylmethacrylate) has various advantages:

- It is tougher.
- It is less brittle.

As with poly(methylmethacrylate):

- The monomer has a distinctive smell which some patients find unpleasant.
- They are relatively inexpensive but this advantage is offset by the tendency to mix substantially more material than is needed so much of the material goes to waste.

Care should be taken when using the monomer as it should be used in a well-ventilated area, as its fumes are highly flammable and should not be inhaled as they are toxic. The polymer dust is also combustible.

As well as temporary crowns, this material is also indicated for construction of temporary inlays and onlays. A more rigid material should prevent overeruption more effectively than the (light-cured) rubbery temporary materials described later in the chapter. It is therefore indicated when the dentist is concerned about occlusal stability or to afford increased fracture resistance to the prepared tooth.

Clinical technique

A suggested clinical protocol of **refining** a preformed crown form using an acrylic material is presented in Box 14.2. This type of acrylic-based material can be used to construct temporary crowns and bridges using blowdown splints made of thermoplastic **resin**.

Box 14.2 Preformed crown form and refining using an acrylic material

1. Complete the preparation.
2. Select a crown form that approximately corresponds to the tooth being temporized.
3. Trim this crown form (using an acrylic bur for a polycarbonate crown form and crown shears for a stainless steel crown form) so that the margins approximate those of the preparation. Roughen the internal surfaces of the polycarbonate crowns.
4. Mix the acrylic material to the consistency of wet sand.
5. Fill the crown form by running the material down the sides to ensure no air bubbles are incorporated inside the crown form.
6. Allow the excess monomer to evaporate and watch the surface until it turns from a shiny to matt finish (Figure 14.7).
7. At this point fully seat the temporary crown onto the moist preparation and remove the obvious excess using a probe or flat plastic to prevent it setting into the undercuts so that the crown can be removed easily later.
8. Remove and reseat the crown several times to reduce the effect of polymerization shrinkage.
9. Place in hot water to accelerate the setting reaction.
10. Trim the margins using an acrylic bur and reseat on the preparation to verify the margins.
11. Check the occlusion and adjust if necessary.
12. Polish if necessary.
13. Lute the crown using a temporary luting cement.

This technique involves the temporary prosthesis being waxed up on a study cast, and then a vacuum-formed splint constructed from this. The splint can then be filled with a higher methacrylate material and inserted intraorally as described above once the preparation has been completed.

> **Thermoplastic:** a polymer which softens when heated and hardens when cooled. Extreme heating will turn the polymer to a liquid.

Commercially available products

With the development of the dimethacrylate composites, many clinicians are now in favour of using them as first choice temporary materials over the higher methacrylates as they exhibit superior properties. See Table 14.3 and Figure 14.8.

Table 14.3 Some higher methacrylate materials currently available on the market

Product	Manufacturer
Dentalon Plus	Heraeus
Duralay Temporary Crown and Bridge	Reliance
Snap	Parkell
Trim*	Bosworth
Trim II*	Bosworth
Unifast III	GC
Unifast Trad	GC

*Trim and Trim II are chemically identical but Trim II is available in more shades.

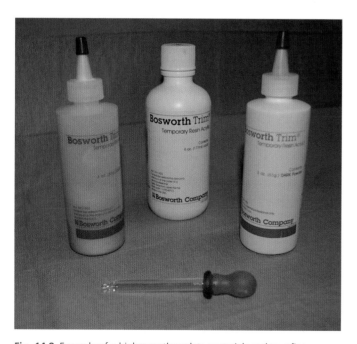

Fig. 14.8 Example of a higher methacrylate material used to refine temporary crown forms (Trim II, (Bosworth).

COMPOSITE-BASED MATERIALS

These materials are examples of **dimethacrylate composites** (see p. 219; sometimes known as **bisacryl composites**) and are constructed using the resin replica technique (see p. 226) or they are used in a custom made vacuum-formed splint.

Chemistry and setting reaction

These more modern materials are based on the resin composite technology described in Chapter 7. These are two subtypes of these materials. The first consists of some form of **dimethacrylate** resin (frequently **bis-GMA** and **triethylene glycol dimethacrylate**) and a filler. In most materials the inorganic filler contains **zirconia** and **silicon dioxide**. This filler forms only 40% by weight of the material as the rest is made up of the resins. Within the resin there may be prepolymerized blocks or beads of resin, which improve the homogeneity of the material and stiffen the paste.

The other type of temporization material uses composite-type technology which is based on the **ethylene imine derivative of bisphenol-A**. This is catalysed by an **aromatic sulphonated ester**. This technology is very similar to that used in the polyether impression material (see Chapter 15). Filler is added to this type of material to increase its strength. These multifunctional methacrylates produce a relatively high cross-link density early on in the setting reaction. This means that a rubbery stage is achieved, so allowing the partially set restoration to be removed without distortion or damage.

Properties

With all of these materials, the presence of filler or prepolymerized resin decreases the amount of polymerization shrinkage as the resin monomer volume is reduced, the shrinkage is reduced in proportion. Therefore the polymerization shrinkage of these materials is closer to 2%. The setting reaction is exothermic with a temperature rise of less than 5°C reported.

These materials are supplied as a base and catalyst (Table 14.4)

Table 14.4 Chemical constituents of dimethacrylate composite temporary materials

Base	Catalyst	Function
Difunctional methacrylate	Difunctional methacrylate	Resin matrix
Inorganic fillers: strontium glass Highly dispersed silicon dioxide Barium glass	Inorganic fillers: strontium glass Highly dispersed silicon dioxide Barium glass	Increases strength Deceases resin monomer volume and therefore shrinkage
Vinyl copolymers	Vinyl copolymers	Assist in cross-linking the resin
Benzoyl peroxide	Tertiary amine	Allows the curing process to start. The initiator in the catalyst modifies the setting reaction to vary the handling properties
Stabilizers such as hydroquinone		Prevent premature setting
Pigments, including titanium dioxide, ferrous and ferric salts		Shade modification

Table 14.5 Comparison of properties of higher methacrylates and dimethacrylate composite materials

Property	Higher methacrylates	Dimethacrylate composites	Comment
Exothermic reaction	Higher	Lower	Primarily due to volume of filler
Polymerization shrinkage	Higher	Lower	Primarily due to volume of filler
Flexural strength	Lower	Higher	Greater cross-linking
Wear resistance	Lower	Higher	Primarily due to volume of filler
Toughness	Lower	Higher	Primarily due to volume of filler
Brittleness	Lower	Higher	Primarily due to volume of filler
Impact resistance	Higher	Lower	Greater cross-linking
Cost	Cheaper	More expensive	Production costs higher

Stage	Mixing, filling the impression and inserting in the mouth	Setting in the mouth	Withdrawal from the mouth	Complete setting (final hardening) done outside the mouth
Time (s)	45–60	45–90	30–60	90 s–4 mins

Fig. 14.9 The working time line of a typical dimethacrylate composite from the start of mix to complete (extraoral) curing. The range of times given reflect the differences in the times between commercially available products and give an indication of the relative times of each stage. Variations in temperature and humidity will also have an effect on the setting time.

and their properties are compared with higher methacrylates in Table 14.5.

The working 'time line'

To aid understanding of the relative timings of the dimethacrylate composite temporary material from start of mix to final set, Figure 14.9 sets out the material's working timeline visually.

Advantages and disadvantages

The advantages and disadvantages of dimethacrylate composites as temporary restoratives are set out in Table 14.6.

Indications

The indications of dimethacrylate composite materials are:

- Temporary inlays
- Temporary onlays
- Temporary veneers
- Temporary crowns
- As a refining material for temporary crown forms
- Short temporary bridges (three units maximum).

Table 14.6 Advantages and disadvantages of dimethacrylate composites

Advantages	Disadvantages
Good aesthetics	Expense
Good colour stability	There may be insufficient thickness for strength interocclusally
Available in a range of shades including a bleach shade	Must be protected from light while in the unset state
Good flexural strength	Can stain with certain foodstuffs
Hard	
Moderately good wear resistance	
Moderately low exothermic reaction	
Polishable due to small filler particles	
Good tissue biocompatibility	
Non-irritant to the soft and hard tissues	
Generally radiopaque	
Replicates occlusal surface	
May be repaired	
Minimal shrinkage	

Commercially available products

Table 14.7 shows a representative group of dimethacrylate materiels which are commercially available.

Table 14.7 Some dimethacrylate composites currently available on the market

Product	Manufacturer
Cool Temp	Coltène Whaledent
Elite Acrytemp	Zhermack
Fill-In	Kerr Hawe
Integrity (also Mini-Syringe)	Dentsply
Prevision CB	Heraeus
Protemp 3 Garant	3M ESPE
Protemp 4	3M ESPE
Protemp II	3M ESPE
Revotek LC	GC
Structur 2 SC	Voco
Telio CS C&B	Ivoclar Vivadent
Temphase Regular (also Fast)	Kerr Hawe
Unifast LC	GC

Presentation

Generally these products are supplied as a two-component auto-mixed paste/paste presentation (Figure 14.10). The advantages and handling of this presentation are discussed in Chapter 1. Some products are presented in a single paste form (Figure 14.11), which is then light-cured when the desired final shape has been achieved.

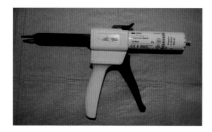

Fig. 14.10 Example of the paste/paste bisacryl composite materials (Protemp 4, 3M ESPE).

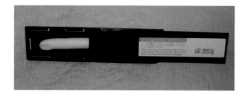

Fig. 14.11 Example of the single paste, light-cured dimethacrylate composite material (Revotek LC, GC).

Clinical manipulation

When a dimethacrylate composite material is to be used, a preoperative impression is made to create a matrix into which it is placed. On reinsertion of the impression and material into the mouth, a temporary restoration is formed which replicates the original tooth surface morphology and is closely adapted to the preparation. This has been termed the **resin replica technique** (see Box 14.3).

- Any residual unpolymerized resin must be removed from the preparation if the temporary restoration has been constructed using a dimethacrylate composite and an addition silicone impression material is to be used to make the definitive impression. Failure to do so will inhibit the set of the impression material as the oxygen inhibited layer will react with the addition silicone.
- Alcohol softens and degrades resin-containing materials and so its use with these materials is undesirable. Some manufacturers misguidedly suggest that unpolymerized resin on the surface may be removed by swabbing the surface with alcohol on cotton wool. This will leave a surface which is weakened and likely to degrade rapidly.
- Cores constructed from resin-based composite or resin-modified glass ionomer cement should be coated with a separating medium such as petroleum jelly. Failure to do this will result in the dimethacrylate composite material bonding to the resin component of the above materials. It is then important to ensure that the petroleum jelly is thoroughly removed prior to the cementation of the temporary restoration.
- Dimethacrylate composite materials tend to take up surface stain easily. It is advisable to always warn the patient to avoid drinking red wine or eating curries otherwise a maroon or yellow coloured temporary restoration may result respectively (Figure 14.12).

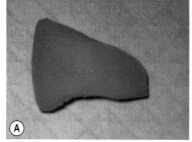 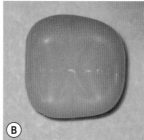

Fig. 14.12 Two temporary crowns made using a dimethacrylate composite material stained with (A) red wine and (B) curry. Note the red and yellow hue taken on by the material respectively. For a comparison with the original colour see Figure 14.13.

Box 14.3 Resin replica technique

1. Take a preoperative impression to construct a matrix of the tooth to be temporized, including at least one tooth on either side of the tooth to be prepared, either in the mouth or on a study cast. The clinician may choose to modify the shape of the crown to be temporized prior to impression taking (for example, building it up to increase the strength of the temporary crown). Inlay wax or resin may be used for this. The impression may be adjusted using a scalpel blade to open up the interproximal areas to increase the bulk and hence strength of the temporary restoration.
2. Select the shade of the temporary material to be used (if applicable).
3. Carry out the tooth preparation.
4. Syringe the first portion of material mixed on the bracket table to check set and consistent mix (and to ensure that the material has fully mixed).
5. Syringe the mixed material into the matrix, keeping the nozzle within the body of the expressed material to avoid incorporating air into the mix.
6. Reseat the matrix on the preparation.

(Continued)

Box 14.3 Resin replica technique (Continued)

7. Monitor the setting material (on the bracket table) and remove it when it has reached a rubber stage, usually 30–90 seconds depending on the material and mouth temperature and humidity. Do not delay any longer or the set material will lock into any undercuts.

8. Remove the matrix impression and allow the temporary restoration to self-cure for 4–5 minutes then remove it from the impression. This process may be accelerated by placing it in hot water.

9. Trim the flash (using a tungsten carbide or diamond burs as the material is more like resin-based composite than acrylic, so composite cutting instruments are preferable to acrylic trimmers) and reseat on the prep(s).

10. Check the occlusion and adjust if necessary.

11. Wipe the surface with a cotton wool roll to remove the oxygen inhibition layer.

12. Polish the completed restoration using polishing instruments (e.g. discs, burs, etc.).

13. Lute the crown using a temporary luting cement.

Note: as there is some variation between different products, the dental team is advised to follow the working timetable for stages of set found in the directions for use.

When using the resin replica technique, a putty impression material should be used to make the preoperative matrix. It will tend to tear less than an alginate impression so that if the first attempt is not satisfactory, the same impression can be used again. Furthermore, due to its good dimensional stability, the putty matrix can be retained and reused if the patient has a problem with the temporary restoration requiring it to be remade some days or weeks later. This would be impossible if alginate was used. The relative merits of putty versus alginate is set out in Table 14.8 and the properties of these materials can be found in Chapter 15.

Table 14.8 Comparison of a putty and alginate matrix for the construction of dimethacrylate composite temporary restorations

Putty	Alginate
Multiple use	Single use
Dimensionally stable	Dimensionally unstable, especially if not stored correctly
Remake of temporary easy	Not possible
Stored with patient's records	Not possible
Increased tear strength	Poor tear strength
Easier to disinfect	Problems with disinfection (degradation and dimensional change)
Longer time to set	Shorter time to set
More expensive	Less expensive

How to repair a dimethacrylate composite material

Resin-based composite materials can bond to the dimethacrylate composite. This allows the repair of small non-load-bearing defects and voids to be filled, margins refined or contacts improved using a flowable resin composite. The preparatory work depends on whether the restoration has been newly placed or has already been in clinical use.
- For newly placed material, remove any contamination (e.g. saliva or dust) with water and dry it with air from the three-in-one syringe. Add the flowable composite and cure in no more than 1 mm increments.
- If the restoration has been in use, the surface should be roughened first before the above procedure is carried out.

COMPOSITE-BASED CROWN TEMPLATE

One manufacturer (3M ESPE) has launched a preformed, malleable composite-based crown called the Protemp Crown (Figure 14.13). This crown is designed to temporize a single unit and is claimed to save much time as it combines the advantages of both composite-based chemically cured temporization with the advantages of pre-fabricated crowns. The filler loading is at a level much closer to that found in resin composites (78% by weight), aiding the handling properties and making the crown form handle as if dealing with wax. The crown form is trimmed to shape and then fully cured using a curing light. It can then be luted in situ.

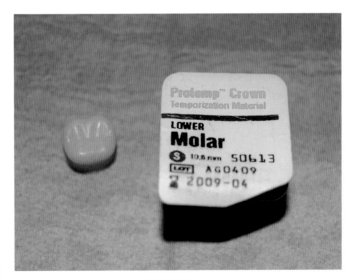

Fig. 14.13 A Protemp Crown (3M ESPE).

LIGHT-CURED TEMPORARY RESIN MATERIALS

Light-cured temporary materials are available for the temporization of intracoronal preparations. These are rubbery in consistency and are retained in the cavity mechanically as they do not bond to the cavity walls. This property is advantageous as it facilitates their subsequent removal. Any material that bonds either chemically or micromechanically to the preparation will have to be cut out. This will damage the preparation and result in a poorer fit of the cast restoration because:

- The bur may cut into the preparation leaving a gap at the margins
- The temporary material may be retained on the preparation walls thus preventing the full seating of the cast.

The above is an important factor when choosing the material to temporize an inlay or onlay preparation. The light-cured temporary materials are reasonably easily removed at the fit appointment using a scaler or excavator. The preparation remains in the state it was at the end of the preparation appointment. This saves much time as no cleaning is necessary prior to trying in the definitive prosthesis.

This type of material is only suitable for use in the short term and should not remain in the oral cavity for more than a month because it slowly degrades and wears (Figure 14.14). This will permit movement of the opposing and adjacent teeth with the consequent need for adjustment of the final restoration. These crowns also have a tendency to develop a malodour due to bacterial activity over time.

Constituents

These materials are based on resin composite technology and consist primarily of a monomer matrix and fillers (Table 14.9). The monomer matrix may also have other chemicals such as plasticizers and diluents added to it to modify its properties. For example, to make the material more flexible and easy to remove. Additionally, pigments, stabilizers and initiators for light curing are included. Frequently, chemicals are incorporated so that the materials will also harden in the presence of moisture. Commonly, addition of calcium sulphate will result in the material hardening in the presence of water in the saliva.

Some manufacturers have added chemicals that have an antibacterial effect. **Triclosan** is one such chemical and it inhibits the growth of cariogenic bacteria during the lifespan of the temporary restoration. Other manufacturers have added a fluoride-releasing agent such as **sodium fluoride** with the intention that the material will impart some caries resistance to the surrounding tooth tissue. For either of these chemicals to be released, the resin must take up water before they will diffuse out. The time scale for this is lengthy and there is some doubt as to the benefit these additions produce.

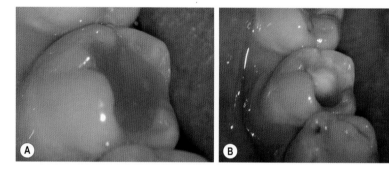

Fig. 14.14 (A) Tooth 47 occlusal cavity temporarily restored using Systemp Inlay (Ivoclar Vivadent) prior to the fit of a gold inlay. Note the discolouration of the material after 3 weeks of use. (B) The material has been removed using an excavator; note the clean cavity. The definitive restoration can now be easily tried in and luted into the cavity. (Note: Systemp Inlay is no longer available and has now been superseded by Telio CS inlay.)

Table 14.9 Main constituents of light-cured temporary materials with examples of commercial products

Generic part	Chemical example	Reason for inclusion	Example product
Monomer matrix	Polyester urethane dimethacrylate	Forms resin matrix	Telio CS Inlay
			Telio CS Onlay
	Ethyl glycol methacrylate		Telio CS Onlay
Filler	Silicon dioxide	Increases strength	Telio CS Inlay
	Copolymers		Telio CS Onlay
	Zinc oxide	Alters viscosity and therefore handling	Duo Temp
	Zinc sulphate		
Chemicals necessary in the curing process	Methacrylate resin	Enables a command cure	Duo Temp
Fluoride-releasing agents	Sodium fluoride	Cariostatic effect	Duo Temp
Antibacterial agents	Triclosan	May have bactericidal effect on surface of dentine	Telio CS Inlay
			Telio CS Onlay
Stabilizers	These may include hydroquinone	Prevents premature set	Telio CS Inlay
			Telio CS Onlay
Pigments	Titanium dioxide and ferrous and ferric salts	Provide tooth colour match	Telio CS Inlay
			Telio CS Onlay

Light-cured temporary materials can interact with other methacrylate-based products (for example, light-cured cavity liner materials) by bonding with them. It is therefore advisable to use a separator such as glycerine to prevent bonding or inadvertent removal of the lining with the temporary.

Chemistry and setting reaction

The setting reaction of these temporary materials is primarily by **light curing** and as such they offer the many benefits of a command set. This is a polymerization reaction with the material shrinking by 1.6–3%. Some materials have prepolymers added to them to decrease polymerization shrinkage. As this shrinkage is relatively low, the formation of marginal gaps, microleakage and discolouration of the material is reduced. The depth of cure of the material is less than 4 mm and as with all purely light curing materials, it is important that it is fully cured. The lower filler loading materials means less heat production, and this will not cause pulpal damage unless the material is left for a long time, in excess of 5 minutes in situ during setting.

Some of these materials set by a dual-cure reaction, so if the light cannot reach the base of the cavity, the clinician is reassured that the material will come to a full set in a matter of minutes. The dark-cure reaction is catalysed by the exposure of the material to moisture, which reacts with calcium sulphate contained in the product. This reaction can take up to 2 hours. This is also made possible by the material absorbing water when in clinical use (**water sorption**) and as a result, some of these materials expand slightly during the setting process. The cavity should be kept moist before applying these materials. The water uptake explains why these materials have a tendency to discolour with use (Figure 14.14A).

Since many of these materials rely at least in part on a setting reaction that requires moisture, their storage is of particular importance. Ensure that they are stored as delivered: the immediate outer covering should not be removed until ready for use (see Chapter 5).

Properties

Of the purely light-cured materials, two viscosities are available (Figure 14.15). The difference in viscosity is related to the amount of filler used. The low-viscosity materials are designed for inlay preparations, whereas the more rigid ones are designed for onlays where the cavity size is larger. The more flexible materials are stickier in their unset state and are difficult to manipulate as they tend to stick to the instrument and pull back from the cavity. It is recommended that the material is placed into the cavity and the gross excess removed prior to light curing. If necessary, the surface can be finished using rotary instrumentation.

The stiffer materials offer higher strength and reduce drifting of adjacent and opposing teeth. The handling of these materials more closely resembles that of putty materials. They are therefore easier to manipulate into the cavity as they can be condensed into place.

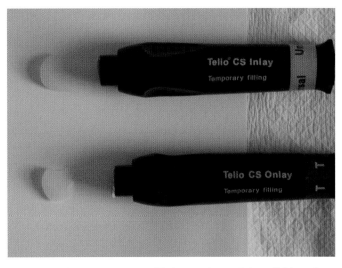

Fig. 14.15 The two viscosities of light-cured materials available: Telio CS inlay (Ivoclar Vivadent) above and Telio CS onlay (Ivoclar Vivadent) below.

If the lower viscosity material is sticking to instruments, an unfilled resin such as a bonding agent can be sparingly used on instruments to act as a separating agent to facilitate manipulation of the material.

Presentation

These materials are presented in two shades; translucent and universal. None of the available materials have ideal aesthetics, but they are radiopaque and easily identified on a radiograph.

Manipulation

Some clinicians do not use a temporary cement to lute these materials in situ but simply light cure them into the cavity, other dentists prefer to use these materials in conjunction with a temporary luting cement. If this is the case, a eugenol-free temporary cement should be used as these materials contain resin and phenolic substances such as eugenol, which will inhibit their polymerization.

Some manufactures supply a desensitizer, which can be applied to the preparation walls prior to placement of the temporary material. The aim is to seal the cut dentinal tubules, so reducing postoperative sensitivity. The material also contains a disinfection agent (glutaraldehyde) to reduce bacterial growth. This material is toxic and should be used with considerable care. Additionally, it is advisable to avoid skin contact when manipulating these materials as sensitization may occur due to the resin contained in the product. It is questionable how effective these agents are and also what effect they have on the dentine. This may also present a problem when a resin luting cement is used for the final restoration as the pretreatment may alter the effect the primer/conditioner has on the dentine, negating any bonding which might occur.

Indications and contraindications

The indications and contraindications for light-cured temporary (inlay) materials are shown in Table 14.10.

Table 14.10 Indications and contraindications of light-cured temporary (inlay) materials

Indications	Contraindications
Temporary dressings for inlay preparations	Allergy to one of the constituents
Temporary restoration of (retentive) cavities	Large (multisurface) cavities
Inter-visit access cavity sealants during an endodontic procedure	Crown or bridge material
Relining prefabricated temporary crown forms and bridges made of methacrylates or polycarbonate	Subgingival preparations
Sealing implant screw access openings	Should not remain in the oral cavity for more than 6 weeks

The higher filled (more viscous preparations) are designed for use in larger-sized cavities and where a shallower cavity is present.

Commercially available products

Table 14.11 and Figure 14.16 show examples of the currently commercially available product. Note the difference in appearance in comparison to the Telio CS products (Figure 14.14).

Table 14.11 Some light-curing temporary dressing materials currently available on the market

Product	Manufacturer
Cimpat LC	Septodont
Clip	Voco
Clip F	Voco
DuoTemp	Coltène Whaledent
Telio CS Inlay (formerly Systemp/Fermit)	Ivoclar Vivadent
Telio CS Onlay (formerly Systemp/Fermit)	Ivoclar Vivadent
Tempit (Light Cure)	Centrix
Tempit Ultra	Centrix

Fig. 14.16 An example of a light-cured temporary material (DuoTemp, Coltène Whaledent). This material also sets in the presence of moisture.

PUTTIES

The last family of materials used for temporization are the **putties**. They are based on **zinc oxide** and **zinc sulphate**. Putties are radiopaque and are placed into the cavity in their soft unset state. They harden in the presence of moisture from saliva and expand during setting. The basic setting reaction is the hydration of calcium sulphate to form a plaster, gypsum. Their wear resistance is poor but they create a good seal and some products are claimed to adhere to dentine. Their indications are to:

- Seal endodontic access cavities between visits
- Temporize inlay cavities
- Temporize retentive cavities.

Typical compositions are shown in Table 14.12.

Table 14.12 Chemical constituents of temporary putty materials

Component	Percentage	Reason for inclusion
Zinc oxide	30–50	Filler
Calcium sulphate	1–30	Setting component
Barium sulphate	0–20	Radiopacity
Ethylene diacetate	10–20	Filler
Talc	0–20	Filler
Zinc sulphate	5–10	Setting component
Poly(vinyl acetate)	1–5	Viscosity controller

Commercially available products

Table 14.13 shows some of the currently available commercial putty materials.

Table 14.13 Some temporary putty materials currently available on the market

Product	Manufacturer	Indication
Cavit	3M ESPE	Endodontic access cavities, inter-visit
Cavit-G	3M ESPE	Very easy to remove, recommended to temporize inlay preparations.
Caviton	GC	General temporization, especially endodontic access cavities inter-visit
Cavit-W	3M ESPE	Easy to remove as softer
Cimpat N	Septodont	General temporization
Cimpat S	Septodont	General temporization
Coltosol F	Coltène Whaledent	General temporization
Tempit (Regular)	Centrix	Endodontic access cavities inter-visit

TEMPORARY LUTING CEMENTS

Purpose

The function of temporary luting cements is to grout the gap between the preparation and the temporary restoration. They are also indicated in some cases to temporarily lute the definitive prosthesis to allow the patient and/or clinician to assess the restoration or restorations during function. Materials used as temporary luting materials are softer, so they have poorer strength. They should not be relied on to retain the temporary prosthesis if the preparation has inadequate retention as this will lead to the loss of the restoration. A temporary luting cement has the following properties:

- It is soft for easy removal, as failure to remove all the cement will compromise the gingival health and seating of the final restoration
- It is strong enough to hold the restoration in situ until the fit appointment.

Eugenol-free products

Eugenol and eugenol-free products are oil-based cements, with **zinc oxide non-eugenol** products using oils other than eugenol such as **ortho-ethoxybenzoic acid**. Zinc oxide eugenol containing temporary cements are covered in Chapter 12.

With the increasing use of resin composite, there has been a move away from eugenol-containing materials as eugenol inhibits the set of resin composites, causing the resin composite to plasticize. Eugenol-free products should therefore be used in the following instances:

- Construction of acrylic temporaries: as eugenol may also interact with acrylic
- Bonding the definitive restoration with a resin composite is envisaged: as eugenol may also contaminate the dentine surface which will affect bonding
- Use of addition silicone impression materials is envisaged: as eugenol interacts with this impression material, it should therefore not be used on a surface contaminated with a eugenol-containing cement.

A temporary cement should not be relied on to retain anything other than a well-fitting temporary restoration as the forces during function will be concentrated in this layer, leading to fracture of the cement lute and loss of the restoration.

Zinc oxide powder (for example Kalzinol, Dentsply) should never be mixed with a zinc oxide temporary cement to try to thicken it in an attempt to retain the temporary restoration. If this is done, the physical properties of the material would become unsuitable for its use as a temporary cement. A well-made, close-fitting temporary restoration on a retentive preparation should instead be relied on. This again highlights the importance of not mixing components of different materials together.

Non-eugenol cements should be used:
- If the patient has an allergy or sensitivity to eugenol
- If acrylic temporaries are to be used after the cement has been used
- If an addition silicone impression material is to be used after the cement has been used
- If resin composite is to be used as the definitive bonding agent or a resin-containing luting cement.

Modifier

Some materials are supplied with a third tube which is called the modifier (Figure 14.17). The purpose of this paste is to further soften the cement to facilitate removal of the temporary restoration at the fit appointment. It will also reduce the hardness and strength of the final set cement. A clinician fitting a well-constructed temporary will invariably need to use the modifier. Without it, the temporary may be very difficult to remove.

If no modifier is available then petroleum jelly such as Vaseline (Unilever) may be used as an alternative depending on the clinician's requirements. Increasing the petroleum jelly content will increase the softness of the cement.

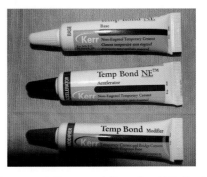

Fig. 14.17 A temporary luting cement (Temp Bond NE, Kerr Hawe). The three tubes contain the base, catalyst and modifier, respectively, from top to bottom.

Table 14.14 Contents of the tube in the variations of the temporary luting cement TempBond (Kerr Hawe) and a summary of their function

Base	Accelerator	Modifier	Cement reaction
TempBond			
Zinc oxide Corn starch	4-allyl-2-methoxyphenol eugenol (oil of cloves) Resin Carnauba wax	Zinc oxide petrolatum jelly	Simple zinc oxide eugenol-setting reaction. Addition of petrolatum jelly slows or inhibits set
TempBond NE			
Mineral oil Zinc oxide Corn starch	Resin Ortho-EBA Carnauba wax Octanoic acid		Form of EBA cement with wax added to weaken the cement, reducing the amount of ethoxybenzoate salt formed and weakening the cement, which will break up on removal
TempBond Clear			
HEMA Dibutyl phthalate Tripropylene glycol diacrylate Inert mineral fillers	Dibutyl phthalate Tripropylene glycol diacrylate Inert mineral fillers Cumene hydroperoxide		Cold-cure resin setting reaction using plasticizer to prevent complete polymerization

HEMA, hydroxyethylmethacrylate; EBA, ethoxybenzoic acid.

Chemistry

The contents of each tube are listed in Table 14.14. In the case of the non-eugenol products, the presentation of these cements is a two-paste system: a base and an accelerator (catalyst). The base consists of **zinc oxide** mineral oils and the catalyst **ortho-ethoxybenzoic acid**. The setting reaction is similar to an ortho-ethoxybenzoic acid (EBA) cement (see Chapter 12). The consistency is slightly less brittle than that of eugenol-containing materials, with the result that the material is less likely to break cleanly when removed from crown margins. It has certain advantages over eugenol-based materials (Table 14.15).

Mixing

The sequence of mixing a paste/paste luting cement is set out in Box 14.4.

Table 14.15 Comparison of a eugenol-free and a eugenol-containing temporary luting cement

Non-eugenol materials	Eugenol-based materials
Do not inhibit setting of resin-based permanent cements	Breaks cleanly, making clearing up easier with no smearing
Do not react with acrylic temporary restorations	Obtundent effect on pulp
Film thickness: 20 µm	Film thickness: in region of 25 µm
Set in 2–2.5 minutes	Set in 3 minutes

Box 14.4 Recommended sequence of mixing a paste/paste temporary luting cement, in this example Temp Bond NE (Kerr Hawe)

Step 1

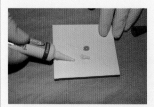

Equal amounts of the base and catalyst pastes are placed in close proximity on a mixing pad

Step 2

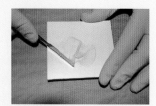

The pastes are mixed for 30 seconds, until the mass becomes a uniform colour. Care should be taken to prevent the incorporation of air

Step 3

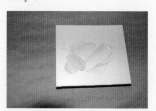

The mixed cement ready for use

Step 4

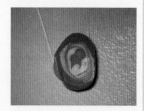

Coat the internal surface of the temporary crown with the mixed cement and seat the crown on the preparation

Temporary cement removal

Some of the cement is often retained on the preparation as a smear when the temporary prosthesis is removed (Figure 14.18). This should be removed using flour of pumice and water slurry on a rubber cup or bristle brush in a slow handpiece prior to try in and cementation of the definitive restoration (Figure 14.19). On no account should prophylaxis paste be used for this purpose as the oils contained in this product may compromise the surface for subsequent luting and in particular when bonding using a resin-based composite material.

One manufacturer has produced a bur specifically designed to remove temporary cement from preparations. Kerr Hawe's OptiClean is made from an abrasive addition silicone compound mounted on a latch grip bur (Figure 14.20). This has the advantage of being small and so can more easily gain access to the whole preparation, especially the approximal surfaces, than a bristle brush or rubber cup.

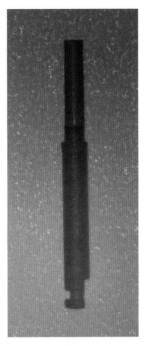

Fig. 14.20 Kerr Hawe's OptiClean bur, designed for removing temporary cement from preparations prior to trying the definitive prosthesis in situ.

The dentist should wait for the cement to fully set before attempting to remove it. Taking a shortcut here will lead to the removal of partially set or unset paste, which tends to smear everywhere and complicating its complete removal. Removal of the fully set material is much quicker as it can be fractured away (Figure 14.21).

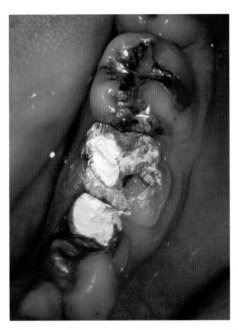

Fig. 14.18 Teeth 36 and 35 immediately after the removal of the temporary crowns; note the temporary cement residue on the preparations.

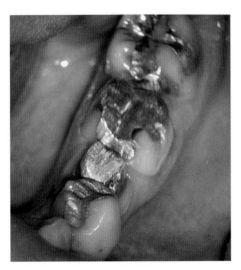

Fig. 14.19 Teeth 36 and 35 after the removal of the temporary cement, using flour of pumice and a bristle brush.

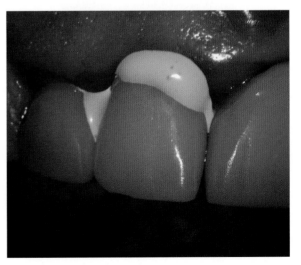

Fig. 14.21 Temporary crown on tooth 11 cemented with Temp Bond NE (Kerr Hawe). Note the material has set and the excess can now be removed much more easily as it will chip off cleanly.

Variations in temporary cement products

A number of modifications have been made to temporary cements for use under certain conditions. These include:

- Availability in an auto-mix presentation (Figure 14.22) as well as the traditional paste/paste system in two tubes (TempBond NE, Kerr Hawe). This facilitates mixing.
- Availability as a clear cement (Figure 14.23) for use in situations where aesthetics demand it. The speed of set can be accelerated by light curing (TempBond Clear, Kerr Hawe).

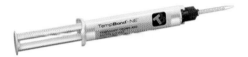

Fig. 14.22 Temp Bond NE auto-mix presentation (Kerr Hawe).

- Available in sachets (Figure 14.24) which can be given to patients in case their temporary restoration comes out between appointments. This is of benefit for patients who cannot return easily to the clinic, for example if they are going on holiday. From a cross-contamination perspective it is superior to the traditional tube or bottle presentation as the sachets contain a unit dose and therefore may be discarded after single use.
- Availability as an addition-cured silicone (Figure 14.25). This is claimed to
  - Have superior marginal integrity
  - Be easier to clean up as it peels off
  - Have no residue on the preparation or inside the temporary restoration.

Care should be exercised when removing temporary cements as their retention may be excellent, and hard and soft tissue damage may result from the clinician's attempts to lever the restoration off the preparation. Furthermore the core may be damaged if a mechanical crown and bridge remover such as Kavo's Corona Flex is used too zealously.

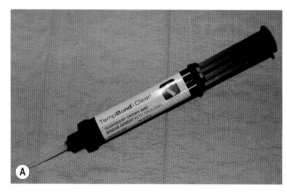
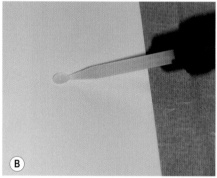

Fig. 14.23 Temp Bond Clear (Kerr Hawe) in auto-mix mixing syringe (A) and the material being extruded (B). Note that the material is almost transparent.

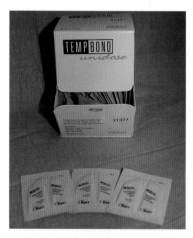

Fig. 14.24 Temp Bond Unidose (Kerr Hawe). This product is presented in unidose sachets.

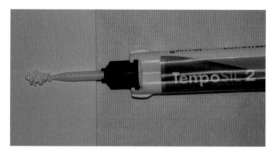

Fig. 14.25 Example of an addition-cured silicone temporary cement (TempSIL 2, Coltène Whaledent).

Temporary cements used as definitive lute

Some clinicians advocate the use of temporary cements to cement definitive restorations in situ. This can be safely done although thorough and conscientious follow-up is indicated to check for wash out of the material as it is more soluble and may be lost with time.

In implant cases, temporary cements may be used as a 'safety net'. If the screw retaining the crown loosens, the crown may be more easily removed to gain access to tighten it if a temporary cement has been used.

Some of these cements smear after setting on the temporaries or soft tissues such as gingival tissue or lips. The use of Orange Solvent Spray on a cotton wool roll or gauze will facilitate its removal (Figure 14.26). This is natural orange oil derived from the rind of oranges.

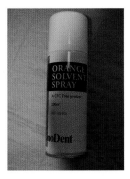

Fig. 14.26 Orange Solvent spray used to remove temporary cement and other materials such as articulator paper markings from teeth and the oral (and facial) soft tissues.

Commercially available products

Table 14.16 shows some of the commercially available temporary luting cements.

Table 14.16 Some temporary luting cements currently available on the market

Product	Manufacturer
Freegenol Temporary Cement	GC
Hy Bond Temporary Cement	Shofu
NoMix Temporary Cement	Centrix
Prevision Cem Cement	Heraeus
Provicol	Voco
Telio CS Link	Ivoclar Vivadent
Rely X Temp E	3M ESPE
Rely X Temp NE	3M ESPE
Temp Bond	Kerr Hawe
Temp Bond Automix	Kerr Hawe
Temp Bond Clear	Kerr Hawe
Temp Bond NE	Kerr Hawe
Temp Bond Unidose NE	Kerr Hawe
TempGrip	Dentsply
TemposcellCimpat	Septodont
TempoSIL	Coltène Whaledent

Most temporary cements are based on zinc oxide eugenol reactions. Those claiming not to contain eugenol are either based on the setting reaction of calcium sulphate or are methacrylate based.

NON HARDENING TEMPORARY CEMENTS

Non-hardening temporary cements are also available. These are indicated where the retention of the preparation is excellent and only for a short time (for example a week) to allow the patient an opportunity to assess the restoration(s) for function, speech and aesthetics. This is particularly true when extensive crown and bridgework is being carried out (Figure 14.27).

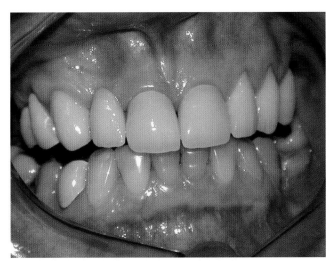

Fig. 14.27 Teeth 15–24 restored with metal ceramic units, luted with a non-hardening cement for a short period of time to allow assessment of function and the aesthetics.

These cements work by grouting the gap between the preparation and the inside of the casting by producing a gasket of soft, rubber-like material. An example on the market is Opotow Trial Cement (Teledyne Water Pik; Figure 14.28). It is based on zinc oxide eugenol and is presented as a two-paste system: a base and a catalyst. This material effectively seals the microgap between the dentine and the casting, but permits easy, non-traumatic removal of the casting at the end of the assessment period. Unfortunately, as this material contains eugenol it cannot be used prior to the use of resin composite materials.

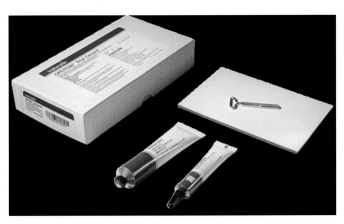

Fig. 14.28 Opotow Trial Cement (Teledyne Water Pik).

SUMMARY

- Good temporization is an important factor in the construction of good quality indirect definitive restorations.
- There are many materials and techniques available, both directly and laboratory made.
- The general principle is that a close fitting restoration is constructed, which is grouted in situ using a soft temporary cement.
- Acrylic derivatives in combination with a preformed crown form or dimethacrylate composite materials are used to make temporary crowns utilizing a direct technique.
- Light-cured materials are available to temporize intracoronal restorations.
- Putty materials can also be used in this instance, as well for sealing endodontic access cavities between visits.
- Bespoke temporary luting cements are available to retain temporary restorations, these are usually based on zinc oxide either with or without eugenol.

SELF-ASSESSMENT QUESTIONS

1. Why is necessary to place temporary restorations?
2. What are the requirements of a temporary restoration?
3. Compare in terms of properties the materials which could be used to construct a temporary crown for an upper left permanent incisor.
4. Some temporary luting cements come with a tube of modifier. What is in this tube? What effect does it have on the set cement? Why would the dentist choose to use a modifier?
5. What materials are available to temporize an inlay preparation? What is the clinician trying to achieve and how does this influence their selection?
6. What precautions should be taken when using a eugenol-based temporary cement?

Chapter | **15** |

Impression materials

INTRODUCTION

For the construction of an indirect restoration or dental appliance (e.g. a fixed restoration such as crown or bridge and removable appliances such as an orthodontic appliance or an occlusal splint), accurate information about the oral cavity or the dental arches needs to be given to the dental technician. This information is usually gathered by **making** (**recording** or **taking**) an **impression**, which involves placing a material into the mouth in an unset or fluid state and which then hardens (Box 15.1). This impression is then cast, so creating a model of the dental or oral structures. More recently, techniques have been developed which use computer-operated optical imaging to create the impression, and the cast is constructed from this information. The impression is a negative, with the model or cast being the positive, and the technician constructs the device/restoration using this cast.

For the device to fit well, it is necessary that the impression accurately reproduces the fine details and dimensions of the oral structures and their relationship to one another. There are many types of impression material available, with the material choice being based on the type of device to be made and the oral conditions. In general, a more accurate impression is required for the construction of a fixed restoration than for a removable device. This chapter describes and discusses the impression materials available to the dentist in order to construct an indirect restoration or appliance together with the allied materials that are used to facilitate the taking of a good impression.

DESIRABLE PROPERTIES OF AN IMPRESSION MATERIAL

While the choice of material is dependent to some extent on the degree of accuracy of reproduction required, all impression materials should have the following desirable properties:

- Easy to handle
- Compatible with oral fluids
- Reproduce detail accurately
- Have good tear resistance
- Have no adverse effects on the patient
- Have a pleasant taste
- Easily removable from the mouth especially from undercut areas
- Be able to be adequately disinfected
- Remain dimensionally stable after removal
- Compatible with all model construction materials.

Inaccuracies can occur at any stage in the process of constructing any dental device. The inaccuracies at each stage must compensate for each other so that the final restoration will fit accurately. Therefore, an impression that is too accurate may not work as the inaccuracies in the other stages in the process are not taken into account. This is called a **total process chain**.

All the impression materials which are available to the dentist have various degrees of accuracy and the indication of the material will depend on the need for detail on the working cast. All of these impression materials require to be supported in an **impression tray** and be retained there until after casting.

Box 15.1 Typical sequence of construction of a dental device

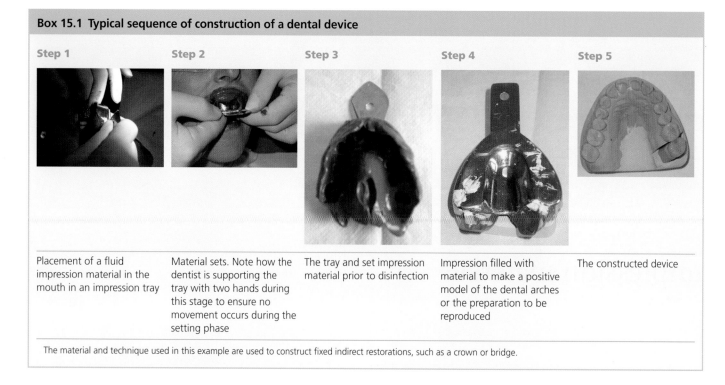

Step 1	Step 2	Step 3	Step 4	Step 5
Placement of a fluid impression material in the mouth in an impression tray	Material sets. Note how the dentist is supporting the tray with two hands during this stage to ensure no movement occurs during the setting phase	The tray and set impression material prior to disinfection	Impression filled with material to make a positive model of the dental arches or the preparation to be reproduced	The constructed device

The material and technique used in this example are used to construct fixed indirect restorations, such as a crown or bridge.

IMPRESSION TRAYS AND TRAY SELECTION

The impression material must be adequately supported during the impression process by an impression tray. There are several types of tray available, and these fall into two broad categories:

- Stock trays
- Special trays.

Stock trays

Stock trays are supplied in a range of average sizes and shapes of arch form. They may be made of **plastic** or **metal** (Figure 15.1). To obtain a satisfactory impression, a stock tray must:

- Be rigid and non-flexible under load when taking the impression
- Extend sufficiently to support the impression material in the region being reproduced
- Fit loosely around the dental arch and not touch the soft tissues
- Have adequate means of retaining the impression material in the tray
- Have a robust (integral) handle
- Be able to be adequately disinfected (if not meant for single use).

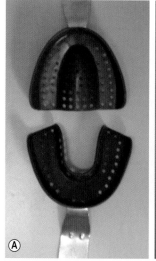
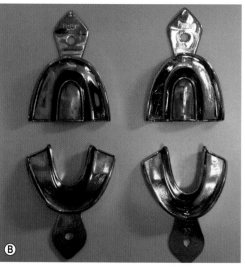

Fig. 15.1 Examples of (A) plastic and (B) metal stock trays.

Plastic stock trays

Plastic impression trays are frequently injection moulded from a high-impact **styrene**. Good trays have a moulded periphery, which takes account of the anatomy of the mouth. They may be either **dentate** or **edentulous** and **perforated** or **non-perforated** (Figure 15.2). Perforations aid in the retention of the impression material.

Adequate extension

It is important that the stock tray is extended adequately to support the impression material, otherwise distortions are likely in any unsupported regions. Figure 15.3 shows a poorly extended stock tray that would be inadequate if a full sulcular impression is required.

Correct size and shape of the dental arch

The tray also needs to approximate to the size and shape of the dental arch. If the tray selection is incorrect, the ill-fitting tray will be unable to support the impression material properly, leading to inaccuracies in the impression (Figure 15.4).

Importance of rigidity

It is very important that the tray is strong enough to withstand the force of the impression material being placed in the mouth. It must not flex, as this will result in stresses being formed within the impression material, and the clinician will be unaware of this. Flexure of the tray under load causes the tray to distort and the impression to flex. The sides of the impression tray will bow out

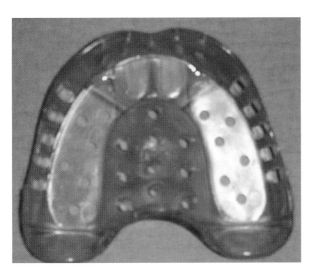

Fig. 15.2 Example of a dentate, perforated plastic stock tray.

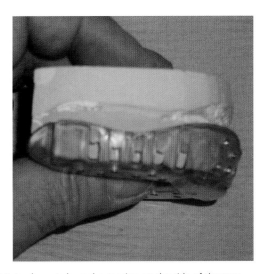

Fig. 15.3 Inadequate buccal extension on the side of the tray.

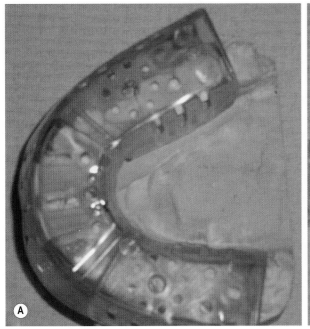

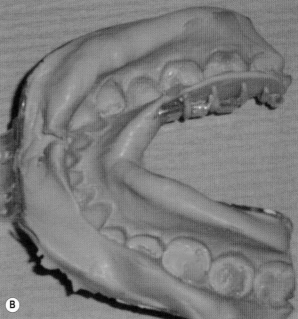

Fig. 15.4 (A) Tray touching the soft tissue on the lingual side (B) Absence of impression material at the site where the tray contacts the tissue leads to inaccuracies in the impression.

in the mouth (Figure 15.5). Once the pressure is released as the impression is removed, the tray will return to its original shape. This will mean that the impression will be narrower buccolingually than the actual buccolingual width in the oral cavity.

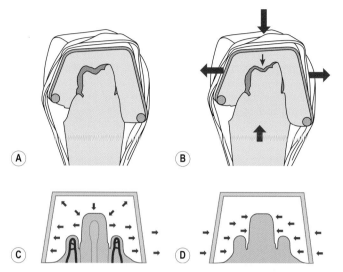

Fig. 15.5 The effects of pressure on the impression while the tray is in the mouth. (A) A flexible tray will distort. (B) If the tray is too flexible, pressure on the occlusal surface of the tray will lead to the lingual and buccal sides being displaced outwards by the impression material. (C, D) Once the impression is removed and the pressure released the tray returns to its original shape leaving the impression distorted.

Tray distortion during impression making will then lead to the cast model being inaccurate and finally the constructed prosthesis not fitting in the mouth. This is seen especially with the higher viscosity impression materials, such as the putty presentation (see p. 261). Some plastic stock trays have strengthening features to maintain rigidity (Figure 15.6).

Triple Tray

One type of plastic tray available is called the Triple Tray (Figure 15.7). This tray system is used when the **double arch** or **dual bite impression technique** is being employed to record an impression for a crown. This technique uses an accurate (usually elastomer) impression material to record both the tooth preparation and the opposing teeth. Although this is a popular technique in North America and can provide good results, its success depends on the patient's ability to close their teeth together without any interference by the tray; thus it can only be used in specific indications. By definition, this technique cannot reproduce the complete dental arch, which can lead to serious occlusal discrepancies. The details of the technique are beyond the scope of this text and the reader is referred to an operative dentistry text for further information.

Metal stock trays

To overcome many of the shortcomings of plastic trays, such as lack of rigidity, many clinicians prefer to use metal trays. These are also supplied as **dentate** or **edentulous** and **perforated** or **non-perforated**. Non-perforated metal trays have a locking rim peripherally

and undercut retention, which holds the impression material in the tray. Metal trays are expensive to purchase but may be disinfected by autoclaving and are therefore reusable.

> ✓
>
> Dentists should get their details engraved on their metal stock trays so that the trays are correctly returned from the laboratory and not misappropriated elsewhere! It is advisable to use laser etching for this if possible, so that the surface is not damaged, which may make cleaning of the tray more difficult.

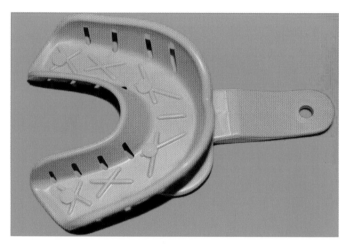

Fig. 15.6 A plastic stock tray with reinforcing ribs to prevent distortion during the impression process. Note also the rigid handle and extensive retentive features.

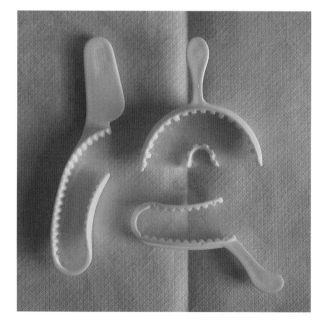

Fig. 15.7 Examples of Triple Trays.

Special trays

A special or **customized** tray is one which is made specifically for one patient. A preliminary impression (using a stock tray) is made and sent to the dental laboratory. A model is cast and wax is laid down on the model, the thickness of which corresponds to specific spacing. This spacing is determined by the impression material to be used in the final impression. The equal thickness of the impression material used means that dimensional change will theoretically be the same in all directions, so decreasing inaccuracies in the impression. Special trays are usually constructed from polymethylmethacrylate (Figure 15.8).

In addition, special trays may be modified, such as the creation of a window. This is done so that an impression material of a lower viscosity can be injected into the tray for accurate recording of displaceable tissues such as flabby ridges.

> **Flabby ridge:** A flabby ridge is one which becomes displaceable due to fibrous tissue deposition. It occurs most commonly in the upper anterior region, opposing the natural lower incisors. Its presence can affect denture stability.

The advent of putties has made the use of customized trays much less common. The putty, forming the bulk of the impression, shows very little dimensional change and supports the light-bodied material which gives fine detail. This has led to an increase in the types of stock tray available on the market.

TRAY ADHESIVES

It is very important that the impression material is retained securely in the tray. This may be done mechanically through perforations as described earlier or by the use of an adhesive. Ideally both these means should be used together as the use of each type alone can lead to failure. For example, the addition of a tray adhesive is helpful where the mechanical retention is not so effective. Figure 15.9 shows the modes of failure of a rim-lock tray and of a perforated tray where no adhesive is used. These discrepancies can potentially lead to distortion of the impression material and failure of fit of the prosthesis. The addition of a tray adhesive will reduce this as it addresses the area where the mechanical retention is not so effective.

All tray adhesives are based on contact adhesive technology. This means that they should be applied to the tray and allowed to dry in advance of the impression being taken. Failure to let the material dry will adversely affect the union between the tray, adhesive and impression material. The adhesive should be applied sparingly to the internal surface of the tray and extended just over the margin of the tray to the external surface to ensure that the periphery of the impression material remains attached to the tray. Pooling of excess adhesive is undesirable as the solution will not dry and will weaken the bond between the impression material and the tray. For the most effective use, two thin coats should be applied with the first coat being allowed to dry before the application of the second. None of the available adhesives is particularly effective and it is unwise to rely on adhesive alone in the tray.

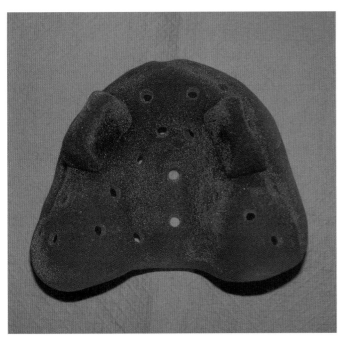

Fig. 15.8 An upper perforated, edentulous special tray constructed of polymethylmethacrylate.

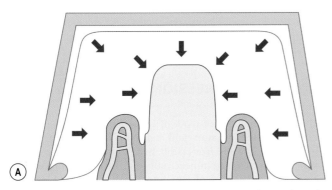
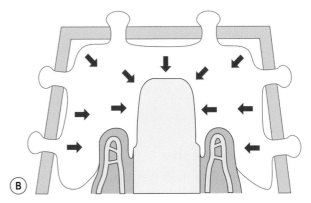

Fig. 15.9 (A) A rim-lock tray, where the impression has pulled away from the tray as a result of the polymerization shrinkage. (B) A perforated tray, where the impression material has pulled away from the tray wall between and despite the presence of perforations. Additional perforations will reduce this but not eliminate it completely.

Most tray adhesives are provided in screw-top bottles with a brush affixed to the lid (Figure 15.10). Invariably, as the adhesive lasts for long periods of time, the excess adhesive from each application gets deposited around the neck of the bottle. This means that the seal on the lid becomes less secure with time, leading to evaporation of the solvent and the consequent thickening of the adhesive. Application of adhesive to the tray thus becomes more difficult and the adhesive layer deposited is thicker than desired, leading to reduced performance.

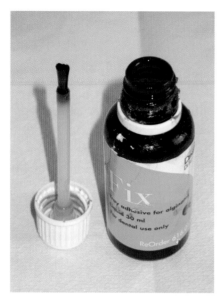

Fig. 15.10 Example of a tray adhesive. Note the brush attached to the lid and a residue of excess adhesive deposited around the screw thread at the neck of the bottle. This compromises the seal of the bottle, causing deterioration of the adhesive with time.

- A paint-on presentation of tray adhesive is preferable to the spray-on presentation. Spraying on the adhesive will result in pooling of the adhesive, which will not dry so decreasing its ability to bond. However, from a cross-contamination perspective, the dental nurse should not dip the brush back into the adhesive if it has been applied to a tray which has been tried into a patient's mouth. Decanting some adhesive into a dappen dish and using a cotton bud will circumvent this consideration.
- The tray adhesive should not be applied in a thick layer as it is unlikely to set prior to impression placement. Multiple thin coats may be used but each should be dry before the next is applied.
- The tray adhesive should be dry before the unset impression material is placed into it. To facilitate this, it is wise to select the impression tray at the start of the appointment. The tray adhesive may then be coated onto the tray. While the preparation is being done, the tray adhesive will dry.

Types of tray adhesive

Most tray adhesives are specific to each generic group of impression materials (Table 15.1). It is important that the correct type of tray adhesive should be used with its corresponding impression material. All adhesives contain a solvent, which evaporates leaving a film of adhesive which will then bond to the impression material.

Table 15.1 Chemical constituents of tray adhesives with their corresponding impression materials

Adhesive	Impression material
Butyl rubber or styrene acrylonitrile dissolved in chloroform or a ketone	Polysulphide
Ethyl acetate in propanol or acetone	Polyether
Poly dimethyl silicone to react with the impression material and ethyl silicate to bond physically to the tray. Ethyl acetate and naphtha are frequently included	Addition silicone
Poly dimethyl silicone to react with the impression material and ethyl silicate to bond physically to the tray	Condensation silicone
10–12% toluene in 45–50% isopropanol (isopropyl alcohol acts as a volatile solvent)	Alginate

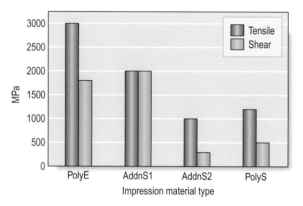

Fig. 15.11 Bond strength between tray/adhesive and impression material: the best adhesive is that supplied with the polyether rubbers.

While the adhesives are adequate in holding the impression materials firmly in the tray the bond between the tray and the impression material varies with the material used. Figure 15.11 shows the bond strengths between the tray and impression material for the four common elastomeric impression materials. The strongest bond is achieved with the polyether adhesive.

The correct type of tray adhesive should be used with its corresponding impression material. They are not interchangeable.

TYPES OF IMPRESSION MATERIAL

There are a number of types of impression material. They may be broadly divided into **non-rigid** and **rigid**. The former group consists of the **reversible** and **irreversible hydrocolloids** and the **elastomeric** materials (which are synthetic rubbers). The rigid impression materials include **impression plaster**, **impression compound (compo)** and zinc oxide and eugenol-based **impression paste**. These are generally restricted in use to record those areas where no undercuts are present, and mainly in the construction of removable dentures.

NON-RIGID IMPRESSION MATERIALS

Hydrocolloids

A hydrocolloid is a colloid in which the continuous phase is water. A **colloid** is a substance which is distributed evenly through another material. A colloid is generally made up of two phases: the **dispersed phase**, which is distributed in the other phase, the **continuous phase**. The two phases are not readily detectable even under microscopic examination. The dispersed phase has particles below 300 nm in size. A colloid exists as either a viscous liquid (**sol**) or as a solid (**gel**). The hydrocolloid impression materials may either be **reversible** or **irreversible**.

Table 15.2 Chemical constituents of agar impression materials

Constituent	Purpose	Per cent of composition
Agar*	Disperse phase of the colloid	13–17
Potassium sulphate	To counter adverse effect of borax on setting reaction of model plaster	1.0–2.2
Borax or borates	To strengthen the gel	0.2–0.6
Alkyl benzoate	To prevent mould growth in impression during storage	0.1–0.2
Wax	Filler	0.5–1.0
Thixotropic materials	Viscosity regulators and thickeners	0.2–0.4
Colours and flavouring	To enhance the taste and appearance of the material	<0.1
Water*	Provides the continuous phase of the colloid. The amount present determines the flow properties of the sol and the physical properties of the gel phases	79–85

*Active ingredient.

Reversible hydrocolloid

Reversible hydrocolloids are based on **agar**. As well as being used as a dental impression material, agar is used as a base for jellies and microbiological cultures. It is non-toxic and non-irritant.

Chemical constituents

Agar is a mixture of **polysaccharides**, **agarose** and **agaropectin**, which are subunits of the sugar **galactose**. These components are extracted from certain types of seaweed, specifically some red algae. The material used as a dental impression material also has other chemicals added to improve the properties and handling of the material. A generic formulation for these materials is set out in Table 15.2.

The gel alone is insufficiently strong to make the material viable as a dental impression material. Borax is therefore added to strengthen the gel. Unfortunately, borax retards the set of the model material (which contains gypsum) and this has an adverse effect when the positive cast is poured from the impression. Potassium sulphate is therefore added in an attempt to compensate for this, and while it reduces the problem it is not eliminated.

Setting

The change in the state of the dental hydrocolloid is determined by the temperature of the material. The gel may be converted to its sol state by heating to between 70 and 95°C. This is known as the **liquefaction temperature**. This is of course far too high a temperature for a material to be placed in the mouth of the patient. Fortunately, the **phase transformation** back to the gel stage occurs at a much lower temperature of between 35 and 50°C, which is just above mouth temperature. This allows the clinician to take the gel and heat it sufficiently to permit it to be placed in the sol state in an impression tray. The assembly is then tempered, allowing the temperature to be lowered until the patient can tolerate the material being seated in the mouth in a fluid state. At that point, the impression tray may be cooled to lower the temperature of the sol, which then solidifies.

The process requires a number of pieces of hardware, namely a hydrocolloid bath and metal trays incorporating water cooling coils (Figure 15.12). There must also be facilities to pour the models as soon as possible after the impression has been taken. This is because the dimensional stability of the agar is determined by the relative humidity and temperature at the point of pouring the plaster cast.

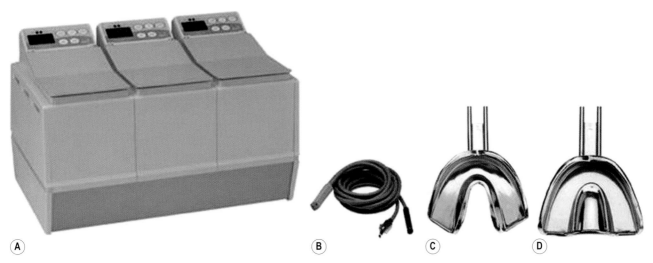

Fig. 15.12A–D (A) Hydrocolloid water bath, (B) tubing for water cooling and (C, D) upper and lower water cooled trays for specific use with agar-based impression material.

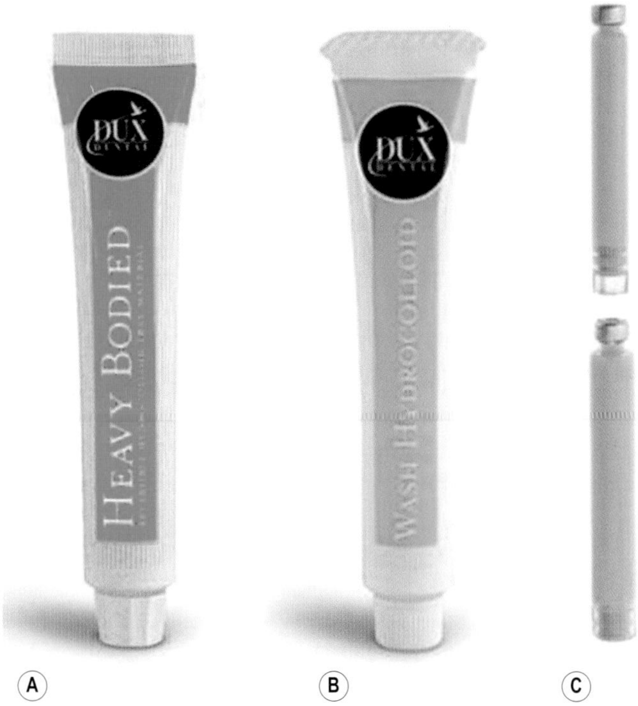

Fig. 15.13A–C Dispensing tubes and syringe cartridges for a reversible hydrocolloid system (CartriLoid, Dux Dental).

The agar impression material is presented in tubes or cartridges for use in a syringe (Figure 15.13).

The water bath consists of three separate chambers. The first is used to heat the agar and is usually set at a temperature near boiling point. Each cartridge or tube is totally immersed in this bath for a minimum of 8 minutes to liquefy the hydrocolloid. The second chamber is a tempering bath, which is used to cool the material to an acceptable temperature. This is generally set at between 43 and 46°C. It is from this chamber that the material is dispensed either into a tray or the cartridges loaded into a syringe. The third bath is primarily a storage bath which is maintained at between 63 and 66°C. A number of cartridges and tubes may be maintained at this temperature in the sol state for several days so that they may be available for immediate use. The complex nature of the preparation means that this type of impression material is more appropriate to the clinician specializing in extensive advanced restorative dentistry.

Material in tubes or cartridges which have not been used may be allowed to cool down. The content will return to the gel state. They may be reused by replacing in the boiling bath, however, they will require a rather longer time to change to the sol state; also, this reheating process may only be repeated up to four times before the material is discarded, because it becomes increasingly harder to break down the agar structure after reheating several times. The material can be sterilized.

Making the impression

The cartridge of material is removed from the tempering bath, placed in a syringe and injected around the preparation(s), ensuring that the nozzle of the syringe remains within the mass of material being injected. The preparation(s) and the immediate surroundings are covered. While this is being carried out, the dental nurse takes one of the tubes from the tempering bath and fills the selected tray with the material. The adhesion of the agar to the tray is poor, so a perforated

tray should be selected. The dental nurse also connects the cooling hose to the tray. The tray is then seated over the syringe material covering the whole of the dental arch. Once the tray has been seated, one end of the cooling system is connected to a cold water supply, and the other is placed to permit the cooling water to drain away to waste. The tray is held steady in the mouth until the mass of hydrocolloid has cooled to below the sol/gel transition temperature. Care is needed at this stage, as the material closest to the tray will cool fastest, with the material at the tooth surface setting last.

> !
>
> - The setting of the material will be slow unless the tray is cooled efficiently
> - The tray should be removed with a snap rather than easing the impression out of the mouth. This is less likely to produce distortion to the structure of the gel.

The reversible hydrocolloid system is probably the only true hydrophilic impression material. It is also the only impression material where the teeth may be left wet intentionally and is probably the most accurate. It is therefore mainly used when accuracy is very important, such as for fixed indirect restorations (crowns and bridges) and it is also used in dental laboratories to duplicate models. However, it must be handled with care to achieve successful results. The viscosity of the material should be such that it is sufficiently thick that it will be retained in the tray but not so viscous that the material will not flow around the teeth as the tray is seated. The impression must be thoroughly washed and all blood and saliva removed before pouring the cast.

Properties

Dimensional stability

After removal from the mouth there is very little distortion, unless the material is in very thin sections. A generous thickness of material is therefore required to limit the deformation which may arise on removal, especially from an undercut. When the impression has been removed from the mouth, the impression should be kept at 100% relative humidity. Failure to do this will lead to changes in dimension as water may be lost. The amount of water which is lost varies with the material type. Furthermore, if the impression is left for a period of time before a cast is made from it, the gel contracts and beads of moisture appear on the surface (syneresis).

> **Syneresis:** the process in which a gel contracts on standing and exudes liquid. An everyday example of this is the separation of whey in the production of cheese.

Similarly if the impression is allowed to dry out and is then immersed in water, it imbibes water but it will not necessarily return to its normal dimensions. This is called **imbibition**. In fact, the impression may take up excess water and swell up, with this swelling being uncontrolled in direction and extent.

> **Relative humidity:** the amount of water vapour in a gaseous mixture of air and water vapour.

Tear resistance

Agar impression material has a relatively low tear resistance and it is only possible to pour one model from each impression.

Practical issues

Agar has its aficionados, who enthuse about the results obtained. However, unless a large amount of advanced restorative work is contemplated, the complexities of heating and storage of the material, together with the need for the tray to be cooled means that the general dentist may find other elastomeric impression materials more convenient to use. The system has significant start-up costs as the hardware needs to be purchased, reflecting the very few agar products available on the market. An example of one such product is CartriLoid (Dux Dental).

Irreversible hydrocolloid

Probably the most commonly used dental impression material is the **irreversible hydrocolloid** called **alginate**. Alginate impression materials change from the sol to the gel state by a chemical reaction, which cannot be reversed unlike the agar-based materials. Alginate impression materials are presented as a powder, to which a measured amount of water is added. This is mixed to a paste and loaded in an impression tray. The paste (the sol phase) then sets, with the sol phase converting to the gel phase. The impression may then be removed.

Chemical constituents

The active ingredients are sodium and potassium salts of **alginic acid**. Alginic acid was first derived from the mucus that exudes from brown seaweed (Figure 15.14). It is now manufactured from synthetic components. A typical alginate powder formulation is shown in Table 15.3.

Table 15.3 Typical chemical constituents of an alginate impression material

Constituents	Weight percentage (%)	Function
Potassium alginate* Sodium alginate*	18	Dissolves in water to form a hydrogel with calcium
Calcium sulphate dihydrate*	14	Reacts with soluble alginate to form insoluble calcium alginate
Potassium sulphate, silicate or borate	7–10	Reduces inhibition of setting of plaster in poured model
Sodium phosphate	2	Acts as a retarder by preferentially reacting with calcium ions. This provides the working time. The material sets once the phosphate ions have been used up
Filler (diatomaceous earth or silicate powder)	56	Filler controlling consistency and flexibility of the set material
Sodium silicofluoride	0–3	Controls the pH of the material. Usually included at the expense of the potassium sulphate fraction
Organic glycols	Small traces	Reduces dustiness of the powder
Oil of Wintergreen, peppermint and pigments	Small traces	Provides pleasant taste and colour

*Active ingredient.

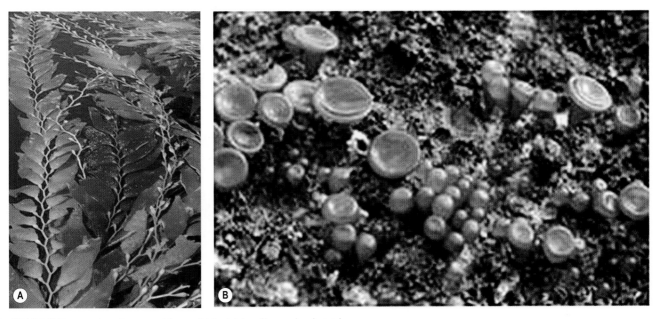

Fig. 15.14A,B Two species of seaweed from which alginic salts may be derived.
(Photos courtesy of Michael D. Guiry, The Seaweed Site) http://www.seaweed.ie/ Seaweed Site from Michael Guiry.

Diatomaceous earth: a soft, siliceous sedimentary rock (Figure 15.15) that crumbles into a fine white to off-white powder. It has a typical particle size between 10 and 200 μm. It is very light as it is highly porous.

Setting reaction

The setting reaction of alginates is a simple **double decomposition reaction**. As well as the alginate salt, the powder also contains hydrated calcium sulphate. On addition of the water, the alginate salt is converted to insoluble calcium alginate and potassium/sodium sulphate. The chemical reaction can be summarized as:

Potassium alginate + calcium sulphate dihydrate
+ water fi calcium alginate + potassium sulphate

Since the reaction starts immediately once the water is added to the powder, sodium phosphate is added to slow the reaction. It can do this as the calcium ions in solution preferentially react with the phosphate ions, forming (insoluble) calcium phosphate. It is only when all the phosphate ions have been used up that the calcium alginate formation will commence. The amount of sodium phosphate will determine the working time of the commercial material. There is a quite marked change in pH during this setting reaction (11 to 7). Some manufacturers include pH sensitive indictors so that the material changes colour during the setting reaction. This can assist in determining that the material has set completely.

As with the reversible hydrocolloids, the set material will retard the set of gypsum-based die material poured into the impression. To overcome this, additional potassium sulphate, silicate or borate salts are added.

Properties

Mixing time

Normally, the mixing time for alginates is between 45 and 60 seconds. Under-spatulation and shortened mixing times will lead to a paste where not all the powder particles have been wetted and consistency will be affected.

Working time

The working time for these materials may be regulated by the amount of sodium phosphate incorporated in the powder – the smaller the amount, the shorter the working time. Manufacturers generally produce material with working times between 45 seconds (fast set) and 1 minute and 15 seconds (regular set).

Setting time

This is manifested by the impression material surface losing it tackiness and showing rebound if indented. The setting times range between 1 and 4.5 minutes, depending on manufacturer and material indication. The very fast setting material can set too quickly. The manufacturer can influence this by increasing the amount of (tri) sodium phosphate added to the powder.

Setting time can also be varied by altering the temperature of the water. Lowering the temperature will slow the set, while increasing the water temperature will shorten the setting time. It is inadvisable to take this to extremes, but is useful clinically for those patients who find impression taking unpleasant or are prone to retching. Using tepid water will increase the setting time and therefore the time the impression is required to remain in the mouth.

✓

It is advisable to retain the impression in the mouth for 2–3 minutes after the initial gel formation has occurred when the material loses its tackiness, as the material increases in elasticity during this period. A longer retention period has adverse effects on the impression and the material may tear. This highlights the importance of following the manufacturer's instructions as they will have determined the optimum conditions for a satisfactory result.

Permanent deformation

Any impression will be compressed in certain areas during the removal from the mouth as it is removed from undercuts. Once removed, the impression should ideally return to its original shape with no distortion. However, most impression materials do not recover completely. A standard requirement for an alginate impression material is that if it is compressed by 20% for 5 seconds, the percentage recovery from this deformation should be in excess of 95%. This means that it could have a **permanent deformation** of 5%. Most commercial alginate impression materials have a recovery from deformation of about 98.5%. Permanent deformation of the impression material will only occur in areas where it was stressed. This, in

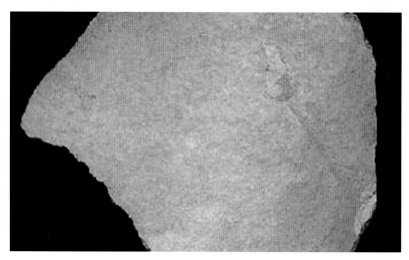

Fig. 15.15 Diatomaceous earth in its original form of soft siliceous sedimentary rock before being ground. *(Photo courtesy of Mineraly a horniny Slovenska) http://www.mineraly.sk/*

turn, means that some parts of the cast produced from the impression will be more accurate representations of the mouth than other parts. Permanent deformation may be minimized by:

- *Reducing the amount of compression*: Increasing the bulk of impression material between the tray and the teeth will reduce the bulk deformation as there will be more material available to be compressed.
- *Reducing the time the impression is under compression*: This may be done by snap removal from the mouth rather than easing the impression out.
- *Allowing longer time for recovery by not pouring the model immediately*: However, to avoid inaccuracies caused by syneresis and imbibition, the model should be made ideally within a hour of the impression being taken.

Strength

The strength of the gel phase of the impression must be optimized to ensure that it will not tear too readily on removal. The clinician has control over many means of altering the gel strength during mixing and manipulation, including:

- *Variation in water volume*: Any reduction in the powder/liquid ratio will weaken the gel.
- *Insufficient spatulation*: This will result in the ingredients not being dissolved sufficiently, leading to the chemical reaction being inconsistent.
- *Over-spatulation*: This leads to disruption of the forming calcium alginate gel and reduces the strength.

The tear strength of alginate is poor and worse than agar.

Advantages and disadvantages

The advantages and disadvantages of alginate impression materials are shown in Table 15.4.

Table 15.4 Advantages and disadvantages of alginate impression materials

Advantages	Disadvantages
Easy flow	Poor dimensional stability
Reproduction of detail adequate	Poor tear strength
Fast set	Distorts if unsupported
Minimal tissue displacement	3 mm minimum thickness required – otherwise distortion occurs where thin sections are found, such as interproximally
Cheap	
Patient tolerance good	Easy to include air

- Too much or too little water weakens the alginate gel.
- Insufficient spatulation results in an uneven set as all the powder does not dissolve.
- Over-spatulation breaks up and weakens the gel.
- Sufficient bulk of material is required for success (minimum of 3 mm).
- Strength of the gel increases with time (doubles in the first 4 minutes) making the material stiffer to remove.
- Retention to tray is poor so use perforated or rim-lock trays ± adhesive.

Indications and contraindications

Alginate is commonly used to make impressions where the reproduction of detail and level of accuracy is not of the highest requirement. This means they are frequently used for:

- Study casts
- Teeth opposing an indirect cast restoration preparation
- Removable orthodontic appliances
- Denture construction, especially partial dentures
- And other dental devices, such as occlusal splints.

Alginate is sufficiently fluid to record detail but it is unsuitable for recording fine detail such as that required for a fixed indirect cast restoration.

Mixing

Manufacturers usually provide dispensing measures for both the water and powder. These are most commonly a measuring cylinder and scoop, respectively (Figure 15.16) and will ensure that the

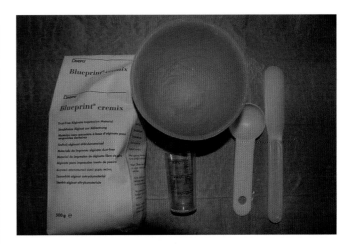

Fig. 15.16 Equipment required to mix an alginate impression material. Note the flexible bowl and straight alginate spatula. A measuring cylinder is used to accurately dispense the water and the scoop is used for the same purpose for the powder. The alginate impression material is Blueprint cremix (Dentsply).

Box 15.2 The correct mixing procedure for an alginate impression material, using Blueprint cremix (Dentsply)

Step 1	Step 2	Step 3	Step 4	Step 5	Step 6
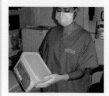	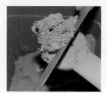		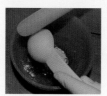		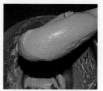

The powder container and its contents should be shaken prior to dispensing the material to fluff the powder and to ensure that the components are well mixed. During storage settlement occurs and the denser constituents will migrate to the bottom of the container and also more powder will be gathered in the scoop, which will affect the powder/liquid ratio

The powder is carefully measured by picking up an excess of the powder in the scoop and then levelling it by using the side of the alginate spatula as shown

The premeasured water is dispensed into the bowl. The water temperature should be between 18 and 24°C

The appropriate amount of the powder is then sprinkled onto the surface of the water and rapidly incorporated to form a paste

Care must be taken to ensure that the surface of all the powder particles are wetted adequately, using a spatula. The paste should be mixed with a figure-of-eight action, compressing the paste against the side of the bowl to eliminate airblows

The material is fully mixed when a creamy paste is produced, which does not drip off the spatula when this is lifted from the bowl. The material can then be loaded into the impression tray

correct volume of water and powder is used. Box 15.2 demonstrates the correct mixing procedure for an alginate impression material by hand. An alterative method involves using a bespoke alginate mixing machine. However, the powder and water should still be handled as directed in steps 1 to 4 in Box 15.2.

- It is important to exercise care when opening the container as the particulate material creates dust, which if inhaled potentially has adverse side effects. This is because a proportion of the particles are of a similar dimension to asbestos fibres, which may lead to pulmonary fibrogenesis.
- The container containing the alginate powder should have a hermetic seal and should not be left open to the atmosphere for any length of time. Water vapour in the air will affect the powder and therefore the properties of the set material.
- It is unwise to vary the stated proportions between the water and the powder as a small variation can adversely affect the properties. A change of only 15% in proportion of powder to water will markedly change both the setting time and the consistency, although some clinicians prefer a slightly runnier mix when making an impression for construction of a denture.

Once the alginate has been mixed, it is loaded into the impression tray. This should be done without delay as the material will be entering its setting phase. A smooth surface should be achieved, which results in better surface reproduction in the impression (Figure 15.17). Some clinicians like to smear some of the alginate over the surfaces of the

teeth using their finger to ensure that the material is properly adapted to the tooth surfaces. In patients with a high palatal vault, the dentist may also place a blob of material in this region prior to the insertion of the tray to ensure that it is recorded properly.

If the surface of an alginate impression is smoothed and wetted under the tap, the material will flow better, with improved reproduction of detail. However, excess water will affect the powder/liquid ratio so weakening the material, which will become apparent when the cast is poured.

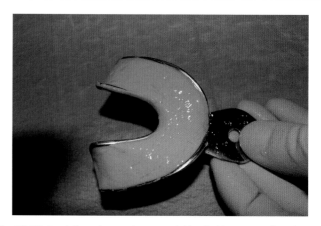

Fig. 15.17 An alginate impression material loaded into a metal stock tray and ready for presentation to the dentist for insertion into the mouth. Note the smooth surface of the impression material, which will result in better surface reproduction in the impression.

When an alginate impression is placed into the mouth, the lip should be everted to displace any trapped air, which would prevent the material from flowing fully into sulcus. The clinician should be careful that they do not pull the impression tray towards their dominant side. This will result in overextension of the impression on the dominant side and an underextended impression on the other side. That is, a right-handed clinician would make an impression which would be underextended on the left and overextended on the right.

It is important to ensure that the patient leaves the surgery without traces of impression material on their face. Alginate is best removed by gently rubbing with a damp tissue.

Disinfection

Disinfection of all impression materials is an essential part of prevention of cross-contamination (Box 15.3). Each impression should be subjected to a disinfection regime before it leaves the surgery. Many dental laboratories will also disinfect all impressions on arrival at the laboratory.

A number of commercial disinfectants are available specifically for this purpose. They have all been tested for compatibility with impression materials and it has also been shown that there are no adverse effects on the dimensionally stability or accuracy of the impression material, provided that the solutions are used according to the manufacturer's instructions. These generally contain disinfectants based on quaternary ammonium compounds.

Alternatively, solutions of sodium hypochlorite may be made up freshly for each impression. It is essential that the material is fresh as the disinfectant effect wears off quickly since the chlorine is used up or lost to the atmosphere. The appropriate concentration of a sodium hypochlorite solution is generally stated to be 1%. This is effective against the majority of bacteria and does not adversely affect the impression materials. It is recommended to label any impression before dispatching to the laboratory to state that the impression has been disinfected and what regime has been adopted. That is, care must be taken to liaise with the laboratory, as use of an over-strength disinfectant may affect the materials used to form the casts made from the impression materials, leading to with roughened and powdery surfaces to the models (Table 15.5).

Box 15.3 Suggested protocol for the treatment of all impressions

1. Immediately after removal from the mouth, the impression should be thoroughly rinsed in cold running tap water.
2. The impression tray (including the handle) and material should be immersed in a bath of a suitable water-based disinfecting solution prepared according to the manufacturer's instructions for the recommended period of time.
3. The impression should then be rinsed gently with tap water. The dental nurse should not forget the impression in the bath otherwise unwanted dimensional change may occur.
4. The impression should then be wrapped in moist tissue/napkin and placed in a polythene bag and sent to the dental laboratory for casting.

Table 15.5 Common failures of alginate impressions

Grainy material	Inadequate or prolonged mixing
	Liquid/powder ratio too low
Tearing	Inadequate bulk
	Premature removal from mouth
External bubbles	Air incorporation during mix
Rough or chalky model	Inadequate cleaning of impression
	Excess water left in impression
	Premature removal of model
Distortion	Delayed pouring of impression
	Movement of tray during impression taking
	Premature removal from mouth of model

Storage and care of alginate impressions

Alginate impressions need to be carefully handled after removal from the mouth otherwise they may be damaged or distorted. If for any reason they must be rested on the bench, they should be placed with the heels of the impression over the sink or edge of the bench (Figure 15.18) and only for the minimum amount of time. This is to prevent distortion of the unsupported alginate, and is particularly pertinent to lower impressions.

The impression should then be wrapped in moist paper towel to prevent syneresis or imbibition. It is important that the correct level of moisture is achieved as too dry or too wet a tissue will affect the relative humidity. As a guide, a paper towel should be wet under a running tap and then wrung out. This damp towel may be wrapped around the impression, which should then be placed in a polythene bag and sealed. A sticker should then be applied to the bag

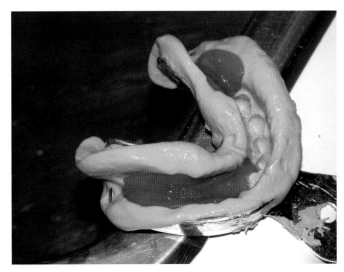

Fig. 15.18 An alginate impression being rested with the heals of the impression hanging freely over the edge of the sink to prevent distortion of the unsupported impression material in this area.

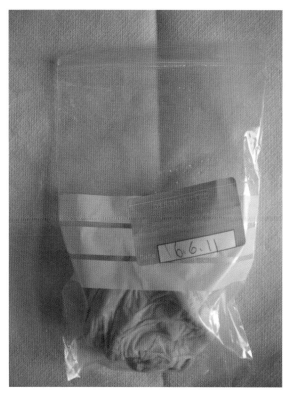

Fig. 15.19 An alginate impression wrapped in a moist paper towel and placed in a sealed polythene bag with a sticker on it, confirming that it has been subject to the appropriate disinfection regimen.

confirming that the appropriate disinfection protocols have been carried out on the impression (Figure 15.19).

Once the impression has been cast, it is advisable to remove the impression shortly after the gypsum has set as the longer the alginate is left, the more difficult it will be to remove as it will dry out.

For the best results with alginate:
- Shake container to ensure that ingredients are properly mixed
- Dispense by metered volumes
- Do not dispense powder free hand
- If possible use a special tray, which should be spaced by 3 mm
- Add powder to water
- Use the correct bowl and spatula
- Mix with figure-of-eight motion
- Swipe the material against the sides of bowl to limit air incorporation
- Hold still in the mouth
- Displace quickly from mouth.

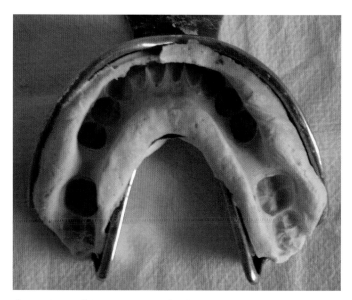

Fig. 15.20 An alginate impression that has dried out. It is now brittle, friable and useless.

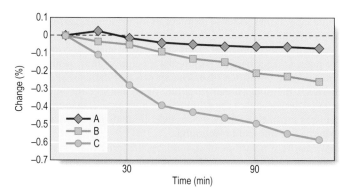

Fig. 15.21 Dimensional change with respect to time of three alginate impression materials.

Long-term accuracy of alginate impression materials

The nature of the setting reaction means that after the material has set there is a risk that any change in water content will influence the dimensional accuracy of the impression by syneresis. The most obvious effect is if the impression is left out in the air for any period of time. There is loss of water and the impression shrinks and if it is allowed to dry out it becomes brittle and friable (Figure 15.20). It follows the behaviour of the material on which it is based, seaweed.

The less obvious effect but one which is equally unsatisfactory is the effect of water uptake, which leads to the gel structure swelling and producing a model that is smaller than the original (imbibition). Alginate impression materials should be poured as soon as is practical after removal from the mouth (after they have been allowed to undergo elastic recovery) (Figure 15.21).

Table 15.6 Some alginate products currently available on the market

Product	Manufacturer	Comments
Alginoplast	Heraeus	Dust-free, regular and fast set
Aroma Fine DF III	GC	Dust-free, enhanced powder wetting
Blueprint Cremix	Dentsply	Lead-free, good powder wettability
CA37	Cavex	Regular and fast set
Cromatic	Vannini	Changes colour as it is mixed and sets
Hydrogum	Zhermack	Dust-free
Hydrogum 5	Zhermack	High stability, short working and setting time
Image	Dux Dental	Dust-free
Impressional Fast Set	Cavex	High definition, dust-free, stiffer
Kromalgin Plus	Vannini	Changes colour as it is mixed and sets
Kromopan – Colour Change	Lascod	Changes colour as it is mixed and sets
Neocolloid	Zhermack	High detail, injectable, ideal for chrome work
Orthoprint	Zhermack	Rapid set for orthodontic work
Palgat Plus	3M ESPE	Fast and slow set, dust-free
Plastalgin	Septodont	Regular set, dust-free
Plastalgin Ortho	Septodont	Fast set, dust-free
Take 1 Alginate	Kerr Hawe	Fast set, colour change
Tropicalgin	Zhermack	Changes colour during the setting process, tropical flavours
Xantalgin Crono	Heraeus	Colour change indicating the stages
Xantalgin Select	Heraeus	Normal set, dust-free

Commercially available products

Table 15.6 lists some of the commercially available alginate impression materials.

Non-aqueous elastomeric impression materials (elastomers)

Alginate materials are not sufficiently accurate to be used for the construction of cast restorations such as crowns and bridges. Agar may be used, although as discussed previously it is not commonly used. Other impression materials need to be used when fine detail and accuracy are required. These are all based on polymeric materials which set by chain lengthening and cross-linking, and are often referred to as **elastomers**. There are three major types of elastomer:

- Polysulphides
- Polyethers
- **Silicones**. These are more accurately described as **vinyl polysiloxanes (VPS)**. They may be divided into three subgroups:
  - Condensation silicones
  - Addition silicones
  - Vinyl polyether silicone (VPES).

Polysulphides

The polysulphide impression materials have been around for a long period of time. They are presented as a paste/paste system to be mixed by the dental nurse, but they have fallen out of favour as they are not very pleasant from the patient's perspective. The material has a distinctive (unpleasant) smell and taste and it takes a long time to set. Some dentists still use and get good results from this type of material.

Table 15.7 Chemical constituents of the polysulphide impression materials

Ingredient	Per cent composition	Function
Base paste		
Polysulphide polymer (thiokol rubber)*	80–85	Polymer, which on initiation will cross-link so setting the impression
Titanium dioxide, silica, copper carbonate†	16–18	Filler (increases with viscosity of paste); particle size is in the range of 2–5 μm
Accelerator paste		
Lead dioxide*	60–66	Oxidizing agent that acts as a cross-linking agent
Dibutyl phthalate†	30–35	Plasticizing agent
Sulphur*	1–1.5	Enhances the reaction
Oleic or stearic acid	1–2	Retarder

*Active ingredient.
†These two components may be found in both pastes, providing materials that are manipulable as well as strong enough for the application.

Chemical constituents

See Table 15.7. The impression material has a distinct dark brown colour due to the presence of lead dioxide. Titanium dioxide (a very

251

strong white colouring agent) is added to the material in an attempt to mask the brown colour but it is only partially successful.

- Polysulphide impression materials have a distinctive and quite unpleasant taste and smell. This is associated with the sulphur content.
- The lead catalyst is a brown colour and is very difficult to remove if inadvertently dropped onto clothes. It leaves a clearly defined brown mark even after washing.

Setting reaction

The setting reaction is a **condensation polymerization** reaction. The accelerator causes oxidation, which increases the length of the polymer chains. This produces a slightly exothermic reaction with a temperature rise of about 3–4°C. Later in the reaction cross-linking occurs between the polymer chains, making the material stiffer and more resistant to permanent deformation. A small amount of water is produced as a by-product of the reaction.

Properties

Polysulphide impression materials are susceptible to environmental changes, namely temperature and humidity. It is also important that the dentist gains excellent moisture control of the preparation as the material is incompatible with moisture. The impression material will contract slightly due to the loss of water in the condensation polymerization reaction. This means that the resulting model will be slightly larger, therefore creating space for the luting cement. Working models should be poured as soon as possible.

Polysulphides should be used in a special tray. No putty version is available as it is difficult to keep it stable in putty form. The material is dimensionally stable and its tear strength is good. Some dentists like to use polysulphide impression materials as the material can be added to for retaking the impression, although this is a risky technique as inaccuracies may be introduced. Polysulphide materials are notoriously difficult to mix, and unmixed catalyst may be left in the material.

Commercially available products

Polysulphide impression materials have all but disappeared from the market, which reflects the fact that they are rarely used in contemporary dentistry. One example of a commercially available product is Permlastic (Kerr Hawe).

Polyethers

The polyether impression materials are very popular among general dental practitioners. The material is the most hydrophilic elastomeric impression material, and this property makes it more likely to capture a preparation margin even when moisture control is not perfect. It is presented as a paste/paste system, one being the base and the other the accelerator, and it is used with a **monophase** impression technique. This means that both the material syringed around the preparation and the tray material is the same. The polyethers are non-toxic and non-irritant.

Chemical constituents

It is not possible to give the exact composition but it normally contains the ingredients shown in Table 15.8. Originally a third tube was presented, which contained a thinner (**octyl phthalate** and about 5% **methylcellulose**) to alter the viscosity of the mixed paste, and addition of these chemicals also addresses the stiffness problem of the polyethers by allowing 'soft' presentations.

Table 15.8 Chemical constituents of the polyether impression materials

Ingredient	Per cent composition	Function
Base paste		
Polyether polymer*	50–60	Polymer which on initiation will cross-link further
Colloidal silica/diatomaceous earth	5–10	Filler
Glycoether or phthalate	10	Plasticizer
Accelerator paste		
Alkyl aromatic sulphonate such as 2,5-diclorobenzene sulphonate*	–	Initiator of cationic ring opening polymerization
Colloidal silica/diatomaceous earth	–	Filler
Glycoether or phthalate	–	Plasticizer
*Active ingredient.		

Setting reaction

The setting is achieved by a cross-linking reaction between the **aziridine** at the end of each polyether molecule. This chain lengthening occurs at the same time as cross-linking between chains occurs by cationic polymerization of the imine groups on the polymer chain. Unlike other elastomeric materials, the base to accelerator paste ratio is not 1:1 but 4:1. There are no reaction by-products, so this material has good dimensional stability.

Properties

Stiffness and tear resistance

Polyether materials are notoriously very stiff. This may present some clinical problems especially difficulty removing the impression from the patient's mouth. Several reformulations have taken place to make the material less stiff on setting and to permit different presentations. One manufacturer produces a 'soft' polyether that is less stiff and so easier to remove. Even with this particular product, polyether materials should not be used in a special tray. Those clinicians who prefer using metal stock trays should take care when using polyether materials. It may be preferable to select a slightly larger tray so there is extra bulk of material to permit movement within the material, facilitating its removal, particularly if deep undercuts are present. The stiffness of the material may present problems with thin dies, as these may fracture when the impression is removed from the casts. This problem may be circumvented by constructing the dies out of another material such as epoxy resin (see Chapter 20).

- It is advisable to place soft (modelling) wax or caulk under bridge pontics to prevent the impression material getting under the bridge. Failure to do this may result in the bridge being inadvertently removed when the impression is removed from the mouth.
- The dentist should ensure that there is adequate spacing between tray and teeth and any undercuts should be blocked out otherwise the tray and contents may be difficult to remove after the impression has set.

Polyether impression materials should be stored at room temperature as cold temperatures increase the viscosity of the material. This may present problems in that the pistons of the mechanical impression mixing machines may be damaged. Tear resistance of the polyethers is good.

Dimensional stability

Polyether materials are dimensionally stable with only small amounts of polymerization contraction. This means that larger dies are gained so that restorations constructed on them will fit the preparation in the mouth. Its accuracy is good enough for indirect cast restorations such as crown and bridge work.

Models should not be poured immediately, but the impression should be left for at least 30 minutes after removal from the mouth to allow it to undergo stress relaxation.

Water sorption

Polyether impression materials absorb water and must be carefully handled. The preparation should be as dry as possible and after removal from the mouth its immersion in the disinfection bath must not exceed the recommended time. Thereafter the impression should be dried with a three-in-one syringe and stored in a sealed polythene bag, separate from any impressions that need to be kept moist, such as alginate. Soaking a polyether impression material in water will cause it to swell and therefore distort.

Some patients remark on the taste being on the unpleasant side!

Indications and contraindications

Polyether materials are indicated for indirect cast restorations such as crowns and bridges. They are favoured by many restorative dentists who are placing the superstructure on implants where the impression material is used to locate and pick up the implant analogues (Figure 15.22).

They may also be used for **functional impressions** (see later and Chapter 23). They are selected principally as they are more hydrophilic than the other elastomer impression materials and so record details more successfully should the moisture control not be perfect. It is worth considering an alternative impression material when confronted with very small thin preparations that may lead to the model being broken on removal.

Commercially available products

The currently available polyether materials are listed in Table 15.9.

Table 15.9 Some polyether products currently available on the market

Product	Manufacturer
Impregum	3M ESPE
P2 Magnum 360 Dynamix	Heraeus
Permadyne	3M ESPE

Silicones

Elastomeric impression materials are also very popular among restorative dentists. There are two types, **condensation** and **addition**, with the names reflecting their setting reaction. Unfortunately silicone-containing materials are inherently hydrophobic due to the silicone to oxygen bond being hydrophobic in nature. To illustrate this very effectively, silicones are used in situations when water needs to be eliminated, such as sealing sinks and bath units in bathrooms (Figure 15.23). There is

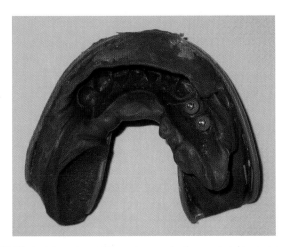

Fig. 15.22 A pick-up impression using a polyether material to construct, in this example, two implant-retained crowns. Note the presence of the implant analogues in the region of teeth 34 and 35.

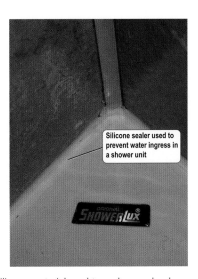

Fig. 15.23 A silicone material used to seal around a shower to contain water within the shower unit.

therefore no such thing as a hydrophilic silicone despite the claims in manufacturers' product promotional literature.

Condensation silicones

Condensation silicones are generally presented as a putty (or paste) and a light-bodied material. The putty is usually mixed using a low-viscosity paste accelerator, and this is kneaded into the mass of the putty.

Condensation silicone impression materials are usually presented as a paste or putty and a liquid/paste catalyst. This means that accurate proportioning of these materials is difficult to achieve, which may lead to variable results.

Chemical constituents

The common chemical constituents of condensation silicone impression materials are shown in Table 15.10.

Setting reaction

Once the two components are mixed together, a condensation reaction takes place forming a three-dimensional silicone matrix. However, this also results in the release of ethyl alcohol. As the alcohol is lost to the atmosphere, the material shrinks quite markedly due to the loss of this by-product. The reaction is slightly exothermic.

Properties

The nature and presentation of these materials means that accurate proportioning of the components is very important. A reduction in the alkyl silicate will reduce the cross-linking. This leads to a weaker material with lowered tear resistance that is more prone to increased permanent set. It is difficult to ensure that the catalyst liquid is incorporated evenly and that none is lost during the mixing phase. This often means that the material behaves erratically. The working and setting times are affected and ultimately the properties of the

material are degraded if the catalyst is lost. The cross-linking agent (alkyl silicate) is susceptible to hydrolysis. The setting of the material will be inhibited if it becomes contaminated with moisture.

The accelerator used with the condensation silicones tends to have a limited shelf-life, as stannous octoate contained therein may oxidize and the ortho-ethyl silicate is not completely stable in the presence of the tin ester.

The putty of a condensation silicone impression material shows minimal shrinkage as the bulk of the material is filler. Shrinkage is proportional to the amount of polysiloxane present, and the small amount present in a putty minimizes shrinkage.

Advantages and disadvantages

This is one of the impression materials which has wide patient acceptance, and for work where the dimensional stability is not critical, it can be the material of choice. It is desirable that the impression is transported to the laboratory and poured as soon as possible.

Indications and contraindications

Condensation silicones are accurate enough to be used to record the preparations that will be restored with indirect cast restorations. However, they are more commonly used in removable prosthodontics, such as for making working impressions for metal-based dentures and for relines. Laboratory putties are mainly condensation silicones.

Commercially available products

A selection of commercially available condensation silicone impression material are listed in Table 15.11.

Table 15.11 Some condensation silicone products currently available on the market

Product	Manufacturer
Coltex	Coltène Whaledent
Coltoflax	Coltène Whaledent
Lab Putty	Coltène Whaledent
Optosil	Heraeus
Oranwash	Zhermack
Protesil	Vannini
Rapid	Coltène Whaledent
Speedex	Coltène Whaledent
Thixoflex	Zhermack
Xantopren	Heraeus
Zetaplus	Zhermack

Addition silicone impression rubbers (vinyl polysiloxanes)

The other type of silicone impression material are the addition silicones. Since their arrival on the dental scene, they have become the most popular materials for use in advanced restorative dentistry. They differ from the condensation silicones in that the setting reaction is an addition reaction and so does not produce any by-product. This means that the material retains its dimensional stability and is more

Table 15.10 Chemical constituents of condensation silicone impression materials

Ingredient	Function
Base paste/putty	
Dimethyl siloxane*	Low-molecular-weight silicone which has reactive terminal hydroxyl end groups
Colloidal silica or micro-sized metal salts such as copper carbonate	Filler to make the paste or putty as the silicone polymer is liquid. Usually the filler particle size ranges between 5 and 10 μm.
Accelerator liquid/paste	
Stannous octoate*	Accelerator
Alkyl silicate*	Accelerator
Colloidal silica	Thickening agent

An exact breakdown of composition is not given as this varies with the consistency of the various putty/paste combinations. Filler loading can be between 35–75%.
*Active ingredient.

accurate. These materials are presented in a variety of forms: **putty** and **heavy-bodied**, **universal (medium) bodied**, **light-bodied** and **extra light-bodied** pastes. As well as impression materials, addition silicone bite registration materials are also available and are commonly used (see Chapter 16).

Chemical constituents

The common constituents of addition silicone impression materials and their functions are set out in Table 15.12. The composition of the two pastes is adjusted such that they have similar consistency to facilitate mixing. This is achieved by varying the amount of filler in each paste. It is not possible to give exact percentage ingredients as this will vary with the type of paste/putty being produced. The amount of filler added will also determine the category of material, i.e. heavy, universal or light-bodied.

Surfactants are added are to address the hydrophobicity of the polysiloxanes. These make the impression material 'wet' the surface of the preparation and the soft tissue better. They also aid in the pouring of the model as the wet stone has an affinity for the hydrophilic surface of the impression. Unfortunately, it takes time for these surfactants to come to the surface to work so their addition only partially addresses the problem and these impression materials remain hydrophobic. The dentist must therefore ensure that the area to be recorded is kept very dry, as any moisture contamination will result in a rolled edge of the preparation margins.

These materials are manufactured commercially by placing all the ingredients in a large vat. The vat is then coupled up to a large mixing machine, which thoroughly mixes and blends all the components to produce the putty (Figure 15.24). It works on the same principle as food mixers with large blades and hook mixers.

Setting reaction

The setting reaction is between the poly methyl hydrogen siloxane in one paste and the vinyl-terminated polysiloxanes in the other. During the addition polymerization, the hydrogen from the hydrogen siloxane backbone links with the vinyl group on the other siloxane chain forming a cross-linked polymer in which no by-product is produced.

Table 15.12 Chemical constituents of the addition silicone impression materials together with their function and approximate percentage

Ingredient	Function
Base paste/putty	
Poly methyl hydrogen siloxane*	Polymer
Siloxane prepolymers*	Cross-linking polymer
Quartz	Filler
Catalyst paste	
Divinyl polydimethyl siloxane*	Polymer
Chloroplatinic salt*	Catalyst
Quartz	Filler
Surfactants and retarders	Regulation of setting and aids to wetting of hydrophobic silicone

*Active ingredient.

! One clinically significant problem with these materials is that any sulphur-containing materials will inhibit the platinum catalyst should they come into contact with the material. Latex gloves often contain sulphur residues from the manufacturing process. If the catalyst is poisoned, a weakened material will result. This is particularly a problem with the putties where the two parts are kneaded together by hand. Latex-free gloves should therefore be used when this is being done.

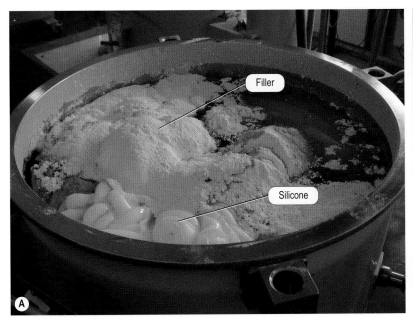

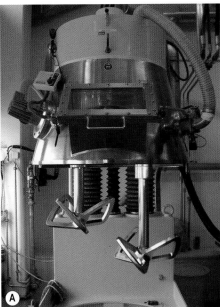

Fig. 15.24 (A) Vat of the contents of an addition silicone impression material prior to mixing. (B) The machine used to mix the material.

Some addition silicones release hydrogen gas as a by-product. This may become incorporated into the model and result in porosity in the die material (Figure 15.25). In an attempt to overcome this, these materials should be left for 30 minutes before pouring the cast in the case of a gypsum material and left overnight if epoxy is to be used to make the die. This is because epoxy takes longer to set than gypsum. Some products have a hydrogen absorber such as palladium to minimize the porosity.

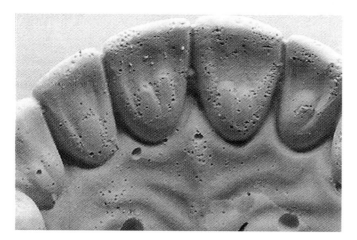

Fig. 15.25 Hydrogen gas released from an addition silicone impression material has caused porosity on the model surface as it has been poured too quickly.

Properties

As mentioned earlier, addition silicone materials are highly hydrophobic. Despite the addition of surfactants, which have a limited effect, moisture control must be excellent otherwise an inaccurate impression will result, often seen as a rolled edge seen in the impression.

Their dimensionally stability is very good. More than one model may be poured from the same impression usually without any problem. Their accuracy may be too good, as it may not be compensated for during the investment and casting process. This will result in a too small a die being produced. A small cast is therefore produced, which may not fit the preparation in the mouth. To circumvent this, extra layers of die spacer may be placed to produce a larger die, so the restoration will fit the prepared tooth.

The materials all show an increase in stiffness from the time that they are defined as being clinically set for a period of up to 2–3 hours. This is a result of further cross-linking after the clinical set has occurred. It has been suggested that the impression may be left in the mouth for a longer period than that recommended by the manufacturer as additional cross-linking will make the material stronger and more resistant to tearing although it is becoming stiffer during this time. This is a benefit as the addition silicones have a poor tear resistance.

The addition silicones may react chemically with the oxygen inhibition layer found on the surface of resin-based composite restorative materials and bonding agents. If a resin-based composite restoration has been recently placed or a core build-up has been done, a layer of separator should be applied to prevent the addition silicone impression material reacting with it.

Table 15.13 Advantages and disadvantages of addition silicone impression materials

Advantages	Disadvantages
Good detail reproduction	Hydrophobic
Excellent dimensional stability	Too accurate
High patient acceptance	Tear strength less good
	Expensive

Advantages and disadvantages

The advantages and disadvantages of addition silicone impression materials are shown in Table 15.13. These materials tend to be expensive due to the inclusion of the platinum-containing catalyst.

Indications and contraindications

Addition silicone impression materials are indicated for indirect cast restorations such as crowns and bridges. These materials offer greater dimension stability than other elastomeric materials, which may be useful if the dental laboratory is some distance from the dental surgery and therefore some time will elapse between making the impression and pouring the model.

There are now some materials based on this technology which may be substituted for alginates. These do not have the same level of accuracy as the conventional addition silicone materials but they are suitable for temporary restoration impressions, impressions for study casts and to record the opposing arch for an indirect cast restoration. They have a much more detailed surface and have long-term dimensional stability. Additionally, they can be used to pour multiple models. One such product is Position Penta (3M ESPE).

Commercially available products

Commercially available products are show in Table 15.14. One company has introduced an impression material coloured silver or gold (Affinis Precious, Coltène Whaledent). This is claimed to be easier to read as it reduces light scatter on the impression surface.

Vinyl polyether silicone

A new material on the market claims to offer all the benefits of both a polyether and an addition silicone, such as high elasticity and tear strength, being hydrophilic and with good flow properties. It is a combination of both silicone materials and has been termed **vinyl polyether silicone**. Two products have been launched: EXA'lence (GC) and Identium (Kettenbach), supplied by Optident in the UK. It reacts with latex gloves and retraction cord solutions and it should be not be used with any hardware that has been in contact and therefore contaminated with polyethers. It should not be stored in a warm place. As with any new material, it is the clinical performance over time which will determine the exact benefits of this combination material.

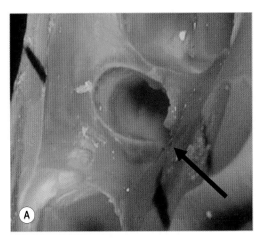
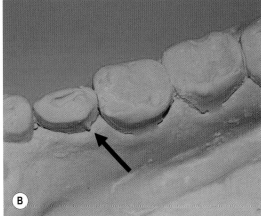

Fig. 15.26 (A) An impression showing defects as a result of inadequate flow of the impression material. (B) A similar defect reproduced on a stone model after an impression has been cast.

Table 15.14 Some addition silicone products currently available on the market

Product	Manufacturer	Comments
ACP	Codent	
Affinis	Coltène Whaledent	May be autoclaved at 134°C
Alginot	Kerr Hawe	
Aquasil Ultra	Dentsply	
Dimension	3M ESPE	
Elite HD+	Zhermack	
Exafast	GC	
Exaflex	GC	
Exajet	GC	
Examix NDS	GC	
Express 2	3M ESPE	
Extrude	Kerr Hawe	
Flexitime	Heraeus	
Fresh	Panadent	
Honigum	DMG	
Hydrorise	Zhermack	
Imprint II Garant	3M ESPE	
Perfexil	Septodont	
Position Penta	3M ESPE	Indications as alginate
President	Coltène Whaledent	
Provil novo	Heraeus	
Status Blue	DMG	
Take 1	Kerr Hawe	
Virtual	Ivoclar Vivadent	
Zerosil	Panadent	

Common properties of the elastomeric materials

Viscosity

Viscosity when mentioned in connection with impression materials refers to the rigidity of the material. These materials are available in a number of presentations from the most viscous to the least: putty, heavy-bodied, medium (or regular/universal-bodied), light-bodied and extra light-bodied. The thixotropy of the material (or as they say 'how it flows and stays where it has been placed without dripping') is also mentioned in promotional literature. This is better referred to as **structural viscosity**. Very few impression materials show true thixotropic properties as they do not thin as they are stressed. Some manufacturers now produce so-called 'soft' putties, which have a lower viscosity than the regular putties.

Frequently the manufacturer reports on the viscosity of the material measured at 45 seconds after the commencement of mixing. This is approximately the time at which the material is being injected into the mouth after mixing by hand but before substantial cross-linking has occurred. The viscosity of all the materials is affected by temperature. Once the material is in the oral cavity the viscosity will immediately start to increase. Here the polyether and both silicones show a very rapid increase with respect to time at 37°C. This must be taken into account with any extensive preparations as the syringing of the light-bodied material has to be quick and also the clinician must ensure that the material has flowed all over the preparation. Failure of the impression material to flow will cause irregularities in the impression (Figure 15.26). The materials are all available in differing viscosities (Table 15.15). These different presentations are designed to allow the restorative dentist a

Table 15.15 Available presentations of elastomeric impression materials

Material	Putty	Heavy bodied	Universal/ regular	Light bodied
Polysulphide	X	√	√	√
Polyether	X	X	√	X
Condensation silicone	√	X	X	√
Addition silicone	√	√	√	√

choice of impression materials depending on the impression technique indicated:

- *Putty and light-bodied wash in a stock tray*. The majority of dentists use the **putty and wash** technique. This technique utilizes two different viscosities of the same material. The light-bodied material is sufficiently fluid, in that it will reproduce the fine detail of the preparation and may be syringed around the preparation and other key areas where accuracy is required such as the occlusal surfaces of the other teeth in the arch. The putty provides support for the light-bodied material which on its own would distort under load during the pouring of the model. A stock tray is selected and filled with the dense putty. The area in the mouth to be replicated is coated with a thin layer of the light-bodied material to provide high detail and the putty and tray is seated over the top of this. The light (perfecting) material and putty bond together, making the impression which can be removed when both viscosities are fully set.
- *Heavy and light-bodied material in a stock or customized tray*. This is very similar to the putty and wash technique with the exception being that the putty has been substituted for a heavy-bodied material. There are many advantages for using a heavy-bodied presentation over a putty:
  - As the viscosity of a heavy body is lower than a putty when the impression is placed over the teeth there will be no displacement of the teeth, which may occur with a very viscous putty. Displacement of the teeth may result in an inaccurate impression. This is particularly the case with teeth that are periodontally compromised.
  - The higher viscosity of a putty may cause deformation of a non-rigid tray (see p. 239) and this will cause distortions in the impression, leading to inaccuracies in the working model.
  - A material of high viscosity will very often displace the light-bodied material from around the preparation, forcing it into the sulcus where accuracy is not required. The ability to capture surface detail of the putty is not as good as the light-bodied material and this is not desirable. A heavy-bodied material due to its lower viscosity is less likely to do this.
  - There may be some folding of the putty, leaving a defect like a seam in the impression.

The heavy- and light-bodied pastes are frequently presented as two different colours to facilitate viewing the final impression.

- *Universal or regular viscosity material in a customized tray*. In this technique, the universal viscosity material is injected around the preparation and also used to fill the tray. The loaded tray is then seated over the syringed material. The detail reproduction of the universal paste must be sufficient to provide an adequate representation of the preparation. This is called a monophase impression and a non-perforated tray should be selected when using this technique. This is commonly used with the polyethers as already described above.
- *Two-stage technique*. The preceding techniques are all **one-stage techniques** in that the impression is taken only once. In the **two-stage technique**, a preliminary impression is taken with putty alone in a stock tray. This is then removed from the mouth. After thorough washing the impression is dried, and vents are cut in the area of the site where detail is required. The impression is then reseated after the light-bodied material has been syringed around the preparation. The excess light-bodied material is extruded out of the vents. Some clinicians modify this technique by placing a sheet of polythene over the putty prior to insertion of the arch. The set putty then acts like a special tray. The sheet is then removed, the light-

bodied material syringed around the preparation and the tray containing the putty reseated. This technique requires considerable care in the reseating of the tray. It is also essential that neither material is contaminated with saliva or the two materials will not bond.

For details of other modifications to these techniques and other impression techniques, the reader is referred to an operative dentistry text for further information.

Working and setting times

All these materials have a clinically suitable working and setting time, however, some are substantially faster at setting than others. This may also be affected by the ambient temperature and humidity. If many preparations require to be recorded, the dentist may choose an impression material which has a longer working time. A short working time may mean that the material has started to set before all the preparations have been covered and so stresses and strains may be incorporated within the impression material, leading to distortions and inaccuracies. Table 15.16 shows a time-line illustrating the sequence from the start of mix to pouring of the working cast.

Figure 15.27 shows the variations in working and setting times at both ambient temperatures such as the surgery working area and in the mouth for representative examples of all four elastomers. It is readily apparent that the polysulphide rubber has a much longer working and setting time than the other three common materials, which show similar working and setting times. However, there is considerable variation between the same generic material from different manufacturers. Additionally different consistencies of the same material frequently show differing working and setting times.

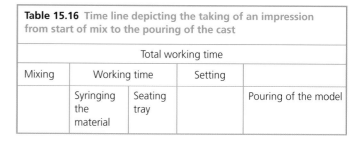

Table 15.16 Time line depicting the taking of an impression from start of mix to the pouring of the cast

Total working time			
Mixing	Working time	Setting	
	Syringing the material	Seating tray		Pouring of the model

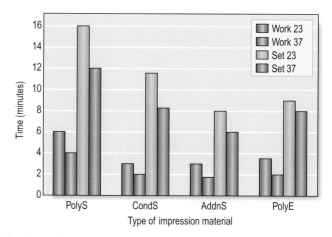

Fig. 15.27 The variations in working and setting times at ambient temperatures (Work23/Set23) and in the mouth (Work37/Set37) for representative examples of all four elastomeric impression types.

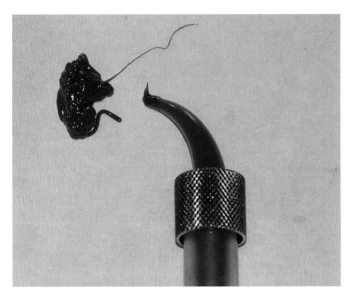

Fig. 15.28 The first bit of the mixed material, which is left on the bracket table as an indicator of final set of the impression material in the mouth.

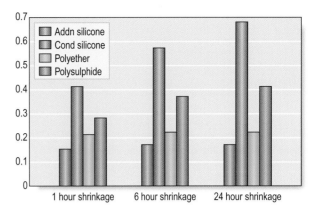

Fig. 15.29 Typical percentage shrinkage of four light-bodied elastomeric impression materials at 1, 6 and 24 hours after impression taking.

In selecting an impression material, it is essential to review the claimed working and setting times to ensure that these are appropriate for the dentist's clinical technique. The dentist must wait for the prescribed time to ensure that all of the impression material has fully set prior to removal of the impression material. This is best achieved by syringing the first mixed material onto the bracket table. This is left to set and will set at a slower rate than the material in the mouth as the temperature and humidity extraorally is lower than intraorally. Once this expressed material has set, the dentist can be confident that the impression material in the tray is also fully set (Figure 15.28).

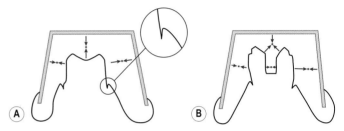

Fig. 15.30 Shrinkage of (A) a full crown impression versus (B) a more complex preparation.

Dimensional change on setting

The degree of shrinkage that occurs with these materials is primarily determined by their setting reaction. Should there be any by-product of the setting reaction then the material will shrink. The most significant shrinkage occurs with the condensation silicones where the production of ethanol continues with time. This means that the impression shrinks significantly, but this shrinkage is not linear with time, with greater shrinkage occurring early after taking the impression. The polysulphide elastomer shows the next greatest shrinkage. The polyether and addition silicones show minimal shrinkage the addition silicone being the most dimensionally stable. One drawback of polyether materials is that their dimensional stability can be disrupted if the impression is stored in water. The impression will absorb water and swell. Storage of these materials during transport to a laboratory is therefore critical and they should be kept dry. The relative amount of percentage shrinkage at 24 hours is shown in Figure 15.29. The effect of this shrinkage is not simple as the material is constrained in the impression tray.

Dimensional change also depends on filler loading, with the higher the loading the smaller the shrinkage. This is because as more filler is added, there is less rubber to shrink and in many cases the shrinkage of the putty is very low indeed as it is up to 75% filler.

The clinical consequences of shrinkage depend on the type of preparation to be recorded. The impression material is initially loaded into the tray. The tray will either have mechanical retention built into it (perforations, rims, or undercut areas) or is coated with an adhesive to retain the impression. This results in different shrinkage vectors. Normally, unconstrained rubber will contract toward the centre of the mass. Constraining one surface (for example against the tray surface) means that the contraction is almost entirely towards the tray surface and the model produced from the set impression will be fractionally larger than the preparation in the mouth. In the case of a full crown, this will not unduly affect the fit of the restoration. The only consequence will be an increased cement lute thickness. However, where there are internal retentive features the contraction patterns are different as isolated sections of the impression will not be constrained by the tray. Here the section of rubber will shrink toward the centre of the mass of that component. Where angled features of the preparation exist this usually leads to curling of the margins. This type of discrepancy is far harder to correct and invariably the prosthesis does not fit the tooth preparation (Figure 15.30).

Recovery from deformation

As with the alginate materials the elastomer impression materials will distort during their removal from the mouth. The concern is that this distortion will not be reversed once the impression is removed. The most forgiving elastomer is the addition silicone, which shows almost no permanent deformation (0.05–0.2%). The next best material is the polyether (1.5–2.0%) with the condensation silicone just behind (1.5–3%). The polysulphides are the most susceptible to permanent deformation (3–5%). However, all elastomers are viscoelastic and should be 'snapped out' of mouth as quickly as possible so that the impression is strained for the shortest time. It the impression is removed slowly, it will flow and strain will be introduced, from which it may not recover.

To remove an impression, use a finger to break the seal at the edge of the impression or blow air or water between the impression and the oral tissues.

Strain

This defines the flexibility of the material. The polysulphides are the most flexible, and the other three materials are less so but similar to each other. When these materials of similar consistency are compared, the condensation silicones are slightly more flexible than the addition silicones while polyether is the stiffest of the four common elastomers.

The clinical significance of the stiffness of the elastomers is most commonly relevant in the dental laboratory. Here, the removal of a very stiff material from the stone die which has been constructed to prepare a prosthesis can damage the model. In particular, the dies of thin narrow preparations such as lower incisors can be broken. This is particularly a problem when using polyethers. Alternative materials may therefore be used for die construction (Chapter 20).

Hardness

The hardness of the impression materials is measured using a **Shore hardness device**. This measures the depth of an indentation in the material created by a given force under a standard load. The values for polysulphide and addition silicones do not change with time but all the other materials become harder.

Impression materials with low flexibility and high hardness values are more difficult to remove from the mouth. To facilitate removal, use a more loosely fitting tray to allow more bulk of material, which may allow some flexure within its body.

Tear strength

It is important that an impression material will not tear (Figure 15.31) at the point in the impression where detail is required for the

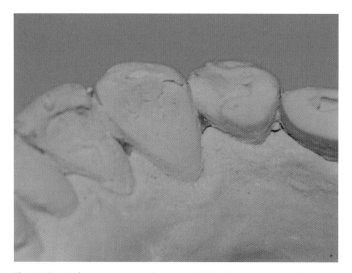

Fig. 15.31 A elastomer impression material that tore on removal from the model, with some of the impression material retained interdentally on the cast. This is more significant if the material tears on removal from the mouth, leaving retained material in situ. The resulting cast will therefore not accurately reflect the intraoral tissues and structures.

construction of the prosthesis. It must therefore be relatively strong in thin sections. All the elastomers have a substantially higher tear strength than the reversible hydrocolloids, which are the alternative for this type of impression.

A high tear strength may cause problems removing the impression from the mouth especially when it has flowed between the teeth or under bridge pontics. It may also have deformed greatly before the material tears, which may be irreversible and lead to an inaccurate model.

When an impression of a post space preparation is required, a material should be chosen which has a high tear strength so that the preparation is properly recorded and any impression material in thin section will be preserved.

Detail reproduction

All the modern elastomers can reproduce the detail of a crown preparation accurately. This is the result of the provision of light-bodied materials with all these elastomers, which contain less filler. The low-viscosity pastes will also flow more readily over the preparation and there is less likelihood of air being trapped between the material and the preparation. The minimum level of reproducibility for each viscosity is set out in the ISO document on elastomers. The requirement is the detailed reproduction of a line of fixed length and certain micrometre thickness. The exact figures vary with the different consistencies of the pastes.

The tip of syringe should be kept in the body of material at all times to prevent air becoming entrapped in the mass of material. The light-bodied material should be applied in a stirring motion to ensure good adaptation to the preparation.

The filler size also determines the ability of the impression material to record fine detail. The smaller the filler particles, the finer the detail the material can record. In order to maximize accuracy, the region which requires the most accuracy should have the light-bodied material syringed over it. This includes the occlusal surfaces of all the teeth in the arch as well as the preparation.

Moisture control

All the elastomers are hydrophobic. It is therefore critical that the site which is to be captured by the impression should be free from any fluid contaminants including saliva and blood. All elastomeric materials should therefore be applied to dry teeth, otherwise the detail reproduction will be inadequate. Good moisture control may be achieved using high-speed suction saliva extraction and isolation of the site with cotton wool rolls or dry guards (see Chapter 2). Under no circumstances should water be allowed to contact the material being syringed around the preparation. If this happens, the moisture will act as a separating medium, preventing the impression material from bonding to the tray, and **delamination** will occur. Some haemostatic agents used to stop gingival bleeding also have an adverse effect on the setting of all impression elastomers.

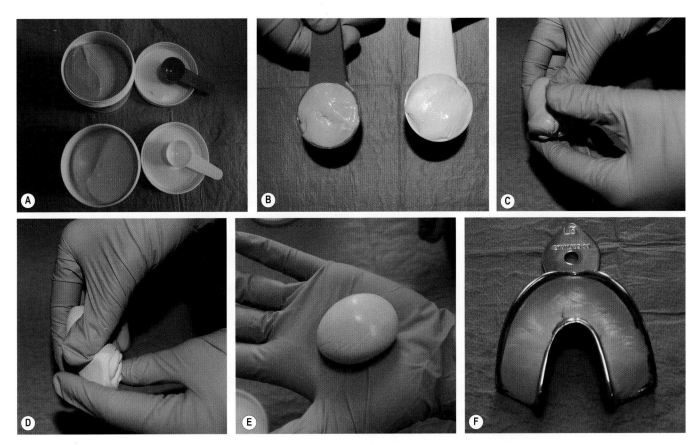

Fig. 15.32A–F The stages of mixing the addition silicone putty Affinis (Coltène Whaledent). (A) This product is presented as a base and catalyst. (B) Note the two distinct colours of the paste to help the dental nurse in determining that the two components are mixed thoroughly. (C) The folding action that reduces the risk of air incorporation; non-latex gloves (vinyl) are worn as latex may theoretically inhibit the set. (D) The dental nurse continues to fold the material until it becomes a homogenous colour. (E) The putty in it mixed form. (F) The putty is then loaded into an impression tray and given to the dentist.

Clinical handling (mixing)

All the elastomeric impression materials with the exception of the polysulphides may be mixed by hand or by mechanical means.

Putty mixing

Currently the materials most commonly mixed by hand are the putties. Handling of these materials is quite critical. Normally they are provided in two tubs containing pastes of differing colours with dispensing scoops of corresponding colours. These are usually of equal volume. The materials are mixed at a one to one ratio by kneading the two putties together until the material is a uniform colour (Figure 15.32). Care must be taken to avoid air incorporation during this mixing phase. These putties are then used with a light-bodied material, which may be mixed by hand or in a cartridge (see later).

When mixing putties, it is essential that powder- and latex-free rubber gloves are worn, as these two components can adversely affect the setting of the silicone.

Mixing pastes by hand

The pastes for all materials are dispensed in two tubes, and equal lengths of material are mixed together. It is important that the dispensation of the length is accurate as variation will alter the mechanical properties of the material. The material is dispensed onto a paper mixing pad of sufficient size to permit the two pastes to be blended together.

The two lengths of material may be dispensed in advance of the material being mixed. Care must be taken, however, that the two lengths of paste do not come into contact with each other prior to mixing. With all the materials, the longer the paste is left on the mixing pad the more likely that the pastes will start to separate. This is observed most commonly with the addition silicones. Here the clear polymer is often seen on top of the length of paste.

To mix two components thoroughly, the two pastes must be blended together with a spatula, ensuring that air is not incorporated into the mix. This is achieved by using the flat surface of the spatula and spreading the mixture across the pad rather in the way that jam is spread across a slice of bread. The spatula should move in a figure of eight. The thicker and more viscous the paste, the harder this process is to achieve satisfactorily.

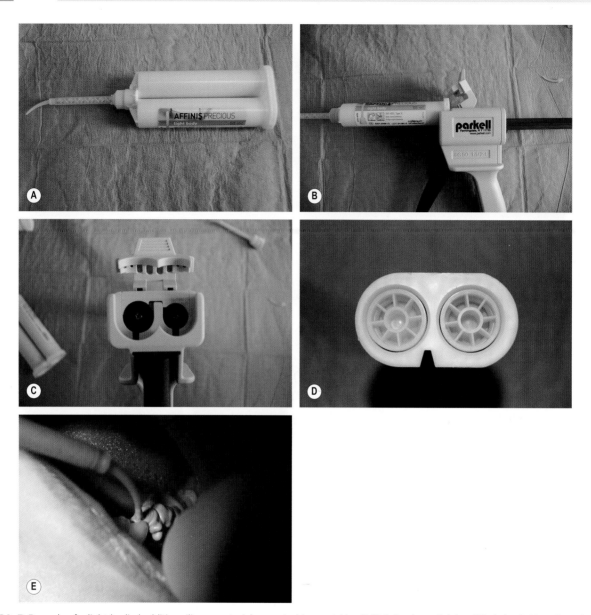

Fig. 15.33A–E Example of a light-bodied addition silicone material presented in a cartridge (Affinis Precious, Coltène Whaledent). Note the ratio of base to catalyst is 1:1 (compared with other ratios for resin based temporary crown materials). This may be syringed directly over the prepared tooth.

The mixing procedure is complicated in that frequently two viscosities are needed for the impression and these must be presented to the operator either simultaneously or within 30 seconds of one another. This usually necessitates the use of two dental nurses for the mixing process to produce an effective result. One mixes the light-bodied material and loads the mixed material into a syringe for injection around the preparation, while the second nurse will mix the heavy-bodied material and loads the tray with it; the tray is then inserted over the light-bodied material.

Mixing by hand is also quite wasteful as excess amounts of paste may be dispensed to ensure that there is sufficient material available for the impression. It can also be difficult to load the syringe with material. Many dental clinics have therefore switched to automated impression mixing, using a bespoke impression material mixing machine.

Mechanical mixing

The limitations of hand mixing have encouraged manufacturers to develop a means of automating the mixing process for elastomeric impression materials. In the case of the two paste systems mechanical cartridge systems are now available with the exception of the polysulphide materials.

The lower viscosity material is presented in a cartridge which contains two tubes with the base paste in one and the activator paste in the other. These are inserted into a gun device with a plunger which expresses the content of each tube down a mixing nozzle with a helical inner spiral inset. Mixing occurs in the mixing nozzle and the extruded paste may be injected directly into the mouth (Figure 15.33) or loaded into a syringe.

Heavy-bodied materials are also available in this formulation, but are more generally mixed by hand or using a mixing machine which can deliver the material directly to the tray (Figure 15.34). (see next section for details.)

Mechanical mixing machines

A number of impression mixing machines now available on the market (Figure 15.35). The original machine was developed by the makers of the polyether rubber in which the mixing process is automated. The impression material is supplied as a paste/paste system (base and catalyst) in foil bags with plastic platens at one end. The cartridge is inserted into a rigid cassette in the mixing machine and a plunger connected to a rotating drive shaft pushes the platens into the foil bags. Equal lengths of the two component materials are extruded from the orifice at the other end into the short mixing nozzle and the mixed material can then be loaded directly into a tray or syringe (Figure 15.36). The advantages of mixing by hand and machine are listed in Table 15.17.

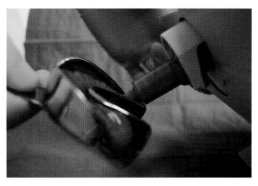

Fig. 15.34 A heavy-bodied addition silicone being loaded into the impression tray after mixing using a mechanical mixing machine.

Table 15.17 Advantages of mixing elastomeric impression materials by hand and by machine

Hand mixing	Machine mixing
No expensive hardware required	Mixing time is reduced
Less bulk for storage	Consistent quality of mix – homogeneous and void free
	Less wastage
	Cleaner
	Less staff intensive

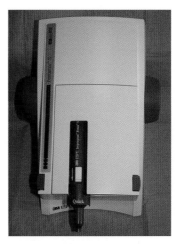

Fig. 15.35 Example of a mechanical mixing machine used to mix impression materials (Pentamix 3, 3M ESPE)

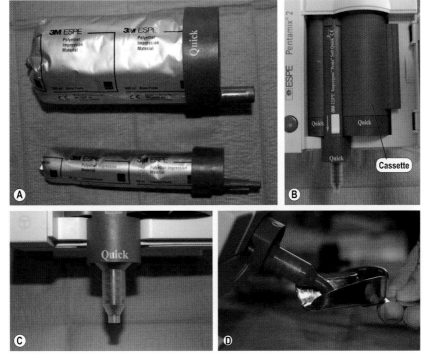

Fig. 15.36A–D Example of a (polyether) impression material (Impregum, Penta Soft Quick, 3M ESPE) supplied in foil bags. The bags are placed into the cassette, the mixing nozzle is attached and the piston then drives the material through this mixing nozzle. The mixed material goes straight into the impression tray.

Partially used cartridges should not be stored upside down (Figure 15.37). Air may become incorporated into them, potentially causing the constituents to separate, so changing the viscosity. The cartridges should therefore be stored horizontally.

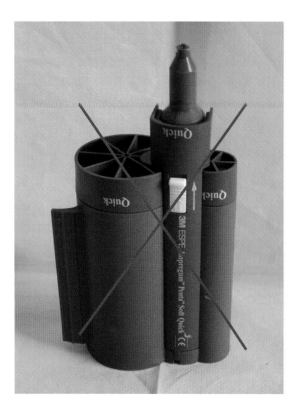

Fig. 15.37 Impression material mixing cartridges should not be stored upside down to prevent air inclusion.

It is particularly important with this type of system that cross-contamination between the two tubes on the cartridge does not occur. To avoid this, the mixing nozzle containing the mixed and unmixed material should be left in situ after use and only removed when the next mix is required. This presents a difficulty with the hand-held mixing gun, if this has been used to deliver the material to the patient's mouth, as there is a risk of cross-infection. This maybe overcome by wiping over with disinfectant wipes.

Under no circumstance should the cap sealing the tubes during transit be used as a regular cover. Continuous replacement will lead to smearing of the two pastes over the individual apertures of the cartridge, causing cross-contamination. This will result in semi-set material blocking the orifices (Figure 15.38).

When a new cartridge is used with hand gun automixing, expel the initial 1.5 mL of material as there may have been some separation of the components within the cartridge and the composition may vary.

Failures in impressions

There are a number of ways in which an impression may fail which are related to material misuse (Table 15.18 and Figure 15.39).

As the elastomer impression materials are rubbery in nature, they are more easily removed by peeling should they be retained on the patient's face. The patient should be instructed to insert their finger nail underneath the material and peel it off.

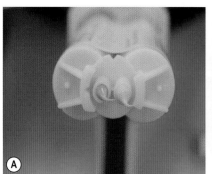 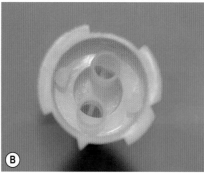 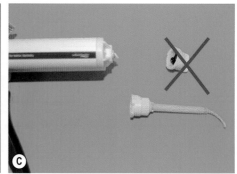

Fig. 15.38A–C The end of the cartridge and the entry to the mixing tube are shown. Excess material can be smeared over the opposing cartridge entrance during tip placement, causing contamination. Replacement of the mixing tip with the transit cap compounds the problem.

Table 15.18 Some impression faults arising as a consequence of material misuse

Mode of failure	Reason for failure
Rough or uneven surface to impression	Incomplete polymerization Premature removal Too rapid polymerization High humidity and temperature leading to premature polymerization
Inadequate flow	Too rapid polymerization High humidity and temperature leading to premature polymerization
Bubbles	Too rapid polymerization Failure to wet surface when using hydrophobic materials Air incorporation Hand mixing Faulty injection technique
Irregular voids	Moisture or debris on preparations Inadequately loaded tray
Rough or chalky cast	Inadequately cleaned impression Failure to wait 20 minutes before pouring
Separation of light- and heavy-bodied materials (delamination)	Too rapid polymerization of material Moisture contamination during impression taking
Distortion	Lack of adhesive on tray Adhesive not dry Using wrong adhesive Lack of mechanical retention from tray Polymerization starts before tray seated Movement of tray during polymerization Premature removal from mouth Incorrect removal from mouth Continued pressure on impression when elastic properties developing Leaving tray unsupported in mouth

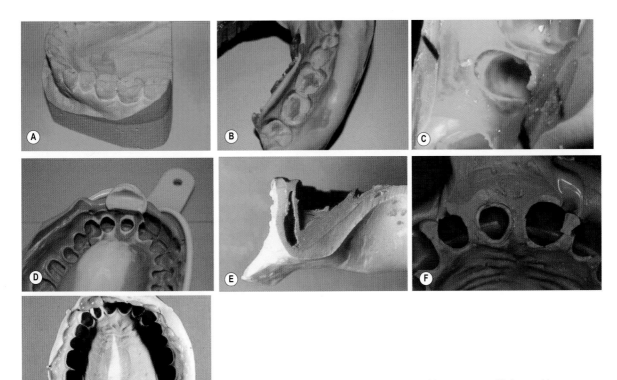

Fig. 15.39A–G (A) Defect on stone model. (B) Separation of light- and heavy-bodied materials. (C) Poor flow of addition silicone. (D) Inadequate material in tray. (E) Airblow beneath surface, (F) Airblow in impression. (G) Incomplete polymerization due to premature removal.

Summary of the properties of the elastomer impression materials

Table 15.19 summarises the properties of the four elastomer impression materials.

RIGID (NON-ELASTIC) IMPRESSION MATERIALS

There is sometime a need for impression materials which are not elastic. There are three major types of material used for this:

- Impression plaster
- Zinc oxide and eugenol
- Impression compound.

These materials are mainly used in the construction of removable dentures.

Impression plaster

Impression plaster is a traditional impression material whose main indication is to record edentulous ridges. It is good for reproducing surface detail and is quite widely tolerated by patients. As it sets rigidly and is very brittle, it must be fractured to release it from undercuts and then pieced back together so that the cast may be poured. As such it displays no recovery from deformation. There is a small setting expansion but the material displays a good dimensional stability. The material is hydrophilic. A mucostatic impression is produced.

> **Mucostatic impression:** an impression where the material is more fluid and does not displace the tissue.

Chemical constituents and setting reaction

The composition of impression plaster is not dissimilar to plaster of Paris (see Chapter 20), being mainly β-calcium sulphate hemihydrate. With impression plaster, more potassium sulphate is included to exert greater control of the expansion. Borax is also needed to retard the set of the materials as potassium sulphate also acts as an accelerator. The setting reaction is the same as for plaster of Paris. When used as an impression material, a higher water to powder ratio is used so that the material is runnier than it needs to be when used to pour models. The setting reaction is exothermic.

Advantages and disadvantages

The disadvantage of impression plaster as an impression material is that some patients salivate excessively and this may damage the surface detail. A small number of patients will not tolerate upper impression taking, as the material flows quite readily during the early stages of the setting reaction. It is usually necessary to construct a special or custom tray when this material is used.

When casting, it is necessary to use a separating medium, otherwise the plaster used for the model will adhere to the impression plaster. The separating medium is usually a solution of sodium alginate painted onto the impression.

Mixing

Mixing is by hand and it is important that correct power/liquid ratio is used, otherwise the consistency and setting time will vary. Ideally the powder should be sifted into water and left for a short time before mixing the water and powder.

Clinical usage

It is essential that the powder is stored in an airtight tin otherwise the water in the atmosphere may start the setting reaction. The material should be used in a 1–1.5 mm spaced special tray. The working time is 2–3 minutes. The tray should be moved from side to side on insertion so that the material can flow. This is called **puddling**.

Zinc oxide and eugenol impression paste

Another traditional impression material used for making the second or working impression of edentulous arches is **impression paste**. This is a zinc oxide and eugenol-based material. It is usually used in thin sections and so may also be used a denture-relining material.

Property	Polysulphide	Polyether	Addition silicone	Condensation silicone
Wettability	√	√	X	X
Surface detail	√	√	√	√
Permanent deformation	X	!	√	√
Patient acceptance	X	!	√	√
Tear strength	√	X	X	X
Dimensional accuracy	!	√	√	√
Disinfection	!	!	√	√
Hydrophilicity	!	√	X	X
Ease of removal	√	X	√	√
Range of viscosities available	!	X	√	√

Table 15.19 Properties of the three common elastomers

√=favourable property; X=unfavourable property; !=material should be used with care under these conditions.

Chemical constituents and setting reaction

The chemical constituents (Table 15.20) and setting reaction of impression paste is essentially similar to the zinc oxide eugenol cement described in Chapter 12. The gum rosin is an important constituent of both pastes and acts as a binder, giving the paste body and reducing the risk of separation of the other components. It also has the property of being thermoplastic so that the impression can be softened in hot water. This aids removal from the plaster model which is subsequently poured. The magnesium chloride and other metallic salts of acetic and hydrochloric acid act as accelerators, so that the material will set in a clinically acceptable time. As with zinc oxide eugenol cements, water catalyses the setting reaction of impression paste.

Table 15.20 Typical chemical constituents of a zinc oxide eugenol impression paste

Constituent	Purpose	Percentage of composition
Base paste		
Zinc oxide*	Reactive component	85
Inert oils such as olive and linseed	Plasticiser and reduces irritation of eugenol	13
Zinc acetate	Accelerator	2
Catalyst paste		
Eugenol*	Reactive component	15
Magnesium or calcium chloride	Accelerator	5
Talc, kaolin, wax or silica	Inert fillers	20
Gum rosin	Binder	45–50
Other oils such as resinous balsam and lanolin	Viscosity and flow regulator	10–15
*Active ingredient.		

Properties

The material produces a rigid impression, which is good at reproducing fine detail accurately. Its lack of elasticity may mean that it breaks or distorts when removed from undercuts. It is used in thin section and should be used in a closely fitting (1 mm spaced) special tray. A mucostatic impression results. Zinc oxide eugenol impression pastes adhere to dry surfaces such as shellac and composition.

There is a small dimensional change as the materials sets with about a 0.15% shrinkage which occurs within the first hour. Thereafter the material is dimensionally stable. As the material is generally used as a perfecting material, if the supporting tray/base distorts, the impression paste will also distort.

Mixing

The impression material is mixed by hand using a paper mixing pad and a Clarident (broad-bladed stainless steel) spatula. It is presented as a paste/paste system with each paste being a different colour to help ensure that the material is mixed thoroughly. Box 15.4 shows a recommended mixing sequence.

The impression paste once mixed sets quite slowly, passing through a thickening phase after which it is to difficult to manipulate. A further phase of hardening occurs before the impression should be removed. It is sometimes difficult to define the setting phase clearly. Once the impression has been inserted into the mouth the setting reaction will accelerate as the increase in temperature and humidity accelerate the setting reaction. As with all impression materials, once the material has set on the mixing pad, the material will also have set completely in the mouth.

The construction of a plaster cast from the impression requires some attention as the only die material that is suitable is gypsum based (see Chapter 20). The impression should be thoroughly washed and dried before pouring the model with plaster or stone. No separating medium is required with this material. Once the stone has set (after at least an hour) the impression and stone model should be immersed in warm water to facilitate the removal of the impression.

Box 15.4 Recommended mixing sequence for a zinc oxide eugenol impression paste

Step 1	Step 2	Step 3	Step 4

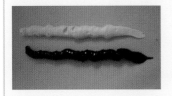 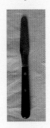 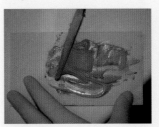 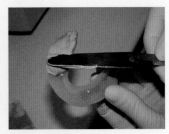

| Equal lengths of both pastes are extruded onto a paper pad | A Clarident spatula is used to mix the pastes together to blend them | Mixing continues using the flat blade of the spatula to spread the mixture until no streaking is seen | The mixed paste is loaded onto the special tray and the impression taken |

- Set impression paste is difficult to remove from instruments. It may be removed from the spatula by warming to a temperature at which the rosin softens. The blade may then be wiped.
- Some patients cannot tolerate the zinc oxide eugenol impression pastes as they often produce a tingling or mild burning sensation of the soft tissues.

To prevent zinc oxide eugenol-containing impression materials from adhering to the patient's extraoral tissues, a liberal amount of petroleum jelly should be smeared on the patient's lips and face.

Commercially available products

Representative examples of the currently commercially available zinc oxide eugenol impression materials are shown in Table 15.21.

Impression compound

Compound or **composition**, or **compo** as it is colloquially known, is one of the oldest impression materials for dentures. They are thermoplastic materials and are supplied in sheets or sticks as (red) compo (Figure 15.40) and **greenstick**, respectively (Figure 15.41). Impression compound is not used so much these days as other materials such as acrylic tray materials have superseded it. However, it is still used for first impressions of the edentulous arch as well as border moulding stock trays to improve their fit or to contain impression material in the tray posteriorly and underextended special trays. It is commonly used to gain some mucocompression in the post dam region for a second impression.

> **Mucodisplacive/mucocompression impression:** the oral soft tissues are recorded under load by a more viscous impression material.

Chemical constituents

The typical constituents of impression are set out in Table 15.22.

Properties

The material is thermoplastic, that is, it softens when heated and hardens as it comes back to mouth temperature. Its transition temperature is about 55–60°C. Above this temperature the material softens

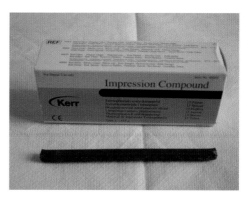

Fig. 15.41 A baton of green impression compound and its packaging (Kerr Hawe).

Table 15.21 Some zinc oxide eugenol-based impression materials currently available on the market

Product	Manufacturer
Impression Paste	SS White
Outline Impression Paste	Cavex
Zoe Impression Paste	Kelly's

Table 15.22 Typical constituents of impression compound

Chemical constituent	Purpose
Resins (such as shellac, rosin, dammar and sandarac) copal resin and waxes (such as colophony and beeswax) carnauba wax	Control consistency
Gutta percha or stearic acid	Plasticizers
Calcium carbonate, limestone, talc	Fillers, control consistency and rigidity Colouring agent

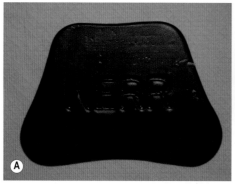

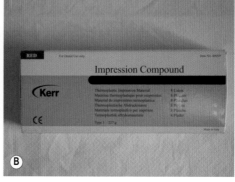

Fig. 15.40 (A) A sheet of red impression compound and (B) its packaging (Kerr Hawe).

and below this temperature it starts to harden again. This transition is achieved by either placing the sheet of compound in a hot water bath or heating in a naked flame. Care must be exercised with the latter method, as excessive heating may cause some volatile components to be lost from the material. Likewise, components may leach out when softening in a hot water bath for a long period of time. It is important that the clinician ensures that the material is completely softened, not just the exterior portions while the central mass is still solid otherwise internal strains will be set up. The material may be **wet kneaded**, whereby the compound is manipulated by hand when wet and this is believed to improve the flow of the material.

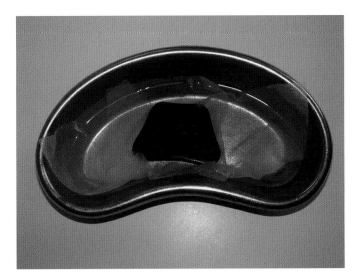

Fig. 15.42 The sheet of red impression compound left in a hot water bath to soften prior to placement in the edentulous stock tray. Note that the dish is lined with gauze to prevent the compound from sticking to the sides of the metal tray. Impression compound is very difficult to remove from the metal surface should it adhere.

Impression compound is a high viscosity material and so poor reproduction of fine detail is achieved and a mucocompressive impression is gained. Its dimensional stability is poor, displaying a 1.5% shrinkage so these impressions must be poured as soon as possible and ideally within the hour.

Clinical use

Red compound

Very hot water should be used in the bath to soften impression compound. A kettle which has freshly boiled is ideal. The water will cool quickly and so will not soften the material adequately. The sheet is placed in the water and left for a minute or so (Figure 15.42).

The impression compound may then be manipulated to ensure that the bulk is fully softened and placed into the impression tray. At this point the loaded tray can be briefly placed back into the bath to soften the material again. The dentist should then remove the loaded tray from the water, check that it is not too hot to be placed into the patient's mouth, and take the impression (Figure 15.43). To check the temperature of the material, place it on an area of the clinician's forearm which has had petroleum jelly applied to it. If it is comfortable and not too hot, it will not burn the patient's mouth. After removal, the impression may then be cooled by placing it under cold running water.

✓
The hot water bath should be lined with gauze to prevent the impression compound from sticking to the sides of the bath. If it does stick it will be very difficult to remove.

Green compound

Greenstick is generally used for border moulding of impression trays and to create a post dam. It is generally heated in a naked flame or

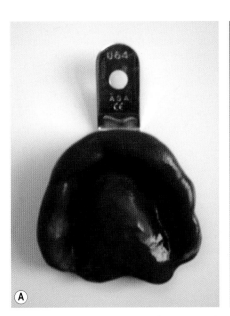

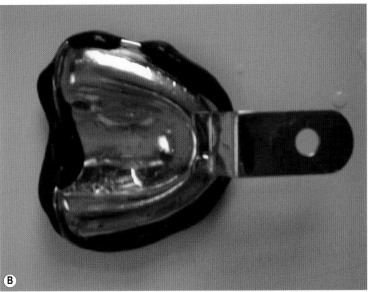

Fig. 15.43 (A) The completed impression of an upper edentulous ridge. (B) Note how the compound has been rolled over the edges of the rim lock tray to retain it in the tray.

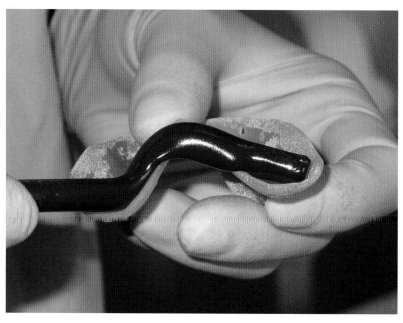

Fig. 15.44 Greenstick (green impression compound) is softened by heating (usually in a flame or warm air device) so that it may be placed on the posterior border of an upper special tray to form a post dam.

hot air stream until it softens (Figure 15.44). Petroleum jelly can be used as a separator on the dentist's gloves to prevent it from sticking to them when hot.

Petroleum jelly should be used to prevent the warmed compound from sticking the dentist's gloved hands.

Commercially available products

Typical commercially available products are listed in Table 15.23.

Table 15.23 Some composition products currently available on the market

Product	Manufacturer	Comments
Impression compound	Kerr Hawe	Greenstick
Impression compound	Kerr Hawe	Red

FUNCTIONAL IMPRESSIONS

Functional impressions involve the insertion of a slow-setting impression material into a denture base. The patient wears the denture with the impression material in it for a day or so and the material sets, thus capturing the shape of the tissues as they are during function. The denture base and impression material can then be sent to the dental laboratory for casting and a more successfully fitting denture should result. Functional impressions are discussed further in Chapter 23.

FUTURE IMPRESSION DEVELOPMENT

There is an increasing interest in direct scanning of the preparation and digitizing the image to produce a model in the laboratory or milling the restoration out of an optimized block of ceramic. These interesting and exciting developments are in their infancy, but show much potential. The technique is described in the ceramics chapter (Chapter 22) where its use is currently applicable.

GINGIVAL MANAGEMENT

In order to properly record all the margins of a preparation, it may be necessary to retract the gingival tissues, so that the impression material will reach the edge of the preparation. A sufficient bulk of impression material is required in this region to give the impression material adequate strength, so that the working cast may be made successfully. Operative dentists therefore need to use some form of **retraction** to expose the margins, particularly in subgingival regions.

Furthermore, the incompatibility of many impression materials with fluids such as water, saliva and blood means that the impression site must be clean and dry. This may be difficult to achieve in areas where good moisture control is a challenge. To gain both adequate retraction and a clean and dry field, a number of retraction materials and systems are available, including mechanical means such as **retraction cord** or chemicals such as **astringents (styptics)** and **vasoconstrictor agents**. Frequently a combination of methods is used, with a chemical used to impregnate the retraction cord.

Mechanical retraction materials

The traditional material used to retract any gingival tissue which is impinging on the margins of the preparation is the **retraction cord**. As the name suggests, this is a thin cord usually made of cotton, which is placed into the gingival sulcus so separating the marginal gingival tissues and the tooth. This pushes the gingival tissues back from the tooth so that the margin of the preparation becomes exposed, visible and accessible.

Different sizes of cord are available corresponding to the variation in the size of the gingival sulcus. Some techniques require a thin cord to be placed first and then a wider cord is placed on top of the first. The cords are left in situ and just prior to the placement of the impression material, the most coronal, wider cord is removed. It is outwith the scope of this text to describe cord placement and techniques.

The cord itself is available as **twisted**, **braided** and **knitted**. The latter two varieties are the most commonly used, in particular the knitted type, which are more effective at retraction as they have a springiness (Figure 15.45).

Retraction cord is used by soaking it in a fluid, either water or a haemostatic chemical (see p. 272), and then it is packed around the preparation using a special instrument. Knitted cords hold and carry significantly more haemostatic chemicals than conventional cords, and are claimed not to entangle in burs unlike other cords. Some retraction cords are coloured to facilitate their placement and some systems are flavoured in an attempt to increase patient acceptance.

Chemicals used with retraction systems

Retraction chemicals that work mechanically

Retraction systems that use chemicals which expand either on their own or in combination with applied pressure are also available. Expasyl (Kerr Hawe) is based on **kaolin**, a type of clay. This material is injected perpendicularly into the gingival sulcus to fill it. The dentist must then wait for a couple of minutes whilst the material expands slightly due to the presence of moisture. It may then be removed by washing away with water from the three-in-one syringe. As well as kaolin, the material contains aluminium chloride and excipients, and may achieve haemostasis by the application of pressure and due to the presence of the aluminium chloride. The material is hydrophilic and popular with those operative dentists using implants. The material may be placed around the implant prior to the impression being taken (Figure 15.46) in preference to the placement of retraction cord which may compromise the gingival cuff around the implant.

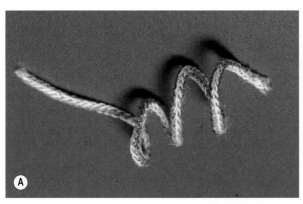
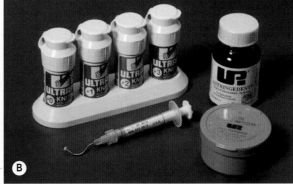

Fig. 15.45 (A) Example of a knitted gingival retraction cord and (B) the astringent solution supplied with it (Tissue Management Kit, Ultradent).

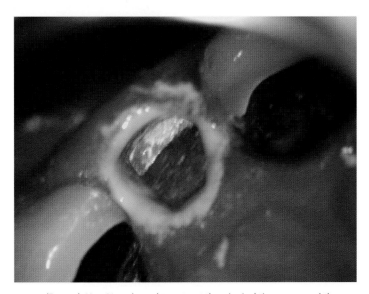

Fig. 15.46 A kaolin-based retraction system (Expasyl, Kerr Hawe) used to retract the gingival tissues around the preparation margins of an implant placed to replace tooth 12.

A mechanical retraction system is contraindicated if periodontal pockets are present. Furthermore, the dentist should make sure that all of the material is thoroughly washed away prior to using a polyether or hydrocolloid impression material to prevent tearing of the impression material.

Other retraction systems are also available (Figure 15.47). Magic Foam Cord (Coltène Whaledent) is an expanding addition silicone which is claimed to expand by 160%. This occurs by bubbles being formed within the material. It is supplied as a paste/paste system and once mixed it is injected around the preparation. Pressure is then applied by the patient biting on a Comprecap, which is a densely packed cotton wool roll. These are available in three sizes.

Haemostatic retraction chemicals

Retraction cord is never used dry; instead it is soaked in a fluid, which may be water but is more commonly a chemical. This chemical is generally a haemostatic agent to control any gingival haemorrhage around the preparation. This will facilitate a clean and dry field which is important particularly if a hydrophobic impression material is being used.

These chemicals are broadly divided into:

- Astringents – such as aluminium trichloride, potassium aluminium sulphate and ferric sulphate
- Vasoconstrictors – such as adrenaline (epinephrine) hydrochloride (this has fallen out of favour as it may have systemic effects on the cardiovascular system which may not be desirable).

Unfortunately, many of these chemicals adversely affect the set of the impression material. It is therefore essential that any residue is removed from the impression site and the area dried after use. An example of an astringent is Racestyptine (Septodont), which if used with a polyether impression material will react with it. Gas is released in the reaction and this will result in bubble defects in the surface of the stone die.

Commercially available products

A selection of currently available gingival retraction systems are listed in Table 15.24 and an example of one such product is pictured in Fig 15.48.

Table 15.24 Some gingival retraction systems currently available on the market

Product	Manufacturer	Notes
Expasyl	Kerr Hawe	Kaolin based
Gel-Cord	Pascal Co Inc.	25% potassium aluminium sulphate
Magic Foam Cord	Coltène Whaledent	Addition silicone with bubbling agent
Racegel	Septodont	Aluminium trichloride plus ethanol
Racestyptine cord	Septodont	Braided cord
Racestyptine solution	Septodont	Aluminium trichloride hexahydrate
Stay-Put	Roeko	Braided cord
Traxodent	Premier	Aluminium trichloride
Ultrapak	Optident	Knitted cord that can be impregnated with 15.5% ferric sulphate

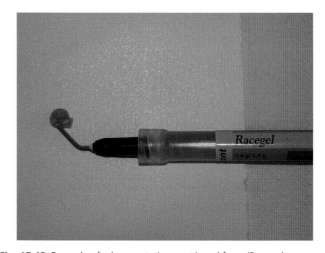

Fig. 15.48 Example of a haemostatic agent in gel form (Racegel, Septodont).

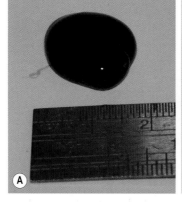
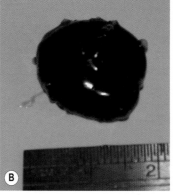

Fig. 15.47A,B An expanding addition silicone retraction system (Magic Foam Cord, Coltène Whaledent). (A) The material at start of mix and (B) after 5 minutes.

Electrosurgery

Electrosurgery (more correctly **radiosurgery**) may be used judiciously by the operative dentist to expose the margins of the preparation prior to impression making. This technique is called **troughing** and removes any gingival tissues from the preparation margins. It may also provide haemostasis. One such product is shown in Figure 15.49.

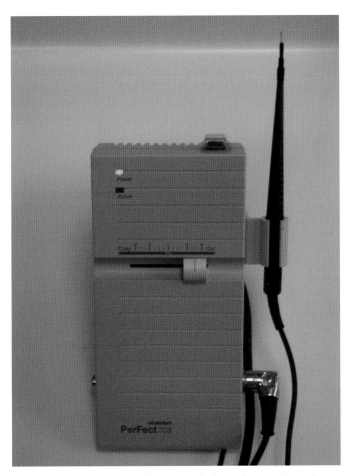

Fig. 15.49 Example of a dental electrosurgical unit that may be used to expose the margins of a preparation by removing the overlying gingival tissue (PerFect TCS, Whaledent).

SUMMARY

- An impression needs to be taken of a tooth preparation or the mouth in the case of a removable appliance, so enabling the dental technician to construct the indirect restoration or device.
- A number of impression materials are available to the dentist, their selection being dependent on the clinical case and the properties of the material.
- These impression materials may be either mixed by hand or by machine.
- Correct impression tray selection is important.
- It is important the margins of the preparation can be accessed by a sufficient bulk of impression material to allow a satisfactory model to be poured. A number of mechanical systems and chemicals may be used for this purpose.
- Computer technology is being developed and some systems are in use to take optical impressions of the preparation, which allows a model to be made by computer-aided design/ manufacture (CAD/CAM) or a restoration to be milled out of an optimized ceramic block.

FURTHER READING

McCabe, J.F., Walls, A.W.G., 2008. Applied Dental Materials, ninth ed. Blackwell Munksgaard, Oxford. (See Chapters 16–19)

Powers, J.M., Sakaguchi, R.L. (Eds.), 2006. Craig's Restorative Dental Materials (twelfth ed.). Mosby Elsevier, St Louis (See Chapter 12)

van Noort, R., 2007. Introduction to Dental Materials, third ed. Mosby Elsevier, Edinburgh. (See Chapter 2.7)

SELF-ASSESSMENT QUESTIONS

1. What criteria should be used for the selection of a tray for fixed prosthodontics?
2. A mix of alginate is stiff and sets too quickly. What may be the cause of this?
3. An elastomeric addition silicone rubber impression is taken and on removal it separates from the tray. How may this be avoided?
4. What are the disadvantages of using an addition silicone impression material for fixed prosthodontics?
5. What are the advantages and disadvantages of using a polyether impression material?
6. What precautions should a clinician take before sending an impression to the laboratory?
7. What methods of gingival retraction are available and what are their advantages and disadvantages?

Chapter 76

Waxes and occlusal registration materials

From this chapter, the reader will:

- Be aware of the various waxes used in dentistry
- Understand their properties
- Be aware of the various applications of dental waxes
- Be aware of the other materials that may be used to construct patterns for cast restorations
- Be aware of the occlusal registration materials available to the restorative dentist
- Know the names of currently available commercial products.

INTRODUCTION

Waxes are a group of ubiquitous materials that play a significant part in both restorative dentistry and in the dental laboratory. They are used extensively in the denture-making process, in making interocclusal records, as a splinting material in denture repairs, for boxing impressions when casting models, and forming the wax pattern in the **lost wax technique** to produce removable and fixed prostheses. A range of waxes with different properties are required to carry out these varying functions. A number of **natural** and **mineral waxes**, **gums**, **fatty acids**, **oils** and **resins** (both **synthetic** and **natural**) are blended together to produce the wax with specific properties required for its intended use (Table 16.1).

> **Boxing an impression:** the placement of a material around the periphery of an impression tray to retain the plaster or die stone until it is set.

CONSTITUENTS OF DENTAL WAXES

The common constituents of most dental waxes are **hydrocarbons** and **esters** with a high molecular weight. The use of natural waxes does

Table 16.1 The natural and mineral waxes used in dentistry

Wax type	Melting temperatures (°C)	Hardness	Role in dental wax
Natural waxes			
Carnauba	84–91	High	Increases melting range and hardness
Ouricury	79–84	High	Increases melting range and hardness
Candelilla	68–75	High	Increases hardness of paraffin wax
Beeswax	62–68	Medium	Common base for many waxes
Japan wax	53	Medium/low	May be substituted for beeswax
Mineral waxes			
Paraffin	40–71	Medium	Common base wax
Ozokerite	65–69	Medium to high	Great affinity for oils and raises melting temperature
Ceresin	77–93	Medium to high	Increases melting range
Montan	72–90	Medium to high	Increases melting range
Barnsdahl	70–74	Medium to high	Increases melting range and hardness and reduces paraffin wax flow

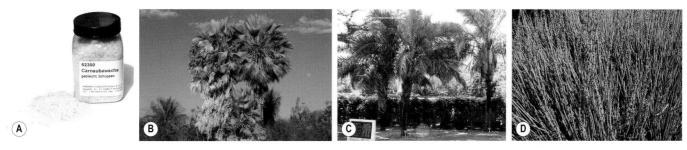

Fig. 16.1 Carnauba wax (A) is derived from the leaf of the Copernicia palm (B) found primarily in Brazil. Ouricury wax is obtained from the leaves of the feather palm (C) by scraping the surface of the leaves while candelilla is sourced from the leaves of a shrub *Euphorbia antisyphilitica* (D).
http://en.wikipedia.org/wiki/en:Creative_Commons. http://creativecommons.org/licenses/by-sa/3.0/deed.en"Attribution-Share Alike 3.0 Unported license wilcopedia.

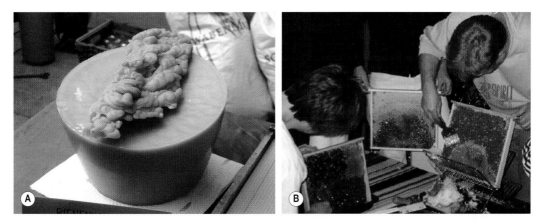

Fig. 16.2 (A) Beeswax cake and (B) beeswax being scraped off the honeycomb.
http://en.wikipedia.org/wiki/en:Creative_Commons. http://creativecommons.org/licenses/by-sa/3.0/deed.en"Attribution-Share Alike 3.0 Unported license Frank Mikley.

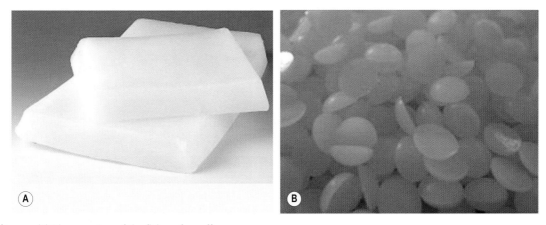

Fig. 16.3 (A) Paraffin wax. (B) Close-up view of the flakes of paraffin wax.

present the manufacturer with a problem as these waxes have variable properties depending on their source and also the time at which they were obtained. The common plant waxes include **carnauba**, **ouricury**, **candelilla** (Figure 16.1) and **Japan wax**. Japan wax is really a fat containing glycerides of palmetic and stearic acid. It is derived from the berries of the sumac tree found in Japan and China and is regarded as a form of lacquer. The animal and insect waxes include **spermaceti** from the sperm whale and **beeswax** (Figure 16.2).

> **Lacquer:** a clear or coloured varnish that dries by solvent evaporation to produce a hard, durable finish.

Mineral waxes are more consistent in their properties and presentations. They are usually derived from the refining of petroleum products. One of the most commonly available is **paraffin wax** (Figure 16.3) with a melting point of 40–70 °C. This wax has a tendency to show substantial volumetric contraction (in the region of 10–16%) during the cooling and solidification process.

The primary source of microcrystalline wax is the heavier oil fractions produced during the petroleum distillation process. These have higher melting points and are formed into plates. They are much tougher than paraffin waxes and show much less volumetric change when changing from liquid to solid. Their properties may be adapted by adding oil, making the wax less hard. The common

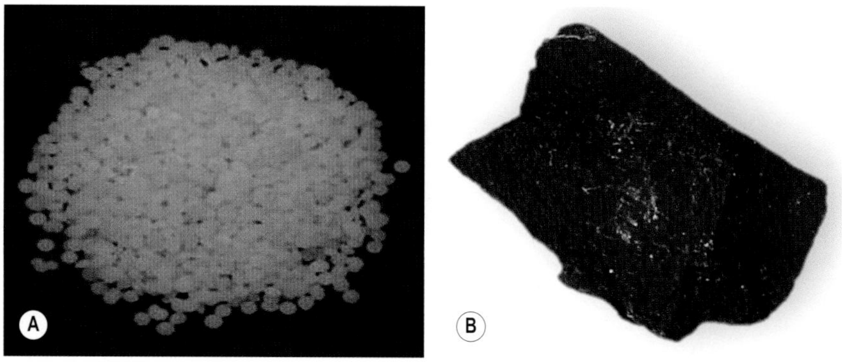

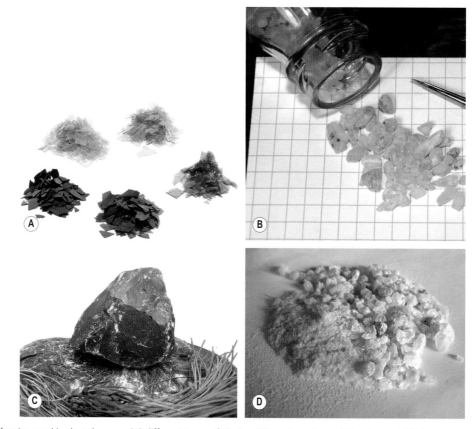

Fig. 16.4 (A) Ceresin wax and (B) ozokerite in its natural form.
http://www.mnfpetroleum.com/New/index.php?option=com_content&view=article&id=99&Itemid=100

Fig. 16.5 Examples of resins used in dental waxes: (A) different types of shellac, (B) sandarac tears, (C) rosin, and (D) dammar.

microcrystalline waxes include **ozokerite**, **ceresin** (Figure 16.4), **montan** and **barnsdahl**. The first three waxes are all derived from shale and lignites found near petroleum deposits. Other waxes which may be incorporated into dental wax include synthetic waxes which have been produced for other purposes, such as **polyethylene waxes** and **polyethylene glycol waxes**. While the use of synthetic waxes in dental waxes is increasing, the natural waxes still predominate.

The handling properties of the individual waxes may be adjusted by the addition of gums, fats and resins. The resins may be either synthetic or naturally occurring. **Dammar**, **rosin** and **sandarac** (Figure 16.5) are three examples in the latter group and are derived from plants. Another common naturally occurring material is **shellac** (Figure 16.6), which is produced by insects. It is commonly

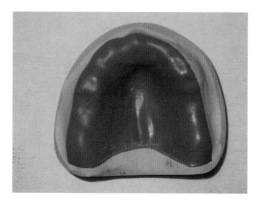

Fig. 16.6 Shellac used to make the baseplate for an occlusal rim.

obtained from India and Thailand. Shellac is a thermoplastic material and is used to make baseplates, which are used in the denture-making process. It is a rigid material when solid and other waxes may be added to it, for example to make occlusal rims. As it is more stable at mouth temperature, it is less likely to distort when used in the mouth.

Occlusal rim: a horseshoe-shaped block of wax on a close fitting rigid base. Also called a bite block.

PROPERTIES

In order to produce a wax which may be used in dentistry, a number of properties need to be considered:

- Melting range
- Thermal expansion characteristics
- Physical properties
- Flow
- Control of residual thermal stressing.

Melting range

It is already apparent that the melting temperatures of the various constituents of the wax will affect the melting range of the final product. By adding waxes of high melting temperatures, the melting range of the paraffin wax-based materials can be increased significantly. This is of importance if the wax is to be used in the mouth as the melting range needs to be higher than mouth temperature. In the dental laboratory the wax needs to change rapidly from solid to liquid to in order to manipulate it. The melting range can be narrowed as well as raised. To manipulate the wax effectively, it must be maintained at the correct temperature. This may be done using a flame or induction coil (Figure 16.7).

Thermal expansion characteristics

The thermal expansion characteristics must be carefully judged as the mode of expansion as well as the amount which occurs is important. In some cases the waxes go though phase changes so that at a given temperature a marked dimensional change will occur or the rate of thermal expansion will change. This must be taken into account in the wax blending to achieve the properties which are suitable for each application.

Physical properties

None of the waxes have particularly high mechanical properties, in fact their compressive strengths and elastic moduli are relatively low. However, within the group of waxes there is some variation with beeswax having the lowest and carnauba wax the highest compressive strength and elastic modulus. The properties are also dependent on the temperature and the composition of the wax mixture is dependent on the intended use.

Flow

The flow characteristics of each individual component wax will vary, with some showing a steady increase in flow with temperature while others show minimal flow until close to their melting point. By blending and varying the composition of the dental wax, its flow can be controlled until a short time before its melting point is reached. This is useful in the dental laboratory when making a wax pattern.

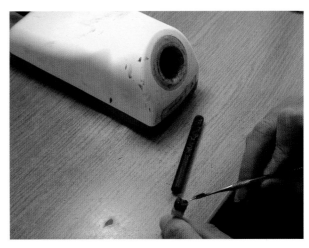

Fig. 16.7 The dental technician using an induction coil to maintain the correct temperature of the wax when a wax pattern is being made so that it can be manipulated effectively.

Control of residual thermal stressing

It is important that once waxes have been formed into a specific shape, they are not permitted to stress relieve by being left for long periods of time between processes in the laboratory. For example, the time between the completion of the wax pattern and investment should be kept as short as possible. Similarly if the wax is compressed into a mould, it may rebound or alter its shape on removal of the pressure if left for too long. Again, the properties of the wax over a given temperature range may be modified by the manufacturer by the blending the constituents of the wax to create a product for a specific purpose.

APPLICATIONS OF WAXES USED IN DENTISTRY

Use of waxes in dentistry can be divided into three distinct areas:

- In the construction of fixed or removal appliances, both of a temporary or permanent nature. These uses include waxes used to form the wax pattern for cast restorations (**inlay waxes**) and wax patterns for cast clasps. Waxes are also used to make baseplates of dentures and occlusal rims. These are sometimes called **pattern waxes**.
- In the construction of auxiliary aids in the manufacture of appliances and implements for both clinical and laboratory use. These uses require **processing waxes**, that is, waxes to extend special trays, box the impression trays and support the plaster during the pouring process and those used to temporarily splint components or fragments of appliances.
- For **occlusal registration**.

Waxes used in prosthesis construction

The pattern waxes may be divided two types:

- Waxes used to make the wax pattern of a fixed restoration and also the prefabricated shaped wax patterns in the shape of clasps for partial dentures
- Waxes used to make a uniform thickness baseplate for a denture.

The nature of the use of the two types of wax means that slightly different properties are required.

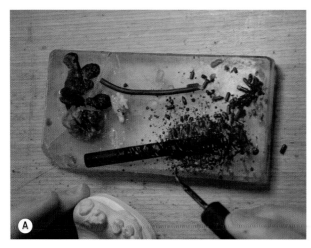
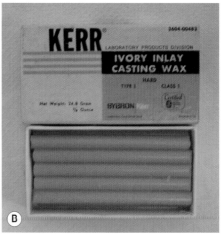

Fig. 16.8 (A) The dental technician's palate, consisting of different colours of inlay wax being used to construct a wax pattern. (B) Inlay wax is also available in ivory for use in diagnostic wax-ups.

Inlay wax

These waxes contain a mixture of paraffin, ceresin, carnauba, candelilla and beeswax. Paraffin wax is usually the major component, forming about 60% of the total composition. The waxes are categorized as **hard**, **medium** and **soft**. Their flow properties are related to this with the harder types generally flowing less. This may be achieved by increasing the content of waxes with lower flow rates such as carnauba. Convention has dictated that these waxes are generally dark blue green or purple but they are also available in ivory (Figure 16.8). This colour is used when diagnostic wax-ups are prescribed so that the wax-up may be shown to the patient. The ivory colour may be visualized more easily by the patient (Figure 16.9) than the use of a non-tooth-coloured wax.

> **Diagnostic wax-up:** waxes laid down to form a pattern on a model to show the intended morphology of the intended restoration.

Since these waxes form the patterns for cast indirect restorations, they must have a high level of detail and dimensional accuracy. Inlay wax used in the laboratory is quite soft and can be carved at ambient temperatures. The thermal expansion has to be modified so that during the investment process, the dimensional change of the investment material may be compensated for. Additionally the wax must not flake or fragments could be lost during the investing process. Similarly the wax must be suitable for use in thin section as the margins of modern crowns generally have fine bevelled edges. This wax may also be used in the mouth.

The flow characteristics of the wax must be such that once the pattern is removed from the model it shows minimal stress relief. Should this occur, it will lead to distortion of the pattern and the final restoration will not fit. This means that the wax needs to be heated sufficiently to melt and adapt to the model surface. To prevent warping, it is recommended that the wax should be heated to between 45 and 50 °C prior to use for a minimum of 20 minutes.

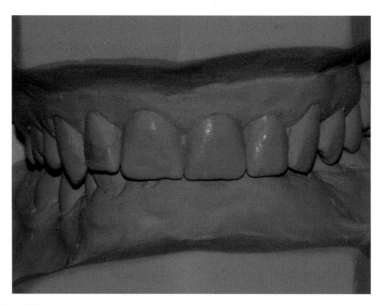

Fig. 16.9 A diagnostic wax-up in ivory inlay wax.

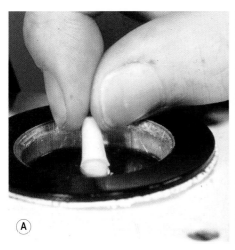
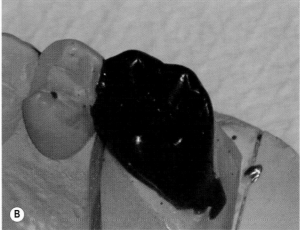

Fig. 16.10 (A) A die being dipped into a heated bath of wax to form a coping prior to the addition of more wax to make the pattern for the crown. (B) The finished wax pattern.

Many technicians achieve this by maintaining a small container at a fixed temperature thermostatically (Figure 16.10). This has the disadvantage that if the temperature is fixed at too high a value, a small fraction of the lower melting point waxes may be slowly lost, which may change the properties of the wax.

The other essential property of these waxes is that they must volatilize without leaving a residue as during the casting process they will be burnt out. Any carbon residue on the surface of the investment will affect the casting surface. Normally the vaporization temperature is set at around 500 °C.

Preformed wax patterns

Casting waxes are generally used for creating specific design features or providing a base of specific thickness on a denture. These are used to establish minimum thickness and shape of parts of a denture, for example large connectors such as lingual and palatal bars. The primary difference between the casting waxes and inlay wax is that the casting waxes are preformed and moulded onto the model which is then invested. Wax is therefore not removed and so the flow characteristics of the wax are less demanding. Generally they are slightly stickier but may still be repositioned easily on the model. They do, however, need to be very ductile as they must be adapted around

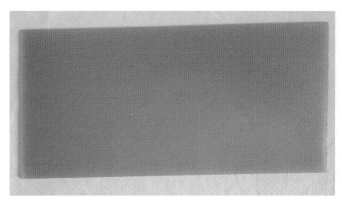

Fig. 16.11 A sheet of baseplate or modelling wax.

teeth and other sharply curved objects on the model without breaking. They must burn out with no residue like inlay wax, below the casting temperature of the alloy used. One special variety of this type of wax is **baseplate** or **modelling wax**, which is so called as it forms the base of a denture (Figure 16.11). Modelling wax is also used to construct occlusal rims or **bite blocks** (Figure 16.12).

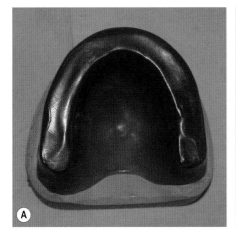
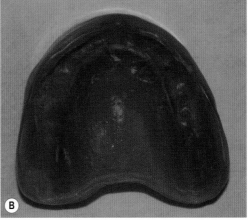

Fig. 16.12A,B Modelling wax is used to construct occlusal rims or bite blocks.

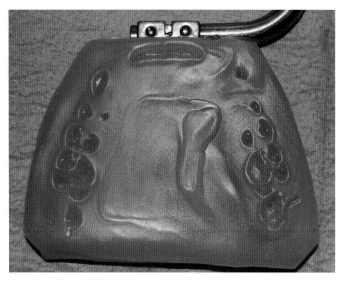

Fig. 16.13 Baseplate wax used on the bite fork of a facebow.

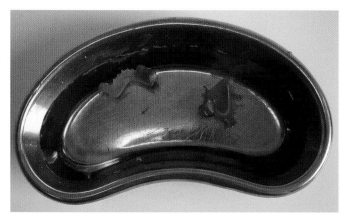

Fig. 16.14 A cold water bath used to chill any wax-based materials when outside the mouth.

Waxes have been used as a means of register the relationship between teeth and jaws, but although they do provide some form of record, their properties do not lend themselves to this application. The problems of flow, stress relaxation and distortion also tend to lead to records in wax being unreliable. The only successful application of wax is in the construction of bite rims to record the jaw relationship. The waxes here usually contain paraffin and ceresin wax with a small proportion of beeswax. Additionally, they may have aluminium or copper particles added as strengtheners or they may be adapted to a shellac baseplate. For any success they need to be used in bulk. This type of wax may also be used to record the indentations of the teeth when a facebow registration is being recorded (Figure 16.13).

 Once the wax bite block or trial denture has been tried in the patient's mouth, the higher intraoral temperature will cause the wax to expand and so its retention may be reduced. Placing wax-based materials in a cold basin of water between the spells of time in the mouth will chill down the wax, causing it to return to its original size and shape (Figure 16.14).

Once the dentist has trimmed the occlusal rim to the desired shape (corresponding to the shape of the final denture), the denture teeth (see Chapter 23) may be positioned into the wax. This waxed-up denture prototype is then 'tried in' the patient's mouth to determine its retention and stability, the occlusion, the occlusal vertical dimension, facial and lip support, and the aesthetics of the denture. For this reason the wax is usually tinted to give a coral pink colour (Figure 16.15).

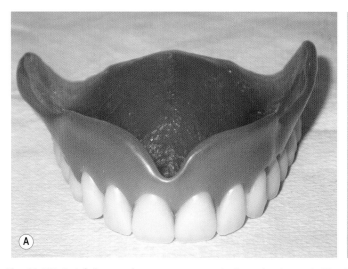

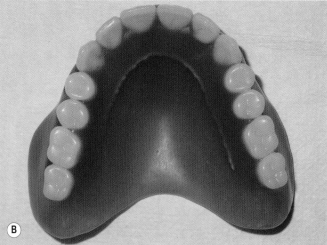

Fig. 16.15A,B A full upper denture set-up to try in the patient's mouth. The denture teeth are set in pink modelling wax.

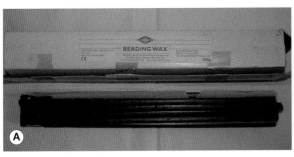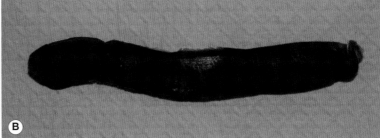

Fig. 16.16A,B Beading or carding wax. Note its softness and pliability.

The primary waxes in the mixture are paraffin waxes (up to 78%). Other constituents are resins, oils and additives such as colouring agents. The common paraffin wax used is ceresin with a small addition of beeswax and some carnauba wax, which act as a hardener. The exact flow characteristics are determined for the climate in which the wax will be used and this means that there are various varieties available worldwide. The dimensional stability of these waxes is not as critical as for inlay wax. The presence of the beeswax permits the surface of the prototype denture to be smoothed and contoured with a warm instrument or fine flame, leaving a smooth surface. The waxes in this case must have a melting point below that of boiling water as the wax after investing will be washed out. Any residue of wax left on the teeth will interfere with complete bonding and interlocking of the resin with the artificial teeth.

Waxes used for auxiliary processing

Boxing, beading or carding waxes

With all impressions, there may be areas where the gypsum will not be retained when it is poured into the impression. There is therefore a need for a material which will temporarily dam these areas in order to retain the plaster in place. Waxes are one of the ideal materials for this as they can moulded easily to the shape required, easily removed after the plaster has set, and are relatively inexpensive. These waxes are known as **boxing**, **beading** or **carding waxes** (Figure 16.16). Their properties relate specifically to their easy pliability at ambient temperatures and also the need to retain their shape up to 35 °C. Waxes of this nature usually contain a high proportion of beeswax.

These waxes are also useful for placing under bridge pontics when an elastomer impression material (in particular a polyether) is being used to prevent the inadvertent removal of the bridge with the impression material as the elastomer cannot get under the pontic.

The term **periphery wax** is also used for a wax designed specifically for boxing impressions or used intraorally as a post dam. Its function in this case is to prevent the loss of the fluid impression material out of the back of the (stock) impression tray. This would be unpleasant for the patient as it may cause them to retch and gag. Periphery wax is white in colour and slightly more viscous than the red beading wax described above. It mainly contains beeswax, paraffin and other soft waxes.

Sticky wax

In an acrylic denture requiring repair, the various components of the broken denture need to be held together temporarily. Wax may be used for this purpose and one such wax has been designed specifically for the purpose, called **sticky wax** (Figure 16.17). As its name implies, the material is sticky when melted and flows to closely adapt to the surface of the fragments to be splinted. However, once it has set, sticky wax is firm and quite brittle so that it fractures rather than flexes. To achieve the required properties various formulations have been produced, but generally these contain a proportion of beeswax mixed with natural resins such as dammar.

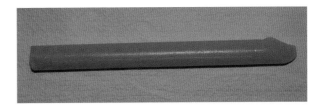

Fig. 16.17 A baton of sticky wax.

Occlusal indicator wax

This is a wax of a specific thickness (usually 1 mm) which is used by a restorative dentist to verify the amount of tooth tissue removed during tooth preparation. This may be done by placing the wax (whose thickness is known) on to the preparation and asking the patient to close together. The wax is then examined; no indentation signifies that there is more interocclusal clearance than the wax thickness and any indentation will indicate that clearance less than the wax thickness is present. This wax contains low temperature softening waxes, which permit its adaptation to the tooth surface at oral temperatures.

Commercially available products

A selection of dental wax products which are currently available are listed in Table 16.2.

Table 16.2 Some dental wax products currently available on the market

Product	Manufacturer	Comments
Alminax	Kemdent	Aluminium-reinforced wax in sheet form
Anutex	Associated Dental	Modelling wax in sheet form
Beauty Wax	Moyco	Hard baseplate wax with a narrow melting range in sheet form
Blue Inlay Casting Wax	Kerr Hawe	Inlay wax
Model Cement	Dentsply	Sticky wax
Occlusal Indicator Wax	Kerr Hawe	Green Indicator wax
Orthodontic Tray Wax	Kerr Hawe	White soft wax
Ribbon/Beading Wax	Kemdent	Soft malleable wax
Sticky Wax	Kemdent	Low melting point beeswax
Tenatex Modelling Wax	Kemdent	Modelling (baseplate) wax
Tooth Carding Wax	Kemdent	Soft malleable wax
W3 Universal Wax	Dentsply	Modelling wax in sheet form

OCCLUSAL REGISTRATION MATERIALS

A number of dental materials are available to the restorative dentist for recording occlusal relationships. Waxes have been used for this purpose for many years but as described earlier, they may distort during function and stress relieve. This may lead to an inaccurate recording and the study casts being incorrectly mounted onto the articulator. As a result, substantial occlusal modification would be required to the restoration. It is therefore critical that these materials are accurate and dimensionally stable. More recently, other materials have been considered and the materials now used are either based on the **addition silicone** or **polyether** elastomers (Chapter 15) and **higher methacrylate resins** (Chapters 14 and 23). However, some wax products are still available for this purpose.

The waxes used for occlusal registration require strengthening to overcome the problems of distortion. This may be done by altering the composition of the wax (Moyco Beauty), the addition of aluminium to the wax (such as Alminax, Kemdent) or by using a metal framework. Unfortunately even with these methods the problem of distortion may not be fully overcome. The way that these materials are used may also introduce inaccuracies. For example, if the patient is asked to close together the wax even when soft resists the teeth and

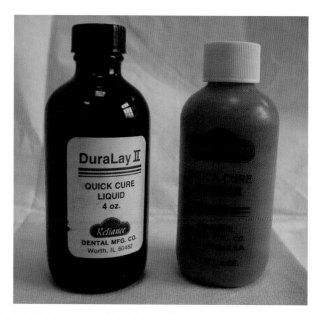

Fig. 16.18 An example of a higher methacrylate resin material (DuraLay II, Reliance) used for many purposes in restorative dentistry.

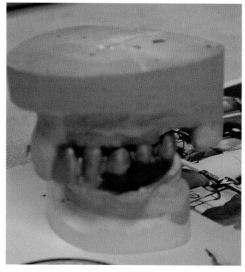

Fig. 16.19 The red occlusal registration material being used to locate the correct occlusal relationship between the upper and lower arches outwith the mouth is DuraLay (Reliance).

the patient tends to bite rather than close together. This will lead to the incorrect occlusal relationship being recorded. For further details of the correct method of occlusal registration, the reader is referred to an operative dentistry text.

The other materials used for occlusal registration are placed on the teeth in a fluid form. They will then set to a solid which can then be removed. **Higher methacrylates** such as DuraLay (Reliance) (Figure 16.18) are more rigid when set but can flow into undercuts and may be difficult to remove from the mouth. For recording the occlusal relationship these materials are mixed into a dough (Figure 16.19).

The dentist may also have asked the dental technician to construct some copings using the same material and these may be used in combination with the dough to record the occlusion. The dough and the coping would bond together, making localization outwith the mouth obvious.

Coping: a thin layer of material that covers the preparation to the margins (Figure 16.20). It may be made of many different materials.

The interocclusal clearance may also be measured using this material. When the preparation has been completed, higher methacrylate dough is mixed and placed onto the preparation. The patient is asked to close together and the material sets. When set the thickness of material may be measured using an Iwannson gauge and this will indicate the interocclusal distance.

The higher methacrylate resins may also be used to build up inlays or post and cores directly in the mouth or indirectly in the laboratory. The **bead-on technique** is used whereby the dentist or dental technician uses a paint brush and dips the brush into the monomer and then the polymer. A bead of material is then formed and this may be applied to the tooth preparation or model. The material also has the advantage that it burns out cleanly during the lost wax technique.

The last group of occlusal registration materials currently used are based on impression elastomers. **Addition silicones** are most commonly used but at least one product that is available is a **polyether**. These materials are easier to remove and manipulate but may present

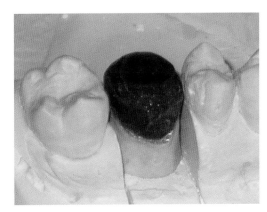

Fig. 16.20 A coping made out of DuraLay (Reliance), which may be used to verify the margins of the preparation. It may also be used to record the occlusion by the addition of unset DuraLay on its occlusal surface. The patient occludes into the unset DuraLay dough, and once it has hardened the occlusal relationship is apparent.

the dental technician with some difficulties as the stone models may 'bounce' slightly as the rubber is not rigid. Attempts to stiffen the rubber have improved this but this bounce phenomenon will still occur. Figure 16.21 shows an example of this material in use.

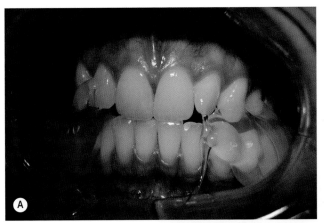
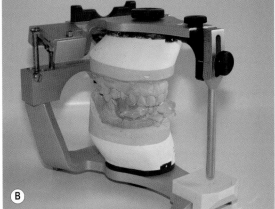
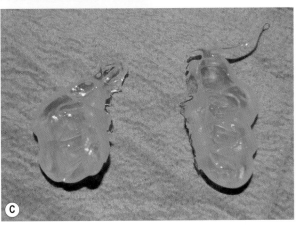

Fig. 16.21 An occlusal bite registration material (Memosil 2, Heraeus) being used to record the patient's protrusive position. (A) Intraoral photograph with the records in situ. The records may then be transferred to (B) the models, which have been mounted on the articulator to permit the angles on the articulator to be set. (C) the bite records removed from the mouth.

Some clinicians also use this material instead of wax to record the maxillary arch on the facebow bite fork (Figure 16.22).

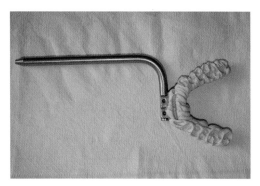

Fig. 16.22 An addition silicone occlusal registration material (Blu Mousse, Parkell Davis) being used in conjunction with a facebow bite fork as an alternative to wax.

Commercially available products

Some of the common bite registration products currently available are shown in Table 16.3.

Table 16.3 Some bite registration products currently available on the market

Product	Manufacturer	Comments
Aquasil Bite	Dentsply	Silicone
Blu Mousse	Parkell Davis	Silicone
Colorbite D	Zhermack	Silicone
DuraLay	Reliance	Polymethacrylate
DuraLay II Inlay Resin	Reliance	Polymethacrylate
Exabite II NDS	GC	Silicone
Exabite II	GC	Silicone
Flexitime Bite	Heraeus	Silicone
Futar-D	Kettenbach	Silicone
Genie Bite	Sultan	Silicone
Imprint Bite	3M ESPE	Silicone
Jet Blue Bite	Coltène Whaledent	Silicone
LuxaBite	DMG	Bis-acrylate
Memoreg 2	Heraeus	Silicone
Memosil 2	Heraeus	Silicone, transparent
O-Bite	DMG	Silicone
Occlufast Rock	Zhermack	Silicone
Pattern Resin LS	GC	Self-curing modelling resin
President Jet Bite	Coltène Whaledent	Silicone
Ramitec	3M ESPE	Polyether
Registrado X-tra	Voco	Silicone
Stonebite	Dreve	Silicone
Take 1 Advanced	Kerr Hawe	Silicone
Virtual	Ivoclar Vivadent	Silicone

SUMMARY

- Waxes are commonly used both in operative dentistry and in the dental laboratory.
- The composition of the wax differs, conveying various properties to it depending on its intended use.
- Waxes may be used to construct patterns which will be cast into metal, for boxing impressions, to hold denture components together while the acrylic is repaired, in the construction of occlusal rims and for setting teeth during the production of dentures.
- Waxes are used for recording occlusal relationships but because they tend to distort, other materials are now more commonly used such as some higher methacrylate resins and elastomers (addition silicone and polyether).

FURTHER READING

Craig, R.G., Powers, J.M., Wataha, J.C., 2004. Dental Materials: Properties and Manipulation. Mosby Elsevier, St Louis (See Chapter 10).

McCabe, J.F., Walls, A.W.G., 2008. Applied Dental Materials, ninth ed. Blackwell Munksgaard, Oxford (See Chapter 4).

Powers, J.M., Sakaguchi, R.L. (Eds.), 2006. Craig's Restorative Dental Materials (twelfth ed.). Mosby Elsevier, St Louis (See Chapter 14).

SELF-ASSESSMENT QUESTIONS

1. A wax-up of a crown is not invested immediately and left overnight. The crown after casting does not fit. What may have caused this?
2. An inlay wax is left in a heating pot to maintain it in liquid form. What are the problems associated with this?
3. What type of wax is appropriate for constructing a bite rim? What precautions should be taken to ensure the rim is stable?
4. What materials are available for occlusal registration? What are the advantages and disadvantages of each?

Section | IV |

Other clinical materials

Chapter 17

Preventive and periodontal materials, implants and biomaterials

From this chapter, the reader will:

- Be aware of the many preventive products available on the market and be able to prescribe them appropriately
- Have a knowledge of the products which aid in the diagnosis of dental diseases or help identify at-risk patients
- Be aware of the materials used in periodontics, such as local antimicrobials and regenerative materials
- Understand the rationale behind the use of these materials and how to use them to best effect
- Have a working knowledge of the various oral surgical materials
- Understand the materials used in relation to dental implants
- Know the names of currently available commercial products.

INTRODUCTION

The old adage of prevention being better than cure is never truer than in dentistry. As dental tissues do not repair themselves readily, preventive dentistry has a critical role. Many of the vast range of products available on the market have a dual role, in that they are to prevent both dental caries and periodontal disease. This is mainly achieved by the control of dental plaque, by breaking down the biofilm and the killing of microorganisms. However, they may also perform additional functions, for example having a desensitizing effect on hypersensitive teeth. It is therefore not possible to categorize neatly these multifaceted products in a convenient way.

> **Dental plaque:** the complex biofilm that is heavily populated with the bacteria responsible for dental disease.

It is often the case that the sooner the diagnosis is made, the more favourable will be the outcome and **prognosis** for the patient. Of course it would be more preferable to identify patients who may be at a higher risk of developing a disease. This would allow preventive measures to be instigated, or the patient to be referred for specialist monitoring or treatment. A number of products are available on the market which may be used by the dental team at the chairside to this end. These range from disclosing solutions to identify dental plaque to products which stain potentially cancerous or **malignant** lesions.

For those patients with periodontal disease, a condition which still has no cure, products are available which either kill the microorganisms in the periodontal pocket or can be used to aid regeneration of the tissues that have been lost as a result of the disease process. There are many such biomaterials available and these may also be used in other oral surgical disciplines, as well as when placing dental implants to replace and aid regeneration of lost tissues.

> **Periodontal pocket:** a pathologically deepened gingival sulcus, the base of which is apical to the cementoenamel junction.
> **Biomaterial:** a material that interacts with a biological system.

PREVENTIVE MATERIALS

Toothpastes

Toothpastes are also known as **dentifrices** and their main function is to 'clean' teeth. They achieve this by:

- Removing food debris, plaque, pellicle and any extrinsic stain
- Polishing the surface of the tooth to reduce the risk of adherence of debris
- Providing a means of delivering various forms of therapeutic agent.

Composition

The main ingredient is some form of **abrasive**, which will mechanically remove debris and also help in the polishing process. Toothpastes may contain some form of **detergent** to aid the cleaning process and improve the wetting of the surface of the teeth.

Therapeutic agents such as one of the various forms of **fluoride** and whitening agents are added to enhance the enamel surface. **Calculus (tartar) control agents** such as **sodium pyrophosphate** and **potassium pyrophosphate** are also incorporated as well as **desensitizing** agents such as **strontium chloride, potassium nitrate** and **calcium sodium phosphosilicate**. See Table 17.1 for a list of common toothpaste ingredients.

Table 17.1 Typical constituents of toothpaste

Component	Chemical example	Function	Approximate proportion (%)
Binders	Carrageenan	Thickening agents and to inhibit liquid and solid separation. Carrageenan is made from red seaweed, cellulose gum from wood pulp or cotton linters and xanthan gum from glucose or sucrose	3–5
	Cellulose gum		
	Xanthan gum		
	polyvinylmethyl ether/maleic acid copolymer (PVM/MA)		
Colouring agents	Food colourants	Give the toothpaste colour. For example, chlorophyll provides a green colour to toothpaste and titanium oxide makes toothpaste white	1–2
Flavouring agents	Peppermint	Make the taste of the toothpaste acceptable. The flavouring masks the taste of the detergent (particularly sodium laurel sulphate)	1–2
	Spearmint		
	Wintergreen		
	Cinnamon		
Humectants	Glycerine Sorbitol	Give the toothpaste texture and maintain moisture content	20–30
Abrasives	Hydrated silica	Various sizes and hardnesses of abrasives are added to aid removal of plaque and debris and polish the enamel after debris removal	22–55
	Hydrated alumina		
	Calcium carbonate		
	Dicalcium phosphate dihydrate		
	Sodium bicarbonate		
	Mica	A milder abrasive that is sometimes included to assist in the polishing process	2–3
Preservatives	Sodium benzoate	Prevent breakdown of toothpaste	1–2
	Methyl or ethyl paraben		
Detergents	Sodium laurel sulphate	Aid in debris removal	1–2
Preventive additives	Sodium monofluorphosphate	Types of agent that may be taken up by the tooth to increase the fluoride content of the surface enamel	0–1
	Stannous fluoride		
	Sodium fluoride		
	Zinc lactate	Acts to disrupt bacterial plaque metabolism, often used in conjunction with stannous fluoride and sodium hexametaphosphate	
Calculus control agents	Sodium pyrophosphate	Inhibit the formation of calculus	0–1
	Potassium pyrophosphate		
	Sodium hexametaphosphate		
Suspension agent	Water	Suspends the insoluble ingredients for mixing	15–20
Desensitizing agents	Strontium chloride	Work either by occluding the dentinal tubules, disrupting the nerve signal or applying a mineral coating using a bioactive material	0–5
	Potassium nitrate		
	Calcium sodium phosphosilicate		
Antibacterial agent	Triclosan	Antibacterial and antifungal agent. Primarily included for control of gingival disease	0–0.3

More recently there have been attempts to add **antimicrobial agents** such as **triclosan**, an antibacterial and antifungal agent that is effective in preventing gingivitis (Figure 17.1). Chemically, triclosan is a **polychlorophenoxyphenol**. These antimicrobial agents help to control bacterial growth by preventing the bacterial proliferation phase of plaque development. Many dentists recommend a toothpaste to their patients which contains fluoride, triclosan and some form of pyrophosphate for the reasons mentioned above and described in detail later.

Flavouring agents may also include saccharin and xylitol. These are sugar substitutes, and xylitol is associated with caries inhibition. A variety of tooth-whitening agents may also be added. These are generally based on peroxide chemistry. For further details of these bleaching agents, see Chapter 18.

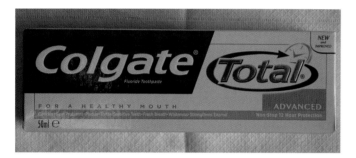

Fig. 17.1 A toothpaste containing triclosan (Colgate Total Advanced).

The factors which influence the effect of a toothpaste on the teeth are shown in Box 17.1.

Box 17.1 Factors influencing the effect of a toothpaste on the teeth

- The composition of toothpaste
- Amount of toothpaste used
- Type of brush and force applied during brushing
- Frequency of tooth brushing and the time taken
- Positioning of the toothbrush and the manner in which it is used
- Type of saliva
- Degree of gingival recession and exposed roots
- Dental materials used to restore the teeth

Mode of action of desensitizing agents

The primary mode of action is by occlusion of the dentine tubules on the exposed root surface. Therefore the tooth is treated with a physical or chemical agent that forms a layer that mechanically obstructs the orifice to the tubule. This prevents tubular fluid movement and leads to a reduction in sensitivity. An alternative method of reduction in sensitivity is by blockage of nerve activity. Potassium ions concentrated within the interior of the dentine tubules are thought to cause depolarization of the membrane of the nerve terminal and this will decrease sensitivity. Unfortunately, with both these approaches, the effects are short term as the abrasive in the toothpaste will not only remove plaque but will also remove some of the outer surface of the root face and the sensitivity will return. In addition, if the patient consumes acidic solutions such as orange or lemon juice or any highly acidic food, there is a risk of tooth surface erosion and loss of the occluding material.

Calcium sodium phosphosilicate, a bioactive glass, has been incorporated into one toothpaste to reduce sensitivity. It undergoes a chemical reaction when which exposed to an aqueous medium such as saliva, provides calcium and phosphate ions. These ions react with tooth tissue to form hydroxy-carbonate-apatite, a mineral that is chemically similar to the inorganic phase of enamel and dentine. This layer has been shown to be effective in preventing further tooth surface demineralization.

Fluoride agents

Three different types of fluoride are used in toothpastes: **stannous fluoride**, **sodium fluoride** and **sodium monofluorophosphate**. In all cases, the formulation of the toothpaste has required considerable care as the interaction between some of the ingredients reduces the fluoride effect. Both the simple fluoride salts are relatively reactive. The addition of stannous fluoride went out of fashion a number of years ago as there were stability problems with the toothpastes and the taste was not particularly pleasant. Some patients also developed intrinsic staining. However, more recently a stabilized form of stannous fluoride has been developed with much better results.

Stannous fluoride is frequently used in combination with sodium hexametaphosphate, providing 1100 ppm fluoride (Figure 17.2). Stannous fluoride has been demonstrated to

- Strengthen the enamel by inhibiting demineralization and promoting remineralization
- Stop the multiplication of *Streptococcus mutans* (one of the bacteria implicated in the development of dental caries).

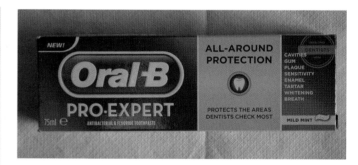

Fig. 17.2 A toothpaste containing stannous fluoride and sodium hexametaphosphate (Pro-Expert, Oral B).

One of the main advantages of stannous fluoride is that it can be used in conjunction with calcium-based abrasives. Sodium fluoride is an alternative to stannous fluoride, but the prime difficulty with its use was the need to change a large number of the abrasives in the standard toothpaste formulations as the use of calcium-based materials leads to degradation of the mixture.

Sodium monofluorophosphate has been used as an alternative as it is more stable and not so susceptible to degradation. Most currently available toothpastes use either 0.45% stabilized stannous fluoride or the equivalent sodium fluoride concentration of 0.24%. Both deliver 1100 ppm fluoride. As well as the well-proven success in reducing the incidence of caries, both these materials also appear to have some beneficial effect on gingival health. Higher levels of fluoride are provided in certain toothpastes, which are recommended for patients with a high caries incidence. These can produce the equivalent of 2400 and 5000 ppm fluoride (Figure 17.3).

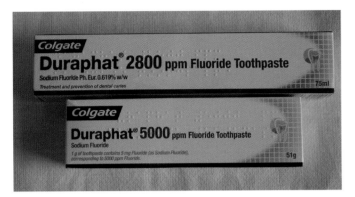

Fig. 17.3 Two dentifrices with higher levels of fluoride for use by patients with high caries risk (Duraphat 2800 and 5000, Colgate).

They should be used with care as overzealous use can potentially lead to **enamel fluorosis** (Figure 17.4) if too much is swallowed. Similarly some toothpastes are available which contain a lower concentration of fluoride and are intended for use by children and infants (Figure 17.5).

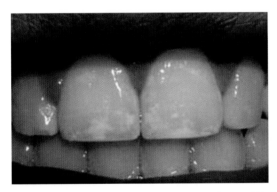

Fig. 17.4 'Mottled' appearance of incisors indicative of enamel fluorosis.

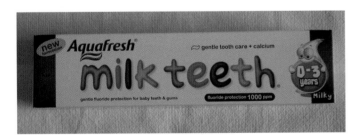

Fig. 17.5 A dentifrice containing a lower concentration of fluoride. This product contains 1000 ppm of fluoride and is meant for the use by children and infants 0–3 years of age.

Anticalculus agents

These are usually either tetra sodium or tetra potassium pyrophosphates. They inhibit growth of hydroxyapatite crystals and this in turn inhibits calculus formation above the gingival margin. Anticalculus agents have a bitter taste and flavourings are added to toothpastes to mask this taste. Sodium hexametaphosphate is a more recent addition to the list of anticalculus agents and appears to be as effective as the older materials.

Abrasives

The abrasives in toothpastes carry both benefits and risks for the teeth. The benefit is that the abrasive helps remove the debris but the risk is that if the abrasive is too effective it will also remove tooth substance. This problem is compounded by the fact that there are three different tooth tissues which may come in contact with the abrasive, all of which have different hardnesses and resistance to abrasion. Enamel is highly resistant to abrasion, dentine is more prone to abrasion while dental cementum is very easily abraded. Fortunately, toothpastes do not need to be too abrasive.

The standard toothpastes use calcium salts with the addition of alumina, whereas those where sodium fluoride is added use silica and mica, a sheet silicate (phyllosilicate) mineral, together with, in some cases, polymer beads, which may also act as an abrasive. The size and shape of the abrasive will influence the abrasiveness of the paste.

Children may be exposed to excessive fluoride if they swallow or ingest toothpaste or eat it. They should therefore put only a pea-sized amount of toothpaste on the toothbrush or even just a smear in the case of a toddler.

In order to maximize the time the toothpaste is in contact with the teeth and therefore the time the active ingredient (fluoride) may work, patients should be encouraged to 'spit and not rinse' after tooth brushing.

Commercially available products

Table 17.2 and Figure 17.6 show representative examples of commercially available toothpastes. It is apparent that many international pharmaceutical companies sell a variety of toothpastes under different brand names. Many are claimed to carry out similar processes.

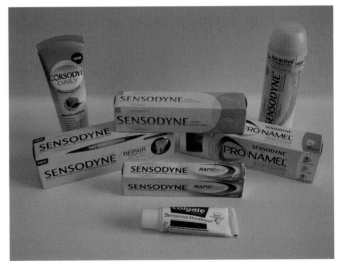

Fig. 17.6 Some of the many toothpaste products available on the market.

Table 17.2 Some toothpastes currently available on the market

Product	Manufacturer	Comments
Aquafresh Big Teeth	GlaxoSmithKline	6 + years; 1400 ppm fluoride
Aquafresh Fresh 'N' Minty	GlaxoSmithKline	
Aquafresh ISO Active	GlaxoSmithKline	
Aquafresh Little Teeth	GlaxoSmithKline	4–6 years and above, 1000 ppm fluoride
Aquafresh Milk Teeth	GlaxoSmithKline	0–3 years and above, 500 ppm fluoride
Arm and Hammer Advanced Whitening	Arm and Hammer	Baking soda base with micropolishing abrasives to polish the surface of the teeth
Arm and Hammer Enamelcare Whitening	Arm and Hammer	Contains calcium phosphate-based remineralizing system
Arm and Hammer Original Coolmint	Arm and Hammer	Abrasive is baking soda, so is less abrasive
Arm and Hammer Enamel Care Sensitive	Arm and Hammer	Addition of calcium phosphate-based agent to coat the foot surface
Colgate Proclincal White	Colgate	0.24% sodium fluoride
Colgate Cavity Protection	Colgate	0.76% sodium monofluorophosphate
Colgate Total Advanced clean	Colgate	Abrasive is silica
Colgate Oxygen Pure Freshness	Colgate	
Colgate Sensitive Pro-Relief	Colgate	1450 ppm as sodium monofluorophosphate
Colgate Smiles Toothpaste	Colgate	
Colgate Total Gum defence	Colgate	Triclosan copolymer added
Corsodyl Daily	GlaxoSmithKline	0.31% sodium fluoride (1400 ppm)
Crest	P&G Oral Health	
Crest Complete	P&G Oral Health	
Duraphat 2800 ppm	Colgate	Over 10 years (POM)
Duraphat 5000 ppm	Colgate	Over 16 years (POM)
Macleans White and Clean ISO-active	P&G Oral Health	
Mentadent P	Unilever	
Oral-B Children's Toothpaste	P&G Oral Health	2–4 years of age 5–7 years of age
Oral B Pro Expert	P&G Oral Health	Over 12 years, stannous fluoride
Pronamel Sensodyne	GlaxoSmithKline	
Retardex	Rowpar Pharmaceuticals Inc.	
Rembrandt Plus	P&G Oral Health	
Rembrandt Sensitive	P&G Oral Health	
Sensodyne Original	GlaxoSmithKline	Fluoride free
Sensodyne Rapid Relief	GlaxoSmithKline	
Sensodyne Toothpaste Gel	GlaxoSmithKline	POM
Sensodyne Total Care Extra Fresh	GlaxoSmithKline	
Sensodyne Whitening	GlaxoSmithKline	

POM, prescription only medicine. These toothpastes therefore should be prescribed by a dentist or doctor.

Mouthwashes

A mouthwash is a liquid solution used to deliver active chemicals to the teeth and the oral soft tissues. They are also referred to as **mouthrinses** and are most effective when used after brushing. They consist of an **active agent** which is dissolved in a carrier such as **water** or **alcohol**. The active agent may be **antimicrobial** or may confer protection against dental caries, in which case it will contain a fluoride preparation such as sodium fluoride. Mouthwashes also contain surfactants to improve the wetting ability of the mixtures as some of the ingredients have a relatively high surface tension. Additionally, flavourings are added to make the mouthwash more acceptable. Some mouthrinses have been specially designed for use in patients with xerostomia.

> **Xerostomia:** a condition in which the mouth is dry and little or no saliva is produced. It is often seen in patients who have had radiotherapy for oral carcinoma or as a side effect of certain medications.

Some products contain alcohol, which acts as a preservative as well as the carrier. However, due to its erosive effects it may cause non-carious tooth surface loss. Similarly, resin-containing dental restorative materials may also be damaged by prolonged alcohol exposure from mouthrinses as the resins may soften. The use of alcohol-containing mouthrinses is unacceptable in child patients and for those whose culture precludes the use of alcohol. They should also be avoided in patients with mucositis as the alcohol will cause a painful 'stinging' reaction on the inflamed mucosa.

The action and therapeutic benefit of some mouthwash rinses is debatable and they should therefore only be viewed as a 'cosmetic' product.

Chlorhexidine

Chlorhexidine gluconate is used extensively to treat periodontal diseases. It has already been discussed in Chapter 13 as many dentists use it during the chemo-mechanical preparation of the root canal system. It is widely regarded as the gold standard active agent in periodontal treatment. It is used in a 0.2% solution and it is bacteriostatic as it inhibits growth of plaque bacteria. It has excellent **substantivity** as it remains active for up to 12 hours after the first application.

Chlorhexidine is so effective that if used long term, it can sterilize the mouth in effect. Furthermore, as it kills bacteria at higher concentrations, the dead bacteria can act as seeding agents in the mouth and increase calculus formation. Its use may also mask the patient's own oral hygiene efforts. For these reasons, unless necessary, one bottle should be used as directed (rinse 10 ml for 60 seconds twice daily) and then the treatment discontinued for a period of 2–3 weeks. However, for certain patients, such as those on radiotherapy or chemotherapy, the long-term use of chlorhexidine products is recommended.

Unfortunately, chlorhexidine has some disadvantages:

- Its main drawback is that is stains teeth quickly because it is adsorbed onto the tooth surface and chemicals which stain are attracted to it. This is more pronounced with certain substances such as tea, coffee and red wine. The margins of resin-based composites may stain as will any rough surfaces. If this occurs then care is required when removing the stain that no damage to the resin composite restoration ensues. If the product is used on a toothbrush rather than as a mouthwash then the staining and unpleasant taste is reduced. To facilitate this, a gel presentation is available (Figure 17.7). Should staining occur, it is reasonably easily removed by a professional cleaning (see Chapter 19 for information on products used for this purpose).

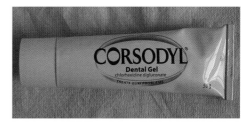

Fig. 17.7 A gel containing chlorhexidine digluconate, which may be applied to the teeth with a toothbrush.

- Its efficacy may be compromised by certain other chemicals added to products. Chlorhexidine is cationic in nature. Anionic compounds, particularly surfactants, such as sodium lauryl sulphate which is used in toothpaste to reduce staining, reduces the efficacy of chlorhexidine.
- It has a very poor penetration of the subgingival biofilm and so its use in anaerobic environments like deep periodontal pockets is limited. Furthermore, it is flushed out from the pockets by crevicular fluid too quickly and neutralized by inflammatory products such as immunoglobulins.
- It has a taste which is very difficult to mask by other chemicals, so preparations containing chlorhexidine may not have a pleasant taste. Many patients complain that it has a slightly metallic taste. Attempts to improve the taste at 0.2% have affected the efficacy.

> If a chlorhexidine-containing product is used after the ingestion of food or drink then the chances of staining will be reduced.

Clearly products containing chlorhexidine should not be used on patients who have a hypersensitivity to chlorhexidine. **Hexetidine** (an oral antibacterial and antifungal agent based on 5-amino-1,3-bis(2-ethylhexyl)hexahydro-5-methylpyrimidine) and **cetylpyridinium chloride** (a cationic quaternary ammonium compound) are also used in mouthrinses but their substantivity is lower than that of chlorhexidine. Rarely parotid swelling may occur with these products.

Commercially available products

Table 17.3 and Figure 17.8 show some of the currently available commercial mouthwashes.

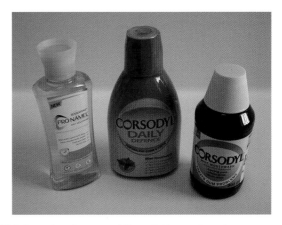

Fig. 17.8 Examples of commercially available mouthwashes.

Table 17.3 Some mouthrinses currently available on the market

Product name	Manufacturer	Active ingredient	Comments
Aquafresh Big Teeth Mouthwash	GlaxoSmithKline	225 ppm sodium fluoride	From 6 years
Aquafresh Extra Care Mouthwash	GlaxoSmithKline	250 ppm sodium fluoride	From 6 years
Aquafresh Extreme Clean Purifying Mouthwash	GlaxoSmithKline	250 ppm sodium fluoride	Adults
Chlorohex 1200	Colgate	0.12% chlorhexidine	
Chlorohex Plus	Colgate	0.2% chlorhexidine	Alcohol-free and 250 ppm fluoride, short-term use (maximum 6 weeks) and not more than 3 times per year
Clinpro	3M ESPE	0.6% stannous fluoride	Gives 240 ppm of fluoride ions when diluted with water
Colgate Veadent Plus Oral Rinse	Colgate	0.5% cetylpyridinium chloride	
Corsodyl Daily Defence	GlaxoSmithKline	0.06% chlorhexidine and 250 ppm sodium fluoride	
Corsodyl*	GlaxoSmithKline	0.2% chlorhexidine digluconate	Original, mint, alcohol-free
Duraphat Rinse	Colgate	900 ppm fluoride	Used once weekly in patients over 8 years, easier compliance
Eludril	Pierre Fabre Oral Care	Chlorhexidine and chlorobutanol	
FluoriGard Daily Dental Rinse	Colgate	0.05% sodium fluoride	Daily use
FluoriGard Fluoride Rinse AF	Colgate		Alcohol-free
Listerine	Johnson & Johnson Ltd.	Alcohol-based (21%); active ingredients include eucalyptol menthol and thymol	pH 4.2, antibacterial
Listerine Advanced	Johnson & Johnson Ltd.	Active ingredients include eucalyptol menthol and thymol	
Listerine Teeth + Gum Defence	Johnson & Johnson Ltd.		
Listerine Zero	Johnson & Johnson Ltd.		Alcohol-free, not for children under 6 years
Listermint with Fluoride	Johnson & Johnson Ltd.		
MacLeans Confidence Mouthwash	GlaxoSmithKline	250 ppm sodium fluoride	
MacLeans Freshmint Mouthwash	GlaxoSmithKline	225 ppm sodium fluoride	
Oral B Anti-Plaque	P&G Oral Health	Fluoride	Alcohol-free, not for children under 6 years
Oral B Sensitive	P&G Oral Health	Potassium nitrate and fluoride	Not for children under 6 years, alcohol-free
Oraldene Ice Mint	McNeil Products Ltd	Hexetidine	
Oraldene Mouthwash	McNeil Products Ltd	Hexetidine	
Periogard	Colgate	0.2% chlorhexidine	Children over 6 years – rinse twice daily with 10 ml for 60 seconds, use usually no more than 7 days
Peroxyl Mouthrinse	Colgate	1.5% hydrogen peroxide	Over 12 years or 6 years with supervision
Plax Multi-Protection Mouthwash	Colgate	Fluoride	
Reach Junior Fluoride Mouthwash	Johnson and Johnson		
Sensodyne Pronamel Daily Mouthwash	GlaxoSmithKline	450 ppm sodium fluoride, potassium nitrate	
Tri-Hydra polymers,	Intended against acid erosion, alcohol-free		
Sensodyne Total Care Gentle Mouthrinse	GlaxoSmithKline	230 ppm sodium fluoride, potassium chloride	Over 6 years and above
Sensodyne Total Care Gentle Mouthrinse	GlaxoSmithKline	Fluoride	

*As well as being available as a mouthwash, Corsodyl (GlaxoSmithKline) is available as a spray or a gel containing 0.2% and 1% chlorhexidine, respectively.

Other fluoride products

Fluoride gels

Fluoride gels are products that are professionally applied in the surgery as their fluoride content is high. These gels are aimed at patients undergoing orthodontic treatment or patients with a high caries risk where individual treatment is more appropriate. Care must be taken in prescribing these, as fluoride levels in the water where the patient lives together with the additional fluoride provide by the product can result in the level of fluoride in the teeth exceeding the recommended level of 1 ppm. This may lead to enamel fluorosis.

Normally, these gels are applied in a tray which is held in the mouth for a period of time or applied to the teeth after cleaning with a normal toothpaste. The residue is then spat out, care being taken to avoid ingestion of the gel. Ideally, the patient should not eat or drink anything for approximately 30 minutes after the application. These gels contain one of three chemicals: **acidulated phosphate fluoride (APF)**, **sodium fluoride** and **stannous fluoride**. These products are based on the work undertaken by Brudevold, who observed that fluoride uptake was increased in an acid environment. He demonstrated that an acid preparation containing both phosphate and fluoride ions minimized the risk of enamel dissolution by the acid and enhanced fluoride uptake. Neutral sodium fluoride (2%) gels for professional use are produced by Dentsply and Colgate markets the Phos-Flur Gel, which contains 1.1% sodium fluoride, and Acidulated Phosphate Gel.

Fluoride gels are also available for home applications. Here, the fluoride concentration is substantially lower, with the most frequently used chemical being a 0.4% stannous fluoride solution. A commercially available product is ClinPro (3M ESPE).

Another gel product, Cervitec Gel (Ivoclar Vivadent) combines fluoride in the form of 900 ppm sodium fluoride and 0.12% chlorhexidine (Figure 17.9). It is indicated to protect exposed root surfaces, treat hypersensitive areas and reduce the bacterial load on the surface of the tooth. It has been shown in clinical trials to be useful to reduce the caries rate in children.

Fluoride varnishes

A varnish presentation is a very convenient method for the application of fluoride to a tooth surface. The sticky nature of the varnish helps to retain the fluoride in contact with the tooth surface for longer than with a toothpaste or mouthrinse. A varnish is indicated in the prevention of caries, especially root caries and is also used to treat dentine hypersensitivity. The fluoride is mixed with an alcoholic solution of resins to form the varnish. This organic solvent then evaporates when applied to the tooth surface and the varnish sets when exposed to moisture. It forms insoluble calcium fluoride globules which occlude the dentine tubules.

The concentration of sodium fluoride is described as a 5% concentration. This means that 1 ml of the suspension contains 50 mg of sodium fluoride, which is equivalent to 22.6 mg fluoride. Due to the high concentration of fluoride in this material, the prescribing dentist needs to be aware of the concurrent use of other fluoride-containing products as overdose may result. The dentist should target the at-risk teeth or early carious lesions as the product should not be applied indiscriminately for the same reason. Usually, two applications a year are recommended for children over 3 years of age and adults. However, if a particular child is causing concern then it may be used up to three to four times yearly.

The best-known fluoride varnish is Duraphat (Colgate; Figure 17.10). This banana-flavoured varnish is presented in a tube or in ampoules for ease of application.

> Some fluoride varnishes contain **colophony**. This is another term for **rosin** (see Chapters 12 and 16). Patients may have hypersensitivity to colophony and so the dentist should enquire about this when taking the medical history if one of these products is being considered for use. Colophony is also contraindicated in patients with bronchial asthma.

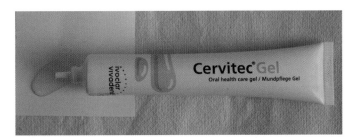

Fig. 17.9 A preventive gel containing both fluoride and chlorhexidine (Cervitec Gel, Ivoclar Vivadent).

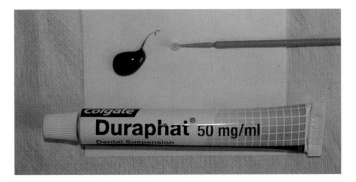

Fig. 17.10 A fluoride varnish (Duraphat, Colgate).

Desensitizing agents

Hypersensitivity to hot and cold foods and drinks may be associated with pain and may be debilitating for the patient. The dentinal tubules are filled with fluid and contain nerve terminal endings. Exposure to hot or cold stimuli causes the fluid to move within the tubules so effecting a neural response. As there are only pain receptors in the dental pulp, this response is interpreted by the brain as pain. As described above, desensitizing agents work in one of two ways:

- Desensitizing the nerve ending
- Mechanically occluding the dentinal tubules to preventing fluid movement.

There are many different presentations of desensitizing products:

- Toothpastes
- Mouthwashes
- Varnishes
- Resin-based materials.

The mode of action of desensitizing toothpastes and mouthwashes has been discussed earlier.

In order to enhance the desensitizing effect of toothpastes marketed for sensitivity, the patient should be advised to place the toothpaste on the affected tooth surface last thing at night after brushing. If the toothpaste is allowed to dwell for a longer period on the surface of the tooth (i.e. during the night) its effect will be seen more quickly.

Desensitizing varnishes

Fluoride varnishes are frequently used by dentists to treat dentinal hypersensitivity. The main indication is to apply high levels of fluoride to a particular surface in an attempt to arrest an early carious lesion. Varnishes are also very effective at reducing dentinal hypersensitivity. Probably the most commonly used product for this indication is Duraphat (Colgate), however, other varnishes are now available which are intended specifically for the treatment of dentinal hypersensitivity. One such product is Clinpro White Varnish (3M ESPE; Figure 17.11),

which also contains fluoride. In most cases, the desensitizing effect is achieved by the occlusion of the tubules and remineralization of the surrounding tooth tissue.

Other water-based varnishes act to occlude the dentinal tubules by forming insoluble calcium and protein precipitates, thus reducing dentinal permeability. VivaSens (Ivoclar Vivadent) is an acid varnish with a base of ethanol. Dimethacrylate and methacrylate modified polyacrylic acids are carried in this vehicle together with some potassium fluoride. The penetration of potassium fluoride is assisted by the presence of the acid, and the dimethacrylates are precipitated out as the alcohol evaporates. The mode of action is primarily tubular occlusion, initially by the varnish and subsequently by calcium salts being released into the tubules together with proteins from the tubular fluid. Another product called Sensitrol (Dexcel Dental) (Figure 17.12), is based on dipotassium oxalate monohydrate in solution.

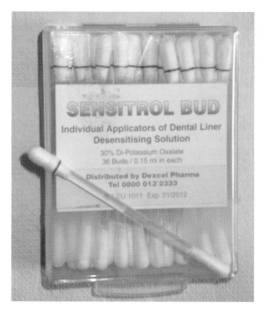

Fig. 17.12 A product based on dipotassium oxalate monohydrate in solution used for the treatment of dentine hypersensitivity (Sensitrol, Dexcel Dental).

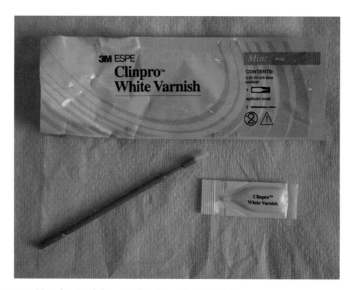

Fig. 17.11 A varnish used to treat hypersensitive dentine (Clinpro White Varnish, 3M ESPE)

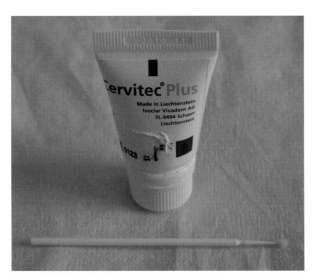

Fig. 17.13 A desensitizing varnish (Cervitec Plus, Ivoclar Vivadent).

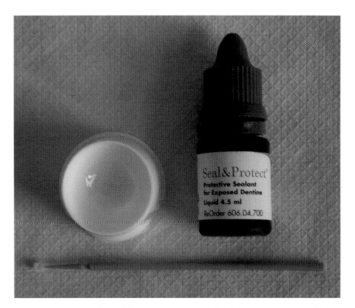

Fig. 17.14 A resin-based desensitizing agent (Seal & Protect, Dentsply).

The oxalate salt is ionized and on application leads to the precipitation of the more insoluble calcium oxalate crystals that block the tubules.

Sensitrol is applied (1–2 drops) using the supplied cotton bud (which is impregnated with oxalate) onto the affected surfaces. The surfaces being treated are gently massaged for 60–90 seconds before being gently air dried for 60 seconds. Acidic foods and drinks should be avoided for 24 hours if possible after application for best effect.

Cervitec Plus (Ivoclar Vivadent; Figure 17.13) contains thymol and works by blocking the dentinal tubules. It has a carrier of ethanol and water which reduces its susceptibility to moisture during application and therefore improves its adhesion to the tooth surface. The product has an antimicrobial effect and is **fungistatic** because it inhibits growth of microorganisms by denaturing proteins and destroying cell membranes.

> **Thymol:** a component of the essential oil gained from the herb thyme.
> **Fungistatic:** material with an inhibiting effect on the growth and reproduction of fungi without destroying them.

Resin-based composite desensitizing products

Some clinicians prefer to use a resin-based composite product which is bonded onto the affected surface to form an insoluble physical barrier. The dentinal tubules are occluded leading to a reduction in dentinal hypersensitivity. Products which fall into this category include:

- Gluma Desensitiser (Heraeus)
- Isodan (Septodont)
- SDI Soothe Desensitising Gel
- Seal & Protect (Dentsply) (Figure 17.14).

Depending on the product, some clinicians prefer not to use these materials as a first-line treatment for hypersensitivity as the preparation stage may involve acid etching of to the tooth surface. The paradox is that this may actually open up more dentinal tubules so exacerbating the problem. Being based on resin composite, these materials are hydrophobic in nature and this may be problematic when they are placed in areas where good moisture control cannot be achieved.

Tooth mousse

Another multipurpose preventive product is tooth mousse. It is indicated for the treatment of dentine hypersensitivity, but may also be used before and after tooth whitening, after professional prophylaxis, during orthodontic treatment and for facilitating remineralization.

Tooth mousse is composed of **casein phosphopeptide (CPP)**, which is a milk protein. This chemical carries calcium and phosphate ions 'stuck' to it in the form of **amorphous calcium phosphate (ACP)**. This forms a complex of **CPP-ACP**, whose proprietary name is **Recaldent**. CPP maintains amorphous calcium phosphate and calcium fluoride stabilized in aqueous solution in the form of calcium phosphate and fluoride ions. It is hydrophilic in nature being water based, and this facilitates its application and usage. CCP is an ideal delivery system for the ions as they are freely available and on application to the tooth surface will precipitate out, resulting in remineralization of the tooth surface. The product binds effectively to enamel, pellicle and soft tissue, giving a longer lasting effect. It also reduces the adherence of certain plaque bacteria and stimulates salivary flow. As the product is based on lactose, it should not be used in those patients who are sensitive to milk proteins and/or hydroxybenzoates.

>
>
> Patients should be asked whether they have a milk protein allergy, as tooth mousse will be contraindicated for this group.

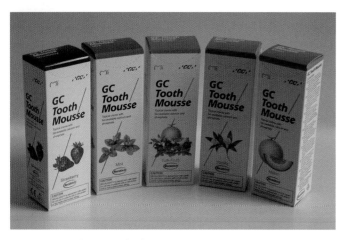

Fig. 17.15 Tooth Mousse (GC).

The product is applied with a finger or cotton bud to the tooth surface at night and/or in the morning. It takes 2–5 minutes for its action to commence. GC Tooth Mousse is an example of one such product and is available in different flavours, namely mint, strawberry, melon, tutti-frutti and vanilla (Figure 17.15).

GC also produces GC MI Paste Plus, which contains 900 ppm fluoride as 0.2% sodium fluoride as well as the CPP-ACP mixture and is claims to enhance remineralization. Recaldent chewing gum is available in some countries but not in the European Union.

Denture care-related materials

Denture cleansers

Good denture hygiene is as important as good oral hygiene. As with the teeth and the oral soft tissues, bacteria and fungi may colonize on the surfaces of a denture irrespective of the material from which it is constructed. These microorganisms exist in plaque, and this plaque, together with food debris, should be removed from the denture surface. Failure to do this may result in infection of the denture-bearing soft tissues, or in the case of a partial denture, damage to abutment teeth in the form of caries.

Many bespoke proprietary denture-cleansing products are available. Ideally these products should be bactericidal and fungicidal. Many products are based on sodium hypochlorite solution, which is effective against both bacteria and fungi. It is also advantageous if a denture cleanser can break down the biofilm and some products may contain citric acid for this reason. Some cleansers in the form of pastes contain the same detergents found in regular toothpaste. Other tablet and powder forms may also contain alkaline compounds, together with detergents and sodium perborate, which when added to water, forms an alkaline peroxide solution. This breaks down to release oxygen, which helps in debris removal.

It is important to be aware that prolonged exposure to any solution containing the chloride ion may cause the (pink) coloured acrylics to bleach white and thus to lose their pigmentation. The instructions for use should be carefully followed, and in the case of sodium hypochlorite solution, a solution of one teaspoon to a tumbler of water should be used for 20 minutes only.

Furthermore, corrosion may occur in dentures containing metal components such as cobalt chrome or stainless steel. These therefore should not be cleaned with sodium hypochlorite solution. Light brushing with soap and water is probably as effective as anything else, unless the denture is heavily contaminated (see Chapter 23).

The use of toothpastes on acrylic dentures should be avoided; the abrasive component of the toothpaste will take the polish off the acrylic surface leading to staining.

Commercially available products

Currently available examples of denture cleaning products are shown in Table 17.4.

Table 17.4 Some denture-cleansing products currently available on the market

Product	Manufacturer
Dentu-Crème	GlaxoSmithKline
Milton Sterilising Fluid	Milton
Poligrip 3 Min Ultra Denture Cleansing Tablets	GlaxoSmithKline
Poligrip Total Care Denture Cleansing Tablets	GlaxoSmithKline
Steradent	Reckitt Benckiser (UK) Ltd

Denture adhesives

Many patients find it challenging to keep the denture in place, particularly a complete lower denture. **Denture adhesives** or **fixatives** are available, which 'glue' the prosthesis to the supporting oral mucosa in an attempt to improve the retention and function of the denture. The amount of food finding its way under the denture during function may also be reduced. Notwithstanding this, a satisfactory denture should not require the use of a denture adhesive and the dentist should ensure that before such a product is recommended, the prosthesis has been properly constructed and is well fitting.

Denture adhesive materials generally contain **gelatin**, **pectin** or a **gum**. They may be thickened by the inclusion of **cellulose** or a filler such as **magnesium oxide**. Some products contain antibacterial agents (one example is **hexachlorophene**) and **sodium lauryl sulphate** is often present to reduce surface tension and ensure that the denture adhesive will flow evenly. Some products may be flavoured. They are presented either as a paste, which is squeezed from a tube and applied to the fitting surface of the denture (Figure 17.16), or as a powder which is sprinkled on. Other products are presented as pads that are placed onto the fitting surface of the denture prior to its insertion into the mouth.

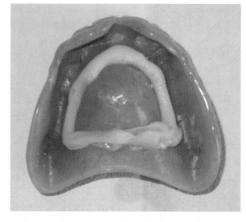

Fig. 17.16 A denture-fixative material applied to the fitting surface of an upper complete denture prior to insertion in the mouth.

Commercially available products

Representative examples of commercially available material are shown in Table 17.5.

Table 17.5 Some denture adhesives currently available on the market

Product	Manufacturer
Fixodent Food Seal	P&G Oral Health
Fixodent Hygiene	P&G Oral Health
Fixodent Neutral Taste	P&G Oral Health
Fixodent Original	P&G Oral Health
Poligrip Flavour Free	GlaxoSmithKline
Poligrip Gum Care	GlaxoSmithKline
Poligrip Super Wernets	GlaxoSmithKline
Poligrip Ultra	GlaxoSmithKline
Poligrip Ultra Wernets	GlaxoSmithKline

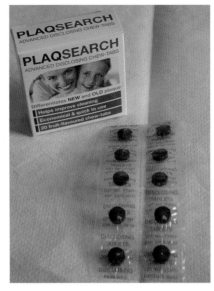

Fig. 17.17 Disclosing tablets used to stain plaque to aid its identification (Plaqsearch, Molar Ltd).

AIDS TO DIAGNOSIS OF DENTAL DISEASES

Disclosing products

These products are designed to highlight the presence of dental plaque. **Disclosing tablets** are composed of a harmless food colouring dye (**erythrosine**) which is taken up by the plaque (Figure 17.17). They may be used in one of two ways, both as a toothbrushing and oral hygiene instruction tool. The first method is that the patient should crunch one of the tablets in their mouth and swill the resulting fluid around. The excess liquid should be expectorated. The patient then inspects their teeth in the mirror for any stained surfaces and is encouraged to use their toothbrush to '**get the stain off**' (Figure 17.18).

Alternatively the patient should first carry out their normal oral hygiene procedures. The quality of the plaque removal can then be verified by using a disclosing tablet to show the plaque remaining. Any stained teeth will clearly show which areas the patient has missed. This will therefore highlight any deficiencies in oral hygiene technique, allowing the dentist and patient to focus on how improvement can be made.

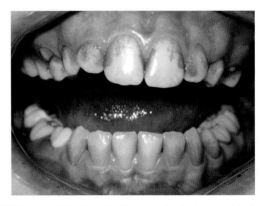

Fig. 17.18 Plaque stained purple after use of a disclosing tablet by a child. The stain is removed by toothbrushing.

Other more sophisticated tests are available, which are designed to be used by the dental care professionals in the surgery. These **disclosing solutions** demonstrate the presence of plaque, such as the Plaque Indicator Kit (GC) and the Plaque Test (Ivoclar Vivadent) (Figure 17.19).

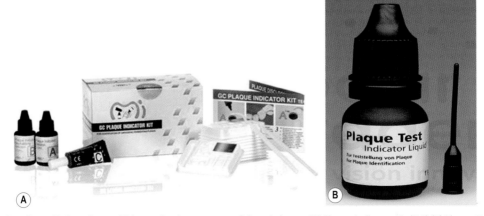

Fig. 17.19 Two professionally applied products which test for the presence of dental plaque: (A) Plaque Indicator Kit (GC) (B) Plaque Test (Ivoclar Vivadent).

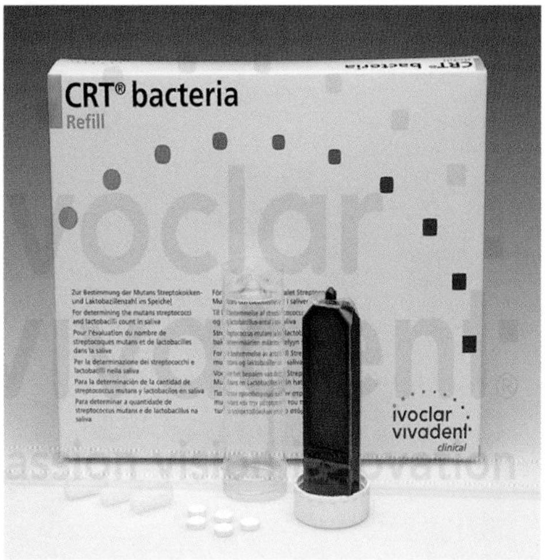

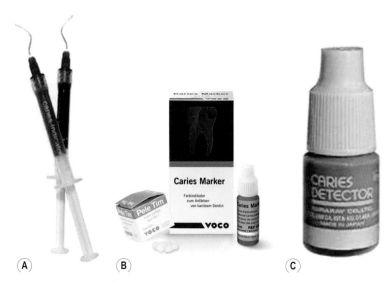

Fig. 17.20 A product that reveals the levels of *Streptococcus mutans* on the teeth (CRT bacteria, Ivoclar Vivadent).

In the latter test the plaque fluoresces under polymerization light, demonstrating its presence. These are usually applied to the surfaces of the teeth on a cotton bud. They are two-toned solutions and can show plaque which has been present for more than 24 hours as the colour varies with the length of time the plaque has been in situ.

Another product (CRT (Caries Risk Test) bacteria, Ivoclar Vivadent, Figure 17.20) reveals the levels of *Streptococcus mutans* on the teeth, one of the most important cariogenic bacteria. It can be used to help the dental team formulate a preventive plan tailored to the needs of the patient.

Dental caries indicators

Some dentists prefer to use an indicating solution during cavity preparation (Figure 17.21). These products contain an indicator dye such as acid red in a propylene glycol carrier solution. They preferentially stain dentine that is demineralized and irreversibly damaged. This stained tooth tissue may then be removed and the dentist reassured that no carious dentine remains. Unfortunately, since the indicators stain both partly and fully demineralized dentine, the dentist may remove more dentine than is necessary, which is clearly undesirable.

Similar products are available which may be used to stain cracks in teeth or to detect root canal orifices. Both of these features may be very difficult to see clinically and the use of a harmless dye such as acid red may aid in their identification.

Dental caries removal solution

One product, launched a number of years ago, offers a chemo-mechanical approach to smooth surface caries removal. The advantage of the product is that it is claimed to be a more conservative technique than the use of rotary instrumentation. Carisolv gel (MediTeam) consists of 0.5% sodium hypochlorite and three amino acids which are supplied as a red coloured gel. The gel is applied to the lesion and allowed to soak in for 30 seconds, and then the softened tooth tissue is removed by scraping with the specially designed instruments. This process is repeated until the gel no longer turns cloudy. The cavity can then be restored conventionally. The product is supplied as a single or multimix presentation and should be stored in the fridge.

The mode of action relies on the sodium hypochlorite combining with the amino acids at a high pH. The chloride ion reacts with amino groups and an *N*-chlorinated form of the amino acid is produced. The loosely bound chlorine is active and can react with the denatured collagen in the carious lesion. The *N*-chlorinated amino acid is unstable and breaks down relatively quickly, so rendering the compound inactive. This ensures that no further denaturing of the collagen occurs after the patient has left the surgery.

Saliva buffering capacity-checking materials

Saliva has an important protective role. As has been explained earlier, saliva buffers acids produced by oral bacteria and neutralizes other acids taken into the mouth such as erosive beverages. An insufficient quantity and quality of saliva severely compromises the ability of patients to protect against harmful intraoral conditions. Salivary flow may be reduced as a side effect of many medications and with increasing age. Furthermore, if the salivary glands have been exposed to radiation as a consequence of radiotherapy for the treatment of head and neck cancers, their function may be significantly compromised.

Fig. 17.21 (A) Syringes with Caries Indicator (Vista Dental Products). (B) Caries Marker (Voco). (C) Caries Detector (Kuraray).

There are at least two products on the market which test the buffering capacity of saliva: CRT (Caries Risk Test) buffer (Ivoclar Vivadent) and the GC Saliva-Check Buffer (GC) (Figure 17.22). Both products can be used for chairside testing for saliva quality, pH and buffering capacity. The results are available in a matter of minutes.

The release of lactic acid is a more reliable indicator of cariogenic potential than quantitative measurement of bacteria. Another test which is used to identify patients at risk of dental caries measures the lactic acid formation rate. A high reading will allow a targeted preventive regimen to be instituted. The Clinpro Cario L-Pop (3M ESPE) system involves a lactic acid indicator swab sample being collected from the dorsal surface of the tongue. The biofilm found on this region of the tongue is comparable with that on the tooth surface. The reading of the colour change of the swab may be compared with the shade card provided and a risk assessment made. The test takes 2 minutes.

Products to treat xerostomia

Xerostomia or dry mouth is, unfortunately, a common problem in the adult population. Available preparations aim to supplement natural saliva and to provide the missing enzymes and proteins found with hyposalivation. The products may be in the form of moisturizing mouthrinses, gels and toothpastes. The mouthwashes tend to be fluoride-containing and alcohol-free. Non-stick, sugar-free chewing gum is also available to help stimulate saliva production. This will not adhere to dentures and is sweetened with xylitol. Products to treat xerostomia also tend to contain lactoperoxidase, lactoferrin, lysozyme, and immunoglobulins, thus providing many of the missing salivary components.

GlaxoSmithKline produces such a range of products with the proprietary name of Biotène (Figure 17.23) containing a salivary LP3 enzyme system similar to that found in normal saliva. Bio-X Healthcare offers a product range called bioXtr.

Oral cancer testing

With the incidence of oral cancer on the increase and the knowledge that early diagnosis will improve outcomes, manufacturers have produced a test which may easily be carried out in a primary care setting. Vizilite Plus with TBlue (Zila Tolmar) is supplied as a mouthwash which stains suspicious lesions blue. Chemically, it is tolonium chloride (toluidine blue), a vital stain which is preferentially taken up by rapidly dividing cells. The product is supplied in three bottles. The second of the bottles contains the stain, with the other two being pre- and post rinse solutions of acetic acid. Any mucosal tissue which stains blue should be reviewed after 10–14 days and the test repeated. Any tissue persisting to stain blue should be referred on for further specialist investigation.

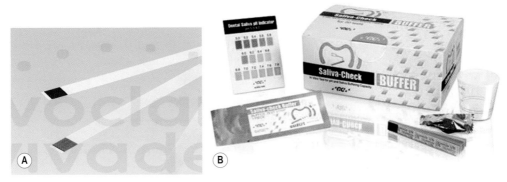

Fig. 17.22 Products to test the buffering capacity of saliva: (A) CRT buffer strips (Ivoclar, Vivadent) and (B) Saliva-Check Buffer (GC).

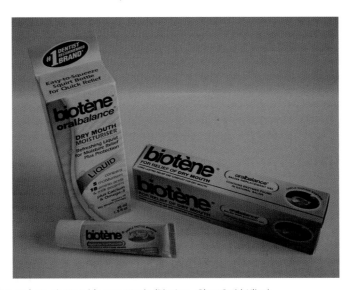

Fig. 17.23 Artificial saliva products for use by patients with xerostomia (Biotène, GlaxoSmithKline).

Another product is VELscope (LED Dental), which is a hand-held device that emits a blue light. Any abnormal tissue will fluoresce when the light is shone on it (Figure 17.24).

Definitive diagnosis is by biopsy and confirmation by histopathological examination.

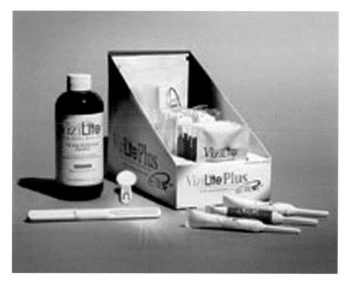

Fig. 17.24 A product for chairside oral cancer testing (VELscope, LED Dental Ltd).

MATERIALS USED IN PERIODONTICS

Topical antimicrobials

The role of bacteria in the aetiology of periodontal disease is well recognized. Antimicrobial agents may be used locally (at the site of disease) as an adjunct to non-surgical periodontal therapy. Their use is controversial among periodontists and clinicians should satisfy themselves that a product will appropriate for the patient. It is not within the scope of this text to debate the merits or otherwise of their use, but rather to describe the products which are available should the clinician wish to consider adjunctive antimicrobial therapy.

The available products are supplied in the form of gels or other presentations which are placed into the periodontal pocket after root surface instrumentation. The intention is that they release the active antimicrobial agent in toxic levels to kill any periodontal pathogens in a sustained manner. This creates a more favourable environment for subsequent repair. It is important the levels of the antibiotic/antibacterial do not reach toxic levels when used at a therapeutic dose in the pocket.

Gels

These products are designed to be of a sufficient viscosity to be syringed into the periodontal pocket and be retained there to be active for a period of time. There are three commonly available products for this purpose. All of them should be used in periodontal pockets equal or greater than 5 mm and in conjunction with root surface instrumentation. This process was formerly known as subgingival debridement or root planing. The gel should be syringed into the

pocket until it is seen to overflow the pocket margin. No excess force should be applied to the syringe as this will disrupt the apical tissues.

Two products are derivatives of tetracycline and contraindicated in patients who are sensitive to this drug and in children under 12 years of age. Atridox (Geistlich Biomaterials) is 8.8% doxycycline and Dentomycin Periodontal Gel (Blackwell Supplies) is 2% minocycline (Figure 17.25). These products should be stored in the refrigerator. The former product is supplied as two gels which, when mixed together, forms a flowable gel that can be placed gently into periodontal pockets.

Another similar product contains 25% metronidazole. It is supplied as a paste with 1 gm metronidazole benzoate equivalent to 250 mg of metronidazole. This drug has a narrow spectrum (unlike tetracycline) and is effective against the anaerobic bacteria found in the periodontal pocket. Elyzol Dental Gel (Colgate) forms a viscous gel when it comes into contact with gingival crevicular fluid and is biodegradable (Figure 17.26). It is applied twice at an interval of a week. The bioavailability of the material is about 70%. This product should be stored at room temperature.

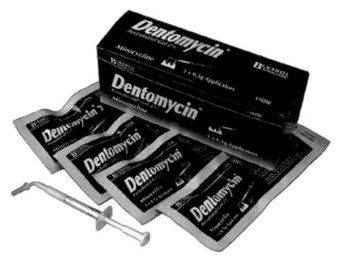

Fig. 17.25 An antibiotic periodontal gel containing 2% minocycline (Dentomycin Periodontal Gel, Blackwell Supplies).

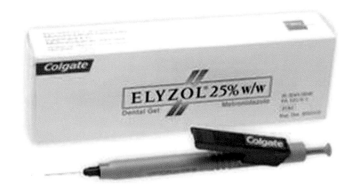

Fig. 17.26 An antibiotic periodontal gel containing 25% metronidazole (Elyzol Dental Gel, Colgate).

Other vehicles for antimicrobial delivery in periodontal cases

Other presentations are also available, which can be placed into peri-odontal pockets over 5 mm in depth to gradually release antimicrobial agents. As with the gels these products should be used only as adjuncts to non-surgical therapy for chronic periodontitis in adults.

The active ingredient in Perio Chip (Dexcel Dental) is chlorhexidine digluconate (2.5 mg), and the benefits of this drug have been discussed previously. The drug is embedded into a solid hydrolysed gelatine with a cross-linked matrix which gradually degrades. Chlorhexidine at the correct bactericidal levels is released as the matrix degrades, for 7–10 days. It is essential that the whole chip is placed and not sectioned, because the dosage of chlorhexidine will be reduced as the material is distributed throughout the gel. Perio Chips are contraindicated in children and adolescents and in those who are hypersensitive to chlorhexidine or other agents contained in the product. They should be stored at room temperature. Some periodontists have concerns that some attachment loss may occur with the use of this product.

Bacterial photo-dynamic therapy is also now being used to kill bacteria in periodontal pockets. Periowave Photodynamic Disinfection (Oraldent) is a bespoke system for this purpose, although the other system mentioned in connection with bacterial PDT in endodontics (Chapter 13) may also be used for this indication. The periodontal pocket is unlike a root canal and the environment of the periodontal pocket is more challenging as it is not an enclosed system. It may be filled with fluid, pus, blood and gingival crevicular fluid. These fluids may have a dilutional effect on the photo-sensitizer, which may have difficulty dwelling in the pocket so there may be benefit from the addition of colloidal silica to thicken it to enable its retention at the site of use. The addition of the thickening agent will, however, have a limiting effect on the spread of the photo-sensitizer, which will reduce the effects of the system.

Regeneration

When bone loss has occurred as a result of periodontal breakdown, it is desirable that these tissues be replaced to restore the supporting structures of the tooth back to normal. This will improve the prognosis of affected teeth and decrease their mobility. Various techniques are available to the periodontist, such as the use of chemicals or membranes which encourage hard and soft tissue to form. Membranes is discussed in the next section.

The use of amelogenin proteins has gained popularity in the last 15 years or so. Amelogenin proteins are enamel matrix proteins that are derived from the epithelial root forming cells. These enamel matrix proteins possess the ability to stimulate both hard (bone and cementum) and soft (periodontal) tissue cell proliferation and differentiation. They may also stimulate angiogenesis.

The amelogenins form an insoluble intracellular matrix that remains on the root surface for 2–4 weeks. This allows selective colonization, proliferation and differentiation of cells. A surface suitable for cementum forming cells (cementoblasts) is created and so new periodontal ligament and bone may be regenerated. Mesenchymal stem cells from the healthy part of the periodontal ligament that are capable of differentiating into specific cell types spread and multiply over the affected area, attaching and populating the surface of the root. They then increase their cellular activity, producing growth factors. Cell metabolism is increased and intracellular signal substances are activated. Growth factors are released and the cells begin to produce collagen and acellular cementum at the root surface. At a distance away from this, the collagen which has been formed starts to condense, and mineralization commences to form alveolar bone. The cells closest to the root then differentiate into cementoblasts, which can lay down the matrix in which the collagen is embedded forming the periodontal ligament. This is an example of tissue engineering using a substrate which is both biocompatible and encourages bioactivity. Emdogain (Straumann) (Figure 17.27) and PrefGel (Biora) are examples of this material available on the market. They are indicated for:

- One-, two- and three-wall intrabony defects
- Class II mandibular furcation defects
- Recession defects.

Another Straumann product is Emdogain PLUS, which is specifically indicated for wide defects, furcation defects and exposed roots at extraction sites. This product also contains Straumann BoneCeramic and Straumann PrefGel. The latter product contains 24% ethylene diamine tetra-acetic acid (EDTA) root surface conditioner, which removes the smear layer so that the enamel matrix proteins can interact and precipitate onto the clean root surface.

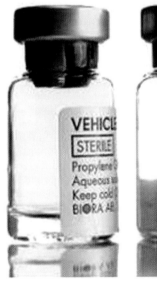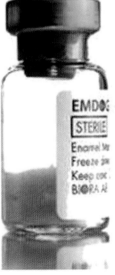

Fig. 17.27 A material containing amelogenin protein (Emdogain, Straumann).

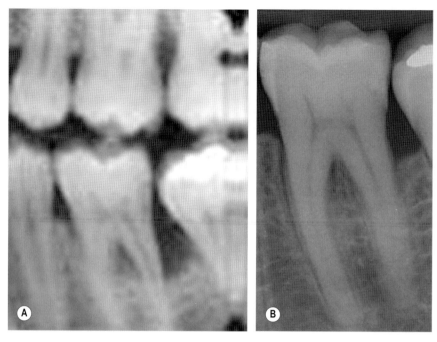

Fig. 17.28 Repair of intrabony defects with a class II lingual furcation (bone loss in the furcation of the tooth on the lingual side but not extending right through) using a material containing amelogenin protein (Emdogain, Straumann). (A) Preoperative view and (B) 2 years postoperatively. Note the infilling of the bony defects, both in the furcation area of tooth 36 and between teeth 36 and 37.
Images courtesy of Dr. D. Nisand, Paris (Straumann)

The product is easy to handle as it may be simply syringed into the pocket to be treated. The product contains propylene glycol alginate and water, which act as a carrier for the active ingredient. There should be no bleeding from the pocket when using this material. On placement the rise to body temperature and change in pH encourages the precipitation of the material onto the root surface. The results can be impressive (Figure 17.28).

Guided tissue regeneration

Another method of regeneration of lost periodontal tissues is **guided tissue regeneration**. This involves the use of a **membrane** which is cell occlusive to prevent the formation of a long junctional epithelium, so allowing the regeneration of cementum and a functional periodontal membrane. Some membranes will allow the passage of fluids and nutrients.

Membranes may either be resorbable or non-resorbable.

Non-resorbable products

ePTFE (polytetrafluoroethylene) membranes are an effective and standard technique. However, the membrane, which is often used in combination with autogenous bone or bone substitute to achieve guided bone regeneration, particularly prior to implant placement is non-resorbable. and is held in situ during its time of action by PTFE sutures. The main manufacturer of this material (Gortex) ceased production in late 2011 due its decreasing popularity.

Resorbable products

Resorbable membranes are made of either synthetic polymers such as lactide/glycolide co-polymers, or polylactic acid blended with a citric acid ester, or natural biomaterials such as collagen. These latter products are often derived from cows (**bovine**) or pigs (**porcine**). The advantage of resorbable membranes is that no re-entry procedure is required to retrieve the membrane.

The patient should be asked whether they have a religious or other objection when materials derived from animals are being contemplated.

Most resorbable products are supplied in a sterile condition and will maintain a functional barrier for between 4 and 9 months before resorbing away. Some products can be moulded to the desired shape, and others are supplied with sterile stencil patterns to facilitate tailoring of the membrane. Shapes of membranes can vary depending on their site of application. For example:

- 'Square forms' are the basic shape
- H shapes are used for interdental defects
- U shapes are used for intraosseous defects
- 'Apron forms' are indicated for dehiscence or recession defects.

Membranes may be used to encourage growth of new tissues in other oral situations, such as an alternative to using a soft tissue autograft (for example palatal tissue), or for soft tissue augmentation. They are usually retained in place for between 4 to 38 weeks to maintain structural integrity, and cover the bone replacement material, protecting it from the faster growing connective tissue which may encroach into the area. Some membranes are a bilayer made from collagen types I and III. This consists of a compact occlusive cell layer which acts as a barrier and prevents the in-growth of soft tissues into the defect. The other layer is porous (collagen) and promotes the integration of newly formed hard tissue. Good cell adhesion at the surface encourages wound healing and minimizes dehiscences. When it becomes saturated with blood the membrane adheres to the defect. The barrier has a high tensile strength and tear resistance and is usually maintained for 4–6 months, allowing undisturbed bone regeneration to take place.

Table 17.6 Some membrane products currently available on the market

Product	Manufacturer	Type of membrane	Comments
AlloDerm	BioHorizons	Processed human dermal matrix with epithelial cells removed, leaving a form of collagen matrix	Regenerative tissue matrix
Bio-Gide	Geistlich Biomaterials	Porcine collagen	Implant use
Bio-Gide Perio	Geistlich Biomaterials	Porcine collagen	Bilayer composed of a rough surface, which is placed against the defect, and a soft surface, which is placed against soft tissue
Bio-Oss Collagen	Geistlich Biomaterials	90% deproteinized cancellous bovine bone embedded in 10% biodegradable porcine collagen matrix	Collagen addition resorbs in 4–6 weeks, does not act as a barrier
Cema	Fortoss	Calcium sulphate	Bacteriostatic for 4–6 weeks
Collagen Membrane	BioSorb	Bovine collagen	
Mem-Lok	BioHorizons	Collagen	Highly purified type I collagen claimed to give predicable resorption period of between 26 and 38 weeks
Ossix Plus	OraPharma	Porcine collagen	Forms unified matrix of cross-linked collagen fibres

Commercially available products

Some of the currently commercially available products are shown in Table 17.6. Some graft membranes are recommended to be used with resorbable pins to hold them in situ for the time of their action so that they remain 'tented' and do not collapse into the defect. An example is Resor-Pin (Geistlich Biomaterials).

Grafts to replace missing bone

Where bone is missing it is often desirable to repair and fill this bony defect. Bony defects can be encountered in various areas of dental practice:

- In periodontology, infrabony periodontal defects are filled in an attempt to replace the bone lost around the tooth. This may or may not be done in conjunction with guided tissue regeneration products.
- In endodontics, repair of large periradicular defects such as cysts and periradicular granulomas could involve using bony grafting materials. These may be used to pack materials (such as mineral trioxide aggregate (MTA)) against them in order to repair the defect in the root (root perforations or open apices).
- Bony grafts are used extensively in implantology to fill dehiscence or fenestration defects adjacent to endosseous implants, again in conjunction with guided tissue regeneration products. Where insufficient bone is present in which to place an implant or implants, bony grafts are indicated to either augment the alveolar ridge, or to create new bone (as with the maxillary sinus floor lift procedure).
- Extraction sockets may be filled up to maintain alveolar ridge height in order to facilitate subsequent implant or prosthetic treatment.

Dehiscence: the premature rupturing of a wound along a surgical suture. This can be within the bone or soft tissue. It is a surgical complication that results from poor wound healing.
Fenestration: an opening, occurring naturally or created surgically.

Box 17.2 Ideal properties of a grafting material

- Non-toxic
- Sterile
- Non-antigenic
- Biocompatible
- Osseoconductive (osteoconductive)
- Osseoinductive (osteoinductive)
- Easy to use
- Readily available
- Have a predictable and reliable outcome

A number of biomaterials are available for these indications (Box 17.2). The graft acts as an osteoconductive scaffold for the ingrowth of blood vessels and a source of osteoprogenitor cells and bone inducing molecules. The graft itself is eventually absorbed by the body and lost as part of normal bone turnover.

Osseoconductive: a graft which acts as a matrix or scaffold for new bone growing from the bones being bridged.
Osseoinductive: a graft which actually forms new bone itself.

Natural bone

Natural bone may be harvested from human or animal sources.

Human bone

The gold standard material for a (bone) graft is one that is taken from the same patient. This is called **autogenous bone** and the graft is termed an **autograft**. Intraoral sites are often used in dentistry for harvesting bone (for example the mental or retromolar region of the mandible) as these sites are convenient and the dentist is familiar with the anatomy. Bone obtained from the hole cut to accommodate a dental implant may also be used. If a larger amount of bone is required then extraoral sites may need to be considered such as the iliac crest, but harvesting in this region is associated with increased morbidity.

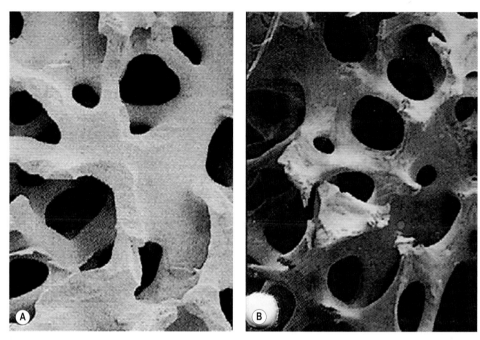

Fig. 17.29 (A) Histological appearance of a bone replacement material, corraline hydroxyapatite (Proosteon implant 500) and (B) normal human cancellous bone.
Images courtesy of Technicare.

Iliac crest: the superior border of the wing of the ilium, one of the bones of the pelvis.

Another potential source of human bone is freeze dried or decalcified freeze dried bone, which is harvested from cadavers and stored in a bone bank. This is termed an **allograft**, i.e. the graft is derived from the same species. Allografts must be carefully selected, harvested and processed to maximize safety and to reduce any potential for infection. This may be described as **homologous** bone, i.e. it has an identical structure to freshly harvested human bone in an autograft.

Animal bone

Natural bone may be derived from a different species and this is called a **xenograft**. **Bovine** and **porcine** products are most commonly used. Xenograft bone is mainly derived from bovine sources, with collagen products derived from porcine sources. The harvested material is treated to remove any proteins, thus rendering them purely mineral grafts. They are chemically and physically identical to human bone and so are not recognized as foreign when implanted. They are effective when mixed with the blood of the patient and no hypersensitivity reactions have been reported.

> **!**
>
> Like membrane products, some patients may, for either religious or animal welfare reasons, object to xenograft products being used on them. It is important to discuss this with the patient during the consent conversation and treatment planning.

Artificial grafts

Artificial (synthetic) grafting materials are also available. These are referred to as **alloplastic graft materials**. They reduce the risk of cross-contamination but may not be structurally and chemically as

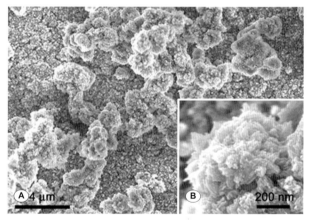

Fig. 17.30 A scanning electron microscopic image of Bioglass 45S5 after incubation in simulated body fluid, showing crystalline carbonated apatite layers on the glass.
http://aiche.confex.com/aiche/2006/techprogram/P59557.HTM

ideal as 'real' bone. They do, however, perform satisfactorily. The commonly used alloplastic graft materials are:

- **Hydroxyapatite.** Unlike human bone, this is composed of large and irregular crystals (Figure 17.29). It exhibits relatively few macro- and micropores and no true trabeculae.
- **Glass granules.** These are irregular fragments with a lack of trabeculation and significant porosity. The bioactive glasses contain silica, sodium and calcium oxide and diphosphorus pentoxide of differing sized granules. A common material is Bioglass (Figure 17.30). The key features of the composition of this glass are that it contains less than 60% of the molar weight of silicon dioxide, high sodium oxide and calcium oxide, as well as a high calcium oxide/phosphorus pentoxide ratio. This makes the glass highly reactive to the aqueous medium and bioactive. The glass is quite soft and can be machined. It will also absorb fluid.

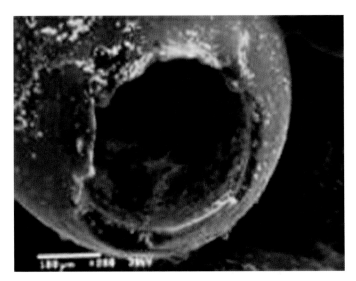

Fig. 17.31 Histological structure of a hollow polymer bead coated with barium sulphate.

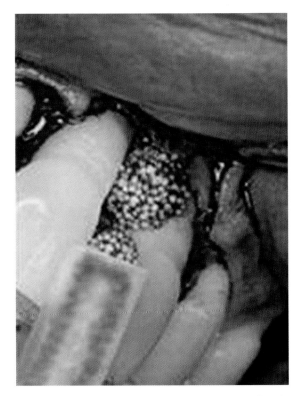

Fig. 17.32 Bioplant HTR-40 placed in the bony defect around teeth 21 and 22 after debridement and root curettage. The graft material has been hydrated with blood gained from the bone marrow prior to use.
Image Courtesy of R.T. Mat, Belgium. http://www.rtmat.com/start_en.htm

- **Polymer beads**. These structures are made up of some or all of the following constituents: polymethylmethacrylate (PMMA), hydroxyethylmethacrylate (HEMA) and calcium hydroxide calcium carbonate (Figure 17.31). The beads are packed into the defect as shown in Figure 17.32.
- **Tricalcium phosphate hydroxyapatite** combinations.

All the above materials are claimed to be bioactive and to encourage bone regeneration. Some are totally resorbable while others remain for long periods of time before being resorbed. Most materials are provided as small granules or blocks which may be trimmed to the size of the defect. The method of placement varies with the material used but with all the products, the allograft should be saturated in the blood of the patient either by aspiration into a syringe containing the graft material or by packing into the cavity before blood clotting has occurred. All materials have to be retained in the defect either by another synthetic material or by achieving closure of the lesion with the available soft tissue, which is sutured over the top.

Depending on the size of the defect, titanium mesh trays containing an autograft or allograft material are used to form a scaffold for the graft.

Commercially available products

Some of the currently available bone grafting products are shown in Table 17.7.

Periodontal dressings

When an open wound results from the surgical procedure (for example with some types of gingivectomy), or if a wound requires to be protected or stabilized, a periodontal dressing may be indicated. This covers the wound, is bacteriostatic and facilitates healing while protecting the exposed wound from the hostile oral environment. The dressing should not contain eugenol as this may cause local necrosis. Two products are available on the market, Septo-pack (Septodont) and Coe-Pak (GC) (Figure 17.33).

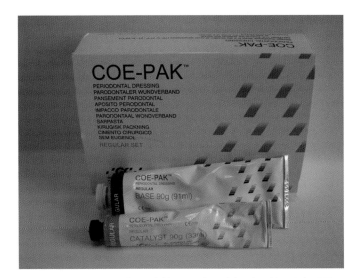

Fig. 17.33 A commercially available periodontal dressing (Coe-Pak, GC).

 Plaque may grow under the pack and so it should stay in place for as short a time as possible.

These products are supplied as a two-paste presentation which is mixed together. The consistency is such that it is very sticky and difficult to mix and to place. The use of water or petroleum jelly such as Vaseline (Lever Fabergé) may facilitate handling as it acts as a separator. GC now produces Coe-Pak in an automix presentation.

Table 17.7 Some bone grafting products currently available on the market

Product	Manufacturer	Type of material	Comments
Bio-Oss spongiosa	Geistlich Biomaterials	Mineral portion of bovine bone	The bony structure will encourage the growth and infiltration of cells and lead to steady bone deposition. The smaller bony canals lead to more rapid new bone formation
Bioplant	Kerr Dental	Biocompatible polymers with a calcium hydroxide coating	Used for anterior socket grafting, periodontal applications and voids around implants
Bioplant HTR (hard tissue replacement) Synthetic Bone Alloplast	Kerr Dental	Granules with a PMMA core, polyHEMA and barium sulphate middle layers and coated with calcium hydroxide-carbonate	Designed for small bony voids. It is claimed to adhere to both bone and metal. No membrane barrier is required and epithelial migration does not occur
Easy-graft	Degradable Solutions AG	β-TCP and polylactide	Hardens when in contact with body fluids to form a porous bone substitute material. It resorbs in nine to fifteen months
Grafton DBM (demineralised bone matrix)	Osteotech	Demineralized bone	Can be used alone, mixed with autogenous bone graft or marrow or combined with other allograft forms. Putty presentation
Grafton DBM Flex	Osteotech	Demineralized bone	Gel form of the above product
Interpore 500	Interpore Orthopaedics, Inc	Porous hydroxyapatite from the coral exoskeleton of *Porites goniopora*	Pore size 600 μm and pore interconnectors 250 μm
MinerOss	BioHorizons	Blend of mineralized allograft cancellous and cortical chips	
Ostim	aap Implantate AG	Synthetic hydroxyapatite nanoparticle paste	Hydroxyapatite sintered to give a high specific surface which is easily resorbed. Supplied as an aqueous paste in a syringe, it does not harden and is rapidly vascularized leading to rapid bone formation. It is osteoconductive and should not be placed where inflamed or necrotic tissues are present
ProOsteon 500	Biomet, Inc	Coralline hydroxyapatite	
R.T.R (resorbable tissue replacement)	Septodont	Syringe is synthetic whereas cone is β-TCP granules with a matrix of highly purified bovine collagen fibres	A cone or syringe which soaks up blood so its consistency changes from a dry rigid to cohesive and malleable gel. It should be inserted into the socket when fully blood soaked otherwise dissociation of β-TCP particles may result during packing. The implant may be placed after 4.5 months
Resorb	Fortoss	β-TCP granules	Resorbed in 6–9 months
Straumann Bone Ceramic	Straumann	Biphasic calcium phosphate (a combination of 60% hydroxyapatite and 40% tricalcium phosphate)	A source of calcium and phosphate ions; initiates mineralization. Hydroxyapatite maintains the supporting scaffold for bone-forming cells and bone deposition. It is supplied in a sterile package and mixed with sterile saline solution or uncontaminated patient's blood or autogenous bone prior to application. It is essential not to compress the material as this will damage the structure. It is therefore applied loosely into site and left for 6 months for the tissue to regenerate. A membrane may be required. Its pore size is between 100 and 500 μm and is 90% porous
Vital Bone Regeneration	Biocomposites	β-TCP in a hydroxyl sulphate matrix	Resorbed and replaced by bone in 4–6 months. It is bacteriostatic with no additional membrane being required

TCP, tri-calcium phosphate; PMMA, polymethylmethacrylate; HEMA, hydroxyethylmethacrylate.

ORAL SURGICAL MATERIALS

Achieving haemostasis

In the vast majority of oral surgical sites, haemostasis is achieved very quickly and uneventfully. However, some wounds do require further means to establish haemostasis. This may be undertaken prior to the patient being dismissed, or may be carried out some hours later if bleeding recommences. The surgeon usually sutures the site (see p. 308) and may also place a haemostatic sponge (Figure 17.34).

These sponges are made of resorbable gelatin containing colloidal silver and are supplied in sterile packaging. They are resorbable, which is advantageous as the patient does not need to return to the clinic to have the material removed.

Intraoperatively, bone wax may be used as a haemostatic agent to control bleeding from bone, but must be fully removed prior to closure of the wound as it is non-resorbable. It has an adverse effect on osteogenesis and causes a mild inflammatory reaction. Its mode of action is purely mechanical. Bone wax is a sterile mixture of beeswax, paraffin and isopropyl palmitate, the latter agent being included to soften the material. Ethicon manufactures one such product.

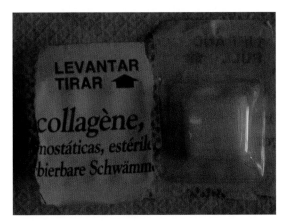

Fig. 17.34 Haemostatic sponge used to stop the bleeding from a dental socket (Hémocollagène, Septodont).

Commercially available products

Table 17.8 shows some of the haemostatic sponges available commercially.

Table 17.8 Some haemostatic sponges currently available on the market		
Product	**Manufacturer**	**Notes**
Gelatemp	Roeko	Foam gelatine sponge with colloidal silver which remains active to prevent infection
Gelitaspon	Gelita	Made of Alpha-Gelatin. It is a purified protein obtained by the partial acidic hydrolysis of collagen
Hémocollagène	Septodont	Sponge impregnated with freeze dried denatured bovine collagen
Surgicel	Johnson and Johnson	Oxidized cellulose

Treatment of infected (dry) socket ('fibrinolytic alveolitis')

Occasionally after the removal of a tooth, the blood clot that forms immediately after the extraction breaks down. The socket may then become infected. A 'dry socket' is a very painful condition necessitating the patient to return to the surgery for further treatment. Usually, this involves irrigation of the socket with chlorhexidine or sterile saline with or without curettage. Some clinicians prefer to dress the socket after wound toilet. This works in two ways:

- Sedative action on the denuded exposed bone
- Occlusion of the socket, preventing further food particles and debris from collecting.

The most widely used preparation is Alvogyl (Septodont) (Figure 17.35). This contains buty-paramino benzoate iodoform and eugenol as the active ingredients, with excipients that include olive oil, spearmint oil, sodium lauryl sulphate, calcium carbonate, penghawar and purified water. The mode of action is through antimicrobial effects induced by iodoform, anaesthetic effects produced by the buty-paramino benzoate and analgesia as a result of the eugenol present in the paste. Some clinicians do not advocate the use of materials containing eugenol or other oils, as they can create a superficial necrosis of bone and nerve endings, which leads to further tissue damage and delay in healing.

> **Excipient:** an inactive substance used as a carrier for the active ingredients of a medicament.

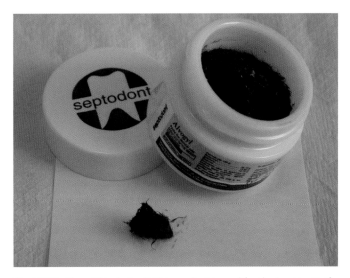

Fig. 17.35 Alvogyl (Septodont). This product is used for the treatment of infected sockets.

Sutures

Depending on the size and position of the wound (i.e. whether there is a pull from a muscle attachment), **sutures** or – in layperson terms 'stitches' – are used to close the surgical site. The objective is to appose the two edges of the tissues in very close proximity so that they may heal. This should be undertaken with care by the surgeon, following the surgical principles of suturing as it will impact on the rate of healing of the wound, with a better technique associated with reduced scarring and reduced postoperative pain.

Depending on the task in hand, a wide range of sutures are available to the surgeon. Considerations affecting choice are the healing rates of tissue, the different tissues being handled, the surgeon's preference and cost. For the purpose of this text only suture materials commonly used in surgical procedures in the oral cavity will be discussed.

Types of suture material

Sutures may be classified as **absorbable** or **non-absorbable**, as well as **monofilament** or **multifilament**.

- **Absorbable** sutures may be divided into those of a **biological origin** or those made using **synthetic polymers**. Those in the former category are gradually digested by tissue enzymes, whereas the synthetic polymers are broken down by hydrolysis in tissue fluids. It is clearly obvious that the surgeon needs to know the time taken by each type of suture material to absorb or to be broken down by the host (absorption rate). Suture strength will decrease during this process and sufficient strength needs to be retained for enough time to serve its function. Absorbable sutures tend to be placed in deep wounds, or for convenience in oral mucosal wounds so that the patient does not need to return to the clinic for an additional appointment to have them removed.
- **Non-absorbable** sutures are made from a variety of non-biodegradable materials. These are encapsulated or walled off by the body's fibroblasts and remain buried within tissues. However, if used for skin or oral mucosal closure, they must be removed. Fine bore, non-absorbable sutures are preferred for vascular anastomoses.

Any (foreign body) tissue reaction elicited is important, as inflammation will result at the site and so increase the incidence of scarring. Sutures used to close oral wounds should have high biocompatibility as there is a high load of microorganisms present in the oral cavity. The suture will naturally attract bacteria and colonization at the margins of a wound may introduce infection, delayed healing and postoperative pain.

As the name suggests, **monofilament** means a single strand or filament, whereas **multifilament** involves several braided or twisted stands or filaments. Braided sutures are stronger than monofilament sutures of the same material and thickness.

Sutures are available is varying diameters. The small number denotes a thicker suture, i.e. 3-0 suture is thicker than a 6-0. It is obvious that the thinner the suture, the lower the tensile strength of the material. The choice of thickness of the suture will depend on the intended use. Finer sutures are used in microsurgical techniques.

Commercially available products

Example of suture product currently available are shown in Table 17.9 and Figure 17.36.

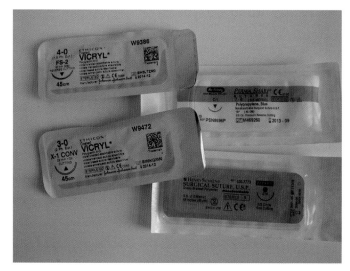

Fig. 17.36 Some packaged suture products. Note the detailed labelling, which conforms to international standards.

Table 17.9 Some suture products used in oral surgical procedures currently available on the market

Product	Manufacturer	Type	Absorbable	Tissue reactivity	Filament	Comments
Coated Vicryl	Ethicon	Poliglecaprone 910	Yes	Mild	Braided	
Coated Vicryl Plus Antibacterial	Ethicon	Poliglecaprone 910	Yes	Mild	Braided	Contains triclosan
Coated Vicryl Rapide	Ethicon	Polyglactin 910	Yes	Mild	Braided	
Mersilk	Ethicon	silk	No	Moderate	Braided	
Monocryl	Ethicon	Poliglecaprone 25	Yes	Mild	Mono	
Perma Sharp PGA	Hu-Friedy	Homopolymer of glycolic acid	Yes		Braided	
Perma Sharp PGA Fast	Hu-Friedy	Homopolymer of glycolic acid	Yes		Braided	
Perma Sharp Polypropylene	Hu-Friedy	Polypropylene	No	Low	Mono	

DENTAL IMPLANTS

The increasing availability and development of dental implants has revolutionized restorative dentistry. The concept of implanting titanium into bone was first postulated by the Swedish orthopaedic surgeon, Per-Ingvar Brånemark. The increasing versatility of implant systems has expanded treatment options. Dental implants may be used to restore a single tooth or even to support dentures (perhaps together with other implants). More recently, orthodontists are using them to as anchorage units in fixed appliance therapy.

The reason behind their success is the structural and functional connection created between the implant surface and the surrounding healthy bone. This is termed **osseointegration**, which is really a functional ankylosis and takes up to 6 months to occur. Osseointegration permits occlusal forces to be transmitted to the underlying bone so supporting the restoration and restoring function. A space of 100Å between the bone and implant surface is seen histologically (Figure 17.37).

> **Functional ankylosis:** osseointegration of the implant with the bony infrastructure which permits occlusal loading.

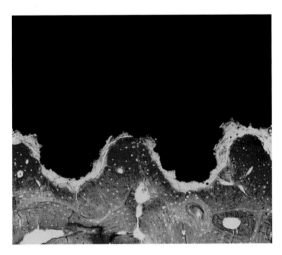

Fig. 17.37 Histological section of bone integrated to the titanium surface of a dental implant (black).
(Courtesy of Robert Gougaloff Wikopedia website)

For osseointegration to occur, close contact between implant and bone is essential. Clearly, a sufficient quality and quantity of bone is essential, although in cases where this is not available grafting techniques may be used (see above). In order to prevent loss of bone after tooth extraction, implants may be placed immediately after tooth extraction.

The success rate of dental implants is higher than with other restorative options although implants can fail for no apparent reason. In this respect, it is unwise to guarantee satisfactory outcome. There is some evidence that failure occurs more frequently in those patients with a previous history of periodontal disease. Often the technique is more conservative to tooth tissue than other treatment options as adjacent teeth need not be involved (prepared), unlike in the provision of a bridge.

Different designs of dental implants have been used in the past, but in contemporary practice one design has predominated. This is the **endosseous** implant which, as the term suggests, involves the placement of the implant into the alveolar bone. The implant osseointegrates with the bone and the suprastructure can be placed on

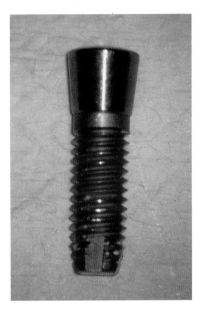

Fig. 17.38 A dental implant made from titanium alloy.

to this fixture. The gingival tissues form a cuff around the implant at the gingival margin. The restorative component – crown, bridge or denture – is subsequently attached either by being cemented or screw retained. This arrangement should yield a good emergence profile.

> **Emergence profile:** the manner it which the crown appears is positioned in relation to the gingival tissues

Implant materials

Implants (Figure 17.38) have been constructed of many materials such as **commercially pure titanium (CPTi)**, **titanium alloys**, **zirconium** and some **ceramics**. CPTi is the most commonly used material, and on which most work has been carried out. Ceramics will osseointegrate but have the disadvantage of being too brittle. Some implants have been treated by a plasma spray technique to coat the surface of the implant with a 50–100 µm thick layer of ceramic. This aims to combine the high strength of the alloy with the good bonding potential of the ceramic. However, there is a risk that this layer may debond or is damaged during placement, leading to eventual failure.

CPTi is not completely pure. It is, in fact, a 99.75% high purity titanium but with some minor impurities including oxygen, carbon, hydrogen, and nitrogen. The metal is highly reactive and oxidizes passively almost immediately when bought into contact with air or tissue fluid. This is of particular benefit as it minimizes the risk of corrosion biologically. The oxide layer formed is about 10–15Å (1/10 billionth of a metre) thick and forms within 0.001 of a second of exposure of the freshly cut surface. This has the added advantage that if the metal is scratched, it 'heals' again quickly as a new oxide layer is formed.

In normal use passivation of the metal is increased by exposing it to nitric acid. This then leads to a thicker durable oxide layer. The metal has a high strength to weight ratio and is not as stiff as stainless steel or chrome cobalt alloy. However, it is about six to nine times stiffer than bone. Although biocompatible, there is evidence of release of titanium ions into the surrounding bone and major organs, but this does not appear to be sufficient to cause any untoward host reaction. Adverse reactions that have been observed are frequently attributed to contamination of the implant surface. The titanium alloys used for implant fixture construction contain 6% **aluminium** and 4% **vanadium** by weight. The alloying process makes the material stronger.

Clearly the surface of the implant is critical as it is this which will osseointegrate with the surrounding bone. The surfaces of many implants are modified to achieve more rapid osseointegration or to perform better mechanically. This may be done in a number of ways:

- The composition of the alloy of which the implant is made may be changed
- The surface of the implant may be coated with **hydroxyapatite**
- A biochemical (such as **bone morphogenic protein**) may be used to encourage bone formation
- The surface of the implant may be **roughened by sandblasting or acid etching**
- The titanium surface may be chemically modified, firstly by being microroughened and then treated with fluoride. With this method, a textured titanium oxide surface results.

Any roughening of the implant surface increases the surface area available for osseointegration. It has also been claimed to offer increased bone formation and stronger bone-to-implant bonding as textured surfaces accelerate initial healing. This occurs by the roughened surface adsorbing and accumulating proteins, activating platelets and retaining fibrin. These factors all contribute to increasing the amount of bone surrounding the implant.

The thickened oxide layer on the implant surface is advantageous as this layer affects differentiation of progenitor cells into mature osteoblasts, leading to subsequent mineralization. This improves implant stability and a porous oxide surface may enhance integration.

A brief description of the restoration of dental implants

Following implant placement, the construction of the superstructure on the implant is carried out in a manner that is quite similar to the construction of a crown on a natural tooth. Of the many dental implant systems now available on the market, some systems require preparation of the coronal portion of the implant after it has osseointegrated. This preparation may be adjusted to slightly alter angulation (if required) and create a finishing shoulder. This preparation is done with the use of a **tungsten carbide** bur under copious water spray. Once preparation is complete a conventional rubber-based impression may be made and a temporary restoration placed. If gingival retraction is required, a material such as Expasyl (Kerr Hawe) (Chapter 15) should be used as all other methods of gingival retraction are likely to cause damage to the implant/soft tissue interface and are contraindicated.

Other systems utilize an **impression coping** to record the position of the implant. The internal part of the implant has a screw thread and it is by this means that the restoration is retained. To restore this type of implant, an impression coping (plastic analogue) is screwed down into the implant. Often this incorporates an internal hexagon to resist rotation during function and to confirm localization of the suprastructure. A locating impression is then taken usually using a polyether impression material. The impression coping is then unscrewed from the implant and replaced into the impression prior to being sent to the technician.

A special model must be constructed by the technician, which has a base metal replica of the implant (**laboratory analogue**), and a silicone-based gingival mask (such as Gi-Mask, Coltène Whaledent) is placed to reproduce the gingival contours more precisely. This material has a good dimensional stability and facilitates better contouring of the final prosthesis during fabrication (see Figure 20.20, p. 357).

The choice of suprastructure is determined by the site, extent and nature of the implant. Abutments may be made of ceramic, CPTi, gold alloy, zirconium and titanium nitride (for further information on these materials, see Chapters 21 and 22). The 'core' part of the system is then screwed into place and tightened using a torque wrench to prevent excessive rotational force being placed on the implant. The definitive restoration may then be luted into place using a temporary or definitive luting cement.

There are too many systems (and manufacturers) currently available to discuss the exact mechanisms of each, or indeed to list the indications and clinical procedures. The reader is therefore recommended to consult a bespoke implant text for further information.

Teeth restored with dental implants should be subject to the same dental preventive measures as other teeth. However, it is inadvisable to probe a fixture as this may introduce bacteria from the gingival margin and potentially initiate peri-implantitis. Bespoke scalers are available, constructed with titanium or plastic for cleaning the implant surface, although many dental implantologists prefer a no-touch approach, opting instead for subgingival irrigation with chlorhexidine.

SUMMARY

- Dentifrices contain detergents, abrasives and therapeutic agents for the prevention of caries and periodontal disease.
- Fluoride-containing materials such as gels, mouthwashes and varnishes can help in the prevention of caries. Care must be taken in their use so as not to exceed the appropriate fluoride levels in the mouth.
- Periodontal materials can be used to stimulate reattachment.
- Bone replacement materials are effective at filling bony periodontal cavities.
- Bone replacement materials may be produced from denatured animal bone or a range of synthetic alternatives and are used to form a scaffold for new bone formation.
- Implants usually containing biocompatible alloys such as those of titanium.

SELF-ASSESSMENT QUESTIONS

1. What fluoride preparations are available and when would these be prescribed?
2. A patient has had radiotherapy for an oral carcinoma. What preventive products should be prescribed and why?
3. What features of dental implants enhance osseointegration?
4. Which ingredients would influence recommendation of a particular type of dentifrice?
5. Describe the diagnostic products that can help in the diagnosis of a high caries risk patient.
6. What are the similarities and differences between autografts and xenografts?

Chapter | 18 |

Dental bleaching systems

LEARNING OBJECTIVES

From this chapter, the reader will:

- Be aware of the various dental bleaching products
- Understand the risks and benefits of these products
- Have an appreciation of the various techniques that are currently used to lighten teeth
- Understand the legal position for the practice of tooth whitening in the UK
- Know the names of currently available commercial products.

INTRODUCTION

Over the past 20 years, the general public and therefore dental patients have become much more conscious of the appearance of their teeth. Their awareness of the treatment options dentists can offer has also increased owing to the increased media attention to dental health and cosmetic dentistry: there are many television programmes showing patient transformations using cosmetic surgery including cosmetic dentistry; and the public is bombarded with photographs of models with very white teeth in advertisements and glossy magazines. Although these photographs are very often 'adjusted' with the use of digital software tools, the perception that white, straight, perfect teeth are the norm and therefore desirable, has in many countries, contributed to a cultural shift, particularly in the USA. The market for cosmetic products and treatments has greatly increased, and it is now very common for patients to enquire about whitening their teeth during their dental appointment. Tooth bleaching is now the most commonly requested cosmetic service. Frequently, this appears in the patients' minds to be more important than the treatment of dental disease. Beauty salons and hairdressers are also offering tooth whitening treatments although there are legal issues (in the UK) concerning non-dental care professionals carrying out any form of dental treatment.

Successful tooth bleaching can greatly improve the patient's self-image, self-confidence and physical attractiveness. This can then lead to improved employment prospects and increased social confidence.

Many products which are designed to lighten teeth can now be bought over the counter (OTC) from pharmacies and chemists and sometimes even in supermarkets. Other products are available only to dentists. Treatments with these products need to be carried out under professional supervision either directly by the clinician or by the patient carrying out the treatment at home, and returning to the dental clinic from time to time to allow the dentist to monitor their progress. Some treatment regimes combine both processes.

Products and techniques are available to lighten both vital and non-vital teeth. This chapter discusses the materials which are used to bleach teeth and the issues which surround their use.

CHEMICAL REACTION: AN OXIDIZING PROCESS

The currently available products used to bleach teeth are based on **hydrogen peroxide**. This is a chemical which, on decomposition, produces species which can take part in an **oxidizing** reaction on tooth tissue, that is **oxygen-free radicals** and **water**. Many products also contain **carbamide peroxide** or **sodium perborate**, which both break down to release hydrogen peroxide.

Carbamide peroxide is a compound of **hydrogen peroxide** and **urea**. In the presence of water, carbamide peroxide breaks down into its two main constituents. Carbamide peroxide products have been shown to be active even after 10 hours of use so enhancing their efficacy. Carbamide peroxide is also referred to as **urea peroxide**, **perhydrol urea** and **carbamyl peroxide**.

Carbamide peroxide is inherently unstable and starts to decompose as soon as it has been manufactured. This decreases its oxidizing power and whitening effect. It is highly recommended therefore that tooth whitening products are stored in a refrigerator at the recommended temperature prior to use to maximize the product's shelf-life. Some products are now supplied in refrigerated packs to achieve the same end (e.g. Evolution ICE, Enlighten).

Sodium perborate reacts with water to form **sodium borate** and **hydrogen peroxide**. The amount of hydrogen peroxide produced using sodium perborate is less than that from a similar amount of carbamide peroxide.

Mode of action

The free radical oxygen species produced by these compounds pass through the pores in the enamel and later the dentine by diffusion that is, moving from areas of high concentration to areas of low concentration until equilibrium is achieved or the source of the species is exhausted. This starts within a matter of 15 minutes of applying the product. It is possible that the active ingredient may eventually reach the pulp. To reduce this risk only a small quantity of the material should be used as the active species penetrates all coronal tissues. The diffusion process in the cervical region of the tooth is more rapid as dentine is more porous in this region. Penetration beneath restorations may occur and there is now some evidence of interactions between amalgam and the active species, leading to mercury release.

The free radical oxygen species break down the high molecular weight coloured complex organic molecules which cause staining. The smaller molecules so produced reflect less light from or they are lost from the tooth tissue with the result that the tooth tissue appears lighter in colour. Generally speaking, after an hour's clinical use these breakdown products are rendered inactive (Figure 18.1).

The concentration of hydrogen peroxide in products varies, depending on whether the product is available to the public as an OTC product or is licensed for use under the direct supervision of a dentist. Concentrations range from 3% to 38%, respectively. The concentration of carbamide peroxide in any commercial product is three times the concentration of the hydrogen peroxide liberated, i.e. 10% carbamide peroxide will break down to release 3.3% hydrogen peroxide.

The degree of shade change depends on:

- The concentration of hydrogen peroxide (greater concentration=greater shade change)
- The time it is in contact with the teeth to be bleached.

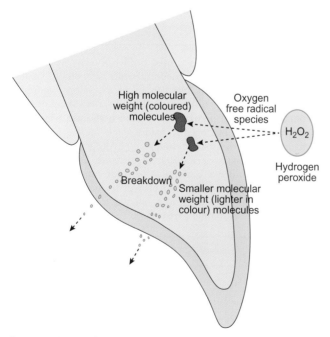

Fig. 18.1 Diagram illustrating the free radical oxygen species entering the tooth, the chemical reaction therein and the products of the reaction leaving the tooth.

COMMON INGREDIENTS IN TOOTH WHITENING PRODUCTS

Besides the active ingredients discussed previously, several other chemicals are included in bleaching products by the manufacturers. See Table 18.1.

Table 18.1 Common chemical ingredients in tooth whitening products

Chemical	Reason for inclusion
Hydrogen peroxide	Active ingredient
Carbamide peroxide	Source of hydrogen peroxide
Sodium perborate	Source of hydrogen peroxide
Urea	Stabilizer, and increases the pH, which is less irritant to soft tissue
	Increased antibacterial effect
Glycerine	Increases viscosity, so that the product is retained in the bleaching tray
Carbopol (polyacrylic acid polymer)	Increases viscosity, decreases breakdown in saliva and slows release of oxygen
Alcohol ethoxylates or sodium xylene sulphonate	Surfactant – promotes wetting by lowering surface tension or to solubilize one of the ingredients, such as an insoluble fragrance
Amorphous calcium phosphate (ACP)	Decreases sensitivity by occluding the dentinal tubules with calcium phosphate
	Improves enamel smoothness and restores lustre
Potassium nitrate	Decreases sensitivity by altering nerve conduction
Fluoride (e.g. sodium fluoride)	Decreases sensitivity by occluding the dentinal tubules
	Promotes remineralization
	Provides caries resistance
Neutralizers	Alkaline substances to create neutral pH
Flavourings	Increases patient acceptability
Carotene	Converts light energy to heat so increasing the activation of hydrogen peroxide by speeding up its dissolution into free radicals in products intended to be exposed to light energy

INDICATIONS AND CONTRAINDICATIONS

Clearly the main indication of tooth whitening products is to lighten teeth which have darkened physiologically or due to smoking or staining by chromogenic materials. The treatment is much more effective in those stains that are just below the enamel surface. Staining caused by some dental conditions is also amenable to bleaching:

* Mild tetracycline staining
* Mild fluorosis
* Mild hypocalcification
* Combination staining.

At the concentrations supplied, bleaching products are safe to use, but as with any treatments tooth whitening procedures are contraindicated in some instances:

* Pregnant women
* Nursing mothers
* Children under 14 years of age
* Patients with kidney disorders or on kidney dialysis
* Patients allergic to hydrogen peroxide or other ingredients contained in the bleaching product
* Heavy smokers, unless they abstain from smoking for the duration of the treatment and subsequently
* Amalgam stains in tooth tissue. Such stains are resistant to bleaching
* Deciduous teeth
* Teeth displaying pathology such as dental caries, deficient restorations or periradicular disease.

SIDE EFFECTS, RISKS AND HAZARDS

No medical or dental treatments are without risk. Tooth bleaching is generally a safe treatment, but there are some associated side effects:

* (Transient) thermal sensitivity
* Gingival and soft tissue irritation
* Gastric irritation
* Altered taste sensation
* Cervical resorption
* Risk of mutagenic effects
* Adverse structural changes in enamel
* Increase in translucency of enamel, especially incisally
* Adverse effects on restorative materials.

Thermal sensitivity

The most common side effect of bleaching treatments is sensitivity to thermal stimuli and occurs in between 25% and 50% of patients. As mentioned earlier, the oxygen species diffuse slowly through the hard dental tissues, eventually reaching the pulp. The volume reaching this site is dependent on the initial concentration and amount used. Many patients experience peak sensitivity on day 3 of treatment. The sensitivity tends to be transient and usually abates 2 days after discontinuation of treatment. Sensitivity has been reported more commonly in the lower than the upper arch, probably because of with relatively smaller size and volume of the tooth crowns. For this reason, many clinicians treat the upper arch before embarking on the lower. This also allows the clinician and patient to see what final result may be achieved (Figure 18.2). Long-term studies have shown no detrimental effects of this sensitivity after a period of 7 years.

Some products have desensitizing chemicals included in their formula. Some clinicians advocate the application of desensitizing agents (such as sensitive dentifrices or mouthwashes containing potassium nitrate or neutral sodium fluoride) alternately with the bleaching chemicals in an attempt to reduce sensitivity.

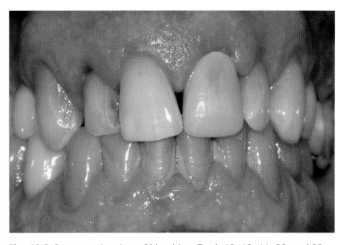

Fig. 18.2 Postoperative view of bleaching. Teeth 13, 12, 11, 22, and 23 were bleached prior to the placement of ceramic veneers on 13 and 12 (after the original failed ceramic veneers had been removed from 13 and 12). Note the colour difference between the bleached upper teeth and the lower arch, which was not treated. Also note that the Directa (Svenska Dental Instrument AB) temporary crown rebased with Trim II (Bosworth) has reacted with the bleaching agent 16% PF Carbamide Peroxide gel (White Dental Beauty, Optident) and turned orange (see p. 314).

Some patients have to discontinue treatment due to sensitivity although they are small in number. Simple analgesics such as paracetamol or ibuprofen will control any symptoms. Sometimes a reduction in the frequency or length of time of application may allow patients to continue with treatment. Likewise, changing the product to one with a lower concentration of active chemical may also help.

Gingival and soft tissue irritation

The next most common side effect is that of irritation of the oral soft tissues, occurring in 33% of cases. It is more commonly associated with self or home treatment. It is usually caused by the patient placing too much bleaching agent in the tray, which is displaced from the tray on insertion, or the bleaching gel may leach out of the tray during use. Both these result in the gel contacting the gingival tissues. Any soft tissue damage usually resolves uneventfully a few days after discontinuation of the treatment. The fabrication of a well-fitting bleaching tray should help to reduce gingival irritation together with careful placement of gel within it.

Gastric irritation

If a large amount of the bleaching gel is inadvertently swallowed, gastric irritation may occur due to release of large volumes of gas and gastric bleeding. Ingestion of large amounts of both hydrogen peroxide and carbamide peroxide can be fatal and these products should be stored securely and out of the reach of children.

Altered taste sensation

Some patients have reported a metallic taste during treatment. The strong oxidizing effect of the active species will cause mucosal changes and may have an effect on the tongue mucosa, altering the taste for short period of time. It may also be associated with a reaction between restoratives and the oxidizing agent. This is observed most commonly when the tray is removed in the morning after overnight bleaching. The taste usually disappears after a couple of hours. Many of the products used for bleaching are supplied in various flavours and the exposure to different flavours may also compromise the ability to taste other foods.

External cervical resorption

The aetiology of external cervical resorption is still not fully understood. There is a higher incidence of this condition in teeth that have undergone tooth whitening treatment. The prevalence is between 6% and 8% and it usually only affects non-vital teeth or those which have a history of trauma. The risk increases as the concentration of hydrogen peroxide rise above 30%. Clearly, if cervical resorption does occur, it will potentially compromise the prognosis of the tooth and should be treated without delay.

Patients should be warned of the possibility of external cervical resorption prior to starting treatment.

Risk of mutagenic effects

There has been some suggestion of an association between dental bleaching and an increased risk of developing neoplastic changes either in the oral cavity or elsewhere. The aetiology of this is that hydrogen peroxide may initiate or promote mutagenic change; it is known to be genotoxic in vitro but not in vivo. The experimental studies which showed these changes used artificially high concentrations of the chemical. The extreme effects produced by these high concentrations are of low significance considering the low concentration of hydrogen peroxide used to whiten teeth. Together with the short application time and short duration of treatment, this risk is very low, even in patients who smoke or drink alcohol, both known risk factors for the development of oral cancer.

Neoplastic change: abnormal new growth of cells.
Mutagenic change: a change induces by a physical or chemical agent to genetic material, usually the DNA of an organism.
Genotoxic change: a damaging action on a cell's genetic material, which affects its integrity.

Adverse structural changes in the dental hard tissues and changes in translucency of enamel

Carbamide peroxide at a low concentration has no effect on the surface or surface microhardness of enamel or dentine when used in a formulation with a neutral pH. However, some studies have shown that exposure to 10% carbamide peroxide for a significant part of the day over a month resulted in the enamel losing its aprismatic layer. Carbamide peroxide at a higher concentration is able to alter the enamel structure but its effect is not as damaging as that caused when enamel is etched prior to bonding.

If used over the longer term, bleaching may increase the translucency of some areas of enamel, especially towards the incisal edge. This is another reason why dental bleaching should be closely supervised by a dentist.

External cervical resorption: a lesion seen under the epithelial attachment where the cementum has become damaged allowing colonization by osteoclasts, which then resorb the root.
Microhardness: a value achieved using an indentation test on the surface under evaluation where the load applied is less than 1 kg.
Aprismatic enamel: amorphous layer of surface enamel with no structural characteristics.

Effects on restorative materials

The active ingredients can affect other restorative materials and these interactions are summarized in Table 18.2.

There is no evidence of any adverse effect of tooth whitening agent use on the bond strength of established bonded restorations.

Antioxidant: a molecule which inhibits the oxidation of other molecules.

Table 18.2 The potential effects of bleaching agents on some restorative materials

Amalgam	Resin composite	Cements	Bonding systems	Temporization materials	Porcelain
The tooth tissue will turn green if the bleaching agent reacts with the amalgam	No effect as the material does not bleach but may be affected by acid nature of the peroxide	Washout of some cements such as glass ionomer cement	Immediate reduction in bond strengths by 25%	Discolours – material turns orange (see Figure 18.2)	No effect as the material does not bleach, except that some superficial stains may be removed
Significantly more mercury released during bleaching					
Removal of the passivation layer					
Oxide layer removed					
Colour change from black to grey					

Wherever possible, bonding using any resin-based composite to teeth which have been bleached should be delayed for at least 2 weeks (and preferably longer if possible) for the following reasons:

- During the bleaching treatment the tooth tissue is saturated with oxygen species. If bonding is attempted, the bond strengths gained are decreased in the order of 25% due to the presence of this oxygen. Allowing the residual oxygen to dissipate out of the tooth for a few weeks will permit higher bond strengths to be gained. The reduction in bond strength is more marked when an acetone-based product is used instead of an ethanol-based one. The primary reason for reduction in bond strength is that the polymerization of the resin is inhibited by oxygen. Some clinicians have advocated the application of **sodium ascorbate** immediately prior to etching to reverse this inhibitory effect. Sodium ascorbate is an antioxidant. After etching, the bonding procedure is carried out as normal. This assumes that the effects have been achieved in the short period of time during application. Since diffusion through the enamel must occur, the time for contact is critical. Short applications may have a superficial effect.
- There will often be some reversal of shade lightening, the tooth slightly darkening once the bleaching treatment is discontinued. A delay will allow the shade of the tooth to stabilize before matching any restorations to bleached enamel.
- When power bleaching has been done in the clinic and when the mouth has been open for the duration of the treatment (at least 30 minutes), teeth become dehydrated. As a result their colour becomes lighter. A delay will allow the teeth to rehydrate and the normal colour to return. The dentist will then more accurately and predictably be able to select the correct shade for a perfectly matched restoration.

FACTORS AFFECTING OUTCOME

Duration of application and patient compliance

The longer the bleaching gel is in contact with the tooth, the more rapid the whitening will be. This is similar to sun tanning, the more one is exposed to the sun's rays, the quicker the tan will be achieved. Some patients find that wearing the bleaching trays overnight is not acceptable. This may be overcome by using an alternative regimen, such as wearing the trays for 2 hours in the evening or whenever they are able to without social embarrassment. Changing the gel every 2 hours decreases treatment time. Faster bleaching is associated with increased side effects, particularly tooth sensitivity. The mouth's response to the chemical will limit the time the patient can tolerate exposure to the bleaching solution.

Most bleaching systems usually produce a favourable outcome within 3 weeks when used as directed, although in some cases desired result may be gained more quickly and others take longer. Overexposure to the bleaching chemicals should be avoided as the intrinsic colour of the tooth will be lost with increasing contact time. Continuing degradation of the organic matrix of the tooth will result in the total loss of the enamel matrix protein, not only leading to a compromised result but also damage to the tooth tissue.

Type of darkened tooth tissue

The inherent colour of darkened tooth tissue will influence the outcome. Generally speaking, teeth with yellow or brown preoperative discolouration are more amenable to a successful outcome with bleaching than those with blue or grey discolouration. Teeth darkened due to age changes are the most amenable to treatment. Younger patients tend to show a greater initial improvement compared with older patients. Opaque enamel tends to become more opaque with bleaching.

Patients with tetracycline staining may find that that although their teeth lighten, a grey shade persists postoperatively and ideal results are not achieved. These cases are the most resistant to treatment, and it may take significantly longer, even up to 6 months, to achieve a satisfactory result. Despite this, significant improvements can be obtained.

It is fair to say that most patients experience some lightening of their teeth although the amount of change or the time taken to lighten are unpredictable. The only way to ascertain the effect is by attempting treatment.

Patients should be warned at the outset of care that there is no guarantee of a successful outcome or of the treatment time.

BLEACHING SYSTEMS AND PRODUCTS

Over-the-counter products

Bleaching strips

Flexible, polyethylene strips impregnated with hydrogen peroxide at concentrations ranging from 6% to 14% in an adhesive gel are manufactured by Procter and Gamble and sold in the USA as Crest Whitestrips (Table 18.3). They are applied after brushing the facial

Table 18.3 Crest Whitestrips products currently available in the USA

Name	% hydrogen peroxide	Applications per day	Duration per application (minutes)	Number of days of treatment	Comments
3D White Advanced Vivid	9.5	One	30	14	
3D White Gentle Routine	6	One	5	28	
3D White Professional Effects	10	One	30	20	
3D White Stain Shield	10	One	5	28	
3D White Vivid	10	One	30	10	
Supreme	14	Two	30	21	Sold only to dental professionals

surfaces of the maxillary and mandibular teeth to be whitened, typically the incisors and canines. They should only be worn during waking hours, except when the patient is eating. The hydrogen peroxide concentration of the strips is not stated on the packaging. Patients can use the 5-minute 'Gentle' product if they have tolerability issues with the higher concentration products.

Paint-on gels

These products have been available since 2004 and as their name suggests, consist of a gel which can be painted on to the teeth to be whitened. This obviates the need to construct a tray and facilitates the bleaching of single teeth. The method of application is similar across the products in that the teeth are dried and the gel is applied twice daily for 14 days.

Commercially available products

Some of the currently available paint on gels are lsited in Table 18.4 and Figure 18.3.

Table 18.4 Some paint-on gel tooth-whitening products currently available on the market

Product	Manufacturer	Active ingredient
Crest Night Effects	Proctor and Gamble	19% sodium perborate
Mentadent Xtra White	Unilever Oral Care	6% hydrogen peroxide
Polapaint	SDI	8% carbamide peroxide
Simply White Clear Whitening Gel	Colgate-Palmolive	16.4% or 18% carbamide peroxide depending whether the product is for sale in Europe or the USA, respectively. This product has now been discontinued in the UK
VivaStyle Paint On Plus	Ivoclar Vivadent	6% hydrogen peroxide

Whitening toothpastes

Many dentifrices are marketed to whiten teeth. While these products are effective at removing extrinsic stain, they cannot affect the colour of the tooth as this is determined by the underlying dentine. There is a concern that increased efficacy of stain removal may be associated with increased abrasiveness, and removing the outer surface of the enamel is clearly not desirable. See Chapter 17 for a fuller discussion of toothpastes.

Professionally supervised techniques

When any cosmetic treatment is being considered, it is imperative that the dentist fully assesses the patient and their mouth. A full history is essential followed by a clinical examination. This will allow a diagnosis to be made, help direct the clinician to the most appropriate bleaching product for the treatment appropriate to the individual's needs, and also indicate the likely prognosis of the treatment.

The oral hard and soft tissues must be in good condition prior to the commencement of cosmetic treatment. Any routine dental care should be completed prior to any cosmetic treatment. Teeth should be examined for caries and integrity of restorations. Any leaking restorations should be replaced. Any periodontal condition must be treated and the patient placed on an appropriate preventive regime. The clinician will also consider other investigations such as a radiographic examination, particularly when treatment of non-vital teeth is envisaged. Sensitivity tests on any suspect teeth will also be required. A tooth lightening procedure should only be part of an overall treatment plan with other cosmetic procedures being considered after the bleaching such as replacement of resin composites or ceramic restorations to improve the final appearance of the other adjacent teeth.

> **!**
>
> It is essential that informed consent is gained prior to cosmetic dental treatment. Patients should be fully counselled of the stages of the procedure, the risks, benefits, likely outcomes and, of course, associated costs.

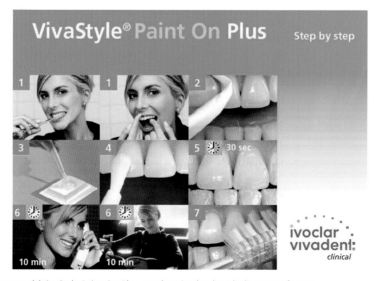

Fig. 18.3 A tooth whitening paint-on gel (VivaStyle Paint On Plus, Ivoclar Vivadent) with directions for use.

Home bleaching

This technique is sometimes also referred to as **nightguard bleaching**, as it requires construction of a thin bleaching tray out of **soft polyvinyl**. This method has been shown to be one of the most effective bleaching techniques. The dentist makes an impression of the arch to be treated, usually in an alginate impression material. The impression is disinfected and sent to the dental laboratory. Once the technician has cast up a model, a thin layer of resin composite material (LC Block-out, Ultradent) is painted onto the teeth on the model corresponding to the teeth to be treated (Figure 18.4).

The painted resin will result in **wells** or **reservoirs being** formed in the tray into which the bleaching gel can be placed by the patient. The need for reservoirs in the tray is determined by the viscosity of the gel, the more viscous the gel the greater the need for reservoirs. The presence of reservoirs increasing the efficacy of the treatment. Larger reservoirs are used for in-office bleaching.

The tray is then constructed by **vacuum forming**. A sheet of clear thermoplastic resin is placed over the model and positioned in a vacuum chamber containing a small heater. As the vacuum is applied the warm plastic sheet is sucked down onto the model forming a snugly fitting tray. Excess material may be trimmed away after the process has been completed (see Chapter 23). The tray is trimmed to correspond with the gingival margins of the teeth (Figure 18.5).

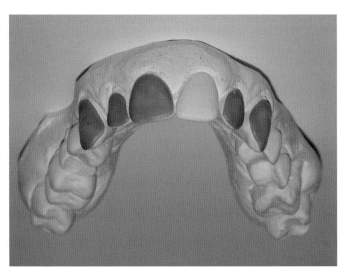

It is important that the bleaching tray fits well so that excess bleaching gel is not displaced from the tray on insertion or during wear.

Fig. 18.4 The working model to construct a bleaching tray. Note the blue light-cured resin composite additions (LC Block-out, Ultradent) to the labial surface, which when the vinyl is sucked down by vacuum over the model makes the reservoirs that will accommodate the bleaching gel and hold it against the teeth.

Prior to commencement of treatment, thorough prophylaxis is carried out. This is followed by a preoperative shade and clinical photographs being taken. These photographs should preferably show the selected shade tab for comparison. After preparation of the tray and preliminary evaluation at the next visit, the patient is instructed to wear the tray with the gel for 2 hours every evening or overnight; as they are administering the bleaching solution to their own teeth, they can take 'ownership' of the results. The patient is recalled for review after a short period of time to allow the dentist to supervise the shade change.

Once a satisfactory result has been achieved a postoperative photograph should be taken and the details of the new shade recorded in the patient's clinical notes.

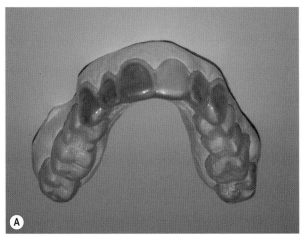

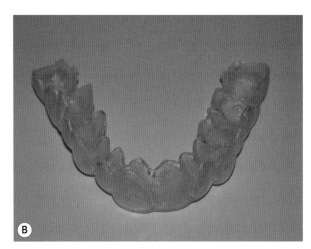

Fig. 18.5 The finished tray (A) on and (B) off the model.

Bleaching of vital teeth

When many vital teeth are to be treated, a technique called **nightguard vital bleaching (NGVB)** is used (Figure 18.6). The concentration of carbamide peroxide used with these products is 10%, which provides a balance between optimal results and minimal side effects, particularly for extended treatment. Usually one arch is done at a time to allow for:

- Comparison of the treated arch with that of the other
- Determination of prognosis/treatment outcome
- Minimizing side effects.

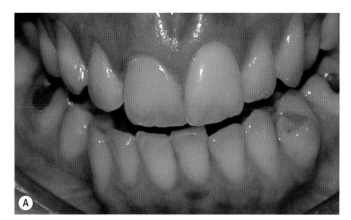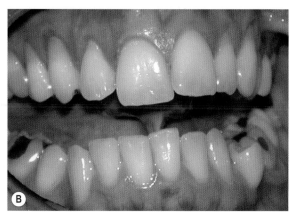

Fig. 18.6 (A) Pre- and (B) postoperative photographs of the lightening of both arches using 16% PF Carbamide Peroxide gel (White Dental Beauty, Optident). All teeth were vital and this result was achieved in 3 weeks. Note that the shade of the cervical resin composite restorations in teeth 15 and 14 has not been affected by the bleaching process.

Many clinicians recommend treating only the upper arch, as the lower teeth are not so noticeable, being largely hidden by the lower lip. The decision to treat one or both arches will be made by the patient and clinician, with usually the patient being the final decision maker.

Treatment for a single vital discoloured tooth is illustrated in Figure 18.7.

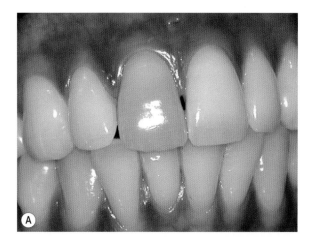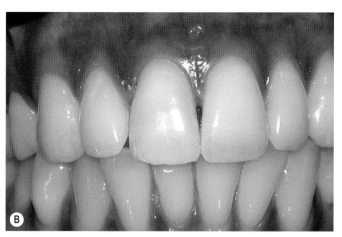

Fig. 18.7 (A) Pre- and (B) postoperative photographs of a vital discoloured tooth (11) lightened using 16% PF Carbamide Peroxide gel (White Dental Beauty, Optident). This result was achieved in 4 weeks.

Bleaching of non-vital teeth

Non-vital teeth are usually discoloured as a result of degradation of blood pigments leaching from the pulp tissue, which leads to the brown colour. Although these teeth are generally amenable to treatment, they have a more uncertain prognosis. To enhance and facilitate the passage of the solution through the tooth tissue, some clinicians advocate the removal of the restorative material in the access cavity.

This technique has been described as **inside-outside** bleaching (Figure 18.8). Severely darkened or stained dentine may be removed at this stage although the clinician must be aware that any removal of tooth tissue will have a detrimental effect on the strength of the tooth. If tooth tissue removal is considered desirable, it should be kept to a minimum. The gutta percha must be sealed using a glass ionomer or resin-modified glass ionomer cement to:

- Prevent bacterial ingress into the root canal system
- Prevent passage of the oxygen species into this region of the tooth, the root filling material and the periradicular tissues.

The patient must be shown how to syringe the bleaching gel into the palatal defect of the tooth. Some patients find it easier if a friend does it for them. The gel may be changed every 2 hours to hasten the bleaching effect. Products containing 10% carbamide peroxide are most commonly used although products with different concentrations are available. While higher concentrations will produce more rapid results, this must be balanced against decreased compliance due to the increased chances of intra-treatment discomfort.

Once the desired result has been achieved (Figure 18.9), the access cavity may be restored using resin composite. Many clinicians elect to use a lighter shade to enhance the lightening effect, and to allow distinguishing between the tooth and restorative material, should the material need to be removed in future. This decreases the risk of sound tooth being removed due to difficulty in differentiating between the restorative material and tooth tissue.

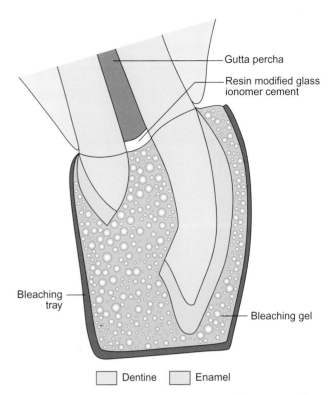

Fig. 18.8 Inside-outside bleaching: the bleaching gel has access to the inside and outside parts of the tooth. Note that the root canal obturating material has been sealed off by the placement of a resin-modified glass ionomer cement to prevent the bleaching chemicals accessing the root canal system.

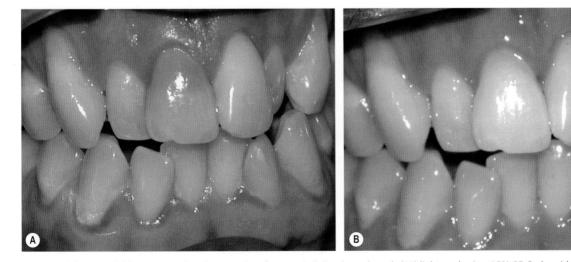

Fig. 18.9 (A) Pre- and (B) postoperative photographs of a non-vital discoloured tooth (11) lightened using 16% PF Carbamide Peroxide gel (White Dental Beauty, Optident) after the palatal access restorative material was removed. This result was achieved after 3 weeks' application of the bleaching solution in a tray externally and internally.

Table 18.5 Some products for home use under professional supervision currently available on the market

Product	Manufacturer	Active ingredient	Comments
10% h.p white	Ultradent	10% hydrogen peroxide	Preformed tray
15% PF Carbamide Peroxide Gel	Ultradent	15% PF Carbamide Peroxide Gel	With potassium nitrate and sodium fluoride
Evolution ICE	Enlighten	10% or 16% carbamide peroxide	
Illuminé Home	Dentsply	10% or 15% carbamide peroxide	
NiteWhite ACP	Discus Dental	10%, 16% or 22% carbamide peroxide	With ACP
Opalescence	Ultradent	10% carbamide peroxide	
Perfect Bleach	Voco	10% or 17% carbamide peroxide	
Perfecta Bravo	Myerson	9% hydrogen peroxide	
Poladay	SDI	3%, 7.5% or 9% hydrogen peroxide	
Polanight	SDI	10%, 16%, 22% carbamide peroxide	
Ramp	Enlighten	11% and 16% carbamide peroxide then 6% hydrogen peroxide	
Rembrandt	Denmat	10% carbamide peroxide	
VivaStyle	Ivoclar Vivadent	10% or 16% carbamide peroxide	
White Dental Beauty	Optident	10%, 16% or 22% carbamide peroxide or 6% hydrogen peroxide	

Commercially available products

Some professional home use bleaching systems available are shown in Table 18.5 and Figure 18.10. One system (Ramp, Enlighten) advocates a three-step process, whereby the concentration of peroxide is increased as the treatment progresses. This is claimed to maximize results as there is a gradual increase in permeability of the tooth tissue to oxygen without significant thermal sensitivity. In this system, 11% carbamide peroxide is applied for 5 nights, then 16% carbamide peroxide for another 5 nights, followed by a 'blast' of 6% hydrogen peroxide.

In-office techniques

'Walking bleach'

This traditional technique was advocated for the treatment of non-vital teeth. All gutta percha is removed coronal to the amelocemental junction and is sealed with a cement such as glass ionomer cement to prevent ingress of the bleaching active ingredients into the radicular parts of the tooth. The active ingredient sodium perborate (e.g. Bocasan powder, see below) and 30–35% hydrogen peroxide are mixed together. A pledget of cotton wool saturated with the solution is placed into the access cavity in the tooth and sealed into the pulp chamber using either glass ionomer cement or a putty temporary material. The patient is recalled 4–7 days later and the cotton wool pellet replaced with a new one infused with the chemicals. This process is repeated until a satisfactory result is obtained. During the treatment period the patient is free to go about their business, hence the term '**walking bleach**'. The results with this technique have been mixed, some cases responding well and others less satisfactorily.

The inclusion of hydrogen peroxide potentiates the effects of the sodium perborate by accelerating the release of oxygen and so produces a better effect. This technique is not used that frequently these days as other methods have proved to be more effective. In addition, sodium perborate is more difficult to obtain in the UK now that

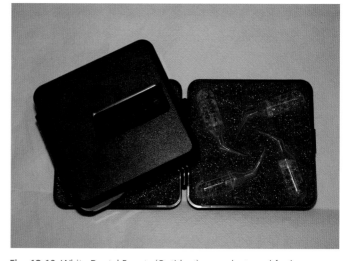

Fig. 18.10 White Dental Beauty (Optident), a product used for home dental bleaching.

Bocasan power (Procter & Gamble) has been removed from the *British National Formulary*. This was a powdered formulation which was added to water immediately before use. The active ingredient, sodium perborate monohydrate generated hydrogen peroxide as well as molecular oxygen upon contact with water. Other (inactive) ingredients included sodium bitartrate (buffer), saccharin (sweetener) and flavours. When mixed with water as directed, the concentration of hydrogen peroxide in solution was approximately 1.3% (assuming quantitative conversion of perborate to peroxide). This is similar in concentration to currently marketed peroxide-containing mouthrinses. Hydrogen peroxide, upon contact with oral fluids and blood, generates molecular oxygen which causes both a chemical and mechanical cleaning action.

Assisted bleaching

This is essentially an extension of home bleaching, but it is done in the clinic using higher concentration of chemicals. It may also be used as a supplement to home bleaching. The main advantage of this technique is that due to the increased concentration of the bleaching chemical, the time of application to achieve the final result is decreased. The disadvantage is the increased cost to the patient as clinic time needs to be used. The chemical is in contact with the teeth to be bleaching for about 30 minutes before it is carefully removed. High concentrations of hydrogen peroxide are caustic so are a potential irritant to the oral soft tissues. The operator must be aware of this and be careful when using this chemical and they should isolate the oral soft tissues from the teeth during treatment. The progress can be assessed and perhaps repeated if indicated a week later. Some of the products available on the market are listed in Table 18.6.

Some operators advocate warming the bleaching chemicals as increasing the temperature will increase efficacy. An increase of $10\,^{\circ}C$ will double the rate of dissociation of hydrogen peroxide as the rate of dissociation is time dependent. As mentioned earlier, an increase of intrapulpal temperature of $3\,^{\circ}C$ will cause irreversible pulpal damage so this should be done with caution.

Power bleaching

The surgery technique of tooth whitening with the application of high-intensity light from either a xenon plasma-arc curing light or a laser has been termed **power bleaching**. The whitening process is accelerated by the energy applied. Consequently the treatment time is decreased but does involve clinic time and the patient has no control over the final result. As with assisted bleaching, treatments usually last 30 minutes and are reassessed and repeated if necessary after 7 days.

High intensity lights were used with the aim of applying heat, so speeding up the procedure as mentioned earlier in the chapter. This was inefficient and unpredictable and resulted in an increased incidence of tooth sensitivity. Other systems have since become available and are initiated and catalysed by light energy from a variety of sources ranging from high-speed halogen curing lights to lasers. Two examples are shown in Figure 18.11.

Table 18.6 Some products for use in the dental surgery for assisted bleaching currently available on the market

Product	Manufacturer	Active ingredient	Comments
Evolution ICE	Enlighten	9% hydrogen peroxide	
Illuminé Office	Dentsply	30% hydrogen peroxide	
Life-Like	Life-Like	44% carbamide peroxide	
LumaArch Whitening System	Quick White	Non-peroxide sodium chlorite/stabilized chlorine dioxide	
45% PF carbamide peroxide	Ultradent	45% carbamide peroxide	With potassium nitrate and sodium fluoride
38% hydrogen peroxide	Ultradent	38% hydrogen peroxide	
Polaoffice	SDI	35% hydrogen peroxide	
Polaoffice +	SDI	37.4% hydrogen peroxide	
Polazing	SDI	35% carbamide peroxide	
VivaStyle	Ivoclar Vivadent	30% carbamide peroxide	
White Speed	Discus Dental	35% carbamide peroxide	
Yotuel Dental Office	Biocosmetics	30% carbamide peroxide	

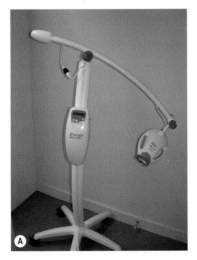
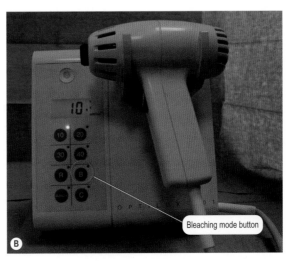

Bleaching mode button

Fig. 18.11 Two lights which can be used in conjunction with a bleaching solution: (A) Zoom! Advanced Power (Discus Dental) and (B) Optilux 501 (Kerr), a high speed halogen curing lamp with a bleach mode.

Due to the high concentration of chemicals used, it is essential that the procedures should be carried out with the teeth isolated from the rest of the mouth. Rubber dam is advisable although syringed liquid rubber dams are now available, which can be applied to the gingival tissues and light cured. This has the effect of masking the soft tissue and thus protecting them. Examples of these products are listed in Table 18.7.

Table 18.7 Some liquid rubber dam products currently available on the market

Product	Manufacturer
Opal-Dam	Ultradent
Paint-On-Dam	Den Mat
Quite White Paint-On-Dam	Denmed

Commercially available products

Some of the currently available power bleaching systems are listed in Table 18.8.

Table 18.8 Some products for power bleaching currently available on the market

Product	Manufacturer	Active ingredient	Comments
36% White Dental Beauty	Optident	38% hydrogen peroxide Potassium fluoride	Can be used without the light
Hi-Lite	Shofu	35% hydrogen peroxide Ferrous sulphate Manganese sulphate	Dual-activated (chemically and light-activated)
LumaArch Whitening System	Quick White	Non-peroxide sodium chlorite/ stabilized chlorine dioxide	Best results gained with the application of light energy
Opalescence Boost	Ultradent	38% hydrogen peroxide Potassium fluoride	Can be used without the light

Use of light

After isolation of the teeth, the selected bleaching gel (see Figure 18.6) is applied to the teeth to be treated and the light positioned as directed by the light manufacturer. Then the light is switched on and the tooth is exposed to the light for the treatment time advised.

Bleaching lights should be used with care as heat is emitted and this may cause thermal injury to the dental pulp.

It has been postulated that the most important factor is the concentration of the active ingredient of the bleaching product and not the light. Some clinicians acknowledge that the use of a light is not necessary to the success of the procedure but is done to add flare to the procedure.

When the bleaching mode button on the Optilux 501 (Kerr) curing lamp is pressed the light can be applied to the teeth to be treated, usually for 30 seconds per tooth. This is both time consuming and tedious for the dentist. The Zoom light illuminates both arches simultaneously so reducing the clinician's time and input (Figure 18.12).

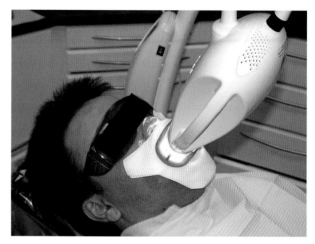

Fig. 18.12 A patient receiving power bleaching treatment under the Zoom light.

Commercially available lights

Some of the lights recommended for power bleaching are shown in Table 18.9.

Table 18.9 Lights for power bleaching currently available on the market

Product name	Manufacturer	Type of light
Velopex Diode	Medivance Instruments Ltd	Diode laser
Luma Arch	DMDS	Xe-Halogen
Optilux 501	Kerr Hawe	High speed halogen
Zoom	Discus Dental	Metal-halide

LONG-TERM PROGNOSIS

The success rate of tooth lightening treatments has been reported to be approximately 90%, particularly when supervised by a dentist. Physiological tooth discoloration (darkening with age) is due to the thickening of the dentine layer due to the continuing deposition of secondary dentine throughout the tooth's life. This may require the bleaching procedure to be repeated to bring the shade back. On average, there is relapse (also called **rebound** or **regression**) of darkening after 1–3 years of the bleaching treatment. If re-treatment is undertaken, the treatment duration is much shorter, a matter of days, but it can cause adverse effects. In some patients, the teeth undergo permanent lightening which requires no re-treatment.

LEGAL POSITION IN THE UK

In September 2011, the European Union (EU) Commission ruled that less than 17% carbamide peroxide and between 0.5% and 6% hydrogen peroxide can be used to whiten teeth provided that it is pre-scribed and administered by a dentist (i.e. the dentist has examined the patient, formulated a treatment plan and given the appropriate warnings and instructions). Products containing or releasing greater than 6% hydrogen peroxide will remain illegal. The UK has to enable this legislation within 12 months but at the time of writing it was still to be done. Until then, the use of peroxide-containing tooth whiten-ing agents packaged and solely intended for this purpose is illegal in the UK. This is not because any concerns have been raised about the safety or efficacy of the various techniques available but due to the European legal ruling some years ago (see next paragraph), which remains relevant until the above legislation is passed.

The UK Cosmetic Products (Safety) Regulations 1996 are derived from the EU Directive (76/768/EEC) passed in 1976 with the aim of protecting the public through control of cosmetic products. Under this legislation, tooth whitening products are defined as cosmetic products and as such are not permitted by the regulations to contain or release more than 0.1% hydrogen peroxide. Trading Standards are responsible to police this act and a prosecution would be made under the Consumer Protection Act 1987. Anyone found guilty of supply-ing or processing goods with the intention of supply is liable to a fine of £5000 and/or up to 6 months' imprisonment. Some companies have challenged this, arguing that tooth whitening products are med-ical devices, as they are classified in the remainder of the European Union. Furthermore, they are used under the supervision of a dentist and therefore should not fall under the Cosmetic Regulations. A few products introduced to the market after these regulations came into force contain sodium perborate and whose use is considered legal. An appeal heard in the UK House of Lords ruled that that tooth whiten-ing products were indeed cosmetics and a change would be required to the EU Cosmetics Directive to allow higher concentrations of hydrogen peroxide to be used for dental bleaching. This has now been done as stated above, although the UK still has to pass the legislation.

The passing of the new legislation will improve the situation for those dentists in the UK who wish to offer their patients a non-invasive and safe treatment option. Interestingly, the new legislation only affects the treat-ment of vital teeth, so that non-vital teeth can be treated without legal risk even now. It would be prudent therefore for these dentists to consult their medical defence organization for up-to-date advice. Dentists should note that not all of these organizations indemnify their members against per-forming such treatments and clearly this would need to be clarified prior to proceeding. While there is anecdotal evidence of Trading Standards turning a blind eye to dentists performing this treatment, the legislation is in place if the organization decided to prosecute other individuals such as hairdress-ers or beauty therapists carrying out dental bleaching should they so wish.

Current advice from one defence organization is to obtain full written informed consent by warning patients of the side effects and risks (listed earlier in the chapter) and that there is no guarantee of any specific outcome of treatment. The whitening treatment should be done in the context of a course of treatment where other issues are addressed such as caries and any periodontal treatment required. In other words, patients should not be recruited solely for a tooth whitening treatment, particularly where dental pathology exists. However despite this, it must be noted that should a complaint be made, with the current legal framework a case would be difficult to defend. It is also interesting to note that at the time of writing, the only cases of successful prosecution in the UK have been non-dental professionals.

SUMMARY

- Tooth whitening techniques are commonplace in modern dentistry and patient demand is increasing.
- Tooth whitening can be carried out by the patient at home or in the dental surgery under close supervision of the dentist; the product used at home having a lower concentration of the active ingredient than those used in the clinic.
- Products containing 10% carbamide peroxide are most commonly used and are the most appropriate for use in extended treatment.
- While higher concentrations will produce a more rapid result, this must be balanced against decreased compliance due to discomfort and greater risk of pulpal damage.
- While outcomes of treatment are usually good, the results can be unpredictable and there may be side effects which the dentist must explain to the patient at the outset to gain informed consent.
- It is important to note that tooth whitening is not illegal in the UK.
- However, practitioners in the UK should be aware that it is illegal to supply of products that are packaged and solely intended for the purpose of tooth whitening with instructions that contain or release more than 0.1% hydrogen peroxide.

FURTHER READING

Greenwall, L. (Ed.), 2001. Bleaching Techniques in Restorative Dentistry: An Illustrated Guide. Martin Dunitz, London.

Haywood, V.B., Heymann, H.O., 1989. Nightguard vital bleaching. Quintessence Int. 20 (3), 173–176.

Kelleher, M., 2008. Dental Bleaching. Quintessence Publishing Co., London.

McCracken, M.S., Haywood, V.B., 1996. Demineralization effects of 10 percent carbamide peroxide. J Dent 24 (6), 395–398.

SELF-ASSESSMENT QUESTIONS

1. List the factors that affect the outcome of a tooth lightening procedure.
2. What is the primary chemical used to lighten tooth tissue? Describe how it works.
3. What effects do the bleaching chemicals have on tooth tissue and what are the clinical ramifications for this?
4. What are the risks associated with the use of hydrogen peroxide in the mouth?
5. Why should any bonding of resin composite to tooth tissue be delayed after a bleaching treatment?
6. Describe the role of light in power bleaching.

Chapter | 19 |

Cutting instruments

INTRODUCTION

Cutting instruments are, of course, not dental materials per se, but the effect they have when used with dental materials and on tooth tissues is of great clinical significance. This chapter discusses the equipment used to cut and polish both dental materials and tooth tissues. Other techniques such as sandblasting, air abrasion and laser cutting, which have found many indications in modern dentistry as they are much less invasive, are also described.

The removal of a variety of materials can be very demanding. It is remarkable that it is possible to remove tooth tissue (enamel and dentine) and all restorative materials (including ceramics, metals and plastics) using the same implement, the dental **handpiece**. In other walks of life, specific dedicated machines are used to cut different substrates.

DENTAL HANDPIECES

Working at high speeds (in excess of 180 000 rpm)

Two types of dental handpiece (drill) are available to work at a high cutting speed, for example, to cut through enamel and to remove existing restorations.

- **High-speed** handpiece, also known as an **air rotor** or **air turbine** (Figure 19.1). As its name implies, it is driven by a supply of compressed air.
- **Speed-increasing** handpiece (Figure 19.2). These are generally driven by an electrical motor. They achieve their speed by using a gearing mechanism much like a gear box in a car.

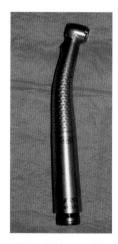

Fig. 19.1 A high-speed dental handpiece (W&H).

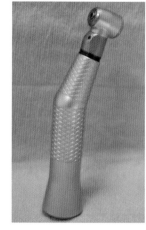

Fig. 19.2 A speed-increasing handpiece (Bien Air). Note the red ring on the proximal end of the instrument. This denotes that the internal gearings increase the speed of the instrument.

Box 19.1 How to correctly insert a friction grip bur into a handpiece

Step 1	Step 2	Step 3	Step 4
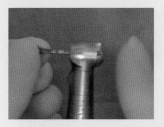	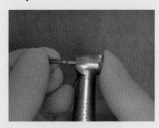	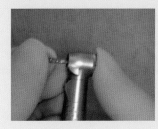	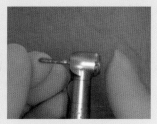
The selected bur should be inserted into the bur hole	The push button on the back of the handpiece head is then depressed	The bur is firmly pushed home	The push button is released and following a security check, the handpiece is ready to use

Both the air driven high-speed instrument and the speed-increasing handpieces use **friction grip (FG)** burs, the **bur** being the cutting component of the system (Figure 19.3). The bur is slid into the jaws of the chuck while these are open and then the jaws are released to grip the bur shank. Box 19.1 illustrates how a friction grip bur should be inserted correctly into a high-speed or speed-increasing handpiece.

A high-speed or speed-increasing handpiece should never be run without fully inserting the bur into the chuck. If the bur is only partly inserted into the chuck, it may be released during use and cause intraoral soft tissue injury or be lost into the patient's oropharynx. In addition, any eccentricity in the running of the chuck will be exaggerated. This will damage the chuck and the bur. If the bur is too short to access the operating site, it should be changed for one of a greater cutting length (see fig 19.31, p. 335).

Strictly speaking, handpieces, particularly those running at high speeds, should not be run without a bur. However with a quality, well-balanced product, there will be no damage if this is done inadvertently.

High-speed handpiece

Internal structure

The turbine is powered by **compressed air**, which passes up the central lumen of the instrument. The air pressure is usually **3 bar** (43.5 psi) although this varies depending on the handpiece manufacturer's advice. This column of air then strikes the blades of a windmill in the handpiece head, causing it to rotate. The chuck is at the centre of the windmill. As the windmill rotates, so does the bur. The internal components of a high-speed handpiece are shown in Figures 19.4 and 19.5.

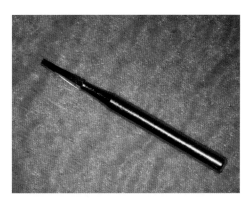

Fig. 19.3 A friction grip bur used with both high-speed and speed-increasing handpieces. Note the long smooth cylindrical portion of the bur, which is held in the jaws of the chuck by friction.

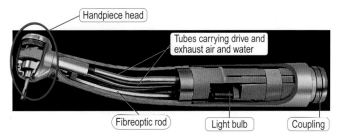

Fig. 19.4 A cut away view of a high-speed handpiece with the primary components identified.
Reproduced with kind permission of W & H.

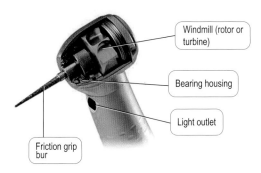

Fig. 19.5 The head of a high-speed handpiece with its components labelled. The blades of the windmill are driven by the compressed air.
Reproduced with kind permission of W & H.

Surrounding the chuck is the **bearing housing**, which is held centrally within the **head** of the handpiece by a plastic ring. This housing must be made to very precise tolerances to prevent the bur running eccentrically. Failure of the bur to run centrally will cause:

- The bur to judder. This leads to vibration that is then transmitted to the material being cut, causing cracking and crazing. This vibration may also be unpleasant for the patient. It can cause the bur to break as it may snatch against the cutting surface.
- Eccentric cutting. This will result in irregular removal of the tissue being prepared so more tissue is removed than is necessary.
- Less control for the dentist due to the irregular cutting.

Inside the bearing housing are seven or eight **ball bearings**, which run freely inside a cage called a **ball race**. The ball bearings are surrounded by a **phenolic resin** that lubricates their movement in the same way as oil lubricates the moving parts of a car engine. The race holds the shank of the bur, allowing it to rotate smoothly along a central axis with minimal friction. These ball bearings are made of either **stainless steel** or a **ceramic material**. There has been a move in recent years towards ceramic ball bearings, primarily because ceramic, is a harder material than stainless steel and wears less. It is also lighter in weight.

Cooling

As significant heat is generated during cutting due to friction, it is critical that effective cooling is provided over the whole cutting surface of the bur. Water is generally used to cool the bur. It is transported to the handpiece head via fine tubes within the body of the handpiece and exits via a number of small outlet holes, which are aligned to deliver the water onto the bur (Figure 19.6).

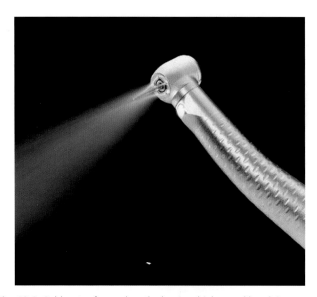

Fig. 19.6 Cold water focused on the bur in a high-speed handpiece to dissipate frictional heat generated during cutting.
Reproduced with kind permission of W & H.

It is desirable to have at least four holes, preferably more. This is because during use the position of the handpiece may prevent one or more holes directing water to the bur. The water may be also deflected

away from the bur by the surface being cut. This compromises the supply of water to the bur and hence the cooling efficiency (Figure 19.7).

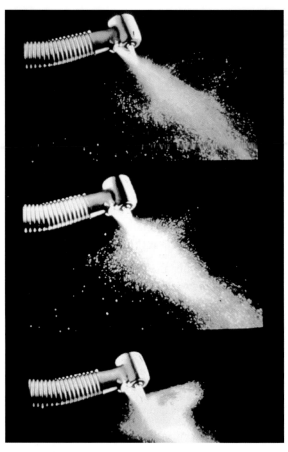

Fig. 19.7 The effect of water and air spray directed from the two apertures on the handpiece head simultaneously. Once air is incorporated, the water does not touch the bur at all. The water flow is disturbed and the air becomes the coolant, but this is ineffective in dissipating the heat.

Illumination

Many modern handpieces now have a light in close proximity to the bur. This is directed at the cutting surface so that the area being worked on is illuminated directly rather by reflection via a mouth mirror, increasing the dentist's clarity of vision. The original lights were small **halogen** bulbs, with the light being transmitted to the handpiece head using a **fibreoptic rod**. Halogen bulbs deteriorate with time in use and have relatively a short life. They are also expensive to replace. Furthermore, the glass fibreoptic rod was prone to breakage if the handpiece was dropped, and deteriorated with time due to repeated decontamination cycles in the autoclave. Many manufacturers have now moved onto using low-power **light emitting diodes (LEDs)**. The resulting light is whiter, more intense and the working life is much longer. LEDs are also relatively stable in wavelength over their lifetime and low-power LEDs produce little or no heat. The rapidly developing LED technology may well see considerable advances in product design and usage featuring these components in future.

Balance

The balance of the handpiece is important from two perspectives:

- Ergonomics
- Precision of use.

A badly balanced handpiece will compromise the accuracy of the dentist's work and increase operator fatigue. Other factors such as the type of the tubing housing, the services (air, water and electrical cabling) to the coupling and how it is arranged on the dental unit will also contribute to the balance of the handpiece. When the handpiece is held in the working position the balance should be neutral or slightly toward the handpiece head.

It is largely the clinician's preference whether a heavy or lighter handpiece is selected. A heavier handpiece will lead to operator fatigue more quickly than a lighter one. The materials used to manufacture the instrument influence the weight of the instrument. Materials such as **peek** (a fibre-reinforced composite material) are being used by some manufacturers to construct the internal components of the handpiece so reducing the handpiece's weight. **Brass** is commonly used to construct handpieces but will make the instrument heavier. **Stainless steel** is also used for handpiece manufacture and lies between these two materials with respect to weight.

Grip

Handpieces are either **knurled** or **smooth** in their external design and this is very much personal preference. Many practitioners prefer the knurled finish as this provides more stability and control of the handpiece. This is especially so when wearing gloves as the dentist's grip on the handpiece is enhanced. It is important that the **knurling** is not too deep or close together to avoid compromising cleaning and sterilizing of the instrument (Figure 19.8).

Size of head

In the past, the larger the head of the handpiece, the greater power could be generated. This needed to be balanced against the decrease in access to the site to be worked on as the dentist's vision was perhaps compromised. Smaller heads overcome these disadvantages but as a consequence, **torque** of the instrument was reduced in the early designs. Technology has now evolved such that it is no longer necessary to compromise the head size for torque.

The importance of torque

One of the critical properties for any dental handpiece is torque (along with concentricity and noise). This is the ability of the bur to continue to rotate and therefore cut when pressure (approximately 70 g) is applied to the substrate. The **free running speed** of a turbine is in the order of 300 000–400 000 revolutions per minute (rpm). As the bur is applied to the tooth the bur slows to a **cutting speed** of between 180 000 and 200 000 rpm. The optimum cutting speed is approximately **one half** of the free running speed.

To allow the bur to continue to rotate, the power must be maintained. The relationship of power, torque and speed are illustrated in Figure 19.9. Power is difficult to maintain with an air supply as the air pressure is not supplied at a constant level and may fluctuate depending on the draw down of air from the compressor. This

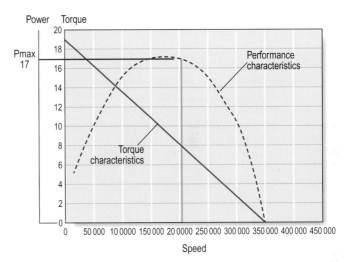

Fig. 19.9 The parabola shows the performance characteristic, i.e. the relationship of speed of rotation of the bur to power. As cutting speed increases so does the power up to a point past which the power starts to decrease. The maximum power is equivalent to half the free running speed and this is therefore the ideal cutting speed. The torque decreases linearly as rotational speed increases, i.e. the bur requires more power to continue to rotate it at the same speed as the pressure applied to it increases. This is due to the increasing drag on the bur.

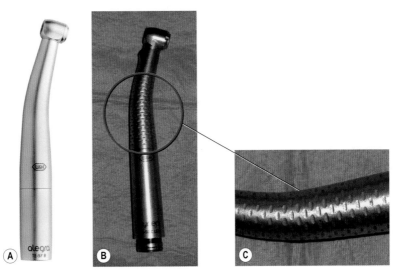

Fig. 19.8A–C Two W&H high-speed handpieces, one with a smooth outer casing and the other lightly knurled.
Image (A) reproduced with kind permission of W & H.

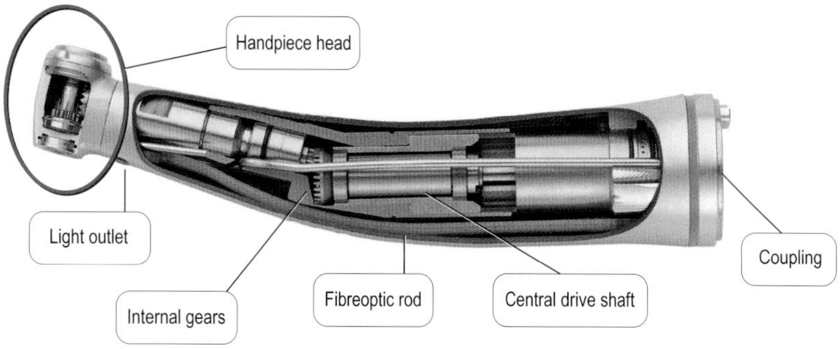

Fig. 19.10 A speed-increasing handpiece with its components labelled.
Reproduced with kind permission of W & H.

Handpiece head

Light outlet

Internal gears

Fibreoptic rod

Central drive shaft

Coupling

will have an effect on the speed of the bur and hence the torque. The air pressure should be set at 2–3 bar (29–43.5 psi) and should be confirmed using an air gauge. There may be significant fluctuations in air pressure due to the various demands on the compressor due to demand from other clinics in a multi-clinic practice.

Indications for using an air rotor handpiece

The indications of an air rotor dental handpiece are:

- Cutting of enamel and gross tooth tissue
- Removal of direct restorative materials
- Gross shaping and polishing of cured direct restorative materials
- Tooth preparation for an indirect prosthesis
- Cutting material used in the construction of indirect prostheses when these need to be removed
- Sectioning of teeth (such as in hemisections).

> **Hemisection:** a dental procedure in which a (lower) molar is divided into parts with individual roots by sectioning.

Speed-increasing handpiece

The speed-increasing handpiece (Figures 19.2 and 19.10) is driven by an electrical motor, also called a **micromotor**. The handpiece is placed onto the coupling of the micromotor on the dental unit (Figure 19.11).

The power to drive the handpiece is provided by the micromotor and the internal gearings in the handpiece cause the bur to rotate at a constant speed and torque.

Torque

The importance of maintaining sufficient torque during cutting has been discussed previously. The free running speed of a 1:5 speed-increasing handpiece is the same as its cutting speed at approximately 200 000 rpm, i.e. the motor speed of 40 000 rpm multiplied by 5 is a 200 000 rpm bur speed. This is maintained by the electrical motor, which delivers a consistent amount of power so the torque will be maintained when the bur contacts the tooth on preparation. This means that the tissue removal achieved using an electric motor-driven handpiece may be more consistent and usually has a higher torque.

Mode of cutting

A bur in a speed-increasing handpiece runs more smoothly compared with a bur in a turbine The bur in a turbine also moves axially (in and out) during use, resulting in a **pecking** motion being transmitted to the material being prepared. This pecking motion causes a rippling effect on the material, leading to the formation of **microcracks** (Figure 19.12).

To prevent microcracks, many operative dentists are now moving onto using speed-increasing handpieces in preference to turbines.

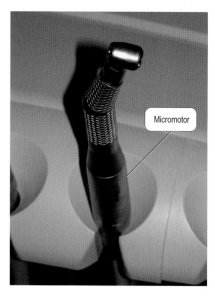

Fig. 19.11 A speed-increasing handpiece coupled onto a micromotor on a dental unit.

Micromotor

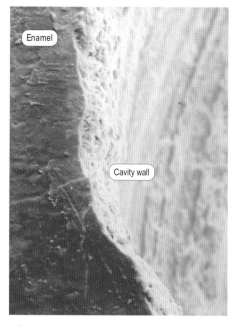

Enamel

Cavity wall

Fig. 19.12 A photomicrograph showing the effect of pecking on the periphery of a cavity. Note the rough edge where chipping has occurred. The outline is irregular as result of the pecking and there is crazing of the surface adjacent to the margin.

This is particularly so when doing work that requires a smoother running bur and precision such as refining tooth preparations, tooth hemisections and polishing. These handpieces also produce less noise and vibration.

Comparison of high-speed and speed-increasing dental handpieces

A comparison of the features of high and low speed handpieces are set out in Table 19.1.

Table 19.1 Comparison of the features of high-speed and speed-increasing handpieces

	High-speed	Speed-increasing
Type of bur used	Friction grip	Friction grip
Power source	Compressed air	Electric micromotor
Torque	Variable	Constant
Motion of bur	Rotation and pecking	Rotation only
Balance	Usually neutral	Motor end heavy

Slow-speed handpieces

Handpieces that operate at a slower cutting speed, that is, between 600 and 250 000 rpm are available as either **contra-angle** or **straight** (Figure 19.13). The internal workings of slow-speed handpieces are essentially the same as previously described for the speed-increasing handpiece as shown in Figure 19.11. The main differences between them are:

- In the internal gearings
- The slow-speed handpiece uses a **latch grip** bur (Figure 19.14) instead of the friction grip bur used in the speed-increasing handpiece.

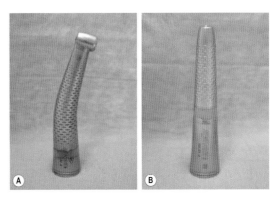

Fig. 19.13 (A) A contra-angle handpiece and (B) a straight handpiece (W&H). A piece of green tape has been placed by the user to differentiate which clinic the handpiece belongs to so that handpieces are not misappropriated after the decontamination procedure.

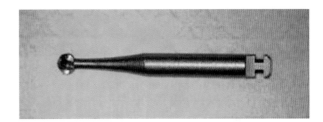

Fig. 19.14 A latch grip bur used in a slow-speed handpiece.

Indications for slow-speed handpieces

Contra-angle handpieces are generally used for operative procedures such as the removal of dental caries and for polishing enamel and restorative materials intraorally. Straight handpieces are used in oral surgical procedures or for the extraoral adjustment and polishing of acrylic and metals. The speed of the handpiece will depend on the task. Table 19.2 lists the cutting speeds for common dental procedures and materials.

Table 19.2 Cutting speeds for some common dental procedures*

Procedure	Handpiece	Gearing ratio	Recommended cutting speeds (rpm; revolutions per minute)
Cavity preparation	High-speed/speed-increasing	N/A/1:5	230 000
Removing existing intracoronal restorations	High-speed/speed-increasing	N/A/1:5	160 000–230 000
Caries removal	Low-speed/speed-decreasing	2:1, 10:1	1500
Fine finishing and polishing	Low-speed/speed-decreasing	2:1	20 000–40 000
Crown preparations	High-speed/speed-increasing	N/A/1:5	160 000–230 000
Mechanical root canal preparation	Speed-decreasing	20:1	Nickel titanium 250–500
Implant placement	Speed-decreasing	20:1	800–1000
Bone removal	Low-speed/speed-decreasing	–	600–2000
Shaping titanium implant abutment	Low-speed/speed-decreasing	–	6000
Prophylaxis	Low-speed/speed-decreasing	4:1	Up to 10 000
Extraoral polishing	Straight handpiece	N/A	6000
Cutting zirconia	speed-increasing	1:5	100 000

*These speeds are influenced by the type of bur being used. Tungsten carbide instruments require lower cutting speeds than diamonds.

Fig. 19.15 (A) Histological section showing the damage in the dental pulp after a cavity has been prepared with no water coolant. The boxed area shows a large number of inflammatory and round cells and the loss of continuity of the odontoblast layer. (B) Normal pulpal tissue is shown for comparison. The boxed area shows the odontoblast layer is undisturbed and columnar in shape with normal tissue beneath.

Most dental handpieces (except air turbines) have coloured rings on the body of the handpiece. These rings denote the handpiece's internal gearings. This feature is illustrated in many of the photographs in this chapter. The colour codes are explained in Table 19.3.

Table 19.3 Ring colour and internal gearing of dental handpieces

Ring colour	Gearing
Red	Increase usually 1:5 but may also be other ratios
Blue	1:1
Green (or double green)	Reduction may be 2:1, 4:1, or 20:1 but not related to a specific ratio

It is advisable to use water cooling even when cutting at slow speeds to:
- Reduce the substantial heat generated by friction. This heat can lead to deleterious effects on the dental pulp (Figure 19.15). Water cooling is more efficient at dissipating the heat than air.
- Excessive heat also has detrimental effects on the substrate, possibly causing it to melt. This melted material can clog the cutting surface of the instrument so resulting in reduced efficiency of the cutting or polishing process. More heat will be generated with larger amounts of the surface area of abrasive in contact with the substrate surface.
- Improve the dentist's vision of the area being prepared, as the water will wash away most debris produced.

Speed-decreasing

Some handpieces are designed to work at slower speeds and are termed **speed-decreasing handpieces** (Figure 19.16).

Indications for use of speed-decreasing handpieces

The main indications of speed-reducing handpieces are:

- *Endodontic canal preparation*. Root canals should be prepared using a slowly rotating file. Many endodontic handpieces also have a design feature to control the torque, with the aim of preventing endodontic file separation during use.
- *Implant placement*. The slow speed of rotation reduces the heat produced by friction so preventing damage to the bone cells that are needed for osseointegration.
- *Prophylaxis*. As the speed is slower, the heat produced and transmitted to the tooth during polishing is reduced. The slower speed also reduces the amount of the prophy paste (see p. 345) being sprayed everywhere! This phenomenon can be further reduced by using a reciprocating prophylaxis handpiece (Figure 19.17).

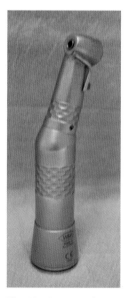

Fig. 19.16 A speed-decreasing handpiece (W&H).

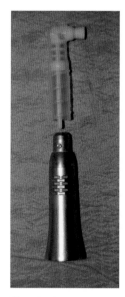

Fig. 19.17 A reciprocating prophylaxis handpiece (W&H).

Particles of prophylaxis paste can ingress into the handpiece and damage the internal workings. It is recommended therefore to use a dedicated handpiece for prophylaxis with a sealed or disposable head. This will preserve the condition and extend the lifespan of other handpieces used for precision procedures.

Reciprocating handpieces

Traditional rotary instruments are not always successful for certain procedures such as the removal of overhangs and ledges particularly in interproximal regions. When a rotating bur is used to polish a surface, there is a tendency for it to create a groove. With each subsequent pass of the bur, it naturally falls back into this groove, so deepening it. For this reason, removal of interproximal overhangs can be particularly difficult. Reciprocating handpieces (Figure 19.18) can move the bur using an oscillating movement, which can overcome the groove forming problem. Flat burs (Figure 19.18) are used to great effect in this situation for fine and coarse polishing and finishing interdentally.

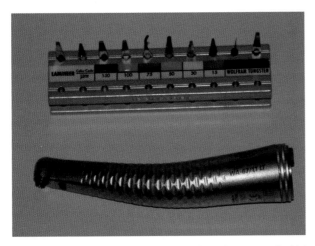

Fig. 19.18 A reciprocating handpiece and the burs that are used with it (W&H and Dentatus, respectively)

The vibration produced during the use of the reciprocating handpiece differs from conventional handpieces and some patients find this unpleasant.

Decontamination of handpieces

It is obviously important that all instruments used directly on a patient can be effectively decontaminated after use. The presence of a large number of tubes and spaces inside handpieces can present challenges for effective decontamination and vacuum autoclaves are recommended to decontaminate these instruments. Many handpieces are manufactured in one piece (**monobloc**) so that debris and microorganisms cannot penetrate into the joints. Instruments intended for surgical use are made of stainless steel. They are designed so that they can be dissembled into their constituent components to facilitate effective decontamination and it is strongly recommended that this is done (Figure 19.19). A recommended decontamination protocol is given in Box 19.2.

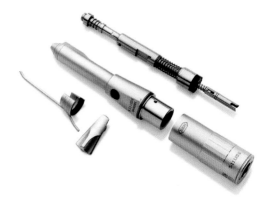

Fig. 19.19 A straight surgical handpiece dissembled into its (five) components to facilitate disinfection.
Reproduced with kind permission of W & H.

Box 19.2 Recommended decontamination protocol for dental handpieces

1. Remove the bur from the chuck in the handpiece head.
2. Rinse under running water (ideally demineralized and cooler than 38°C).
3. Dry with a cloth.
4. Wipe with an alcohol impregnated cloth.
5. Oil, preferably using a bespoke oiling and lubricating machine.
6. If applicable, use a washer-disinfector to clean handpieces, having first verified their suitability with the manufacturer. If a washer-disinfector is used, it may remove all the lubricants during the cleaning cycle and so further lubrication may be required after the cycle has finished.
7. Autoclave either bagged or unbagged depending on the autoclave type.

Recommended personal protective equipment (PPE) should be worn during such procedures to protect the worker.

Some symbols are laser etched onto the side of the instrument to provide the operator with information (Figure 19.20). In addition to this, other information such as CE mark (if applicable) and dot matrix codes may also be included.

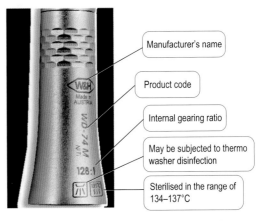

Manufacturer's name

Product code

Internal gearing ratio

May be subjected to thermo washer disinfection

Sterilised in the range of 134–137°C

Fig. 19.20 External handpiece markings labelled with explanation of the codes.
Reproduced with kind permission of W & H.

Handpiece maintenance

To prolong their lifespan and to ensure optimal performance, it is essential that all dental handpieces are carefully maintained. They should be cleaned and lubricated after every use and prior to sterilization. Bespoke machines are available (Figure 19.21), which aid lubrication of the internal workings of the handpiece before they are placed in the autoclave.

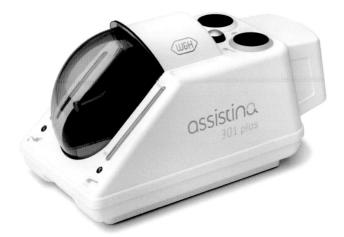

Fig. 19.21 The Assistina (W&H) machine used to lubricate dental handpieces prior to decontamination in the autoclave.
Reproduced with kind permission of W & H.

Like a motor vehicle, each handpiece should also be sent to the manufacturer or repair centre for an annual service.

Dental handpieces – the future

The use of information technology may well play a significant part in the development of dental handpieces in the future. An **information storage card** may be carried by the surgeon and inserted into the base unit prior to the operation. The card could hold information such as the surgeon's preference of cutting speeds and torques, thus simplifying procedures during the operation. Other information on the use of the handpiece during the procedure could also be documented and used as a medicolegal record.

Piezo technology is still in its infancy but it is possible that it will improve with time, and so give the operative dentist other options when cutting is indicated. It is of particular use in the removal of bone, and there is minimal damage to the adjacent bone and to the surrounding soft tissue as no heat is generated during the cutting process.

The cavitation effect produced by the insert (bur) on the tissue fluid means that the site remains clear of fluid and is easy to see. This system requires substantially less pressure to use in hard tissue removal compared with conventional methods. Patients report that there is less postoperative pain which is probably due to the less traumatic cutting effect. There is also no vibration, which reduces the discomfort.

The other piezo application which has been developed is in dental prophylaxis. A range of inserts made from titanium nitride may be used for scaling both supra- and subgingivally and also for root canal preparation and crown margin definition. One of the first companies to use this technology is Mectron s.p.a (via Loreto 15A, 16042 Carasco (GE), Italy).

Piezo effect: the effect of applying a stress to certain types of crystallites. These can be naturally occurring materials (such as quartz) or artificial materials such as ceramics and polymers. Compressing these produces an electromotive force that can be harnessed to drive various devices.

DENTAL BURS

The removal of tissue or material is achieved by the **bur** in the handpiece. 'Cutting' is a misnomer as burs primarily grind or abrade the surface of the substrate. For high-speed instruments, the common materials used for producing cutting burs are **diamond** or **tungsten carbide**. **Stainless steel** burs are used when working at lower speeds. Burs used in straight handpieces tend to be made of tungsten carbide.

Dental burs are produced in a range of shapes and sizes, and their use depends on the material to be removed and the task to be done.

Parts of a bur

A dental bur consists of three distinct parts (Figure 19.22):

- **Shank**: the portion which fits into the handpiece chuck and is of a standard size.
- **Neck**: the connector portion that joins the shank to the head. This is frequently tapered to accommodate the reduction in size of the cutting blades.
- **Head**: the portion of the bur that contains the blades or abrasive material.

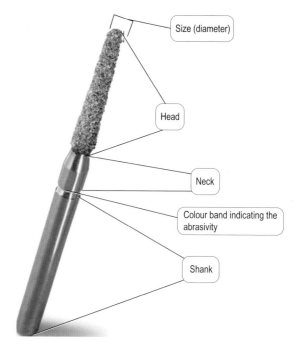

Fig. 19.22 The parts of a (diamond) bur.

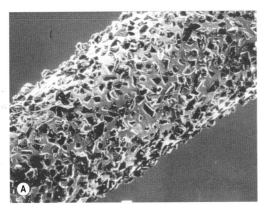
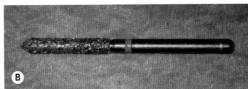

Fig. 19.23 (A) Magnified image of a diamond coated bur and (B) a photograph of a coarse crown preparation bur.

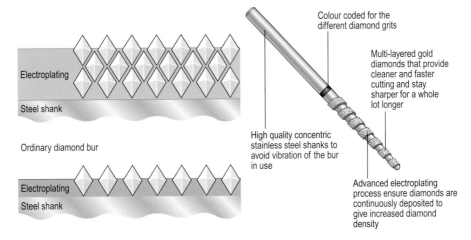

Fig. 19.24 Multi-layered diamond bur where, instead of one layer of diamond being deposited during the electroplating process, a number of layers of diamond grit are built up to give an increased diamond density so enhancing cutting efficiency.

Diamond burs

A diamond bur consists of a central shaft of metal forming the shank. On this is added a **resin** in which fine **diamond** particles are embedded, producing the appearance shown in Figure 19.23.

During what is a **grinding** process, the diamond wears away the tissue. The various layers of diamonds are slowly revealed as the bur wears due to 'plucking out' of the diamond particles (Figure 19.24).

Burs can become magnetized. This may cause them to 'stick' by magnetic forces to other dental manipulation instruments. The dentist may not notice this and the bur may be carried for a distance on an instrument before falling away. Such a bur may inadvertently be lost into the patient's oropharynx and the dental team should be aware of this potential hazard.

Abrasivity

Diamond burs are the dentist's workhorse. Their intended use will depend on the bur's **abrasivity**. The degree of abrasivity is determined by the size of the diamond particles embedded in the resin, which varies from supercoarse to ultrafine. Table 19.4 lists the various degrees of abrasiveness available.

Table 19.4 Colour codes, particle sizes and indications for use of diamond burs

Colour	Name	Size of particle (μm)	Uses
Black	Supercoarse	Above 175	Removal of existing restorations
Green	Coarse	150–175	General tooth preparation and removal of existing restorations
Blue/no ring	Medium	105–125	
Red	Fine	~45	Refining and finishing
Yellow	Superfine/extrafine	25–30	Finishing
Black	Ultrafine	15	

Tungsten carbide burs

Tungsten carbide (WC) is another cutting material but it is very brittle. During use tungsten carbide burs can **snatch** the substrate that they are cutting. The noise so produced has been termed **chatter**. This snatching may cause the bur to shatter. The clinician should be mindful of this as the fragments can displace into soft tissue or the

333

oropharynx. The mode of action is different from diamond burs, in that tungsten carbide burs grind and chip the surface as opposed to the abrading action of diamonds (Figure 19.25).

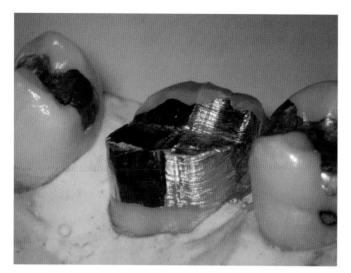

Fig. 19.25 A simulated crown preparation on an extracted tooth. The mesial half (left side) of the preparation has been prepared using a tungsten carbide bur and the distal part was prepared using a diamond bur. The amalgam core surface prepared by the tungsten carbide bur is shiny as it is smoother whereas microgrooves can be seen on the distal part of the preparation corresponding to the coarseness of the diamond bur.

Most tungsten carbide burs (Figure 19.26) consist of a stainless steel shank and neck on which the cutting blade made of tungsten carbide is attached. In some cases the neck is also made of tungsten carbide.

The tungsten carbide is milled to produce the cutting tool. The milling permits adjustment to the **blade angle** and **rake**. The bur blades can be positioned at different angles to the long axis of the bur in order to change the fashion in which the bur behaves in contact with the substrate. More obtuse angles will produce a negative rake angle, which increases the strength and longevity of the bur. The bur may be less efficient in 'cutting' initially. More acute angles will produce a positive rake angle which has a sharper blade, but which dulls more quickly. The milling can also produce **cross-cuts**

(Figure 19.27). The construction of the bur means that if undue pressure is applied laterally to the bur, then there is a risk that the joint between the tungsten carbide and shank will fail, causing the bur head to be detached from the shank (see Figure 19.22).

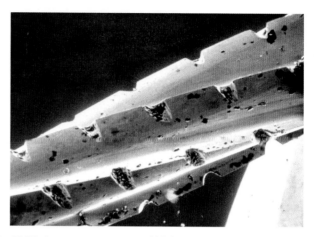

Fig. 19.27 A cross-cut tungsten carbide bur.

The distance the blades are apart (i.e. the number) will determine the bur's cutting power. The more aggressive burs have their blades further apart than the finest of the finishing instruments. Tungsten carbide burs are particularly indicated for cutting metal, for example, when existing extra- or intracoronal restorations have to be removed. As mentioned above they are also commonly used to finish tooth preparations and restorations as they produce a smoother surface than diamond burs. However, they do tend to blunt easily and their relatively high cost can mean that replacing them regularly can be an expensive exercise.

Some clinicians believe that these burs are 'kinder' to enamel in that they preferentially remove dental cements (for example orthodontic cements) than diamond burs so reducing potential collateral damage to natural dental hard tissue. However, this is a subject of much debate.

Cross-cut burs are indicated for cutting metal alloys such as amalgam, gold or nickel chrome. There are more cutting edges contacting the substrate which is being cut and so their cutting is more efficient.

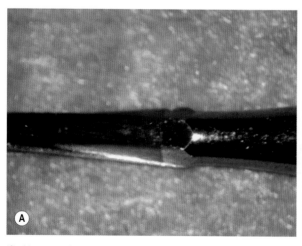
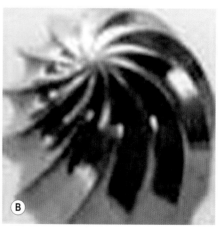

Fig. 19.26 Magnified images of two tungsten carbide burs. (A) A friction grip bur for use with a high-speed handpiece and (B) a bur used in a straight handpiece for trimming acrylic.

The amount of chatter is reduced as is the likelihood of tooth fracture or enamel crazing.

Straight handpiece burs

Tungsten carbide burs are the most commonly used bur type in a straight handpiece (Figure 19.28), an example being to trim acrylic. A recommended decontamination protocol for high-speed burs is given in Box 19.3.

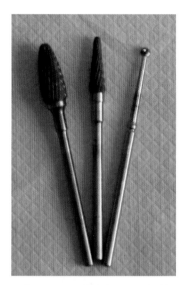

Fig. 19.28 A range of tungsten carbide burs used with a straight handpiece. Note the long shank that fits into the straight handpiece.

There is much controversy as to whether burs can be effectively cleaned of debris and decontaminated. Additionally, stainless steel burs will corrode if left in fluid for a time. For these reasons, many dentists consider burs to be for single use only and therefore discard them after one use.

Stainless steel burs

Stainless steel burs (Figure 19.29) are mainly used at lower cutting speeds, such as for removal of carious dentine or during cavity preparation (for example to create an undercut).

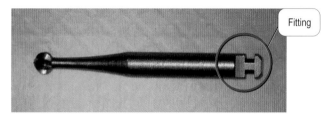

Fig. 19.29 A (round) stainless steel bur. The **fitting** part is where the bur is secured into the handpiece. This is know as a **latch grip** fitting.

As with other types of bur, they come in a variety of sizes and shapes (Figure 19.30). They tend to corrode with prolonged contact with water and so tend to be single-use instruments. Stainless steel burs are supplied with a longer or shorter shank to improve access to the operating site. These are called **short shank** (SS) or **longer length** (L) burs (Figure 19.31).

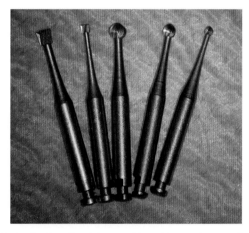

Fig. 19.30 A selection of stainless steel burs. The two burs on the left are two sizes of **inverted cone** burs while the others are **round** burs, again three sizes are shown.

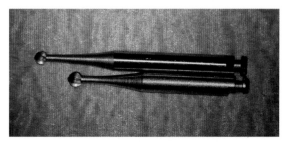

Fig. 19.31 Two stainless steel latch grip burs; the lower one is a normal size and the other is longer length. Shorter shank burs are also available.

Box 19.3 Recommended decontamination protocol for high-speed burs

1. The bur should be rinsed under running water using a brass wire bur brush to remove any contaminants such as debris, blood or saliva. The bur may be also soaked in a container of soapy water or a suitable disinfection solution such as Rotagerm (Septodont). This contains potassium hydroxide, propylene glycol and ethoxyamine alkyls in solution. The bur should not be soaked for more than 2 hours to prevent corrosion.
2. The bur is then placed in an ultrasonic bath for a cycle to loosen debris. The burs should not be allowed to vibrate against each other or another hard surface.
3. Sterilization in an autoclave or dry heat sterilizer is the next stage:
   - Dry heat sterilization at 170°C for 1 hour. This does not cause corrosion or dull the tungsten carbide.
   - Autoclaving at 121°C for 20–30 minutes at 1.1 bar (15 PSI)
   - Autoclaving at 134°C for 3–5 minutes at 2.1 bar (30 PSI) will also be effective although there is some risk of corrosion.
   - Demineralized water should be used for the final rinse cycle so to prevent water marks or discolouration of the bur.
4. The bur should then be visually inspected to ensure the instrument is clean and undamaged or corroded.
5. The bur should be placed on absorbent paper and allowed to dry completely.

It is advisable to keep the burs in a bur block during this process so that the cutting surface does not become damaged. The use of cold sterilizing solution is contraindicated, as these solutions may contain an oxidizing agent, which will weaken carbide burs. As with other decontamination processes, the operator should wear the recommended PPE before handling any contaminated instruments.

Quality products – quality results!

The precision and efficiency of cutting depends on the quality of the cutting instruments – both the handpiece and bur. Use of poor-quality equipment will result in imprecise, traumatic cutting, a short service life and clinician and patient fatigue. For this reason, it is false economy not to invest in good-quality products. Regularly changing blunting burs will further increase cutting efficiency and decrease extraneous damage to the tooth.

In order to optimize cutting efficiency and decrease extraneous damage to the tooth, burs should be regularly changed to prevent them from blunting.

AIR ABRASION

Air abrasion is akin to the technique of sandblasting used in the building industry to clean the surface of stone work. A stream of fine particles of sand is blasted against the metal surface to be cleaned using compressed air, causing any debris and dirt to be slowly blown away (Figure 19.32). This simple technique has been adapted to dentistry. Originally attempts to adapt the technology were carried out in the 1940s but alternatives such as the air turbine were considered

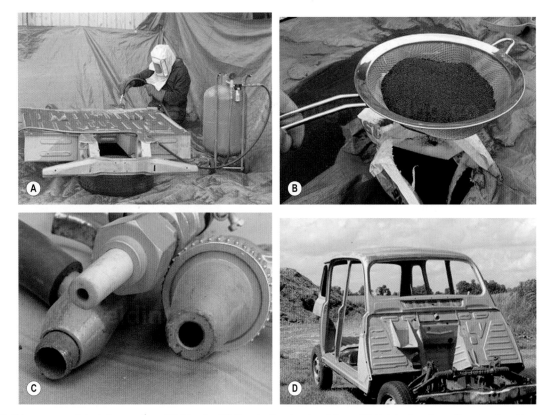

Fig. 19.32A–D (A) compressed air delivery system. (B) Abrasive (C) Nozzles for abrasive delivery (D) Finished surface after abrasion. The components and the technique for sandblasting metal work in industry. Note the protective equipment worn by the operator.

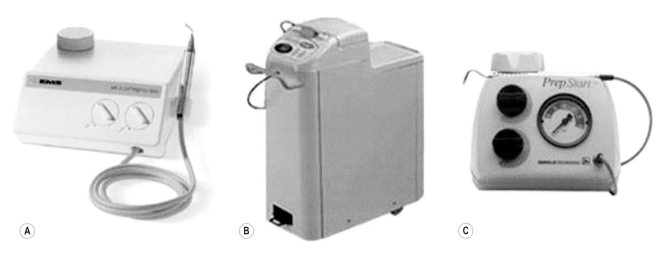

Fig. 19.33 Commercially available air abrasion units. (A) AIR-FLOW® Prep K1 Max (EMS Optident (UK) Ltd), (B) KCP 1000 (American Medical Technologies) and (C) PrepStart H$_2$O (Danville Engineering).

to have greater applications. The currently available machines (Figure 19.33) commonly use 27 μm **aluminium oxide (alumina)** powder, which is directed onto the tooth surface with fine tipped nozzles using compressed air at less than 2.7 bar (40 psi). The removal of different tissues in a controlled manner can be altered by:

- Changing the compressed air pressure
- Altering the size of the nozzle
- Altering the rate of flow of the abrasive
- Using different abrasives. As well as aluminium oxide, quartz and sodium bicarbonate are sometimes used. Some devices also include water.

Advantages and disadvantages

- The main advantage of air abrasion is that microcavities may be prepared so preserving tooth tissue. The use of magnification and dental materials which are capable of restoring tiny cavities make this is a very conservative method of restoring carious lesions.
- There is no need for local anaesthesia and patient acceptance is high as there is no noise or vibration from the device (Figure 19.34).

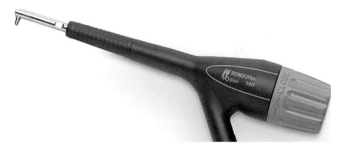

Fig. 19.34 The RONDOflex plus (KaVo). This instrument fits onto a high-speed coupling and the powder particles are directed onto the area to be treated at a speed of 20 m/s.

- The surface gained is better for bonding as its surface area and surface energy are higher. The device can also be used for removing cement residues from inside crowns and bridge retainers.

Unfortunately these machines are unable to remove existing restorations and so their usage is somewhat limited. Greater abrasivity may be achieved by using 50 μm alumina or 27 μm corundum powder, a crystalline form of alumina which is harder (Figure 19.35).

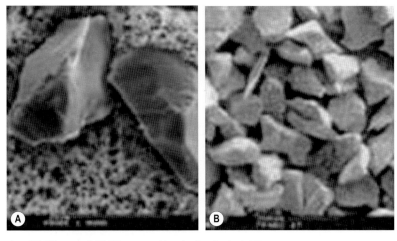

Fig. 19.35 The two sizes of abrasive, (A) 50 μm and (B) 27 μm, used to air abrade dental tissues.

SANDBLASTING

Sandblasting is used primarily in the dental laboratory. However, mini-sandblasters have been produced which may be used judicially intraorally with suitable protection for the patient. This entails the application of rubber dam to provide complete protection of the rest of the mouth and airway together with effective high-speed aspiration of the debris. The process is very similar to that described above for air abrasion. Usually sandblasting is more aggressive, using large abrasive particles at higher pressure. The abrasive used is usually alumina and as previous described, the particle size varies with the required effect.

The effect of applying a jet of alumina on to the surface of metals is to partly abrade (roughen) the surface which aids mechanical retention and increases the surface energy of the substrate. The force of the jet of alumina may also cause the surface to become impregnated with powder particles, which further aids retention. Abrasive size ranges from 20 to 100 μm; more commonly 50 μm alumina is used (Figure 19.36).

It is important that the prepared surface is not contaminated after preparation by saliva or other external contaminants. If used intraorally, the operating site should be isolated from the rest of the mouth with rubber dam. This is to prevent damage to other hard tissues or more critically surrounding soft tissues if the jet of particles is inadvertently misdirected. The other problem associated with this technique is that the particles can be dangerous if inhaled. It is essential that the dentist and dental nurse wear a mask covering their mouth and nose to prevent inhalation. Both the patient and dental team must also wear protective eye wear.

One product, the CoJet Intraoral Adhesive Repair System (3M ESPE) blasts sand which is coated with a ceramic onto the surface to be treated. This results in the treated surface becoming impregnated with this ceramic so enhancing the subsequent bond with silane. This has been termed **tribochemistry**. Subsequent resin composite bonding produces a strong chemical bond to the resin composite material finally placed onto the surface (Figure 19.37). For more information on bonding, see Chapter 11.

> **!**
>
> In most laboratory machines, an enclosed chamber will collect the used alumina. This should not be recycled because it will be contaminated after use.

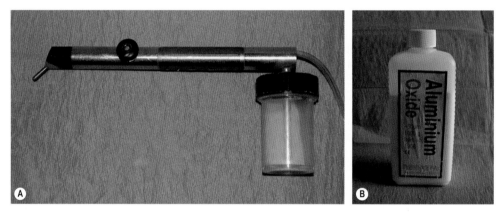

Fig. 19.36 (A) A sandblasting machine (Danville Engineering) which can be used extra- or intraorally. (B) It uses 50 μm alumina, which can be purchased separately.

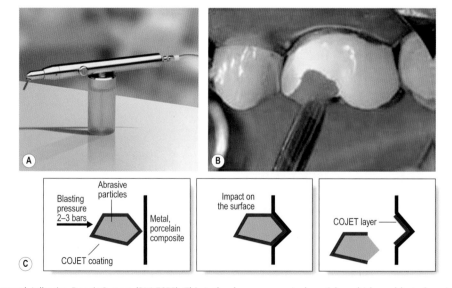

Fig. 19.37A–C CoJet Intraoral Adhesive Repair System (3M ESPE). This technology uses coated particles which are blasted against the surface of a metal. The result is that the coating is retained on the metal surface as the particle falls off leaving a ceramic covering on the metal surface. This may be used to bond further material onto the surface.

(CUTTING) LASERS

Lasers have been used in dentistry almost since their invention in 1963 although they have only recently moved beyond the role of experimental devices. Even now the use of lasers for cutting dental hard tissue still remains in its infancy.

Three types of laser have been commonly used in dentistry:

- Carbon dioxide (CO_2)
- Neodymium: yttrium aluminium garnet (Nd:YAG)
- Erbium: YAG (Er:YAG)

How they work

The laser consists of a lasing medium (for example CO_2) in a lasing cavity surrounded at either end by a concave mirror. One of these mirrors is semi-reflective. To produce the beam of collimated coherent light, the lasing medium is excited, usually by electrical means. This produces a steady stream of photons which pass through the semi-reflecting mirror and are delivered either via a fibreoptic cable or a hollow tube to a handpiece, which can be directed at the material to be operated on (Figure 19.38).

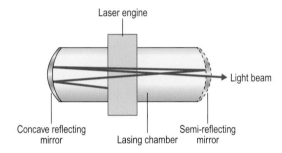

Fig. 19.38 Diagrammatic representation of a laser. The light beam is produced by exciting the lasing medium in the chamber. The photons pass backward and forward within the chamber until they have sufficient energy to pass through the semi-reflecting mirror.

A disadvantage of laser cutting is that the beam of light can either be reflected from the surface it contacts, or, depending on the wavelength, it can pass through the material or it may be absorbed. It is therefore possible that collateral damage may result to surrounding hard or soft tissues as a result of reflection or passage through tissue. Furthermore, unlike a conventional dental handpiece, if the beam is removed from the tooth surface it can still come into contact with some tissue, potentially causing damage to it.

Using lasers in dentistry

The use of a laser to remove hard tissue requires a different approach compared with that of a conventional handpiece. Lasers are designed to precisely remove small amounts of tissue rather than cut out substantial amounts of tooth. This means that the time required to carry out conventional dentistry is longer when using a laser than when using conventional means.

The wavelength at which the laser operates determines the effect it will have on the tissue being removed. For example, the CO_2 laser beam is absorbed at the surface of a tooth and much of the energy is converted to heat. This leads to melting of the enamel with the result that the enamel crystals are converted from hydroxyapatite to apatite. As this occurs at a very high temperature, there are serious concerns that the pulp tissue may be damaged.

Carbon dioxide laser

The CO_2 laser operates in the **infrared** range of the spectrum at a wavelength of 10.60 μm. The cutting beam is therefore invisible. A co-located **helium neon** (HeNe) laser beam is used to identify the position of the infrared beam, and it is this guiding beam which the dentist positions on to the tooth surface. Generally, the beam is focused to produce the most effective cutting and this entails keeping the light source at approximately the same distance from the tissue during the treatment time. The effect of a continuous CO_2 laser beam on the enamel and root surface is shown in Figure 19.39.

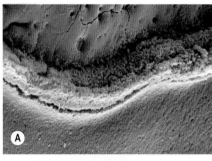
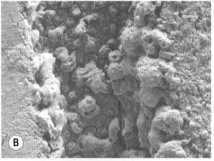
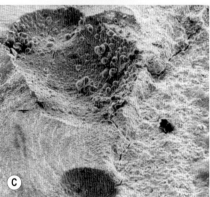

Fig. 19.39 (A) Photomicrograph showing the surface of enamel after irradiation with a CO_2 laser. A crater has been produced with the loss of tissue on the surface of enamel. At the periphery, normal enamel can be seen but then this leads to a cracked surface which follows the outline of the laser beam. Inside this area, there is a changed structure which is amorphous and without crystals. This is fused apatite. (B) This photomicrograph shows the surface of a root. The laser beam has been drawn down the surface and has produced a trough. Again, the surface after lasing is irregular and there are spheres of coalesced debris. There is also cracking and crazing present. (C) This photomicrograph shows the enamel–root interface with a small crater in the enamel. Here the laser power has been reduced and water cooling added. The result is that the crater is defined without cracks. Debris from the lasing process is still adherent to the surface. This is residue from the plume of material which is generated by the laser beam. The plume usually contains both fragments and volatiles from the interaction between the beam and the tooth.

One particular problem with the CO_2 laser is that is difficult to transmit the beam down an optical fibre. Most CO_2 lasers still rely on articulated arms. These are a number of hollow tubes linked by kneel joints and mirrors at the joints, which reflect the beam down the tube to the site of application. Although this laser is still used occasionally it does not appear to be one which will be used routinely for hard tissue cutting in dentistry.

Nd:YAG laser

This was the first type of laser which was produced specifically for the dental profession and has certain advantages. The lasing medium is a crystal of **yttrium aluminium garnet** doped with **neodymium**. This operated at the mid-infrared wavelength at 1.06 μm. As with the CO_2 device, the beam is invisible to the naked eye, and a co-located HeNe beam is used to identify the beam position on the tissue being treated. The advantage of this laser is that its delivery is simpler as the light beam is passed down an optical fibre. Unfortunately the beam produced is absorbed best by dark-stained material or red coloured objects. The absorption of tooth tissue is limited and to achieve tissue removal the tooth has to be painted with a chromophore to allow absorption to occur. Stained carious dentine absorbs the beam and it is possible to remove this with the device (Figure 19.40)

It is apparent that carious dentine may be removed quite successfully although there is the risk of considerable heat being generated during this process. The energy is also absorbed by blood and coagulation can be achieved in surgical procedures. However, this type of laser is now rarely used for hard tissue cutting, with its applications being for soft tissue work.

> **Chromophore:** a coloured dye that absorbs particular wavelengths of light.

Er:YAG laser

The most popular laser now for the removal of dental hard tissue is the **EYAG** laser. The lasing medium is, like the Nd:YAG laser, a crystal of yttrium aluminium garnet, but in this case doped with **erbium**. The laser beam produced is in the infrared waveband at 2.94 μm and also requires a HeNe visible light beam to locate the cutting site.

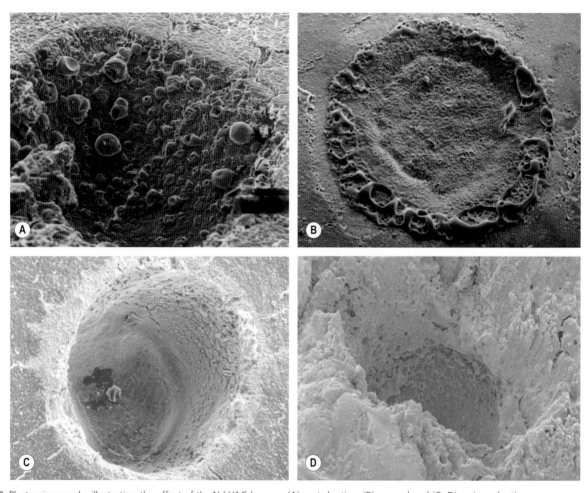

Fig. 19.40 Photomicrographs illustrating the effect of the Nd:YAG laser on (A) root dentine, (B) enamel and (C, D) carious dentine.

Most manufacturers produce a conventional dental handpiece design to deliver the beam to the site on the tooth (Figure 19.41).

The Er:YAG has proved to be the most effective of the commercially available lasers for tooth cutting. The beam is rapidly absorbed by the tissue, particularly water-containing tissues. This water is converted to steam and there is micro-fragmentation of the enamel surface. The enamel fragments break away and a cavity is produced (Figure 19.42). The cutting effect is enhanced by the use of a fine water spray directed at the cutting site.

The beam is pulsed and can emit number of pulses per second. It is interesting to note that when cutting a tunnel (as in Figure 19.42C) the slower the pulse rate, the faster the tissue is removed. This is due to the fact that the debris has to escape from the hole. If the laser pulses too quickly, it will start to hit the fragments as they are expelled from the cavity. This makes the cutting less efficient. It is therefore obvious that the main drawback of this type of laser is that the length of time taken to cut a conventional cavity is longer than it would be using conventional treatments.

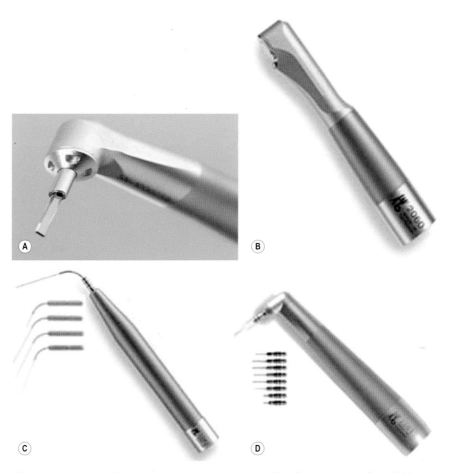

Fig. 19.41A–D The various handpieces used to deliver the laser beam to the tooth surface for a commercially available Er:YAG laser (KaVo).

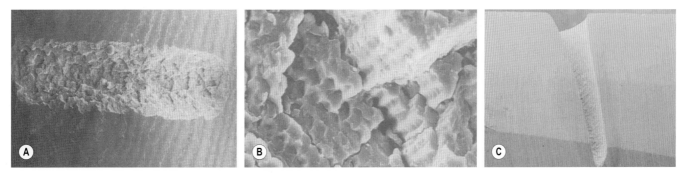

Fig. 19.42A–C Photomicrographs showing the effects of an Er:YAG laser on enamel. (A, B) The cracks along the enamel prisms can be clearly seen. (C) Cross-section through a tunnel preparation through both enamel and dentine. The cut surface is clear of smear and is ready for any necessary restorative treatment.

ABRASIVES AND POLISHERS

It is desirable that all surfaces in the mouth are smooth so that food debris and dental plaque accumulation is reduced and corrosion of metals is prevented. A rough surface is annoying and poorly tolerated by the patient and may inflict damage on the oral soft tissues. Smooth surfaces can be achieved by using various **abrasives** and **polishers**. These all work in a similar fashion by creating finer and finer grooves on the surface of the restoration so as to give the appearance of smoothness. All polishing agents contain an abrasive material but as the polishing materials become finer, the size of the abrasive becomes smaller.

Abrasives

To render a surface smooth, a range of abrasive materials is usually required, with the size of the abrasive being steadily reduced to produce finer and finer lines on the surface. Several factors will affect the process:

- *The hardness of the abrasive.* Abrasives need to be harder than the material being polished in order to be effective. The harder they are the more abrasive they will be.
- *The shape of the abrasive particles.* Again, the abrasives need to be sharper than the material being polished with sharper-edged particles being more efficient.
- *The size of the abrasive particles.* Larger-sized particles cut deeper grooves. By varying the particle size of the abrasive, the size of these scratches is altered to produce a smoother surface.
- *The mechanical properties of the abrasive.* The more brittle is the abrasive, the greater is the number of particles that will break to form a new cutting edge. The newer abrasive systems have particles which wear during use, producing finer particles and an increasingly smoother finish.
- *The speed of movement of the abrasive over the surface.* The slower the movement of the abrasive, the deeper the scratches produced.
- *The direction of movement.* Scratches should be produced in all directions to produce the best result.
- *The amount of load applied to the substrate.* The heavier the load, the more is the risk of generating heat and consequential changes to the structure of the material being polished (see next section). This may also lead to fracture of the cutting instrument.
- *The properties of the substrate.* Brittle materials can be abraded more rapidly whereas malleable and ductile materials will smear instead of being removed.

- Abrasives must be used in the correct sequence of decreasing abrasivity, otherwise the abrasive on the instrument will become clogged and ineffective. Changing from a coarse to a superfine abrasive without going through the medium and fine abrasives will be equally fruitless.
- Some finishing systems depend on the amount of pressure on the substrate the dentist exerts, the higher the pressure the more abrasive their action.

Effect of heat during finishing

Any finishing using rotary instrumentation will generate heat due to friction. This may cause the surface of the substrate to melt and changes to the properties of the surface produced as it flows to fill in any scratches. This is seen particularly with thermoplastic polymers. Care must be exercised with polymeric materials, as excessive heat will cause stress relief and warping. Similarly with resin-based materials, smearing can occur as the polymer approaches its glass transition temperature.

Types of abrasive

A range of abrasives may be used in dentistry. The commonest are **alumina** and **silica**, which are produced in varying sizes to provide a range of abrasivity from coarse to very fine. These abrasives may be mounted on a variety of instruments such as discs, strips and rubber wheels.

Finishing discs

The most popular method of finishing restorations is with the use of finishing discs (Figure 19.43). These are supplied in two sizes and two thicknesses, and a range of degree of abrasiveness. The discs are clipped onto a **mandrel**. They can be used reversibly to polish in front or behind the surface.

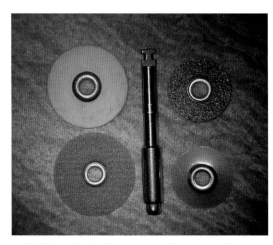

Fig. 19.43 Finishing discs (Sof-Lex, 3M ESPE) together with the mandrel required to attach them to a slow-speed handpiece.

Finishing strips

These are similar to finishing discs, but as the name suggests, they are supplied as strips for working interproximally (Figure 19.44). The strips are backed by polyester with two grits of different fineness on the working side. There is no grit in the middle of the strip to facilitate insertion into the area to be smoothed and to prevent abrading the contact area. They are supplied in two widths.

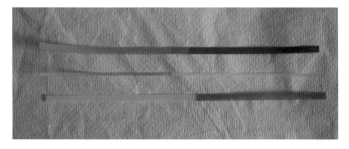

Fig. 19.44 Finishing strips (Sof-Lex, 3M ESPE).

Rubber wheels

Rubber wheels are supplied for polishing purposes in a variety of shapes and sizes (Figure 19.45). The active ingredient is **silicon carbide** or **alumina** bonded with rubber. The darker the rubber, the coarser the abrasive. As previously mentioned, the dentist should begin with the coarsest and work to the finest.

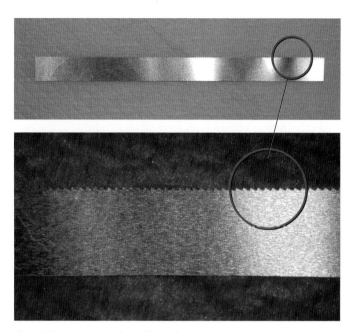

Fig. 19.46 Interproximal saw (Komet).

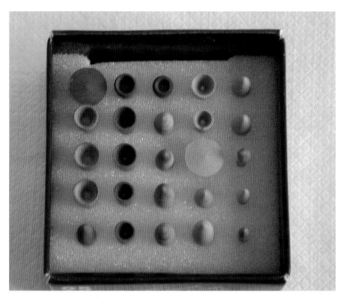

Fig. 19.45 A selection of rubber wheels in differing shapes and sizes.

Usually the dentist should use the darkest colour of abrasive first and move gradually to the lightest as they represent the coarsest abrasive to the finest. However, this is not always the case and depends on the system.

Interproximal saw (serrated strip)

This useful tool is a strip of thin metal with a serrated edge on one side (Figure 19.46). It is particularly useful to work with between teeth where bonding agent or resin composite has joined them together. The clinician should use it carefully as the serrations may damage soft tissue if this has not been fully retracted and guarded during use.

Polishing

The process of polishing is the creation of a smooth reflective surface, which has a lustre to it, using physical or chemical means. Polishing reduces the irregularities to produce finer and finer grooves in the surface.

The microscopic appearance of most materials is of an irregular-shaped surface with ridges and troughs. The polishing process is designed to reduce the height of these irregularities such that the surface is as flat as can be achieved. The process of polishing is achieved by starting with the coarsest abrasive and working through the range of abrasive sizes to reach the ultra-fine. During the process the surface irregularities are reduced to a minimum. A range of instrumentation and materials are available to achieve a high lustre.

The instruments which are used to polish substrates, the abrasives are primarily bonded with a binder to produce various types of finishing instrument. The abrasives are produced by:

- **Sintering** the abrasive. The abrasive is heated so that it softens and the particles bind together. This type of abrasive instrument is the strongest.
- **Vitreous bonding** – using either glass or ceramic. The glass acts a binder, holding the abrasive particle together.
- **Resinous bonding** – the binder is usually a phenolic resin. This is softer than the abrasive and wears quite quickly.
- **Rubber bonding** – this is achieved usually using a silicone rubber. These abrasive instruments will wear very quickly if used on a hard surface.

The last two systems rely on cold or hot pressing to mould the instrument. Hot pressing produces a more durable material which frequently has very low porosity. When using the bonded abrasives, care must be taken in their selection. If they wear to quickly, there is a considerable cost implication for the clinic. If, however, they wear too slowly they will become clogged with the swarf and debris which they have removed. This results in loss of abrasive efficiency and also a risk of heat generation, leading to damage to the substrate.

Polishing stones

These stones are made of alumina that has been sintered and fit into a slow-speed handpiece. They are available in a range of colours which indicate their degree of abrasivity: **pink**, **blue**, **green** and **white** (Figure 19.47). The highly abrasive pink and blue coloured stones are used primarily in the dental laboratory while the less abrasive green and white stones are used more commonly in the oral cavity. They can be used either with or without water spray, which may help to clear away the polishing debris. Their main indications are gross reduction of restoratives such as resin composites and glass ionomer cements.

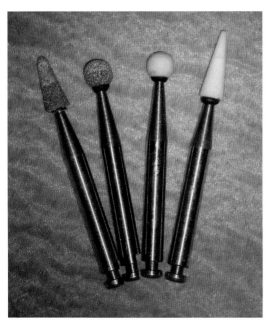

Fig. 19.47 Green and white polishing stones.

Brushes

Conventional brushes

These have bristles that are similar to an extra hard toothbrush and are used in a slow-running handpiece at between 600 and 10 000 rpm. They are usually used to carry a slurry of polishing material to the polishing site. More recently there has been a move to impregnate the bristles with an abrasive rather than to have a separate abrasive material. The abrasive in this case is usually fine grit silicon carbide powder. The risk involved with these finishing instruments is that the bristles themselves can be abrasive; if excess pressure and high speed is used, swirl marks from the bristles will appear on the surface and heat can be generated.

Brushes for polishing resin composite

Small brushes are also available, which fit onto a mandrel and are used in the slow-speed handpiece. Their bristles are made of elastomer and impregnated with diamond grit even at their tips (Figure 19.48).

Polishing materials

Lustre paste

Lustre paste is used to produce a highly polished surface, usually on resin composites. It is composed of diamond or aluminium oxide in glycerin. It comes in different colours, pink and white, representing different grades of abrasive particle contained therein. The pink lustre

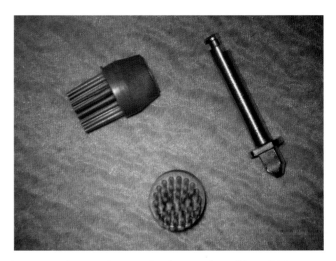

Fig. 19.48 Sof-Lex Finishing Brushes (3M ESPE), used for polishing resin-based composite restorations.

paste is used first, with a prophylaxis cup in a slow-speed handpiece, and this is rinsed off before the white paste is used.

Pumice slurry

Pumice is crushed porous volcanic stone that is a highly siliceous volcanic glass. It is used as a suspension in water to polish acrylics in the dental laboratory and in the surgery it may be used to remove temporary cement from teeth and for polishing them. However, it can abrade some restorative materials so care must be taken when using it. The slurry should be made up with water to a thin paste. After placing in a polishing cup, the abrasive should be moved quickly over the surface at high speed to prevent the build up of heat.

Pumice slurry should be made as follows: a small amount of pumice powder is placed into a dappen dish and water added. Excess water may be absorbed by using a cotton wool roll until the desired consistency is achieved (Figure 19.49).

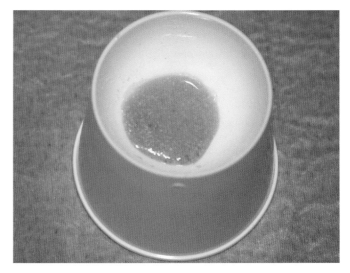

Fig. 19.49 Pumice slurry used for polishing.

Table 19.5 Laboratory polishing materials for dental materials

Name of material	Constituents	Substrate to be polished	Comments
Emery	Alumina and iron coated on cloth or paper	Metal alloys and plastics	Quite abrasive
Garnet	Magnesium aluminium iron silicate on paper discs	Metal alloys and plastic materials	Milder abrasive
Tripoli	Ground porous siliceous rock mixed with wax	Metal alloys and plastic materials	Presented as a brick of material used with a brush/mop
Whiting or precipitated chalk	Calcium carbonate	Acrylics	Used in a suspension in water
Zinc oxide and alcohol	Zinc oxide and alcohol	Amalgam	
Iron III oxide (rouge)	In a soap base	Gold alloys	Should not be used on cobalt chrome alloys as it contaminates the surface, leading to corrosion
Chromium oxide	In a soap base	Stainless steel and cobalt chrome alloys	

Other polishing materials

Other polishing materials are available for different purposes, particularly for polishing in the dental laboratory (see Table 19.5).

Prophylaxis paste

Prophylaxis paste (Figure 19.50) is used to remove stains from the surfaces of teeth. It is composed of an abrasive, usually pumice or chalk (calcium carbonate) within a solution of oils, which acts as a binder. Some products contain fluoride. Most products are flavoured. Table 19.6 lists examples of some of the prophylaxis pastes available on the market.

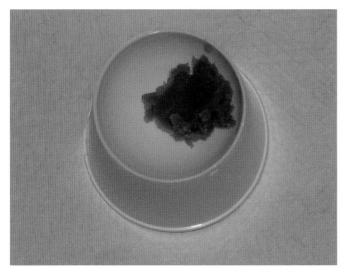

Fig. 19.50 A prophylaxis paste (Nu-Pro, Dentsply).

Table 19.6 Some prophylaxis pastes currently available on the market

Product	Manufacturer
Cleanic	Kerr Hawe
Clinpro Prophy Paste	3M ESPE
Détartrine	Septodont
Nu-Pro	Dentsply
Oraproph	SS White
Prophy Paste	SS White
Proxyt	Ivoclar Vivadent
Zircate Prophy Paste	Dentsply

Prophylaxis paste should not be used on any surface prior to bonding. Due to the presence of various oils in the paste, these can contaminate the surface to be bonded so significantly reducing the bond strength gained.

Some dentists prefer using a rubber cup for prophylactic polishing, as it is less aggressive and less traumatic to the soft tissues inadvertently touched during the procedure. However, whether a rubber cup or a brush is used is very much personal choice.

Electrolytic polishing

Electrolytic polishing is the reverse of **electroplating**. This technique is particularly useful when it is desirable to remove only a minimum amount of the material to be polished. An example of this is the fit surface of a cobalt-chrome denture, where conventional polishing may remove more material than would be desirable, so affecting the fit of the denture to the oral tissues. This is the reason why nickel-chrome alloys that are to be used for crown or bridgework are not polished by this method as the process would compromise the intimate fit of the casting. The alloy to be polished is made the anode of an electrolytic cell. When the current is passed through the cell, the anode is dissolved leaving an altered surface. When this technique is used, the polish gained is maintained for a long period.

SUMMARY

- A number of dental handpieces are available to the dentist, all of which have different indications.
- The type of bur used to cut tooth tissue or dental material will have an effect on that substrate.
- Other techniques may be used to remove tooth tissue or to prepare surfaces prior to bonding, such as air abrasion and sandblasting.

- Lasers may be used to cut dental tissue, and these instruments have a different effect on the dental tissues than other cutting instruments.
- It is desirable that dental restorations are polished to gain a smooth surface which is better tolerated by the patient and reduces plaque adherence. In some cases, it will also reduce the effect of corrosion. There are many different polishing instruments available to achieve this.
- Other agents may be used in combination with rotary instruments for polishing, such as an abrasive in a carrier solution.

SELF-ASSESSMENT QUESTIONS

1. What methods of removing tooth tissue are available to the dentist?
2. Explain what is meant by torque and its importance when preparing dental tissue.
3. What effect does a tungsten carbide bur have on tooth tissue?
4. Describe the disadvantages of using a laser to cut tooth tissue.
5. What are the objectives of achieving a polished substrate?
6. What precautions must be taken when using air abrasion or mini-sandblasting in the mouth?

Section | V |

Laboratory materials

Chapter | 20 |

Model and investment materials

From this chapter, the reader will:

- Be aware of the various materials used in the construction of dental models
- Understand their indications
- Understand the chemistry behind and the properties of gypsum materials
- Be able to correctly manipulate these materials both in the clinic and laboratory
- Be aware of the different types of investment material and each is indicated
- Understand the properties required of an investment material and how to manipulate them to best effect.

INTRODUCTION

The last section of this book deals with the materials used in the process of fabrication of indirect restorations and dentures. In all cases the underlying method of production involves a technique that can be traced back many hundreds of years and which was used extensively in the manufacture of jewellery: the **lost wax technique**. In this technique, a model of the substructure is first prepared. On this the prototype prosthesis is made using materials such as waxes that can be shaped to the required anatomical shape but which can also be destroyed by heating. Once this prototype is prepared it is invested or surrounded in a material which on setting will form the negative of the prototype pattern. The material for the prototype is then removed by heating. This leaves a space in the investing materials, which is filled either by casting or by applying a dough of the material and closing the mould under pressure. The details of this process will be described for each application.

In clinical practice, it is often necessary to make models of the patient's teeth. The models are used by the dentist to (in conjunction with other information) to plan a course of treatment or to preoperatively design a prosthesis such as a bridge. Once the treatment plan has been decided, the teeth are prepared and an impression is taken for a new model, and the restoration is then constructed in the dental laboratory by the dental technician on the second model.

Both the preoperative model and the working cast are constructed out of a material based on **gypsum**. This is commonly referred to as (**dental**) **plaster**. As such, plaster is one of those ubiquitous materials which is used in many types of clinical dentistry and in the dental laboratory. Dental plaster is also traditionally used to make an impression of the edentulous mouth prior to the construction of a complete denture (see Chapter 15). A special form of plaster may be used when metal restorations are to be cast using the lost wax technique. This chapter discusses all the dental materials used in the construction of dental models and those used as investment materials.

TYPES OF MODEL

A **model** may be defined as a replica of the structures in the oral cavity. It is made by pouring a material such as dental plaster into an impression of the area.

- If the resulting model is intended to be used for treatment planning purposes, for example in orthodontics or restorative dentistry, it is known as a **study model** or **study cast**.
- A special type of model may be cast for laboratory construction of a restoration. This is referred to as the **working cast**.
- In the case of a cast restoration such as a crown or bridge, individual teeth may be removed from the rest of the cast so that the restoration can be waxed up and worked on more easily. An individual tooth structure or preparation on a model is known as a **die**.

There are a range of materials that the technician can use, the choice of which depends on the purpose and use of the cast. In certain cases, for example when the framework for a metal denture is waxed up, the whole model is required. This is called a **refractory model** and is made out of a special material – a **refractory material** – so that it may be invested and subjected to high temperature so that the metal framework can be cast on to it. A refractory material retains its shape and strength, that is, it is physically and chemically stable, at high temperatures. This material should also be resistant to thermal shock and have appropriate thermal properties for the intended purpose.

Models may be made out of dental plaster, dental stone or investment material. All these material are based on gypsum but have different properties, which will determine when and how they are used.

DENTAL PLASTER AND DENTAL STONES

Gypsum is **calcium sulphate dihydrate** and occurs naturally at many sites around the world. It is **crystalline** in form (Figure 20.1). To be used as a casting material, the crystalline gypsum is heated at 130°C to remove some of the water contained in it. The product is called **plaster of Paris**, named after the site where this process was first carried out. The plaster is called **calcined** and the chemical produced is **calcium sulphate hemihydrate**. Further heating (up to 200°C) will drive off all of the residual water, leaving behind anhydrous calcium sulphate.

Dental plaster is provided in the hemihydrate form. Once water is added to this, the hemihydrates reverts to the dihydrate with the liberation of heat. It is this reaction which occurs with all dental plasters. The form of the crystalline hemihydrate determines the precise type of plaster which is produced although all types are chemically identical and are dissimilar only in structure and form.

Dental modelling plaster

Conventional dental modelling plaster such as plaster of Paris is produced by heating the gypsum to between 110 and 130°C in an open vessel. The hemihydrate so formed is known as the β-hemihydrate. The powder produced is made up of irregular particles which are porous. These particles are not packed closely together (Figure 20.2). Figure 20.3 shows dental models made out of plaster of Paris.

Dental stone

If the dihydrate is heated under pressure and in the presence of water vapour at 125°C, it produces much more uniformly shaped

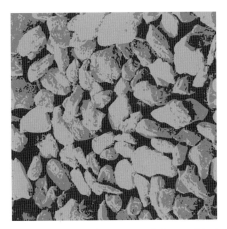

Fig. 20.2 Illustration of the crystal structure of plaster of Paris. Note the large, irregular particles that are loosely arranged and porous.

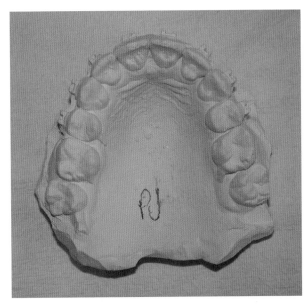

Fig. 20.3 A dental model made out of plaster of Paris. Note its white colour.

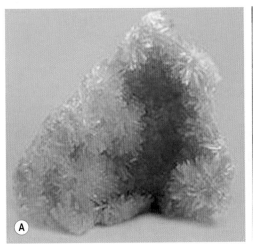
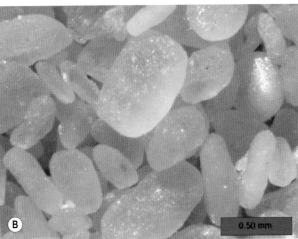

Fig. 20.1 (A) Gypsum stone as it occurs naturally. (B) A micrograph of the microscopic structure of the stone.
http://www.mindat.org/photo-71006.html

349

particles. This material has much reduced porosity (Figure 20.4) and is known as α-**calcium sulphate hemihydrate**. The variant used in dentistry is known as **dental stone**. Figure 20.5 shows dental models made out of this material.

However, most dental casts are constructed of a mixture of plaster of Paris and Kaffir D, usually 50/50 by weight. This resultant mixture is called **orthodontic plaster**.

die stone. This material is produced by dehydrating the gypsum in the presence of calcium or magnesium chloride. The combination of chemicals is boiled together, and then the chlorides are washed away with boiling water. The chlorides aid in separating the gypsum particles and the end result is a powder which is even less porous and much less irregular in shape (Figure 20.6). The powder is also the densest of the three types of hemihydrate. Figure 20.7 shows a dental model made out of this material.

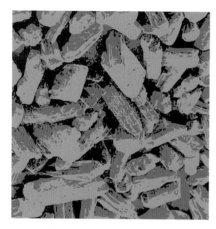

Fig. 20.4 Illustration of the crystal structure of dental stone. Note the more uniformly shaped particles and much reduced porosity.

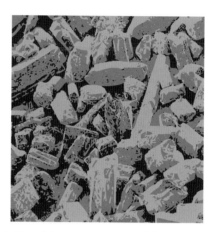

Fig. 20.6 Illustration of the crystal structure of die stone. Note the particles are much more uniformly shaped, smaller and denser than dental stone or plaster of Paris.

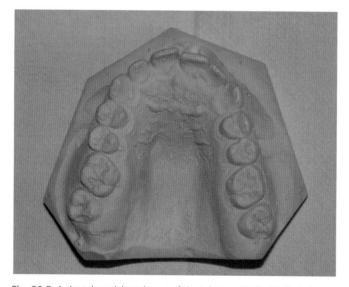

Fig. 20.5 A dental model made out of dental stone (Kaffir D). Note its yellower colour.

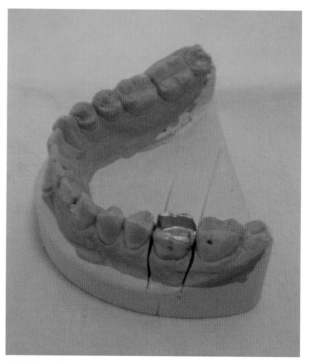

Fig. 20.7 A working cast made out of die stone, in this case to construct an inlay/onlay for tooth 36. The die stone is only used to make the teeth part of the cast, with the base being constructed out of dental stone. This is done for commercial reasons, as die stone is much more expensive than dental stone and accuracy and hardness are not critical in this region.

High-strength dental stone (die stone)

Further treatment of the dihydrate improves the properties of the stone, such as increasing its strength and abrasion resistance. The material produced is called **densite**, **high-strength dental stone** or

Die stones are available in a range of colours (Figure 20.8).

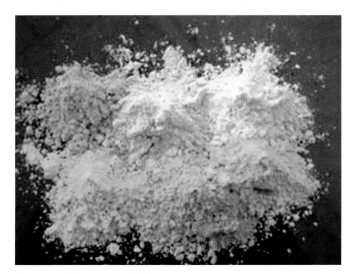

Fig. 20.8 Different types of die stone.

Commercially available products

A large number of companies produce a range of dental stone and die making materials, including Sybron Kerr, Ivoclar Vivadent, Vita Zahnfabrik, Schottlander, Kemdent and Dentsply.

Chemical consituents

As indicated above, the setting reaction for all these hemihydrate materials is initiated by mixing with **water**. The amount of water required to achieve a suitable mix varies with the plaster type. It is possible to calculate the exact amount of water required to mix with a specific weight of water. Due to the porous nature of the powder and its particle irregularities, the amount of water to achieve a suitable mix of plaster of Paris must be increased so that the powder is wetted. The mass of water required for the other two types of stone is reduced in proportion to the porosity of the powder and the shape and density of the particles. The consequence of using more water in the rehydration of the hemihydrates is that the plaster so formed will be weaker and more friable. With all types of dental plaster the amount of water used should be the minimum required to produce a creamy mix that can be effectively manipulated into an impression to produce an air-blow-free model. The manufacturer will provide this information.

Other chemicals may be added to the stone for various reasons:

- **Potassium sulphate** is added to accelerate the setting time. A 2% solution is used as an alternative to water and will reduce the setting time of model plaster from 8–10 to 4–5 minutes. The compound crystallizes very quickly and encourages further crystal growth. A 4% solution decreases the setting expansion.
- **Borax** is used to retard the set. A 2% solution will prolong the setting time of some gypsum materials by up to a few hours. The addition leads to the formation of a calcium salt of the borate. This is deposited on the dihydrate crystals, preventing further crystal growth.
- The addition of **sodium chloride** has the effect of reducing the setting expansion by providing extra sites for crystal growth. This in turn reduces the degree of growth at individual sites so preventing the crystals from being pushed apart.

- **Calcium sulphate dihydrate** provides nuclei of crystallization and therefore it acts as an accelerator. These set particles have a marked effect when used at very low concentrations between 0.5 and 1%. However, its effects above this value are less apparent.

Using specific combinations of these chemicals, the manufacturer can 'tune' the gypsum product to the application for which the material is designed.

Setting process

The setting process was originally described by Le Chatelier and confirmed by van't Hoff in 1907. The process has been described as being the result of differences in the solubilities of the dihydrate and hemihydrates of calcium sulphate.

As the hemihydrate powder is added to the water, some of the powder dissolves. A reaction occurs and this hemihydrate is converted to the dihydrate. The solubility of the dihydrate is very low and a supersaturated solution is rapidly formed. Since the stability of the supersaturated solution is very low, the dihydrate crystals start to precipitate out. This process continues as more hemihydrate dissolves in the water. This is a quite an aggressive exothermic reaction and has potential for tissue damage due to burning if handled incorrectly.

Supersaturated solution: a solution that contains more of the dissolved material than could be dissolved by the solvent under normal circumstances.

Due to the high exothermic reaction of gypsum products with water, care should be exercised when it is being used. This was recently demonstrated by an English schoolgirl who placed her fingers in a bowl of unset plaster. The material was allowed to set with her fingers in it and as a consequence of thermal damage, she suffered serious injuries resulting in the loss of several fingers.

Properties

Compressive strength

The compressive strength of plaster-based materials ranges from 12 to 45 MPa 1 hour after setting depending on the type of hemihydrate used. β-hemihydrate has the lowest compressive strength, that is, greater porosity leads to lower compressive strengths. After 1–2 hours the model appears dry but over a period of time further water is lost to the atmosphere. As this water is lost from the model, the compressive strength rises significantly. Once about 7% water has been lost, the compressive strength reaches approximately 60 MPa.

Surface hardness and abrasion

The hardness and compressive strength are linked in that higher compressive strengths are associated with higher hardness values. After the loss of water to the atmosphere the hardness also increases significantly. However, there is still a risk that dies and models will be damaged during any construction process. Attempts have therefore been made to make the model more abrasion resistant. For example, impregnation of the die with a variety of materials such as **epoxy resin**, **methylmethacrylate**, **glycerin** or hardening solutions containing 30% **colloidal silica**. The last leads to slight improvement in the hardness.

It is important to bear in mind that many of the disinfectants used on dental impression materials may affect the surface and damage the gypsum. It is essential that the impression is thoroughly washed before casting with plaster or plaster-based materials and that the impression material and plaster are chemically compatible.

Reproduction of detail

Gypsum is not idea for producing very fine detail but the ISO requirements for gypsum model materials requires that they reproduce a 0.05 mm line using a specific consistency of mixed material. This is considered to be sufficient to provide the detail required for most dental applications.

Hygroscopic expansion

Hygroscopic expansion will occur if the setting plaster is immersed in water while it is setting. The crystals can grow more freely in water and therefore the degree of expansion is greater. This phenomenon has been utilized in some investment materials to achieve a specific amount of expansion as part of the casting process. The effect on modelling stone is relatively insignificant as, under normal conditions, the expansion is of the order of 0.05% compared with 0.1% after immersion.

Volumetric change on setting

Theoretically it would be expected that plaster should show volumetric contraction on setting, however, a slight setting expansion is always observed. This is attributable to the manner of crystal growth of the dihydrate and the set materials show micro-porosities. An advantage of this is that the models are fractionally oversized and any prosthesis made on such a die will be slightly bigger than the original. The setting expansion is in the order of 0.3–0.4% for plaster compared with 0.05–0.3% for dental stone. The open crystal structure is stable once set but is porous permitting water to be taken up. This can lead to surface degradation of the model.

Working and setting time

The chemical process starts immediately when the powder comes into contact with the water. This means that the formation of crystals of the dihydrate will start to form quite quickly. The working time in this case is defined as the point at which the material cannot be manipulated into the casting ring or impression satisfactorily. The working time is generally around 2–3 minutes and the setting time varies between 2 and 3 minutes for an impression plaster and up to 20 minutes for a refractory investment.

The working and setting times of the various gypsum-based material may be varied by both the manufacturer and also by the dental technician during the mixing process. The manufacturer can accelerate the set and vary the setting expansion of the gypsum by the addition of potassium sulphate, borax, sodium chloride or additional calcium sulphate dihydrate as previously discussed. The technician may vary the working and setting time by altering the powder liquid ratio, temperature of the water and the degree of spatulation of the mix.

Indications

Dental plasters and stones have a number of indications.

- *Construction of study casts for general diagnosis.* Casts are made out of plaster of Paris or dental stone or a combination. They may be

held in the hands to allow the dentist to examine the relationship of the teeth in relation to each other with more ease than in the patient's mouth (Figure 20.9).

- *Construction of study casts for use in orthodontics.* These casts may be for diagnosis but are also made at various stages as the treatment progresses and as a medicolegal record of the final result. Orthodontic models are traditionally trimmed in a specific way by grinding on a **grinder** (Figure 20.10). Thus when the casts are put together and placed on a bench they will not come

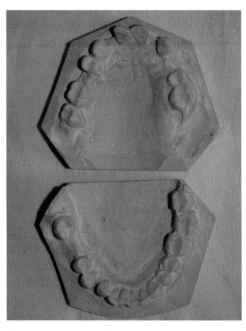

Fig. 20.9 Study casts made out of dental stone.

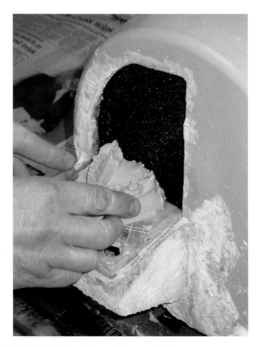

Fig. 20.10 A model being trimmed on a grinder.

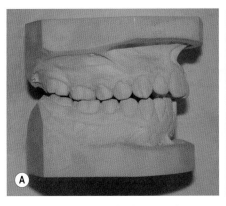 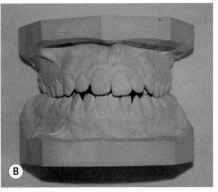 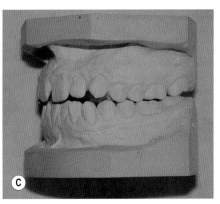

Fig. 20.11A–C Trimmed orthodontic study casts. Note their stability in various positions.

apart. This permits them to be viewed from different perspectives, for example from the front and both sides. This is termed **orthodontic trimming** (or **ortho trimmed** models for short) (Figure 20.11). Frequently, these models are treated with sealer to protect the surface. This can be a **soap solution** or a proprietary material which contains resin in a volatile solvent may be used. This process is known as **soaping**.

- *Construction of study casts for advanced restorative diagnosis.* These models are commonly required for mounting on an articulator (Figure 20.12) to facilitate their examination for this indication. This is done if an occlusal discrepancy is suspected or for a more complex restorative case where multiple units are to be restored. It is sensible that these casts have their occlusal (articulating) surfaces poured in die stone as its abrasion resistance is greater than other dental stones. This should minimize damage to the accurate reproduction of the surfaces when the casts are moved together during examination.

- *Construction of working models.* These models may be used to construct a fixed restoration such as a crown or a removable restoration such as a denture or orthodontic appliance. The model material used will depend on the device being constructed.
  - A cast used to construct a fixed restoration will be made of die stone to maintain its accuracy during the manufacturing process of the cast. This model will require to be sectioned to create the die. This may be done by pouring the model conventionally and placing **Ney pins** into the sections that require to be removed (Figure 20.13).

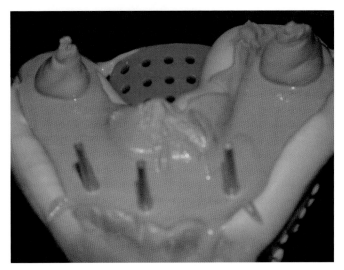

Fig. 20.13 Construction of a working cast for a crown.

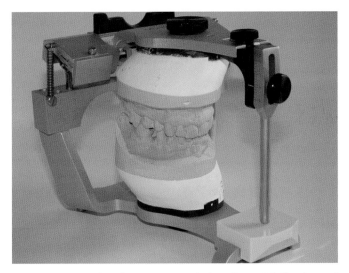

Fig. 20.12 Mounted study casts on an articulator (Denar Mk II) to be used for advanced restorative treatment planning/occlusal analysis. The occlusal surfaces of both casts are composed of die stone.

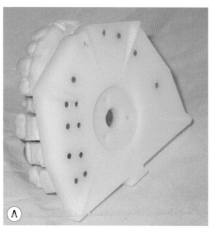 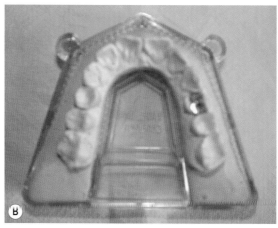

Fig. 20.14 Two bespoke model tray systems used to construct a working cast for a fixed indirect restoration.

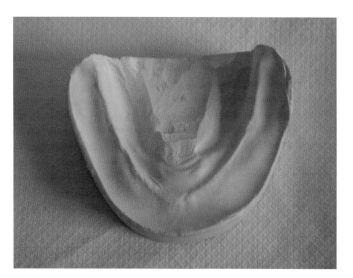

Fig. 20.15 A working cast for a lower complete denture.

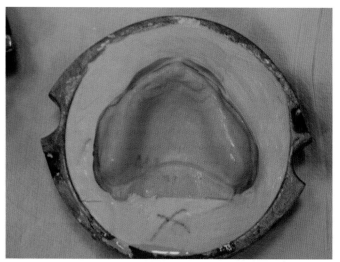

Fig. 20.16 A working cast of a complete denture embedded in plaster of Paris in a flask awaiting acrylic to be pressed into it and cured under pressure.

- Alternatively a bespoke model tray system may be used which allows sections to be removed from the model whilst maintaining their relationship to each other (Figure 20.14).
- A working model for a denture or orthodontic appliance is usually composed of dental stone and does not require any further modification (Figure 20.15).
- *Construction of refractory models.* The material from which these models are made is able to withstand being invested and heated to a high temperature without damage. It is used most commonly in the construction of metal-based dentures and ceramics. The wax pattern is laid down on the working model (except the working model has been poured with a refractory investment material) and wax pattern of the denture is laid down. This can then be invested, the wax burnt out and the alloy forced into the mould to create the casting (see later).
- *As a flasking material.* This is required when a waxed-up denture is to be processed into acrylic. Plaster of Paris is used in the flask to hold the working model and waxed-up denture, so that the acrylic may be pressed and cured under pressure (Figure 20.16).

Compatibility of gypsum-based materials with impression materials

It is important to verify that the impression material and the material chosen to construct the model are compatible. All gypsum-based products are compatible with the commonly used impression materials and so dies may be made from them without problems.

Manipulation

The operator has three variables which may be used intentionally or unintentionally to alter the behaviour of the material. These are:

- Powder to liquid ratio
- Water temperature
- Degree of spatulation of the mix.

Powder to liquid ratio

To achieve ideal results, careful attention should be paid to the powder to liquid ratio. Failure to do this will result in the properties of the material being affected. Ideally, the water should be weighed out according to the manufacturer's instructions as this fixes the powder to liquid ratio accurately. Many manufacturers provide a measuring cylinder for this purpose when die stone is to be mixed (Figure 20.17). Additional water will make the mixing easier but will slow the setting time and produce a weakened plaster. This is because the solution takes longer to become saturated for the precipitation process to take place. The result is that the plaster is unlikely to withstand normal loading.

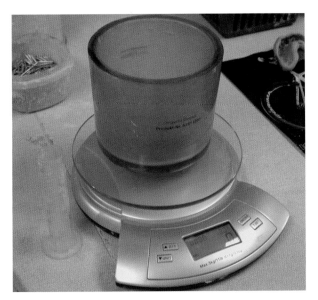

Fig. 20.17 A measuring cylinder used to accurately dispense the correct amount of water to be mixed with the corresponding amount of powder. The cylinder is used with digital balance to ensure the recommended weight of material is dispensed.

The powder should also be accurately dispensed. A scoop is provided by most manufacturers so that the correct amount of powder is added or the material is supplied in a sealed packet containing the correct amount (Figure 20.18).

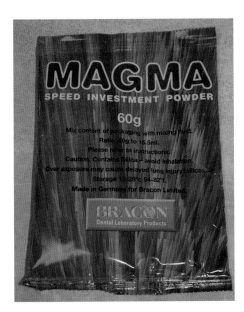

Fig. 20.18 Pre-packed material (in this case investment material) supplied in a packet so that the powder contents are mixed with a fixed amount of water.

Water temperature

Setting time can be influenced by temperature change. Increasing the temperature has two effects. Firstly the solubility of the hemihydrate and dihydrate changes with increased temperature so that at 100°C it is identical for both. This means that if solubility was the only factor, raising the temperature would actually slow the set. However, and, secondly, as with all chemical reactions, the mobility of the ions (in this case calcium and sulphate) increases with increased temperature. The set is therefore accelerated. The result of raising the temperature of the water is therefore a combination of these two factors. In general this usually results in a small acceleration in the rate of reaction and a reduction in setting time.

Degree of spatulation of the mix

It is essential that any plaster-based material is adequately spatulated so the particles are wetted thoroughly and a smooth mix is obtained. However, increasing the speed or time of spatulation generally results in a reduction in the setting time. This is because the crystal nuclei are disrupted, leading to the formation of more crystal sites and more rapid precipitation of the dihydrate. Finally, there is greater setting expansion.

Mixing

Gypsum-based materials should be stored in dry conditions so that moisture cannot penetrate the powder, which can cause a partial premature setting of the material. Box 20.1 shows the correct mixing protocol for gypsum-based materials.

Where the impression material and the model are the same, that is, plaster of Paris, a separating medium should be applied to the impression material to prevent the two components uniting. For further information of the use of plaster as an impression material, see Chapter 15.

Models made of dental stone may fracture and chip if they are not carefully handled. This is especially relevant when models must be posted between the clinic and dental laboratory. They should be well wrapped and tightly packed to avoid their bashing together during transit. Study models form part of the patient records and should be protected from damage. In the UK, models must be retained as a record for 11 years.

Epoxy resin and other die materials

Other materials are sometimes used to construct dies, for example **epoxy resin**. Techniques such as **electroplating** using silver or copper and other materials such as cements and amalgam have been used in the past to construct dies but their use these days is rare.

An epoxy resin is used to construct the die if the preparation is thin or narrow and therefore at a greater risk of breakage. This material is stronger, tougher and more abrasion resistant than die stone. However, it is less accurate and not as dimensionally stable. It shrinks during setting by up to 0.3%, and this shrinkage may continue for 3 days after initial setting. As potentially a smaller cast may be made on an epoxy die, the fit of the cast in the mouth may be compromised if this is not compensated for in the manufacturing process. Epoxy is cured by polymerization and may take up to 12 hours to fully cure depending on the product. The viscosity of epoxy is high and the material is difficult to pour. This means that air may become trapped in the die and porosity introduced.

Box 20.1 Recommended protocol for mixing gypsum-based products

Step 1

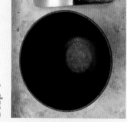

Gypsum based materials should be mixed using a flexible **bowl** and a **plaster spatula**. The water is placed into the bowl and powder should then be sprinkled onto the surface of the water. This attempts to ensure that any compacted material which has agglomerated is quickly broken up

Step 2

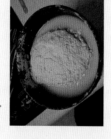

The powder should then be allowed to settle for about half a minute. This reduces the risk of air incorporation in the mix during the initial mixing phase

Step 3

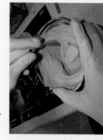

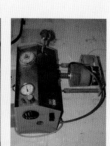

The mixture should be stirred briskly while smearing the mixture against the side of the bowl. It should take approximately 1 minute to produce a smooth mixture which, at this point, is now usable. Alternatively mechanical mixing may be used. This has the advantage that it may be done under a partial **vacuum**

Step 4

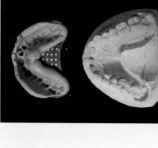

Once mixing is complete, the bowl and its contents should be vibrated and this should be continued during the pouring process. This helps the plaster flow into surface of the impression and eliminates air bubbles that would result in surface inaccuracies on the poured cast.

Step 5

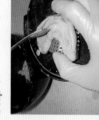

Once the model has been poured the material should be left to harden for up to an hour before the impression and model are separated. In cases where there are thin or narrow preparations, it is sometimes wise to leave the separation for even longer rather than risk the fracture of the model

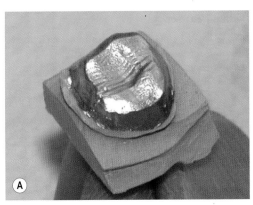
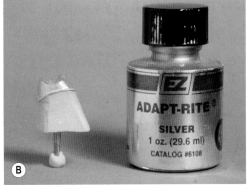

Fig. 20.19 (A) A die painted with (B) a die spacer.

Epoxy resin may react with some of the commonly used impression materials. Condensation and addition silicone and polysulphides are compatible, but the use of a separator is necessary. Polyethers are compatible while agar and alginate are incompatible with epoxy resins. Some chemicals in the epoxy resins may cause allergy in hypersensitive patients.

Die spacers

Fitting a cast restoration onto a preparation requires that it is cemented in situ. If the cast was made on the naked die, it would fit too closely to the preparation and there would not be enough room for the cement lute. This would result in incomplete seating of the cast.

After the die model has been made, the dental technician will paint a number of layers of varnish onto the die to create a space between the casting and the preparation. This space will then be filled by the cement lute, the thickness being determined by the luting material to be used. Each layer of varnish has a theoretical known thickness and so multiple layers will increase the space to the desired amount (Figure 20.19). One such product is Tru Fit (George Taub). Die spacers are required in a range of thicknesses for the different impression materials due to the differences in their dimensional change (Chapter 15). The filler in the die spacer is usually colloidal gold or silver. The use of alternate colours on the die allows the technician to see where the material has been deposited.

Implant fabrication models

Generally most fixed and removal prostheses are constructed on rigid stone casts. However, some casts require some modification. Dental implants are generally constructed on casts that have been modified to include a resilient material to mimic gingival tissue (Figure 20.20).

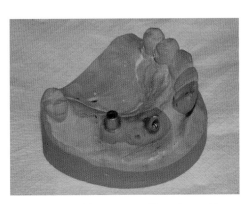

Fig. 20.20 A resilient material incorporated into the working cast prior to the construction of an implant-retained bridge.

This will provide some 'give', so that the correct emergence profile may be established by the dental technician without overcontouring. These materials tend to be addition-cured silicones (e.g. Gi-Mask, Coltène Whaledent).

Mounting plasters

As discussed earlier, dental plaster expands on setting. This expansion may introduce inaccuracies, particularly when accurate study casts are to be mounted on an articulator. Certain products are available which limit the expansion and are mixed with dental plaster when this is used to mount study casts on an articulator.

Cleaning of dental stones

Dental stone can become dirty in appearance especially after multiple handling or visits to the dental laboratory. They may be cleaned successfully by **steam cleaning**. This is especially important if the clinician is presenting the models to the patient to facilitate discussion of their case or if the student is presenting the models as part of an examination.

In the UK, legislation has recently been introduced regarding disposal of gypsum-containing materials as they release hydrogen sulphide when discarded in landfill sites. These products now have to be disposed of as special waste which permits recycling.

CASTING INVESTMENT MATERIALS

The **lost wax technique** is used in the production of inlays, crowns, bridges and denture bases for dental applications. An **investment material** is used to form the mould from the wax pattern. When the wax is burned out, the void so created corresponds exactly to the size and shape of the restoration being cast. A range of alloys may be used to make the restoration depending on its indication (Chapter 21). The melting point temperature of the alloy determines the type of investment material to be used. The wax pattern may be sprued (see Figure 21.13) or laid down on a refractory model made from a refractory investment material. This material can withstand high temperatures without breaking down.

Chemical constituents

Most investment materials have three ingredients:

- A refractory material
- A binder
- Other chemicals which modify the physical properties, such as to reduce the thermal expansion of the investment or to reduce oxides being formed on the metal. These additives include sodium chloride, potassium sulphate, magnesium oxide, boric acid and graphite.

Types of investment material

The composition of the investment material varies with the melting temperature of the alloy to be cast. Base metal alloys demand a higher melting temperature than precious metal alloys. The refractory chemicals are the same for all casting investment materials. These are one of various forms of **silicon dioxide (silica): quartz, crystobalite** or **tridymite**. These chemicals have a major influence on the changes in dimensions during the casting process. The role of the refractory material is to ensure that the investment is stable at the casting temperature. It does not participate in any chemical reaction during the investment process. Instead, it resists the heat of burnout and provides mould expansion by thermal expansion.

The binder holds the refractory material together, conveys strength and contributes to mould expansion by the setting expansion. There are three types of investment material, based on the binder in the material:

- Gypsum bonded
- Phosphate bonded
- Silica bonded.

Gypsum bonded

Gypsum-containing products are used for the precious metal alloys, such as gold-containing alloys, which cast at lower temperatures. The binder is α-calcium sulphate hemihydrate but it cannot be used alone as it is unable to withstand the heat. The addition of silica improves heat resistance but it can only be used up to about 1200°C. Above this temperature, the calcium sulphate reacts with the silica and sulphur trioxide is formed. This gas will cause porosity in the casting and contribute to corrosion. These investments contain approximately 60–65% forms of silica, 30–35% α-hemihydrate calcium sulphate and 5% chemical modifiers.

Phosphate bonded

Phosphate bonded investment materials are used for higher temperature casting, such as for palladium alloys and base metal alloys. The α-hemihydrate calcium sulphate is replaced by a chemical such as ammonium dihydrogen phosphate. Magnesium oxide (the binder) is also frequently added, which may also form phosphate compounds. In these materials, only about 20% of the investment is the binder with the rest being some form of silica filler. The binder provides strength to the investment at room temperature and on heating reacts with the silica to strengthen the investment at higher temperatures. Phosphate investment materials are stronger than gypsum-based ones. Frequently, these materials are mixed with special solutions provided by the manufacturer. These are generally a form of silica sol in water.

Silica bonded

These investment materials contain ethyl silicate or silicate materials and are used for casting at higher temperatures. Again, the filler is quartz or crystobalite plus small additions of magnesium oxide. These investment materials are becoming less popular as the investing process is complex and time consuming.

Properties

Any investment material must achieve the difficult problem of ensuring the casting formed at the end of the casting process is the same dimensions as the wax former from which it was produced at the start. It should also have other attributes:

- Easy to manipulate and apply and to adapt well to the surface of the wax pattern
- A fine particle size so that a smooth surface is gained on the casting
- Hardens quickly
- Strong enough when set so that it can be handled at room temperature. It must also be able to withstand the casting force
- Stable over the full range of casting temperatures. It must not decompose during the heating process
- Its expansion characteristics must be adjusted to take account of the dimensional changes in the wax and casting alloy during the casting procedure
- Any radical changes to the expansion behaviour of the investment should not occur around the casting temperature of the alloy
- Must be porous to permit air and gasses to escape thought the investment while casting is carried out
- Should break cleanly away from the casting after cooling.

Effect of heating the investment

The refractory material produces the necessary expansion of the investment without breaking up and the requirements can be set out as in the following equation:

$$
\begin{aligned}
&\text{Wax shrinkage during investing} \\
&+ \text{alloy shrinkage after casting}
\end{aligned}
=
\begin{aligned}
&\text{Wax expansion during heating} \\
&+ \text{setting expansion of investment} \\
&+ \text{hygroscopic expansion of investment} \\
&+ \text{thermal expansion of investment during heating}
\end{aligned}
$$

These dimensional changes are the result of the inversion of different quartz derivatives during the heating process. The degree of change and the temperature at which this occurs is specific to the different type of quartz which is being used. By adjusting the percentages of the different quartz forms in the investment, a smooth expansion profile can be achieved.

The binder behaves in a similar way. In particular the calcium phosphate-based investments take account of the changes that occur when the hemihydrate is mixed with water. During the mixing process the hemihydrate is converted to the dihydrate. Any excess water is lost during the early heating phase. However, as the temperature rises above 105–110°C, the calcium sulphate starts to lose water, converting to anhydrous calcium sulphate, causing a small contraction that compensated for by the concurrent expansion of the silica constituents.

Table 20.1 Effects of the various variables under the control of the dental technician on the dimensional change of the investment material

Change to variable	Set time	Consistency	Setting expansion	Thermal expansion
Increasing water to powder ratio	Increased	Increased	Decreased	Decreased
Increasing the time of spatulation	Decreased	Decreased	Increased	No effect
Increasing the rate of spatulation	Decreased	Decreased	Increased	No effect
Increasing the water temperature	Decreased	Decreased	Increased	No effect
Changing the location of sprue	No effect	No effect	More critical	Less critical

This rather complex group of changes is very carefully controlled by the manufacturer. However, there are factors outwith their control, for example, where the operator can alter the behaviour of the investment usually to the detriment of the casting (see Table 20.1).

Some modern investment materials compensate so well for the changes in dimension throughout the process that large multiple unit one piece castings have become possible. This obviates the need to solder or laser weld smaller units together (which are the alternative methods).

Manipulation

It is critically important that the water is measured accurately and the material is mixed in a vacuum to eliminate any air inclusions. The casting ring is lined with a ceramic material which helps with expansion of the investment during setting and burnout, and contributes to hygroscopic expansion. A surfactant is sprayed onto the wax pattern to reduce surface tension so that good adaptation is achieved between the investment material and the pattern (Figure 20.21). The investment material is poured and vibrated into the casting ring and around the wax pattern. The size of the casting ring depends on size of the casting (Figure 20.22).

The investment material should then be allowed to fully set before use. The burnout temperature is usually about 500–600°C with the burnout time depending on a number of factors such as the size of ring, the burnout temperature and number of casting rings in the oven. Once the investment ring has been heated to burn out the wax, it should be cast without being allowed to cool as the investment could crack.

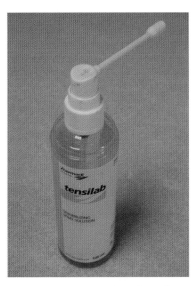

Fig. 20.21 A surfactant spray used to reduce the surface tension on a wax pattern prior to investing (Tensilab, Zhermack).

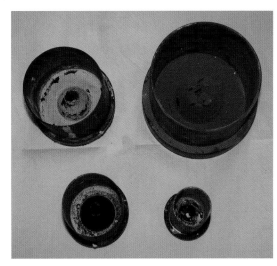

Fig. 20.22 Casting rings of various sizes.

Investments are also used for brazing (see Chapter 21) with gypsum or phosphate-bonded varieties usually being employed.

 The primary cause of investment failure is damage during the heating process. Too rapid heating will lead to cracking as the residual water is converted to steam. Additionally, where the investment has to undergo a phase change, too rapid heating will cause disruption and damage to the investment.

Commercially available products

A large number of companies produce a range of investments for use in the dental laboratory, including Sybron Kerr, Ivoclar Vivadent, Vita Zahnfabrik, Schottlander, Kemdent and Dentsply.

SUMMARY

- A range of plasters are available to produce models suitable for all dental applications, including indirect fixed prostheses construction, study models and denture models.
- Plasters show sufficient hardness and reproduction of detail to provide an effective base for the construction of indirect fixed prostheses.

- Quality of the set plaster is affected by water temperature, spatulation and powder/liquid ratio.
- Investment materials are designed to be stable over large temperature ranges. These temperatures are determined by the casting alloy.
- The composition of the investment is determined by the casting temperature.
- Investment materials can be friable and need support during the casting process.

FURTHER READING

McCabe, J.F., Walls, A.W.G., 2008. Applied Dental Materials, ninth ed. Blackwell Munksgaard, Oxford (See Chapters 3 and 5).

Powers, J.M., Sakaguchi, R.L. (Eds.), Craig's Restorative Dental Materials (twelfth ed.). Mosby Elsevier, St Louis (See Chapter 13).

van Noort, R., 2007. Introduction to Dental Materials, third ed. Mosby Elsevier, Edinburgh (See Chapter 3.1).

SELF-ASSESSMENT QUESTIONS

1. What precaution may be taken to prevent dental stone models fracturing as impression materials are removed?
2. What steps may be taken to protect the surface of a working model to prevent damage during the technical procedures?
3. What particular properties should a manufacturer attempt to produce in an investment material?
4. What effect will changes in the powder to water ratio have on an investment material?

Alloys used in dentistry

From this chapter, the reader will:

- Be aware of the various alloys which are used in dentistry
- Understand the effects each metallic element has on the properties of these alloys
- Understand how the manufacturing processes affect and influence the dimensional stability of dental castings
- Be able to correctly prescribe an alloy for a particular indication
- Understand how alloys may be used as metal substructures to support ceramic material
- Be able to discuss the use of dental alloys in a case with a dental technician
- Know the names of currently available commercial products.

INTRODUCTION

There is a long history of the use of metals in the mouth. These materials have been demonstrated as being the most durable in the oral environment. One of the earliest metals used was pure gold. Its advantages are:

- It is inert
- It does not corrode
- It does not cause adverse tissue reactions.

However, over time, pure gold has been replaced by alloys of gold. The reason for abandoning gold in its pure form is that it is too soft and flexible.

The addition of other metals to gold has produced a series of alloys whose mechanical properties are superior than that of pure gold. Further developments such as the need to have more reactive materials and the inherent cost of gold are other reasons for the production of the range of alloys that are available.

Each group of alloys has been designed for specific purposes and the composition determines the behaviour and reactivity. Dental alloys are usually moulded to specific shapes using the **lost wax**

technique. This means that they must retain their properties despite the fact that they will be heated to a high temperature and the molten material cast into a mould before being allowed to cool. The requirements put considerable demands on the performance of the alloys.

The range of applications for alloys in dentistry is far-ranging:

- In fixed prosthodontics alloys are used for the construction of crowns, bridges, inlays/onlays, posts and implants
- In removable prosthodontics metal alloys are used to fabricate metal-based dentures
- Orthodontists use wires to align teeth and these are also constructed from metal alloys
- Many dental instruments are metallic.

This chapter describes the alloys used in dentistry together with their methods of manufacture, specifically their application and practical aspects of alloy performance.

For a detailed analysis of the metallurgical features of the dental alloys, the reader should consult a metallurgy text.

ALLOYS

Alloying is the addition of one or more metallic elements to the **primary** or **matrix metal**. The incorporation of these additional metals alters and frequently enhances the mechanical properties of the alloy. These properties may well vary substantially from the component metals.

Alloys may be referred to as being **binary**, **ternary** or **quaternary**. This means they have two, three or four metallic constituents, respectively (compare with amalgam; see Chapter 6).

Structure of alloys

Alloys are essentially **crystalline** in structure. The crystals that initially form then grow towards each other until they touch. This is similar to how ice crystals form. At the point where the crystals touch, the water is fully frozen. In the same way, the metallic crystals grow as the alloy

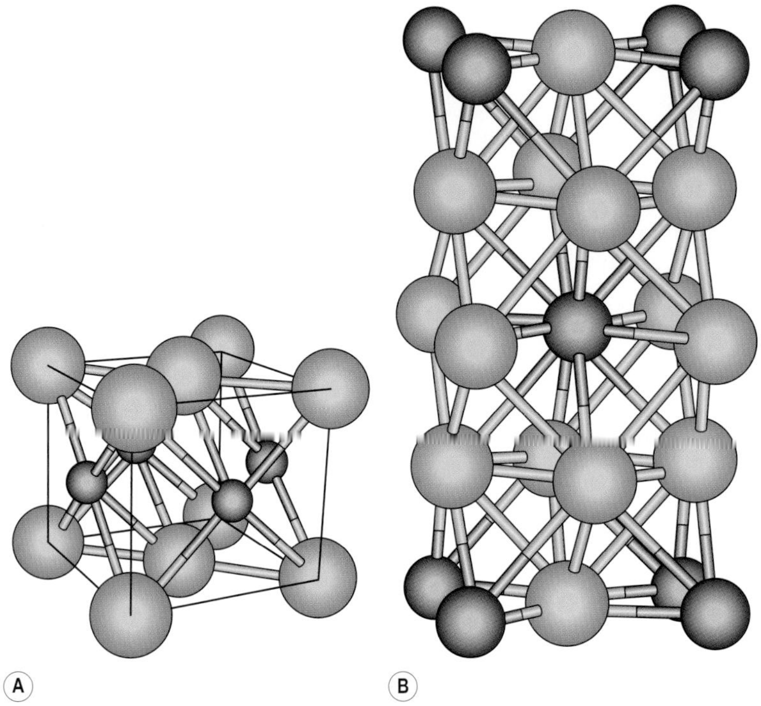

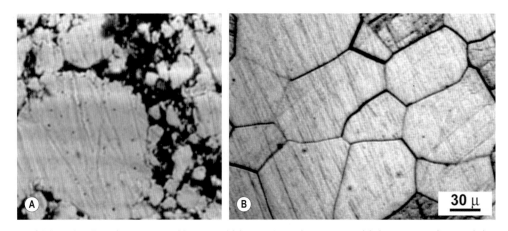

Fig. 21.1 The atomic arrangement of two solid alloys: (A) a gold copper system and (B) an aluminium titanium system. The diagrams show the relative positions of both elements within the alloy.

Fig. 21.2 Microstructure of (A) a solid alloy of iron, zinc and boron and (B) a titanium, aluminium, molybdenum, vanadium and chromium alloy (VT22) after quenching. Note the grains and their junctions (grain boundaries).
(A) Modern Research and Educational Topics in Microscopy. Méndez-Vilas and J. Díaz. (B) http://commons.wikimedia.org/w/index.php?title=User:Edward_Pleshakov&action=edit&redlink=1).

cools (Figure 21.1). The arrangement of the crystals depends on the size of the atoms of the various constituent metals. If these are similar, then atoms of one constituent can replace those of another. If one metal's atoms are much smaller, they may be trapped between the larger atoms, filling the interstitial space between the crystals.

The crystalline structure consists of crystals or **grains** abutting one another. The boundaries between the grains are referred to as **grain boundaries** (Figure 21.2). The size of the grains determines the properties of the alloy. The smaller the grains the better, as more boundaries prevent **dislocations** in the structure. To achieve this, some elements such as iridium or ruthenium may be added to dental alloys, particularly gold-based alloys, to reduce the grain size. These elements are called **grain refiners**.

General mechanical properties

Strength

Clearly, one of the many advantages of metal alloys is that they are strong and able to withstand forces during function without permanent deformation. This allows restorations to be constructed in thin sections, which in the mouth is advantageous as tooth tissue may be conserved by minimal tooth preparation.

- **Yield strength** is the force per unit area (stress) required to permanently deform the alloy. Exceeding the yield strength is clearly undesirable for dental applications. Yield strength is therefore a property used to describe the behaviour of an alloy. It is measured in mega pascals.

- The **yield point** is defined in as the stress at which a material begins to deform plastically. Before the yield point the material will deform elastically returning to its original shape when the stress is removed. Once the yield point is passed a proportion of the deformation will be permanent and irreversible.
- Related to yield strength is **hardness** which increases as yield strength increased. This gives the dentist and dental technician an indication of the difficulty to grind and polish an alloy. Some metal alloys may be heat treated to increase their hardness.
- **Ductility** is the ability of an alloy to deform under tensile stress. This is important when clasps require to be bent and inlays burnished to enhance their fit and marginal adaptation. The **stiffness** of the alloy is determined by its elastic modulus and the design of the casting.

Effect of heat on alloys

As alloys are composed of several individual metals, they have a **melting range**. When an alloy is cooled, some of it will continue to be in the liquid phase while other parts will start to solidify. The converse is also true, in that when the alloy is heated, some parts of the alloy will become molten first. The temperature at which the alloy liquefies on heating is called the **liquidus**, and the **solidus** is the temperature at which it becomes a solid again.

One of the most commonly used fabrication techniques for dental restorations is **casting**. This process is described later in the chapter but essentially an ingot of alloy is heated to above its liquidus and thrown into a mould of the restoration to be constructed. It is important that the dental technician knows the liquidus temperature of an alloy as it must be heated above this point to cast properly. The liquidus temperature determines both the casting temperature and choice of investment material. The dental technician must also know the solidus of the alloy. This is of particular significance when working with a ceramic bonding alloy, as it must be heated to a high temperature so that ceramic may be fired onto it. Clearly it must not be heated near to a point where it starts to become a liquid.

Heat treatments are often utilized in dental technology to enhance the alloy performance. This is described in more detail later in the chapter. However there is a potential disadvantage to this technique. Heating and reheating of the alloy may be necessary during the multiple firings required to add ceramic to the metal substructure. This may be detrimental for the properties of the alloy, particularly with base metal alloys. A good example of this is stainless steel which becomes very ductile and loses its strength when it is heated.

Biocompatibility

It is obvious that metal alloys which are used in the mouth must be resistant to **corrosion** and tarnish. Clinically this may manifest as an unpleasant metallic taste, irritation or allergy. Nickel is added to some base metal alloys and is responsible for a hypersensitive reaction in approximately 12% of females and 7% of males worldwide. Clearly alloys containing a known allergen should be avoided in patients sensitive to it.

> **Tarnish:** a thin layer of corrosion forming on the surface of metals such as copper, brass, silver, aluminium and other similar metals as a result of the surface undergoing a chemical reaction. Tarnish is not necessarily the sole result of contact with oxygen in air. Silver needs hydrogen sulphide in order to tarnish. Tarnish appears as a dull, grey or black film or coating over metal. It is a self-limiting surface phenomenon unlike rust. The outer layer of the metal reacts and the tarnish coating seals and protects the underlying layers from further reaction.

> At least 10% of the population is sensitive to nickel and patients should be asked about it when taking the medical history. Females appear to be more prone to hypersensitivity reactions with nickel and this may be attributable to its extensive use in costume jewellery. Any patient with a history of hypersensitivity to nickel or other metallic elements should be prescribed alloys which are free of the allergen. Noble metal alloys are more likely to be biocompatible than base metal alloys because they are inert.

Economic considerations

Inevitably cost is a consideration when the raw materials are expensive, for example precious metals such as gold. As these elements are traded in the world markets, their prices may fluctuate widely as their value mirrors financial and political global events. Gold is a very safe commodity and in times of economic hardship it is often purchased. In a world of supply and demand, such purchasing practices force the price to rise. This is also true for other commodities. Before the advent of catalytic converters, when the price of gold was high, other elements were being used in dental alloys. One such element was palladium; however, all Japanese car manufactures now require this element to make catalytic converters for engines designed for using lead-free fuel. Russia as the major producer of palladium was able to push its price up to reflect demand. The consequence for dentistry in both examples was that the price of dental alloys increased and therefore the cost of the final restoration. Many laboratories charge the dentist by the weight of the metal plus a fee for the construction of the restoration; other laboratories charge a flat fee irrespective of the metal price. The latter approach may significantly decrease the profit margin of the laboratory when metal prices rise. Dentists working outwith a third party (such as an insurance company or the National Health Service (NHS) in the UK) may be advised to charge the patient the laboratory fee plus a fee for the clinical time so that their profit margin is not affected by fluctuations in the market.

> The cost of the prosthesis may influence the decision made by the patient regarding the restoration that they prefer to have. In order to facilitate this choice, the dentist and their supplying technician must be clear and transparent with their charging policies.

Types of alloy

The metals used in dental alloys may be divided into two categories: noble and base metals. Examples of **noble metals** are gold, **platinum, rhodium, ruthenium, iridium** and **osmium**. Such elements are good for dental use as they are resistant to corrosion in the hostile environment of the mouth. From a chemistry perspective, silver is a noble metal but as far as dentistry is concerned it is not considered so because it corrodes in the mouth. These preceding elements are sometimes referred to as **precious metals** as they tend to be expensive. This term can be confusing as it does not refer solely to cost and therefore should be used carefully. Equally it does not mean noble as in noble elements, as silver and palladium are not dental precious metals. The term is more descriptive of the *physical properties* of the alloy. Nobility of the alloy depends on the sum of the amount of noble elements

Table 21.1 Definition of high noble, noble and base metal alloys according to percentage of noble metals present

Type of alloy	Noble metal content
High noble	Contains at least 40% by weight gold and at least 60% by weight of the noble metal elements (gold, iridium, osmium, platinum, rhodium)
Noble	Contains more than or equivalent of 25% by weight noble metals
Base metal	Contains less than 25% by weight of noble meals

contained in it. The American Dental Association has defined alloys as **high noble**, **noble** and **base metal alloys** (Table 21.1).

Alloys may also be categorized by their major component, for example, a gold-based alloy. They may also be described by their appearance such as yellow or white. White gold alloys are not, of course, white but silver in appearance.

Base metals refer to metals which are not noble, e.g. **titanium**, **nickel**, **copper**, **silver** and **zinc**. These elements corrode more than noble alloys but are alloyed with noble metals as they have a significant effect on the properties of the alloy, such as increasing strength, decreasing flexibility and increasing wear resistance of the alloy.

Casting alloys for tooth restorations

Some cast restorations such as inlays, onlays, some crowns and bridges are composed solely of metal (Figure 21.3). The vast majority of these restorations are constructed out of noble alloys but in certain situations the clinician may prescribe the use of a base metal alloy. Both these types of alloy may also be used for bonding to dental ceramic to construct tooth-coloured restorations. To optimize the union between the alloy and ceramic, the constituents of these alloys may be varied (see later).

High noble and noble alloys

The vast majority of noble alloys are based on gold (Box 21.1). As mentioned earlier, pure gold is too soft to be used alone in dentistry and to achieve adequate mechanical properties it must be alloyed with other elements (see Table 21.2). The four types of gold casting alloy used in dentistry are summarized in Table 21.3.

The properties of noble alloys vary markedly and this is affects their indications:

- Type I gold alloys are soft and are only used for small inlays in low-stress areas

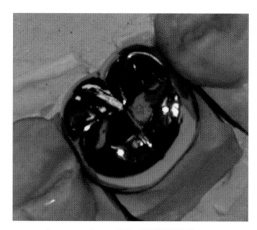

Fig. 21.3 A full metal crown manufactured by casting. This type of restoration may be made out of noble or base metal alloy.

- Type IV gold alloy have increased hardness, tensile strength and yield stress.

Box 21.1 Measuring gold content

- Gold content of an alloy may be measured in **carats**.
- A carat is the percentage of gold multiplied by 24 over 100.
- Pure gold is 24 carat so a gold alloy which is 50% gold is 50%Au/100 × 24 = 12 carat.
- Gold content may also be expressed by its **fineness**. This is the percentage of gold multiplied by 10. Pure gold is therefore 1000 fine.

Addition of copper: order hardening

The increase in hardness is accompanied by a decrease in ductility and corrosion resistance. The element mainly responsible for this is **copper**. Copper conveys **order hardening** to the alloy. This is where the copper atoms form ordered clusters instead of being randomly distributed within the alloy. This ordered atomic structure prevents movement or slippage of the layers of atoms. For this phenomenon to occur the alloy must contain at least 11% copper and so some effect will be seen in type III gold alloys although it is seen more so with type IV. The amount of copper added works only up to a point as the alloy will tarnish if it contains more than 16% copper. Order hardening may be achieved by heating the alloy to 400 °C and holding it in the furnace at this temperature for 30 minutes.

Table 21.3 The four types of gold casting alloy used in dentistry

Type	Description	Elemental composition (%)							Indications
		Gold	Silver	Copper	Platinum	Palladium	Zinc	Others: iridium, ruthenium, rhenium	
I	Soft	80–90	3–12	2–5	0	0	0	<0.5	Single surface inlays (low stress)
II	Medium	75–78	12–15	7–10	0–1	1–4	0–1	<0.5	Inlays
III	Hard	62–78	8–26	8–11	0–3	2–4	0–1	<0.5	Inlays/onlays Crowns Bridges
IV	Extra hard	60–70	4–20	11–16	0–4	0–5	1–2	<0.5	Cast posts and cores Long span bridges Partial denture clasps

Table 21.2 Elements that are alloyed with gold for use in dentistry and the effects they impart to the final alloy

Alloying element	Strength	Density	Melting point	Hardness	Colour change	Corrosion resistance	Tarnish resistance	Coring potential	Other comments
Silver (Ag)	Increases	*	Decreases	Increases	Whitens – may counteract reddening effect of copper	Decreases	Decreases		Increased porosity
Copper (Cu)	Increases	Decreases	Decreases	Increases	Reddens	Decreases	Decreases if included more than 16%	Decreases	
Platinum (Pt)	Increases		Increases	Increases	Lightens yellow gold	Increases		Increases	
Palladium (Pd)	Increases	Decreases	Increases		Whitens	Increases	Decreases silver tarnish	Increases	Cheaper than platinum
Zinc (Zn)	Decreases	Decreases	Decreases	Decreases		Decreases	Decreases		Oxygen scavenger. Improves castability
Indium (In)	Decreases		Decreases	Decreases	Yellows (palladium/ silver alloys)		Increases		
Iridium (Ir)	Increases		Increases	Increases		Increases	Increases		Grain refiner
Ruthenium (Ru)		Decreases	Increases	Increases	Whitens	Increases	Increases		Grain refiner
Rhodium (Rh)		Decreases	Increases	Increases	Whitens	Increases	Increases		Grain refiner
Nickel (Ni)	Increases	Decreases	Increases	Increases	Whitens	Increases			

This book avoids the use of chemical symbols where possible to facilitate understanding. However, the symbols are included in this table and subsequent tables in case the reader is confronted with a data sheet with only chemical symbols on it.
*The metal inclusion has no effect on that property where no entry is made in the table.

A gold alloy may be softened by the same process. The temperature is higher than that used for order hardening and the alloy is cooled quickly by quenching.

Other constituents

Platinum and **palladium** have similar effects on the properties of the final gold alloy. Their inclusion in the alloy leads to a higher melting point. This may be advantageous if the alloy requires to be soldered at some point, for example to join bridge components together if the technician is concerned that a large casting may not be dimensionally accurate enough if cast as one unit.

Zinc is included as a scavenger of oxygen as it will preferentially react with oxygen so preventing oxidation of the other components. It is relatively reactive and pure zinc will take up oxygen to passivate the surface. It is included in noble metal alloys for the same reason as in dental amalgam (see Chapter 6).

Iridium and **ruthenium** are primarily used to assist in corrosion resistance. They are incorporated in very small quantities.

Indications

There are several indications for prescribing a cast gold restoration:

- Gold alloys are very strong in thin section. This means that the dentist may consider providing a gold restoration where there is little interocclusal clearance. More tooth tissue may be conserved as it need not be sacrificed in favour of accommodating the dental material. The minimum thickness of a gold alloy should be 1 mm and 1.5 mm over a functional cusp.
- Cast gold restorations function well in the mouth as their wear resistance is the same as enamel; thus differential wear will not occur on opposing teeth.
- They are durable in function and have a good longevity.
- Gold alloys are dimensionally very accurate as little change occurs in this respect during their construction using the lost wax technique. This minimizes chairside time as less adjustment should be required at the fit appointment.
- If any adjustment is required at the chairside, gold alloys may be relatively easily polished by the dentist prior to fitting. Unlike ceramic, the gold restoration does not need to be returned to the dental laboratory to be finished should any chairside adjustment be required.
- The patient may elect to have a gold restoration for a variety of reasons: the use of gold to restore anterior teeth is more popular in some cultures, or on the recommendation of their dentist for one or more of the reasons listed above.

Contraindications

Although cast gold has many advantages and indications, it is not suitable in every case or for every patient. The contraindications are as follows:

- The primary dental disease should be under control and stable, that is the patient's caries rate/risk must be low and their oral hygiene good. Therefore those patients who have a high caries rate and are unable (or unwilling) to maintain a good level of oral hygiene are unsuitable for gold alloy restorations.
- Gold alloy restorations may be contraindicated in some patients on grounds of cost. To have a gold restoration prepared, constructed and fitted requires a minimum of two surgery appointments and a laboratory bill. The price of gold, even at a low level, can be considerable.
- Many patients decline gold restorations as they do not like the appearance of gold and may prefer a tooth-coloured restoration. This problem can be overcome by sandblasting the 'polished' surface of the gold, which has the effect of decreasing the shine or 'glint' of the gold. This may be a satisfactory solution for some patients (Figure 21.4).

Bonding gold alloys to tooth tissue

Restorations constructed out of gold alloys are usually luted into or onto the preparation. Gold alloy itself has no inherent ability to chemically bond to tooth tissue. However, it may be treated so that it can bond to tooth tissue with the use of an adhesive resin-based cement. If the gold alloy contains more than 16% copper, it may be

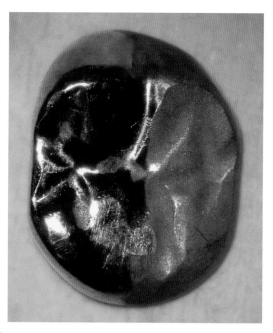

Fig. 21.4 A full gold crown, half (right side) of which has been sandblasted with 50 μm alumina while the other half (left side) has been polished to illustrate the difference in appearance between these treatments. The sandblasted surface reduces the glint of the gold when the patient smiles.

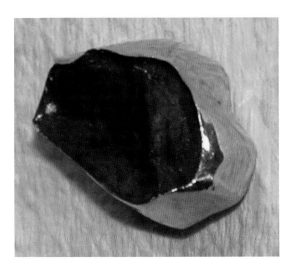

Fig. 21.5 The fitting surface of a gold onlay which has been heat treated so that the restoration may be bonded onto the tooth surface with the use of a resin-based adhesive cement. Note the darkened surface of the gold alloy, which is now rich in copper oxide and which permits chemical bonding.

heat treated by putting it in the furnace at 400 °C for 9 minutes. This forms a surface oxide layer of copper oxide, to which the resin based adhesive may bond (Figure 21.5).

This phenomenon is advantageous as it allows the dentist to bond such restorations as gold veneers or onlays on to tooth tissue particularly where little or no mechanical retention exists. The dentist should specifically and clearly request this treatment on the laboratory prescription form if a bonding technique is going to being employed. Additional, albeit limited, micromechanical retention may be gained by sandblasting the fitting surface of the gold alloy. Both these techniques may be combined to provide the most secure method. In this case, the fitting surface is firstly sandblasted followed by the heat treatment prior to dispatch to the clinic.

When laboratory work is returned to the dental surgery, it will be contaminated with bacteria. It is therefore important that the appropriate disinfection regime is followed prior to trying in of the prosthesis in the mouth of the patient. All metal and metal-ceramic restorations may be placed in the autoclave and subjected to a normal cycle. This will have no detrimental effect on any surface oxide layer created on gold or non-precious metalwork. For wax and plastics and other low melting point materials, alternative means of disinfection such as immersion in a cold sterilization solution should be considered. However, note that pre-silanated ceramic restorations cannot be disinfected by heating as this will break down the silane layer, compromising the bond gained between the ceramic and the resin cement.

Alternative metal alloys used for metal crowns

The more commonly used alternatives to gold alloys are the silver alloys. Cast base metal alloys are infrequently used to construct all-metal restorations unless cost is a very significant factor. Base metal alloys are more commonly used in the construction of resin-retained bridges and as bonding alloys.

Chemical constituents of alternative metal alloys and their functions

- Common alloys used as an alternative to those containing gold are the **silver-palladium** and **silver-platinum-copper** alloys. These usually contain 60–70% silver, 25% palladium and up to 15% copper.
- A **nickel-chromium** or **cobalt-chromium** alloy may also be used as a cheaper alternative.
  - Nickel-chromium alloys have between 60% and 78% nickel and 10–12% chromium, with the difference being made up with molybdenum.
  - Cobalt-chromium alloys usually have about 55% cobalt and 27–30% chromium, and the bulk of the remainder is made of molybdenum as for the nickel alloys.

Properties

Silver alloys have a major disadvantage in that they tarnish and corrode. They have variable properties and care must be taken in the selection as some are quite ductile and are unsuitable for use in load-bearing areas of the mouth.

Base metal alloys tend to have larger grain sizes and do not include grain refiners. They are stronger than the noble alloys. Additionally, they are also harder and their ductility is reduced. This means that they may be used in a thinner section and still possess sufficient strength for function. These alloys may be used in a thickness as low as 0.3 mm. The increased hardness of base metal alloys also imparts greater wear resistance, but it can lead to potential wear of opposing tooth tissue.

Base metal alloys are harder to adjust, finish and polish due to their hardness and lack of ductility. Many dental technicians sandblast the casting to remove any residual investment material and the green oxide layer. This may help to reduce the surface roughness. **Electrolytic polishing** may be used in preference to polishing and finishing these alloys by traditional means (see Chapter 19). However, many technicians believe that base metal alloys may be finished as well as noble alloys even though it takes longer to achieve and requires more work!

If the metal surface of an indirect restoration requires adjustment, measure the thickness of the metal to be adjusted prior to making the adjustment by using an Iwannson gauge. This will prevent inadvertent perforation of the surface being adjusted (Figure 21.6).

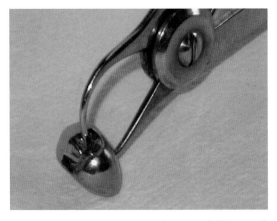

Fig. 21.6 An Iwannson gauge measuring the occlusal thickness of a crown prior to adjustment of the occlusal surface.

Table 21.4 Some commonly used casting alloys of high noble, noble and base metal alloys currently available on the market

Name	Manufacturer	High noble/ noble/base	Colour	Melting range (°C)	Casting temperature (°C)	Comments
Argenco 18	Argen Corporation	High noble	Yellow	874–904	1010	40% gold (type III)
Argenco 60S	Argen Corporation	High noble	Yellow	860–904	1010	60% gold (type IV)
Bodent 60	Charles Booth	High noble	Yellow	860–890	990	60% gold (type IV)
Bodent 75	Charles Booth	High noble	Yellow	890–930	1020	71% gold 12% silver 12% copper 4% platinum (type IV)
Bocast N	Charles Booth	Noble	Yellow	865–940	1040	40% silver 20% palladium 20% gold
Bopal	Charles Booth	Noble	White	970–1080	1140	3.4% gold 46% silver 33.3% palladium 19% copper
CB2	Charles Booth	Noble	Yellow	680–780	860	40% gold 40% silver 9.7% copper 9.8% indium
NPG+2	AalbaDent	Base	Yellow-gold	1068 liquidus	1148	Contains 2% gold

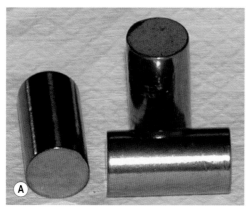
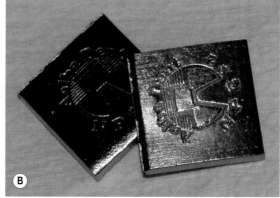

Fig. 21.7A,B Two dental alloys supplied in ingots.

Commercially available products

Table 21.4 show some commonly used casting alloys currently available on the market. It is clear from Table 21.4 that alloys of different composition can have similar melting ranges and casting temperatures. Care needs to be exercised in their selection. It is wise to establish a dialogue between dentist and technician so that the dental team can determine which alloy should be used in any particular case.

Alloys are usually supplied to the dental technician as ingots (Figure 21.7).

Bonding alloys

Cast restorations function well but are not tooth coloured. As there is an ever-increasing demand for aesthetic tooth-coloured restorations,

a metal substructure may be partially or fully covered in ceramic to give the restoration the appearance of a natural tooth. Alloys used for this purpose are called **bonding alloys**. The resultant restoration is called a **metal-ceramic** or **porcelain-bonded restoration**. The composition of these alloys is very similar to the alloys used for metal-only cast restorations, with small alterations made to enhance ceramic bonding. Both noble and base metal alloys may be used for bonding ceramic.

It is important that the alloy and ceramic are matched to one another both in chemical compatibility and in colour. Similarly, the laboratory behaviour including casting and fusing temperatures must be matched so that neither material adversely affects the other.

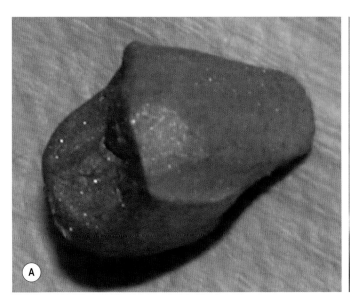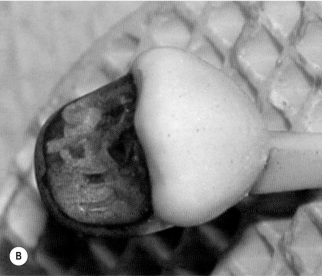

Fig. 21.8 (A) A metal coping forming the substructure for a metal ceramic crown just prior to the placement of the ceramic on the buccal surface. The design of the coping allows the ceramic to shrink fit onto it. Note also the grey matt surface (caused by sandblasting) to afford some micromechanical retention for the ceramic to bond to the metal. (B) The same coping with the ceramic fired on to it.

The coefficents of thermal expansion of both materials need to be similar otherwise expansion and contraction will occur on heating and cooling, and this will cause cracking of the ceramic. If anything, the alloy should contract more. **Delamination** of the ceramic can also occur clinically either **adhesively** (within the ceramic mass) or **cohesively** at the metal/ceramic interface (see Chapter 22).

In the construction of a bonded crown, adequate ceramic and alloy thickness need to be accommodated. Each material requires a minimal thickness to achieve sufficient strength and good aesthetics, respectively. To achieve this, more tooth tissue needs to be removed. This may compromise teeth with large pulps or where the crown width is small. Under ideal circumstances, the minimum interocclusal clearance for a bonded crown is 1.7 mm (0.6–0.8 mm of the metal coping and 0.9–1.1 mm thickness of the ceramic) opposed to a minimum thickness of 1 mm with an all-(noble)-metal occlusal surface.

Bonding ceramic to metal

There are three modes of attachment of the ceramic to the metal substructure:

- **Compression fit**. As the ceramic shrinks when fired, it will shrink fit onto the metal coping (Figure 21.8).
- **Micromechanical retention**. The surface of the metal coping exhibits irregularities and micromechanical bonding of ceramic onto metal will occur as the ceramic may flow during firing. In fact this may be enhanced by sandblasting the metal surface prior to the application of the ceramic.
- **Chemical union**. Chemical bonds will form via the oxide layer so connecting the ceramic and the metal alloy. This may be enhanced by the inclusion of elements such as **tin**, **gallium**, **indium** or **iridium**. These elements tend to be burned out during casting so a proportion of new alloy must be used with every subsequent casting so that a sufficient amount is maintained.

Some alloys used for metal ceramic crowns contain elements that form oxides in air. More recently, base metals have been used for this purpose and these form a thick oxide layer. The disadvantage is that the restoration can occasionally take on the alloy colour, appearing green at the margins, and cohesive failure may occur unless the oxide layer has been removed and re-formed more thinly.

Bonding alloys fall into four catagories:

- **High gold alloys (high noble alloys)**. These contain primarily gold (84–86%) with additions of platinum (4–10%) and palladium (5–7%). The addition of palladium and platinum raises the melting point of the alloy to above the fusing temperature of the ceramic. Failure to do this means that the coping would melt as the ceramic is fired. These alloys unlike other gold alloys do not contain copper as this may discolour the ceramic. It also would lower the melting temperature of the alloy.
- **Gold-palladium alloys (high noble alloys)**. These fall into two groups: those with silver where the gold content is 51–52% with additions of palladium (26–31%) and silver (14–16%); and those where gold (45–52%) and palladium (38–45%) are the only precious metals present. These alloys were introduced to reduce the cost of the alloy. The addition of palladium can also affect the expansion characteristics of the alloy and care must be taken to ensure that the ceramic used is matched in thermal behaviour to these alloys.
- **Palladium-silver alloys (noble alloys)**. There is considerable variation in the composition of these alloys from 53% up to 61% palladium. The remaining percentage is made up by silver and small additions of indium and tin. The alloy is less likely to flex under load and may therefore be more suitable for bridges where flexure under load may occur. However, as the silver content is increased, there is a greater chance of discolouration of the overlying ceramic.

Table 21.5 Example compositions of alloys (high noble and noble) used for metal ceramic bonding

Alloy	Elemental composition (%)						
	Gold	Platinum	Palladium	Silver	Copper	Cobalt	Gallium
High noble							
Gold-platinum-palladium	85	7	5–7	1			
Gold-palladium-silver	77		10–13	9			
Gold-palladium	50–53		36–40				2
Noble							
Palladium-gold	30–35		55–60				5
Palladium-gold-silver	16–32		42–62	6–26			
Palladium-silver			55–60	25–38			
Palladium-copper-gallium	2		74–80		10–15		9
Palladium-cobalt			78–88			4–10	2–8

- **High palladium alloys (noble alloys).** These alloys are primarily palladium with the addition of copper, gallium and cobalt. The percentage of palladium included ranges from 74% to 89%. Copper can be present up to 15% and gallium up to 9%. The addition of copper does not appear to affect the aesthetics of the final restoration although there is a risk that during the ceramic firing process the alloy may creep. This is almost certainly due to the copper influencing the behaviour of the alloy near its melting point.

Chemical compositions of bonding alloys

The differences in the composition of the high noble and noble alloys are summarized in Table 21.5, which gives examples of the alloy compositions. High noble and noble bonding alloys are composed primarily of metals such as **gold**, **platinum** and **palladium**. These are required in the proportion of at least 75% noble metals to convey adequate corrosion resistance to the alloy. Noble bonding alloys based on gold tend to be yellower.

Compatibility of the alloy with the ceramic

Some noble bonding alloys may react chemically with some ceramics, which is undesirable as this may cause discolouration in the ceramic. This is most prevalent with silver- and copper-containing alloys and occurs as some metal vaporizes and reacts chemically with the ceramic. Palladium-cobalt alloys may also have this effect, principally due to the presence of even a small amount of cobalt. This phenomenon is called **greening**, and may also be related to the composition of the ceramic in question.

All the palladium alloys have greater thermal contraction coefficients and should therefore be matched to the ceramic, which show greater shrinkage on firing.

The melting range of a bonding alloy is also significant. There must be an appreciable difference between the firing temperature of the ceramic and the melting temperature of the alloy. That is, the solidus must be considerably higher than the fusion temperature of the ceramic. If these temperatures are too close, permanent deformation of the metal substructure can occur during firing of ceramic. The result would be that the casting will no longer fit the model and therefore the prepared teeth. Platinum and palladium are now used as alternatives to gold as the primary elements in the alloy to accommodate this.

The investment and casting of the bonded alloys must withstand much higher temperatures as the casting temperatures are much higher. Therefore phosphate-bonded investment (see Chapter 20) is used. On removal from the investment the coping is cleaned. The metal surface must be free of grease and other contaminants otherwise imperfect bonding of the ceramic to the metal will occur. This means that the coping must undergo a **degassing procedure**, which is a means of cleaning the outer surface of the alloy by burning off the grease and debris. At the same time the formation of the oxide layer is induced so that after this procedure the coping is ready for the application of the ceramic powder. In most cases there is little or no removal of air/gas from the metal work interior. This treatment is usually carried out at around 1030 °C.

Properties

Bonding alloys have a high modulus of elasticity and a high yield stress to avoid stress being transmitted to the brittle ceramic (see Chapter 22). If the metal substructure was to flex then fracture of the ceramic would occur. Similarly the metalwork margin may be pulled outward as the crown cools if insufficient alloy bulk is present. This can lead to an increased marginal gap. The thermal properties of the ceramic and metal alloy must match closely. Creep is sometimes seen as comparatively low melting ranges are used.

Palladium is added to all bonding alloys to aid oxide formation, which in turn enhances the bond to the ceramic. The high palladium alloys tend to form a much thicker layer of oxide. This can present difficulties for the technician as the layer becomes difficult to mask. The high palladium alloys do, however, have the benefit of **low** specific gravity. Additionally, they are less expensive so the cost of restoration is reduced.

Specific gravity: the ratio of the density (mass of a unit volume) of a substance to the density of water.

Table 21.6 Metals included in noble bonding alloys and the effects they impart to the final alloy

Element	Effect on alloy	Comment
Gold (Au)	Main constituent in high noble alloys	
Platinum (Pt)	Main constituent in noble alloys Hardens (platinum is more effective than palladium) Increases melting temperature	More difficult to mix with gold Increases tendency to core
Palladium (Pd)	Increases corrosion resistance Widens separation between solidus and liquidus	Whitens gold alloys Increases tendency to core
Copper (Cu)	Hardens greatly Strengthens Reduces melting temperature	Imparts reddish colour
Silver (Ag)	Hardens Strengthens Counteracts red tint of copper as whitens alloy Increased tarnish	Probable cause of greening of ceramic Increases thermal contraction
Zinc (Zn)	Reduces melting temperature Oxygen scavenger Improves castability	
Iridium (Ir)	High melting temperature	
Ruthenium (Ru) Rhenium (Re)	Act as nucleating sites during solidification, produces a fine grain size	
Tin (Sn) Indium (In)		Migrate to surface and produce oxides for ceramic chemical bonding

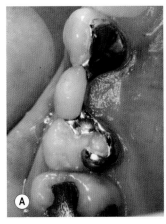 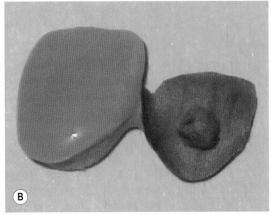

Fig. 21.9 (A) A resin-retained bridge replacing tooth 14 (*Courtesy P H Jabobsen*). (B) A resin-retained bridge whose retention wing has been sandblasted. Note the grey matt surface. These restorations are constructed using non-precious metal alloys because the retention of these alloys to the resin adhesive is superior to noble metal alloys.

Table 21.6 provides a summary of the constituents of high noble and noble alloys and the effects of their inclusion in the alloy.

Base metal bonding alloys

As well as noble alloys the dentist may also prescribe the use of a base metal alloy for metal ceramic restorations. These alloys tend to be chosen for two reasons:

1. Higher bond strengths are gained to resin composite adhesive cements than with noble metal alloys, allowing the restoration to be bonded to the underlying tooth. This property is utilized in the construction of resin-retained bridges and other restorations intended for adhesive bonding, such as when the geometry of the preparation is unfavourable with little or no retention being present (Figure 21.9).

2. On grounds of cost, as the alloy is cheaper than a noble metal alloy, reflecting the price of its constituents. For this reason it may be used as a semi-permanent/long-term temporary prosthesis such as a temporary bridge. As it is strong it will not break during function and is more predictable than a plastic equivalent but yet cheaper than one constructed out of a noble bonding alloy.

Table 21.7 Metals included in base metal bonding alloys

Element	Composition (%)	Reasons for inclusion	Comments
Nickel (Ni)	70–80	Refines grain structure Increases ductility	Potential for hypersensitivity reaction
Chromium (Cr)	10–25 (Ni Cr) 23–32 (Co Cr)	Imparts tarnish and corrosion resistance	Passivation material
Cobalt (Co)	50–65 (Co Cr)	Increases elastic modulus Increases strength Increases hardness	Primary component in Co-Cr alloys
Molybdenum (Mo)	4–10	Decreases thermal expansion	
Tungsten (W)		Used in conjunct with cobalt Decreases thermal expansion	
Manganese (Mn)	0.12–3.1	Increases fluidity and castability	
Silicon (Si)	0.3–11	Increases fluidity and castability	
Beryllium (Be)	Not more than 2	Lowers fusion range Adversely affects ductility	Vapour and dust cause lung tissue damage in technicians so not frequently used
Aluminium (Al)	0.2–4.2	Increases strength	
Carbon (C)	Not more than 0.2%	Increases strength and hardness	Embrittles the alloy

Constituents

The base metal alloys (Table 21.7) are usually either based on **nickel-chromium** or **cobalt-chromium**. In both types, a small percentage of molybdenum is also present. Nickel-chromium alloys usually contain about 11% chromium, approximately 6% molybdenum and the balance being nickel. However, the biocompatibility problems associated with nickel and beryllium have resulted in chrome-cobalt alloys (15–20% chromium, balance cobalt) becoming more popular. The advantage of the additon of chromium is that it is a good passivator, forming a surface oxide layer that conveys corrosion and tarnish resistance to the alloy. Cobalt-chromium alloy are usually about 50–65% cobalt and 25–32% chromium with a small addition (2–6%) of molybdenum.

Properties

The mechanical properties of these alloys are significantly higher than the high noble alloys. Their tensile strength is between 60% and 100% higher, the yield strength is in the region of 60% higher and the elastic modulus is almost three times that of the conventional high noble alloys. The density is about half that of the conventional gold alloys and they are slightly harder. These properties favour the use of this type of alloy in long-span bridges where there is less risk of the bridge sagging or flexing.

Some base alloys are grey or black in colour. This may be problematic in a bonding alloy as it may be very difficult if not impossible for the ceramist to mask this colour out; thus it will affect the aesthetics of the restoration.

Advantages and disadvantages

Table 21.8 sets out the advantages and disadvantages of base metal alloys.

Table 21.8 Advantages and disadvantages of base metal bonding alloys

Advantages	Disadvantages
Good corrosion resistance	Possible allergy as contains nickel
Low creep during firing of ceramic	Toxic due to presence of beryllium (if present) especially when cast and ground
High modulus (0.3 mm minimum thickness)	Difficult to cast High shrinkage on cooling and the thermal contraction differs from ceramic so delamination may result
High yield strength	Difficult to finish and polish due to hardness
Low density	Adhesive failure to ceramic due to thick oxide layer

Chemical bonding

One of the advantages – and the main indication – for base metal alloys is that they may bond to tooth tissue with a resin-based adhesive. By their nature, base metal alloys naturally form a thick surface oxide layer, which can bond chemically with a resin-based adhesive. Unfortunately this oxide layer is too thick and there is significant potential of cohesive failure within this layer causing the prosthesis to debond. Thus, this layer may be removed during the processes when the casting is removed from the investment material and the sprue is removed. An oxide layer will then have to be re-formed. This degassing process involves sandblasting the casting with 50–100 μm aluminium oxide and then steam cleaning it. The steam cleaned casting is put on a firing tray and in a furnace at a low temperature, rising to 650–950 °C without vacuum; this temperature is held for 1 minute.

It is important to stress that the metal surface must also be free of contaminants prior to attempting to bond the ceramic to the metal substructure. For further information on the chemistry and the mode of action of adhesive cements, see Chapter 11.

Acid treatment versus sandblasting

Sandblasting the metal coping with alumina has already been discussed as an effective method of creating a rough surface to facilitate micromechanical bonding (Figure 21.10).

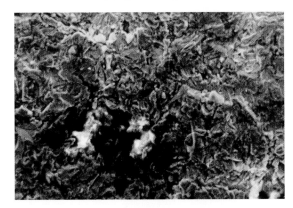

Fig. 21.10 Scanning electron micrograph of the surface of a sandblasted fitting surface of a resin-retained bridge substructure. Note the irregular surface that permits micromechanical bonding (field of view: 150 μm).

The application of an acid to the metal coping is another method to create pits in the surface into which the resin adhesive cement may adhere. This latter method was popularized with the advent of the **Maryland bridge**. A base metal (nickel-chromium) alloy was acid etched in a special bath in the dental laboratory. This etch pattern in the metal allows a resin composite cement to bond to it and therefore to the tooth. These bridges were retained satisfactorily but their delicate acid etched surface was easily and quickly contaminated usually during the intraoral try-in stage, and the bridge has to be returned to the dental laboratory to be re-etched to re-establish the etch pattern otherwise a suboptimal bond was gained, leading to debond. As sandblasting is more convenient and may be done in the dental surgery, the use of acid etched bridges has fallen out of favour. There is an additional benefit in that the bond strength gained by sandblasting appears to be enhanced.

The best etch pattern in Maryland bridges (acid-etched bridges) was seen with alloys containing beryllium. However, concerns about beryllium being carcinogenic and therefore hazardous to laboratory staff handling it means that this element is now rarely used.

Titanium

Titanium is a light weight metal with a low density, and thus the only metal that may be used in an almost pure form. It has a very high melting point (1668 °C) in comparison with the alloys used in dentistry. It has a relatively low elastic modulus and a very low coefficient of thermal expansion. It is highly corrosion resistant at body temperature and is regarded as biocompatible. As such, it is frequently used for the construction of implants. It has the ability to passivate if scratched, as the surface is normally covered by a thin oxide layer. Should this be scratched, a new oxide film is formed immediately. This means that it is resistant to attack by most acids and chlorides. The most frequently used titanium alloy for medical and dental applications contains 90% **titanium**, 6% **aluminium** and 4% **vanadium** (Ti-6Al-4V). Alloying produces an enhanced strength. At the same time there is a risk of corrosion and the casting temperature is very high, causing problems in a conventional dental laboratory.

Alloys for denture substructures

The cobalt-chrome alloys are best known for construction of metal base dentures (Figure 21.11). These alloys offer many advantages for this application. As described above, they have a high elastic modulus, making them stiff and strong. Thus they can be used in thin section and the rigidity of the alloy is maintained in thin components such as clasps. The bulk of the denture may also be kept to a minimum, that is, an equivalent acrylic denture would require a much thicker base to approach the same strength. The alloy is, however, brittle and not ductile, and difficult to cast.

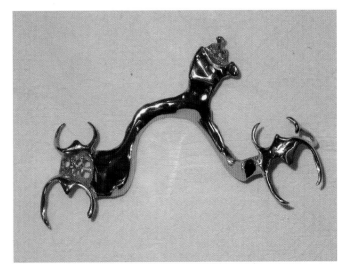

Fig. 21.11 The skeleton denture base of a partial denture that has been manufactured using chrome-cobalt alloy.

Constituents

The composition of these alloys are similar to that described above for casting and metal bonding alloys. The chromium content should not be increased over 29% as this makes the alloy very difficult to cast, as a brittle phase is formed. The role of molybdenum is to refine the grain size so providing more crystal nucleating sites. It therefore conveys a solid solution hardening effect. Carbon is sometimes added in very small quantities (no more than 0.2%) and results in the formation of carbides. These carbides increase the strength and hardness of the alloy but also the brittleness, particularly if excessive carbon is used. Casting porosity may also be introduced, which may lead to fracture of a component of the denture such as a clasp.

Casting and finishing

The low density of chrome-cobalt alloys means that castings are lighter and better tolerated by the patient. This is particularly so when compared with acrylic dentures, which need to be thicker to be of sufficient strength to function.

Induction casting is generally used when working with cobalt-chromium alloys as it requires a melting temperature of between 1300 and 1400 °C. As heat treatment will reduce their yield strength and elongation, care must be taken if the alloy has to be soldered or welded. Heat should be applied for the shortest time possible and at the lowest possible temperature.

Very accurate impressions are required as any distortions will result in the metal base not fitting in the mouth. From this perspective, the alloy is very unforgiving with adjustment more or less impossible. If a cobalt-chromium cast will not fit, the dentist would be well advised to carefully take a new impression and request that the laboratory remakes the casting.

Clasps should be adjusting with care as these may break as the alloy has a poor ductility. Any clasps requiring adjustment should be adjusted a little at a time to prevent fracture. The alloy is difficult to adjust and polish and any adjustments should be made in small increments to prevent heat building up locally due to friction. Generation of too much heat will damage the alloy and any acrylic attached to the metal base. This may result in the acrylic burning. However, when the alloy has been polished, the final polished surface is highly scratch resistant and durable.

Care should be taken when adjusting a metal denture base, as heat may build up locally due to friction. This may burn any acrylic attached to the metal denture base.

Methods of manufacture

Generally speaking, the devices produced from the dental alloys are manufactured by **casting** or by being **wrought** or **swaged** into the desired shape.

Casting

The lost wax technique is commonly used to construct fixed prosthodontic restorations such as inlays, onlays, crowns, bridges, and removal prostheses such as the skeleton framework for metal dentures. The principles are the same for both disciplines. The casting process for a crown is described below. Any variations relating to different alloys will be mentioned at the appropriate stage.

1. A **wax pattern** is made which corresponds to the shape of the object (Figure 21.12). This wax is designed to burn out at a temperature below 600 °C.

2. A **sprue** is then attached to the wax pattern. This sprue is usually made of **wax** but it may also be made of **plastic, stainless steel wire** or even a **hollow metal tube**. The sprue forms a pathway through which the molten alloy will travel. Although most castings require only one sprue, multiple sprues may be required and this depends on several factors such as the complexity of the design of the wax pattern, its width and length. The molten metal will solidify last in the sprue so it is usually of a wide diameter and is short in length. It is therefore also important that the spruing is correct. See p. 379 for principles of sprue placement.

3. The distal end of the sprue is attached to a apex of a cone-shaped rubber mould (Figure 21.13). The objective in sprue positioning is to ensure that the molten alloy will flow directly into all parts of the device without damaging the investment. Frequently there is a **reservoir** (see p. 389) waxed onto the sprue to ensure that there is substantial bulk of molten metal within the sprue otherwise there is risk of the alloy **freezing**, i.e. starting to solidify, leading to a failure of casting.

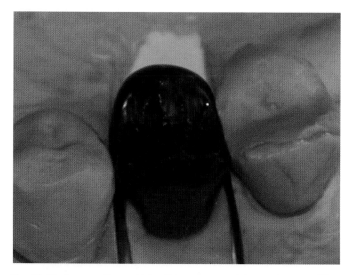

Fig. 21.12 A wax pattern which will become a metal ceramic crown. The occlusal surface will be in metal.

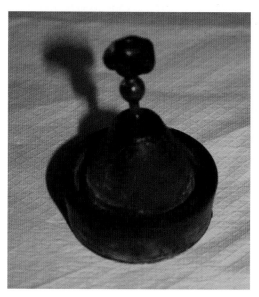

Fig. 21.13 A wax pattern of a full gold crown which has been sprued and attached to the rubber base. Note the reservoir on the sprue, to prevent the alloy freezing.

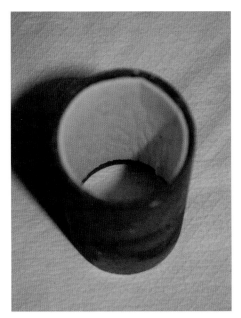

Fig. 21.14 The casting ring lined with a sheet of lining material to counteract the effects of expansion of the investment during the heating and cooling phases.

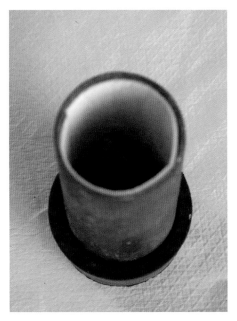

Fig. 21.15 The casting ring slid over the rubber base with the sprue and wax pattern placed in the centre of the ring to assemble the casting ring assembly.

4. A metal casting ring is lined by a piece of lining material, usually an aluminium silicate ceramic or cellulose paper liner (Figure 21.14). During the casting process the investment expands and the liner is compressed. This helps to counteract the effects of expansion of the investment during the heating phases. The casting ring is fitted over the wax pattern–sprue assembly, and into the rubber-cone shaped mould (Figure 21.15), The wax pattern should be situated in the hottest part of the ring called the **thermal centre**. This is to ensure that the alloy is maintained as close to the casting temperature and above the liquidus for the longest possible time so that it will flow. Additionally the wax pattern must not be too high in the casting ring otherwise the air which is forced out through the micro porosities in the investment during the casting will rupture the investment causing a casting failure. Often the wax is coated or sprayed with a **wetting solution** to reduce the surface tension and prevent inaccuracies on the casting surface due to air entrapment.

5. The investment material is then poured into the casting ring (Figure 21.16) taking care that all the air incorporated during mixing is vibrated out otherwise an inaccurate casting may result. The material used is determined by the casting temperature of the alloy to be used.

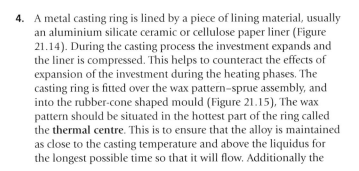

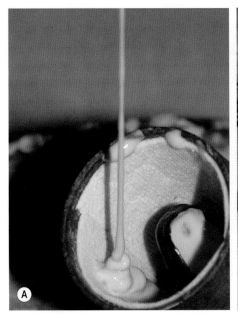

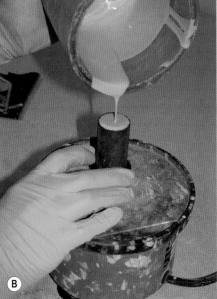

Fig. 21.16A,B The investment material is carefully poured into the casting ring on a vibrating base to ensure that no air is entrapped in the investment material or adjacent to the wax pattern.

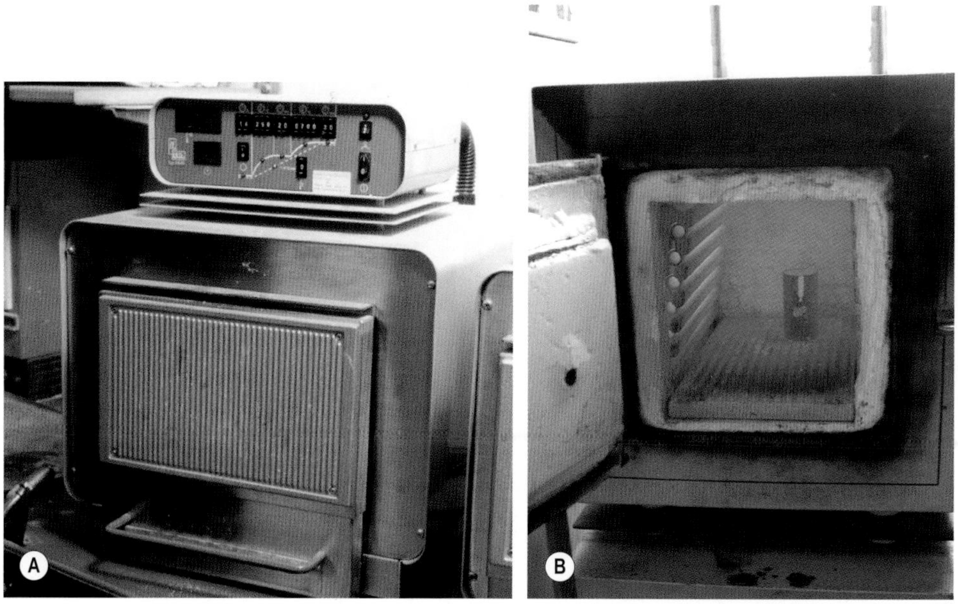

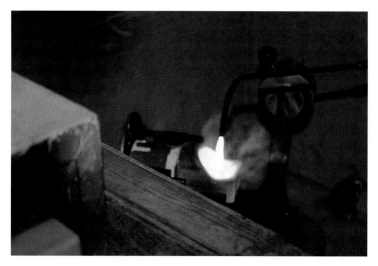

Fig. 21.17 (A) An oven used to burnout the wax pattern. (B) The oven door has been opened to show the casting ring inside.

Fig. 21.18 Ingots of alloys being melted in the casting crucible by the application of heat from an oxyacetylene torch.

6. When the investment material has set, the rubber casting base is removed and the casting ring and its contents are placed in a burnout oven (Figure 21.17) to remove the wax. This burnout phase is carefully controlled both for time and temperature to ensure that the investment material is not damaged by heating too quickly. Initially the residual water in the investment must be driven off. The wax will then melt and as the temperature rises any residual wax will vaporize. It is important that no wax residue remains otherwise the casting may be damaged. The sprue material may be removed at an early stage if it is metallic. The end result of this process is investment material surrounding a void that corresponds to the shape of the wax pattern.

7. The alloy may now be introduced into the void in the casting ring to form the prosthesis. The alloy is heated to the recommended casting temperature either by the application of a naked flame (for example an **oxyacetylene torch** (usually less than 1200°C) (Figure 21.18) or by using an **electric induction casting machine**. The choice of heating method depends on the casting temperature. At higher temperatures oxides may be formed and this is more likely to occur with the oxyacetylene torch. A **flux** (see p. 381) may be used to prevent excessive oxide formation. Electric induction casting tends to be favoured when working at high temperatures, as it is critically important that all of the metal alloy is heated to the correct temperature. See also p. 378. When this point has been reached the molten alloy is then forced into the void in the casting ring, most commonly by using a centrifugal force. The mould may then be left to cool at room temperature or is quenched in cold water. If noble alloys are quenched then the material is left in an annealed state which facilitates burnishing and polishing. The quenching also produces a violent reaction in the investment which becomes granular and causes it to fracture. If a gold-based alloy casting is left to cool at room temperature then a harder, stronger casting results, but this makes the alloy more difficult to finish.

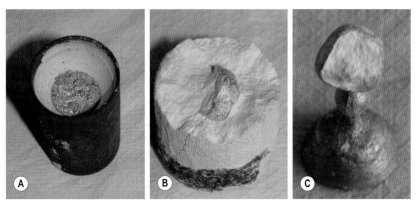

Fig. 21.19 A–C The investment material being removed from around the casting.

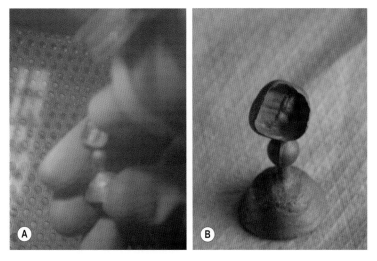

Fig. 21.20 (A) The casting is sandblasted to remove any residual investment material and surface oxides. (B) The sandblasted casting.

8. The casting is then removed from the investment material and ring (Figure 21.19).
9. At this point, it is covered with surface oxides which require to be removed. These days, most dental laboratories sandblast the casting to achieve this (Figure 21.20).
10. The sprue is then removed and the casting may be finished by grinding and polishing until a high lustre is gained (Figure 21.21).

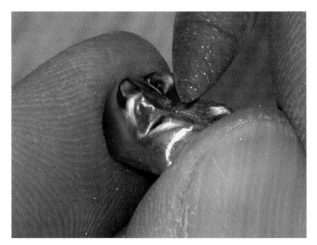

Fig. 21.21 The casting with the sprue removed being ground and polished to a high lustre.

The procedure for casting of a cobalt-chromium alloy is almost identical except that the casting temperature is substantially higher and a larger casting ring is needed to accommodate the larger wax pattern. Additionally, the casting is allowed to cool slowly rather than quenching the casting ring. This is also the case for the palladium-based alloys used for metal-ceramic crowns.

Dimensional accuracy of the lost wax process

The lost wax technique provides a high level of accuracy, there being a dimensional change of less than 0.05%. Clearly during the process, various expansions and contractions occur but these dimensional changes are mostly cancelled out by each other as the manufacturers of the waxes, investments and alloys have worked to achieve a balance in the properties of the systems they produce.

However, dimensional variations may occur. These are usually attributed to excessive expansion or contraction of the investment. To prevent excessive expansion, the recommended casting temperature should be used and the correct type of investment material used (Chapter 20). This should be mixed in the recommended proportions and at the recommended temperature.

• A smaller than expected casting is usually due to the mould not having been heated sufficiently.
• A distorted casting can be due to the wax pattern being damaged during the investing process or by incorrect sprue placement, preventing the metal flowing to the extremities of the mould. Thickening the margins of the wax pattern can reduce this risk to some extent.

Ease of casting

Different alloys possess different properties, depending on their composition, and this affects the ease of casting. A number of factors determine casting ability.

- *Alloy density*: Denser molten alloys are more readily thrown into the mould and so are easier to cast. Base metals are nearly half as dense as gold alloys and so need a higher thrust force to get the molten alloy into the entire investment void. Metal alloys which exhibit good fluidity when molten cast more readily.
- *Casting temperature*: The correct casting temperature is very important. It is critical that the entire alloy is completely molten prior to casting otherwise casting failure will occur. This is easier to achieve when the solidus and the liquidus of the particular alloy are closer together. This is more commonly observed with gold alloys. Normally the noble metals show the correct characteristics, a shimmering blob which moves under the blowtorch flame. This is generally about 40–60 °C above the liquidus. Other alloys such as those containing platinum and palladium have a larger difference between the solidus and the liquidus, and it is more difficult to get a homogeneous solution. This may lead to segregation of the components on solidification.

Density: mass per unit volume.

As already mentioned in the previous section, electrical induction heating tends to be used when working at higher temperatures as the process can be more readily controlled. The alternative is to heat the alloy by gas and air or gas and oxygen. The latter method uses an oxyacetylene torch. With this device the dental technician must carefully control the ratio of oxygen to acetylene. If too much oxygen and acetylene are mixed, as stated above, excessive oxidation occurs with the result that metal carbides are formed. This **embrittles** the resulting alloy with a resulting change in its properties.

If using a flame, the reducing zone of flame and a flux may be used to prevent oxidation.

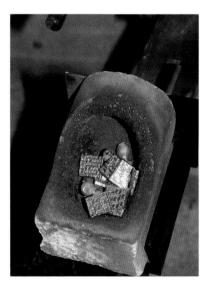

Fig. 21.22 The buttons from previous castings are being reused for a subsequent casting along with new ingots of metal.

Base metal alloys usually require higher melting temperatures in the range of 1200–1500 °C. This is considerably higher than the gold alloys, which melt at about 950 °C. Gold alloys may therefore be heated by a gas and air torch, but other alloys will require either oxyacetylene or electrical induction heating.

Normally the **button** (Figure 21.22) and sprue from previous castings may be reused with subsequent casting to avoid wastage of expensive raw materials. However, elements such as zinc, tin, gallium, indium or iridium may be burned out during the casting process. To ensure that sufficient amounts of the necessary elements are available, there must always be a proportion of new uncast metal present in the crucible mixed with the older button. Clearly the dental technician must ensure that the alloy being used is the same, otherwise the casting will fail.

With high noble metals it is also recommended that borax is added to the semi-molten metal as it is being warmed. This enhances the flow of the molten material.

Coring

The method of alloy cooling also has an effect on its final properties. If the alloy is allowed to cool slowly then the mechanical properties of the resulting cast will be better than if the cast is cooled quickly for example by quenching. If the alloy is cooled quickly then the composition of the alloy will vary at different sites as some premature precipitation can result in different composition within the grains. The first part of the alloy to solidify will be richer in one material and the last to cool will be richer in the other. This is called **coring**. This **cored structure** is usually undesirable as it is more prone to corrosion as electrolytic cells are set up on the surface of the alloy between areas of different alloy composition. If coring occurs, it may be removed by **homogenization heat treatment** – that is, the alloy is reheated and allowed to cool slowly. Coring is the reason why cast posts are weaker than a commensurately sized wrought post (see Chapter 13).

Troubleshooting with casting

Porosity

Porosity can be a common problem with castings. These voids can be irregular or spherical. A number of factors may lead to voids being present in the casting.

Some metal alloys will dissolve oxygen when heated and are molten. When they cool, some of the absorbed gases are liberated, but inevitably some gases become trapped as the alloy solidifies. This is termed **gaseous porosity** and manifests as spherical voids (Figure 21.23).

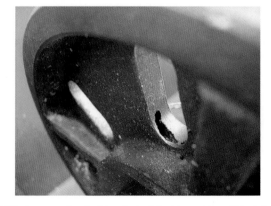

Fig. 21.23 An example of a blow hole defect in cast iron. This defect could have resulted in catastrophic failure with the fly wheel fracturing in service if it had not been detected.

This porosity may affect all parts of the casting. The dental technician may reduce its incidence by carefully heating the alloy so that it is not overheated or is not heated for too long a time period. Another method would be to cast the alloy in an inert atmosphere or in a vacuum. Palladium alloys are particularly prone to this as are those containing copper, silver, platinum or gold.

Sometimes rounded margins or regular large voids are seen in a casting. This is usually due to air being unable to escape from mould through the porosities within the investment causing a back pressure effect. The dental technician may overcome this by:

- Using an investment material of adequate permeability
- Using **vents** to allow air to escape
- Ensuring that all the wax is removed from the mould by doing the burnout for a sufficient length of time and at the correct temperature
- Placing the pattern no more than 6–8 mm away from end of casting ring
- Using a sufficient casting force to ensure the alloy may displace the air inside the mould.

Sprue placement

The correct number, diameter, length and placement of sprue are important. As mentioned above, for more complex designs (for example, a partial denture skeleton) multiple sprues may be needed. This ensures that the mould is completely filled with molten alloy before any of it starts to solidify.

A reservoir is often placed on the sprue near to the casting in an attempt to eliminate irregular voids in the casting. This is a sphere of wax placed on the sprue which when burnt out will leave a spherical void. The reservoir must have a greater cross-sectional diameter than the casting so that the alloy in the reservoir solidifies last and providing molten alloy to offset any shrinkage. To be effective the reservoir needs to be in close proximity to the pattern (see Figure 21.13).

Incorrect placement of sprues may result in the turbulent flow of the molten alloy into the mould, which would cause porosity. Sprues should be placed at the bulkiest section of the pattern to be most effective.

The mould should initially always be heated with the sprue hole downwards so that any particles of investment material which may break away from inside the mould may fall out of the mould. Failure to do this will result in irregular voids and inclusion of particles of investment material within the casting. This positioning of the investment ring will also aid the flow of molten wax out of the mould. Figure 21.24 shows an imperfect casting.

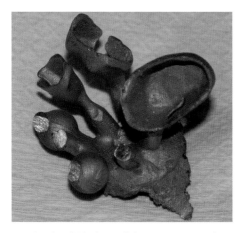

Fig. 21.24 A casting in which three of the seven patterns have not cast perfectly. Note the porosity and insufficient metal in these three remaining copings. (The other four copings have been removed from the button.)

Wrought alloys

A wrought alloy is one whose shape has been mechanically altered. This is done at room temperature in the cold state and is termed **cold working**. The alloy is first cast into ingots and the alloy is then drawn (pulled) into a wire through dies of gradually decreasing cross-section of the required shape – usually round, oval or square. Wrought alloys have a grain structure which has been described as **fibrous** (Figure 21.25).

The advantage of a wrought alloy is that it has an increased yield strength and hardness than a commensurately sized and shaped cast alloy. However, its properties may revert back to those of the original if the alloy is reheated as, for example, during **soldering** (see p. 381).

Wrought alloys are mainly used in orthodontic wires (mainly base metal alloys but also titanium, nickel-titanium alloy (Nitinol) or cobalt-chromium-nickel alloy (Elgiloy)), endodontic files (see Chapter 13) and in denture clasps.

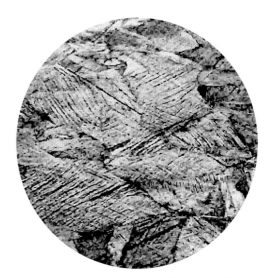

Fig. 21.25 Photomicrograph of a wrought alloy. Note its fibrous grain structure.

Swaging

Another method of cold working a metal alloy is that of **swaging**. This is when the alloy is pressed in a mould of the desired shape. The force applied to the alloy may be controlled (**explosion forming**) or a sudden hydraulically applied pressure (**hydraulic forming**). The resulting alloy form is called **swaged**.

Stainless steel is very often swaged as it has a high value of modulus of elasticity and proportional limit so an adequate rigidity is achieved with a very thin sheet of metal. This is advantageous as the weight of the resulting denture is low.

Other base metal alloys used in dentistry

Stainless steel

Modern stainless steel alloys used in dentistry are based on the addition of chromium to the original carbon steel, a binary alloy of carbon and iron. Carbon steel is formed by the addition of small quantities of carbon to iron. It changes phase on heating above 912 °C to a material known as **austenite**. If austenite is cooled quickly then the austenitic phase is transformed to a structure called **martensite**. This structure is lattice like and highly distorted and strained. This means that the material in this form is a hard, strong and brittle alloy. This is the strengthening mechanism for carbon steel. Martensite can be decomposed to ferrite and iron carbide, which is accelerated by heating. This reduces the hardness but increases the toughness.

To produce stainless steel, 12–30% chromium is added to the carbon steel alloy. Other metals may be added producing a whole range of stainless steel alloys, although the three main metals must be present. Chromium improves the resistance to corrosion and tarnish as it has a passivating effect. The passivating layer is not formed instantaneously as with titanium.

Of the various types of stainless steel available (ferric, martensitic and austenitic stainless steel) the austenitic stainless steels are most commonly in dentistry as they are the most corrosion resistant. Their composition is: 18% chromium, 8% nickel, 0.15% carbon, and the remainder is iron (18–8 stainless steel). 18–8 stainless steel has a high ductility and may be cold worked without fracturing. Substantial strengthening occurs during any cold working. There is very little risk of sensitization, and for this reason, it is used in orthodontic appliances.

The martensitic stainless steel alloys contain 11–16% chromium, up to 2.5% nickel and about 0.25% carbon, with the remainder being iron. These alloys have high strength and hardness and are used for surgical and cutting instruments. However, the reduction in chromium content means that the martensitic alloys are less resistant to corrosion. If any **tempering** occurs, the corrosion resistance is further reduced. The material is also less ductile than the 18–8 alloys.

Tempering

Tempering is a heat treatment technique for alloys. In steels, tempering is done to 'toughen' the metal by transforming the brittle martensite into ferrite. It is accomplished by a controlled reheating of the alloy to a temperature below its lower critical temperature.

> **!**
>
> Metallic instruments should not be heated in a naked flame as the metal will become tempered and damaged as well as discoloured.

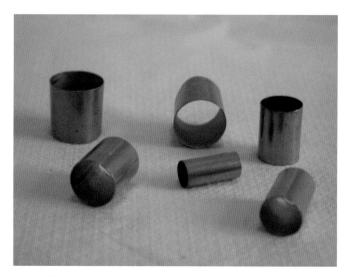

Fig. 21.26 A selection of copper bands which are supplied either **hard** (unannealed) or **soft** (annealed). The hard variety must be heated until cherry red before quenching in cold water. This will anneal them so rendering them malleable prior to use.

> **Lower critical temperature:** The temperature at which an alloy completes its transformation from one solid structure to another, as it cools.

Annealing

Annealing is a process in which materials are treated to render them less brittle, more ductile, more workable. Annealing decreases the possibility of a failure by relieving internal strains. This is achieved by heating the material and then cooling it very slowly and uniformly. Annealing may be used advantageously in the dental surgery when copper bands (Figure 21.26) are to be used as matrices for amalgam restorations. This is done by heating the unannealed (hard) copper ring in a flame until cherry red before being quenched in cold water. The copper band will then be softer and more malleable.

Nickel titanium

Nickel-titanium (**NiTi**) alloy has already been discussed with respect to endodontic files (see Chapter 13). It is also commonly used to fabricate orthodontic archwires (Figure 21.27). These alloys contain approximately 54% nickel, 44% titanium and less than 2% cobalt. They have a relatively low stiffness – of about one-fifth that of stainless steel. The ultimate tensile strength is nearly three-quarters that of stainless steel. This means that the alloy can be used in wires for orthodontic therapy to apply relatively low orthodontic forces when compared with stainless steel wires of the same dimensions. The two advantages of this type of alloy is that it demonstrates shape memory and is also **superelastic**. These phenomena are the result of the fact that the alloy can exist in two stable forms. Transition between the two can be achieved by heating or by the application of strain but the transition is reversible.

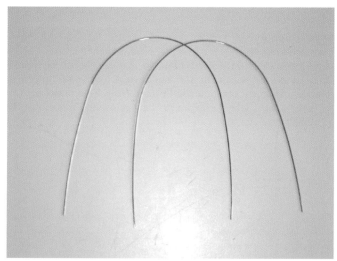

Fig. 21.27 Nickel titanium orthodontic archwires.

Table 21.9 Summary of the various base metal alloys used in dentistry

Alloy	Indications							
	Crowns	Bridges	Metal ceramic restorations	Implants	Partial denture framework	Endodontic files	Orthodontic wires	Preformed crowns
Cast cobalt-chromium	X	X	√	X	√	X	X	X
Cast nickel-chromium	√	√	√	X	√	X	X	X
Cast pure titanium	√	√	X	√	√	X	X	X
Cast titanium	√	√	X	√	√	X	X	X
Wrought pure titanium	√	√	X	√	X	X	X	X
Wrought titanium	√	√	X	√	X	X	X	X
Wrought stainless steel	X	X	X	X	X	√	√	√
Wrought cobalt-chromium-nickel	X	X	X	X	X	√	√	X
Wrought nickel-titanium	X	X	X	X	X	√	√	X
Wrought β-titanium	X	X	X	X	X	X	√	X

Summary of indications of base metal alloys

A brief summary of the indication for base metal alloy uses is set out in Table 21.9.

SOLDERING AND WELDING

Soldering

Soldering is the process whereby two metals may be fused by using an intermediary alloy. **Solders** are special alloys which have a lower melting point than the metals being joined. This fusion temperature must be 50–100 °C lower than the melting temperature of alloys to be joined, otherwise the alloys to be fused will deform. They may be **hard** or **soft**, but the latter alloys are not used for dental applications as they lack the necessary corrosion resistance. Hard solder alloys have higher melting points than soft solders. A flux is used as it cleans the alloys being joined and dissolves any surface oxide on the metal. This oxide layer must be removed to permit wetting and flow of the solder on the alloy surface. **Borax** is the flux used with gold-based solder alloys and **potassium fluoride** is used with base metal alloys and stainless steel.

Solders are presented as liquids, powders or pastes. To work successfully, solders should:

- Be chemically compatible with the alloys being joined
- Have a comparable strength
- Should be the same colour as the alloys to be fused
- Be able to flow well at a low temperature
- Be able to wet the components well
- Be corrosion and tarnish resistant.

Strictly speaking the term soldering should not be used in dentistry. **Brazing** is the same process as soldering but done at a temperature over 425 °C. As this technique is carried out above 425 °C all dental soldering should be called brazing.

Depending on the purpose, the dental technician may choose either a **gold** solder (Table 21.10) or one based on **silver** (Table 21.11).

- Gold solder is predominantly chosen for soldering most dental alloys. It displays good corrosion and tarnish resistance and its target temperature ranges between 750 and 900 °C.

Table 21.10 Common constituents of gold solder alloys used in dentistry

Constituent	Weight (%)	Reasons for inclusion
Gold	45–81	Corrosion resistance
Silver	8–30	Active component
Copper	7–20	Active component and strengthens
Zinc	2–4	Decreases melting range
Tin	1.5–2.5	Decreases melting range Improves flow
Phosphorus (P)	Trace	Decreases melting range Improves flow

Table 21.11 Common constituents of silver solder alloys used in dentistry

Constituent	Weight (%)	Reasons for inclusion
Silver	10–80	Main component
Copper	15–30	Main component
Zinc	4–35	Decreases fusion temperature
Cadmium (Cd)	Trace	Decreases fusion temperature
Tin	Trace	Decreases fusion temperature
Phosphorus	Trace	Decreases fusion temperature

- The fusion range of silver solders is between 600 and 750 °C and their main indication is for joining base metal alloys especially stainless steel and orthodontic appliances. Although their tarnish resistance is poorer, they provide a stronger joint and are easier to use than gold solder alloys.

The alloys to be fused must have uncontaminated surfaces as mentioned in the last section, otherwise imperfect fusion may result. A gypsum-based investment material is used to create a jig to hold the pieces to be fused in close proximity. This is called the **soldering investment**. Flux is spread over the alloy surfaces, which are heated to the correct temperature. The solder alloy is then added and this flows onto the surfaces of the alloys to be joined. The flow is encouraged by capillary action which draws the molten solder into the narrow gap between the two components to be soldered. Any metallic oxides are dissolved as they are formed and this protects the alloy surface from oxidation during soldering. The investment material may then be removed and the joint finished and polished using rotary instrumentation.

Welding

Welding may be defined as the joining of two metals by heating the parts themselves with or without pressure. This has been termed **hot welding**. In **resistance welding** or **spot welding**, the pieces are pressed together between two copper electrodes so allowing an electric current to flow. Welding is not used for gold alloys as these alloys are good conductors of electricity or for **butt joints** as insufficient surface area is available for fusing. It is indicated for **overlapping joints** of stainless steel or other cobalt-chrome alloys.

In contemporary dental technology, welding is done by lasers (**laser welding**) and this has largely superseded soldering of smaller units to construct a larger prosthesis, such as a full arch framework.

COMMUNICATION WITH THE DENTAL LABORATORY

The dentist has a legal obligation to prescribe the full details of the restoration; this includes the design and the materials from which it is made. The dentist therefore must understand the materials that are available and are most appropriate in any given situation. The type of alloy required should therefore be documented on the **laboratory prescription** form (**lab ticket**). The dentist has a legal responsibility to prescribe the alloy as well as the design of the prosthesis.

Dental technicians are very knowledgeable about the materials which they use and the prescribing dentist should not hesitate to contact their technician to ask for advice on the materials that are being considered for use and well as other issues regarding the case such as the design of the prosthesis or prostheses.

METAL-FREE DENTISTRY

The use of metals to construct dental fixed prosthesis has declined in recent years in favour of tooth-coloured restorations. This has become possible due to the advances in science and materials, which has enabled production of restorations with superb aesthetics and which also function very well. This has been driven by the demands of patients who would ideally prefer a tooth-coloured restoration. That said, alloys are still used extensively in dentistry and will continue to be used for the foreseeable future.

SUMMARY

- Alloys are designed for specific application.
- They form three main groups: high noble, noble and base metals.
- Addition of base metals to noble metals enhances mechanical properties but increase risk of corrosion.
- Alloys for metal ceramic restorations must have higher casting temperatures.
- Base metal alloys are less dense than noble metals but present problems with regard to aesthetics.
- Stainless steel alloys of different compositions are used for different applications.

FURTHER READING

Anusavice, K.J., 2003. Science of Dental Materials, eleventh ed. WB Saunders, Philadelphia (See Chapters 19 and 20).

Powers, J.M., Sakaguchi, R.L. (Eds.), 2006. Craig's Restorative Dental Materials, twelfth ed. Mosby Elsevier, St Louis (See Chapters 15, 16 and 19).

van Noort, R., 2007. Introduction to Dental Materials, third ed.. Mosby Elsevier, Edinburgh (See Chapters 3.3, 3.5 and 3.9).

SELF-ASSESSMENT QUESTIONS

1. How would a dentist select a dental alloy for a metal-ceramic crown?
2. What are the benefits of using a noble rather than a high noble metal as a dental alloy?
3. What are the reasons for the addition of silver and copper to noble alloys?
4. What are the means of bonding a ceramic to a metal substructure?
5. Base metal alloys are either based on nickel-chromium or cobalt-chromium alloys. What are the advantages and disadvantages of these alloys?
6. Why should new alloy ingots be used with old casting buttons to ensure a good casting?

Dental ceramics

LEARNING OBJECTIVES

From this chapter, the reader will:

- Understand what constitutes a dental ceramic and the different types of dental ceramic
- Understand their properties and how these affect their manufacture, clinical applications and performance
- Understand how ceramics may be strengthened with other materials, for example alloys, alumina or zirconia
- Understand the principles of preparation when ceramic restorations are planned
- Be aware of the role of CAD-CAM in the construction of all-ceramic restorations
- Know the names of the currently available commercial products.

INTRODUCTION

For many years the term **dental porcelain** described the material which was used to construct aesthetic restorations such as anterior crowns (Figure 22.1). Dental porcelain or **ceramic** is related to other ceramics which are used to make objects such as Chinese porcelain vases, engine mouldings, ballistic protection, roof tiles and the heat-proof tiles on NASA's space shuttle (Figure 22.2).

It is now acknowledged that the term 'dental porcelain' was incorrect. This is because little or no **kaolin** is present in the dental version, unlike the other (decorative) ceramics mentioned above (Table 22.1). Kaolin is a **clay** (chemically **hydrated aluminium silicate**). The reason for the absence of kaolin from dental ceramics is that it is opaque and this influences the optical properties and therefore the aesthetics of the final restoration.

The ceramics now used in dentistry have been specifically produced for dental applications. A **ceramic** may be defined as a material which is an inorganic non-metal solid produced by the application of heat which is then cooled. It may be amorphous and partly or wholly crystalline. Dental ceramics need to be translucent and so **feldspar** and **silica** are incorporated into the material to achieve this. Dental ceramics are therefore really **glasses** called **feldspathic** 'porcelains'. **Pigments** are also included to improve and optimize the aesthetics.

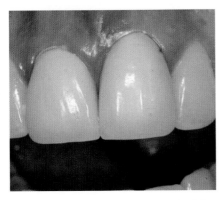

Fig. 22.1 Teeth 11 and 21 restored with crowns made of dental 'porcelain'.

Table 22.1 Comparison of the composition of decorative and dental ceramics

Composition	Decorative ceramic (%)	Dental ceramic (%)
Kaolin	50–70	3–5*
Quartz (silica)	15–25	12–25
Feldspar	15–25	70–85
Metallic colourants	<1	1
Glass	0	Up to 15 depending on fusing temperature

*Note the small amount of kaolin in dental ceramic with a consequent increase in the percentage of feldspar.

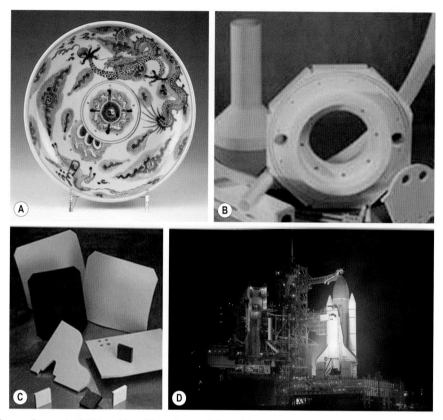

Fig. 22.2A–D Examples of uses of ceramics (A) Fine china, (B) engine mouldings, (C) body armour for flack jackets and (D) heatproof tiles on a space shuttle.

CONVENTIONAL DENTAL CERAMICS

> **Vitreous:** having an amorphous structure.

Conventional dental ceramics are vitreous ceramics made up of a silica network with either **potash feldspar** (potassium alumino silicate) and/or **soda feldspar** (sodium alumino silicate) (Figure 22.3 and Table 22.2). This latter material is also called **albite**. Feldspars are a mixture of both of these materials with the proportions differing to yield different properties. Feldspar is the lowest fusing component and melts and flows during firing, forming a solid mass uniting the other constituents. **Borax** is also frequently included to further lower the fusing temperature.

The **flux**, in the case of a ceramic material, is a material which increases the viscosity of the molten glass and lowers the fusion and softening temperature of the glass. **Binders** act by holding the ceramic particles together prior to firing. As well as conveying opacity to the final product, **cerium** also produces fluorescence. Feldspathic porcelains are also referred to as **opalescent porcelains** as various metallic oxides are added to convey opalescence and provide colour.

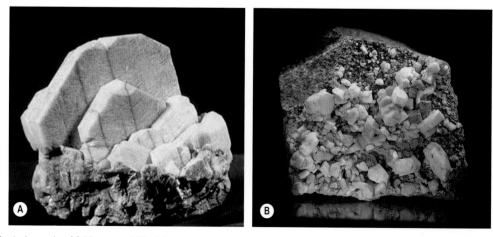

Fig. 22.3 (A) A geological sample of feldspar; and (B) albite.
Wilkopedia Licence for free use.

Table 22.2 Typical composition of two dental ceramics, an enamel and a dentine shade, used in the construction of an all-ceramic crown

Compound	Reason for inclusion	Dentine (approximate %)	Enamel (approximate %)
Silicon dioxide (silica)	Part of the glass-forming structure	66	65
Aluminium oxide (alumina)	Forms part of the glass structure Alters softening point and viscosity	14	14
Calcium oxide Potassium oxide (potash) Sodium oxide (soda)	Fluxes	0 7 4	2 7 5
Boron trioxide Boric oxide	Flux It may also act as glass modifier, lowering the melt temperature and forming its own glass network	6	7
Lithium oxide	Strengthens; can act as a flux	Trace	Trace
Magnesium oxide	Flux	Trace	Trace
Fluorspar	Flux	Trace	Trace
Metallic oxides	Colouring agents	Trace	Trace
Oxides of Cerium Zirconium Titanium Tin	Opacifying agents	Trace	Trace
Starch Sugar	Binder	Trace	Trace

The amounts and constituents vary as to the requirements of the final product. Table 22.3 lists the metallic oxides used together with the colour which their inclusion imparts.

Table 22.3 Metallic oxides convey various colours to the ceramic

Metallic oxide of	Colour
Chromium	Green
Cobalt	Blue
Copper	Green
Iron	Brown
Manganese	Lavender
Nickel	Brown
Titanium	Yellow/brown

Fluorescence: the ability of a material to emit visible light when exposed to ultraviolet light.
Opalescence: the ability of a translucent material to appear blue in reflected light and orange/yellow in transmitted light.

Manufacture of the ceramic powder

The ceramic is supplied to the dental laboratory as a powder. The manufacturers make this powder by taking the raw materials and grinding them to form fine powders. These are blended together and then fired at a high temperature in a furnace. The molten mass thus produced is then rapidly cooled in cold water, which leads to large internal stresses, cracking and crazing of the mass. The resulting fragments of ceramic are known as **frit**, with the process called **fritting** (which is a **pyrochemical reaction**). The frit is then milled to a very fine powder. This powder may now be mixed with distilled water by the dental technician to form a creamy paste and the restoration built up.

Types of dental ceramic

The feldspathic ceramics form **leucite** and a glass phase when heated to a temperature of between 1150 and 1500 °C. The leucite material is **potassium aluminium silicate**, which has almost twice the coefficient of thermal expansion of feldspar. The manufacturer carries out this process to provide the dental technician with a powder with defined amounts of the appropriate components to permit the mass to be fired successfully.

The composition of the ceramic powder is such that a further chemical reaction is not required. Instead the particles of the ceramic powder fuse when it is heated to just above its glass transition temperature. This is called **sintering** (see Chapter 9). It is very important that the powder particles are very closely packed so that a dense compact structure without air inclusions is produced. During sintering, the glass phase will soften and start to coalesce. This is termed **liquid phase sintering**. This process takes time and may be halted at any stage by removing the ceramic from the heating oven. During the heating process, the glass phase will initially soften and a friable matrix is established. As the temperature rises the other components tend to fill the voids within the glass matrix. There is controlled diffusion between the particles, and as this continues, a dense solid is formed.

There is a range of dental ceramics, and these may be defined by the firing temperature: the **ultra low** (fired below 850 °C); **low fusing** 'porcelains' (fired between 850 and 1100 °C); and **higher fusing** ceramic powders, which are used primarily for denture teeth. All these are manufactured under controlled conditions within a factory environment. The ultra low fusing ceramics are used primarily as **shoulder** 'porcelains' (see p. 389), or to correct minor defects and to add surface colouring and shading.

Low fusing ceramics should not be subjected to multiple firings as this is likely to lead to distortion. They must also be supported by a substructure otherwise they are likely to sag (see p. 390).

Dental laboratory procedure

The technical process to construct a ceramic restoration in the dental laboratory is time consuming and requires considerable care to achieve a satisfactory result. This process is described below.

The traditional method involved an impression being cast to produce a working model. The preparation die was then removed from the model and the dental technician laid down a platinum foil onto the die and closely adapted the foil to the surface of the die. The purpose of the foil was threefold:

- It formed a supporting matrix for the ceramic which was laid down to build up the restoration
- Prevented the ceramic powder coming into contact with the die so protecting it from damage
- Provided support during the firing process and ensured that the fit to the model was maintained.

However, more recently, use of platinum foils has fallen out of favour as the ceramic crowns produced were not strong and tended to fracture. This is now overcome by the use of a substructure which supports the overlying ceramic. Until recently, the primary means to provide this support was to fire the ceramic onto an underlying metal coping, usually a gold alloy. This coping also prevents crack propagation. However, more recently, use of alumina, leucite and zirconia core structures has proved fruitful. Like the metal coping, these materials provide strength and prevent crack propagation. They are relatively opaque but modern techniques using glass infiltration of a friable, part-sintered framework has produced core materials which are very much stronger than conventional dental ceramics. The construction of these cores may be carried out by hand in the dental laboratory or may be produced by the computer-aided design–computer-aided manufacture (CAD-CAM) technique from factory prepared blocks of the sintered materials. This is discussed in detail later in the chapter.

Building up the restoration: dentine portion

The ceramic is either built up on a refractory die which itself is placed in the furnace or onto a core or coping by the technician applying an opaque shade to mask the colour of underlying substructure. This is either fired in the furnace or left to dry. The dentine portion of the restoration is then laid down using the appropriate shade of the 'dentine' ceramic powder.

The ceramic powder is mixed with distilled water to form a creamy paste, which is then laid down onto the coping. It is important that the minimum amount of air is incorporated into the powder slurry during this process to avoid porosity and stress concentrations in the final product. To produce minimum shrinkage during the firing process the powder must be condensed to remove water and pull the ceramic particles closer together. This is called **compacting** and is achieved by either vibration, spatulation or smoothing/burnishing with a brush. Once condensation has been achieved, the excess water is blotted away using absorbent tissue (Figure 22.4).

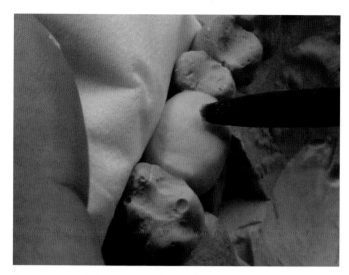

Fig. 22.4 Tissue being gently applied to the ceramic mass to absorb the water coming to the surface as a result of compaction. Note the use of a fine paint brush to apply the powder to build up the restoration.

Building up the restoration: enamel portion

Once the dentine portion of the restoration has been applied, the appropriate shade of enamel is selected and this is built up as previously described. The final built-up mass is substantially oversized than the restoration it will finally become. A combination of the condensation process and firing will reduce the size markedly. At this point, the mass is referred to being in the **green state**, i.e. the prefiring state. It is very fragile and must be handled very carefully (Figure 22.5).

Firing: first bake

The mass is fired to fuse the particles together and form the final restoration, by a series of 'bakes' in the furnace. It is important that the mass is slowly heated initially to eliminate the water from the slurry and allow shrinkage to occur. To achieve this, it is usually held near the entrance to the furnace for sometime before being introduced inside (Figure 22.6).

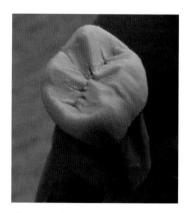

Fig. 22.5 The completed crown form in the green state prior to firing.

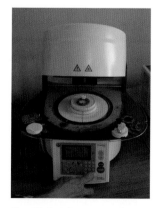

Fig. 22.6 A furnace used to bake dental ceramic. Note that the ceramic mass in the green state is sitting a short distance to the furnace entrance to allow water to be slowly driven off before it turns into steam. If steam was allowed to form, the powder core would break.

During the first 'bake' the water is driven off and the powder particles sinter together. The majority of the shrinkage occurs during this firing and is in the range of 10–20%. The temperature of the furnace is set at about 50 °C below the fusing temperature of the ceramic powder being used. During this time, the binders are burned off and the ceramic particles start to fuse at the points of contact, forming a porous mass. The voids in the porous mass start to disappear as the molten glass flows between the particles, drawing them closer. This is called **pyroplastic flow**. Shrinkage continues to occur until an almost void-free material results. This is often referred to as the **biscuit bake** or **biscuit firing** (Figure 22.7).

It is important that once this firing cycle has been completed, the ceramic is allowed to cool slowly and uniformly. This will prevent stresses forming, as different portions of the material shrink to different extents. Stresses can lead to cracking and a loss in strength due to **thermal shock**.

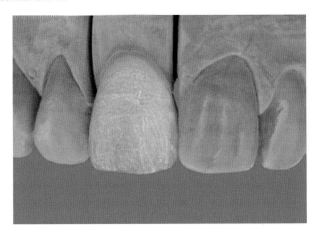

Fig. 22.7 A metal-ceramic crown at the biscuit stage. Note the chalky appearance of its surface.
Image courtesy of Vita Fabric.

Firing: subsequent bakes

If the technician deems that further ceramic is required to complete the restoration, this is added and the restoration fired again. Figure 22.8 shows a crown just prior to firing with the various ceramic powders built up. The different colours help in differentiating the dentine and enamel powders. These colours are lost in the firing.

The firing process is then repeated but in this case the temperature of the furnace is increased. There is a further slight contraction, and the voids between the particles are filled by the molten glass, which is drawn into the spaces between the sintered particles by capillary action to form a solid mass.

Some considerations in firing

- This process must be carefully controlled as the temperature of the furnace and time that the ceramic is in it is critical.
- Overfiring can result in molten glass flowing too much and the restoration losing its shape. Modern furnaces are usually computer controlled and the changes required during the firing process can be programmed into the memory. This may involve firing in air or a partial vacuum, producing an atmosphere about 10% of normal. Some ceramic products come supplied with a bar code which is scanned to input the firing cycles required by that particular ceramic. This is of particular importance as each manufacturer's ceramics have different firing parameters that should be adhered to precisely.
- The size of the particles of the ceramic powder also has an influence on the finished crown. Finer grained powders produce more uniform surfaces than coarser grains. Although the firing process and the densification which occurs will leave a structure which is solid, there is still a risk of small air voids being present. This is the case even when the firing process is carried out under vacuum. Much of the air within the ceramic structure is removed as the vacuum develops. The little that remains will be below atmospheric pressure. Once the furnace temperature has reached to within about 50 °C of the final firing temperature, the vacuum is released and this results in the voids collapsing as the pressure external to the crown is increased by a factor of 10 above the internal pressure in the crown.

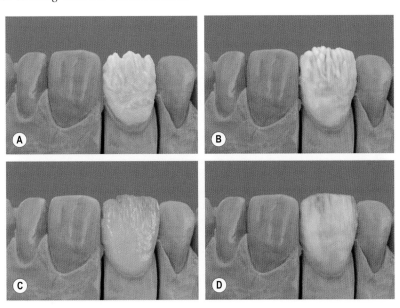

Fig. 22.8A–D (A) An all-ceramic crown being built up to restore tooth 11 using dentine ceramic (pink) and enamel (white). (B, C) The crown has been fired and (D) further 'enamel' ceramic has been added.
Images courtesy of Vita Fabric.

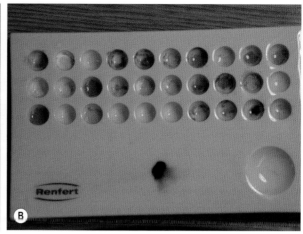

Fig. 22.9A,B Stains may be applied to the ceramic restoration to incorporate characterizations such as hypoplastic spots, occlusal fissures or microcracks.

Staining

Stains may now be applied using a paint brush to characterize the final restoration, such as the staining of occlusal fissures or hypoplastic spots. The staining kit resembles an artist's palate (Figure 22.9). The stains may be applied to the surface of the restoration or become incorporated within the ceramic. If the stain is applied on surface, it may be lost if any adjustment is made or during function. Generally speaking, stains are better incorporated within the structure of the ceramic (Figure 22.10).

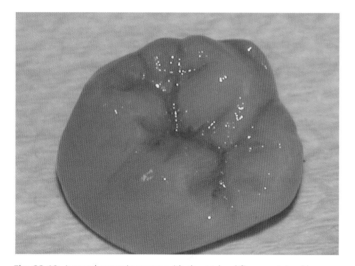

Fig. 22.10 A metal-ceramic crown with the occlusal fissures stained brown.

Glazing

The final stage of the firing process is the **glazing** of the restoration. This produces a glassy smooth surface on the restoration, sealing it. It will also fill in any small areas of porosity at the surface. Glazing is achieved by either very carefully re-firing the restoration to fuse the outer layer of ceramic completely or by using glazes with lower fusing (transparent glass) temperatures which are applied as a thin layer to the outer surface of the restoration. The restoration may then be adjusted with fine diamonds and polishing rubbers (Figure 22.11).

Properties of fired dental ceramics

Aesthetics

It is widely recognized that ceramic is the best dental restorative material with respect to aesthetics. When the shade and any characterization has been carefully prescribed and then replicated into the restoration, the aesthetics can be excellent creating an almost imperceptible result. It can be quite a challenge to notice the difference even for dental care professionals, particularly with all-ceramic restorations. Ceramics are colour stable and achieve a very smooth surface finish and have the ability to retain the finish better than other materials. However, they will be affected by acids. In particular, topical fluoride gels can etch the surface of the ceramic. This etching leads to the surface glaze being disrupted quite rapidly, possibly resulting in surface staining. Bulk colour changes can occur if the tints incorporated during the crown construction are involved.

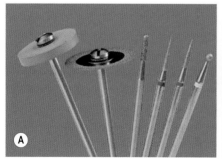
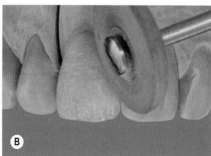
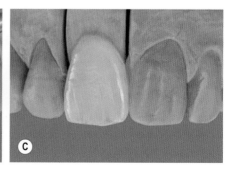

Fig. 22.11 (A, B) A range of cutting instruments which may be used to polish ceramic. (C) The final glazed crown; note the glass-like surface. *Images Courtesy of Vita Fabric.*

Dental ceramics provide a very high level of **translucency**, which is important when matching the restoration to natural tooth tissue. As well as matching the shade of the adjacent natural teeth, dental ceramics must also be able to fluoresce and be opalescent. Natural tooth tissue has this ability, the best example of this is viewing a ceramic crown under ultraviolet light in a nightclub, where it will often appear 'dead' and dark compared to the adjacent teeth.

> **Translucent:** the ability of a material to allow the passage of light but diffusing it so that it is not possible to see any clear outline or structure behind.

Chemical stability

Dental ceramics formed during the firing process are chemically stable (inert) and resistant to chemical attack. They are also biocompatible and have a good soft tissue compatibility. However, strong acids such as hydrofluoric acid can be used to etch the surface of the ceramic. This is used when the ceramic restoration is to be bonded to the tooth surface, for example a veneer or to repair fractured ceramic.

Thermal properties

The thermal properties of dental ceramic and tooth tissue shows a great similarity, i.e. the coefficients of thermal expansion and thermal diffusivity are close to one another. This means that the ceramic restoration will behave in the same way as the underlying dentine with respect to thermal expansion and contraction and will exhibit a slower rate of heat transfer. The restoration will therefore not be stressed during oral thermal cycling. Thermal diffusivity is poor and may present a problem if the dentist carried out a sensitivity (vitality) test on the tooth by applying a very hot or cold material to the ceramic crown. The material will not transmit these extremes of temperature well, making the results of the test difficult to interpret.

Themal shock may be avoided by firing ceramic materials as few times as practicable and allowing them to cool slowly on their removal from the furnace. Soldering of metal components should be avoided after the ceramic has been added for the same reason.

Dimensional stability

While fully fired ceramic is dimensionally stable, this not the case prior to firing, when a large volumetric shrinkage is seen from the early sintered state to the fully fired product. This property makes ceramic a challenging material for the dental technician and restorative dentist to work with. The construction and maintenance of accurate occlusal contacts is difficult if not impossible unlike the lost wax technique, where the wax and metal may be much more accurately worked with. The inclusion of a try-in appointment is invaluable where the restoration is returned to the clinic in the biscuit stage. The occlusion can then be adjusted to create stable contacts prior to the restoration being glazed and fitted.

The large shrinkage seen has prompted the development of **shoulder ceramics**. Shrinkage at the margins of the preparation leads to an open margin and potential for leakage with the attendant

sequelae. Shoulder ceramics shrink much less and so a more accurately fitting restoration is produced. To overcome the problem of ceramic shrinkage, many restorative dentists prefer metal margins but in reality this solution is only helpful in the non-aesthetic zone.

Mechanical properties

Dental ceramics are very strong in compression but are also very brittle and have low flexural strengths. However, in tension and flexure the ceramic behaves as a glass. The best analogy for this is the impact of a cricket ball against a pane of glass. The ceramic must always be supported by an underlying structure or it will fracture under load, particularly if the ceramic is unsupported. Ceramic also has a low fracture toughness, which means crack propagation between defects will readily occur.

Dental ceramics show **static fatigue**, which is the decrease in strength over time even without the application of load. They can also develop **slow crack growth** during cyclic loading in a moist environment, which may, over time, lead to fracture of the ceramic.

Effects of tooth preparation

Ceramics may also fracture during function if the initial tooth preparation was inadequate. If the height of an anterior crown preparation is reduced excessively then a large area of tooth must be replaced by ceramic. If the unsupported ceramic is thicker than 1 mm it will have no support from the underlying tooth structure and therefore is at risk of flexure during chewing and biting, and thus fracture (Figure 22.12).

Vacuum versus air firing

During the firing cycle, if residual air is retained because air voids were present in the unfired ceramic mass, incomplete fusion of the glass particles will occur. These air voids may be quite extensive

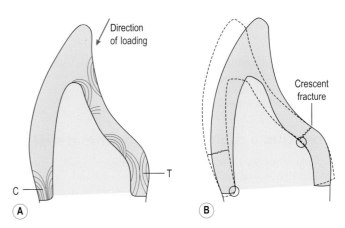

Fig. 22.12 (A) The build-up in stresses in a ceramic crown once it is loaded. (C = compressive stress and T= tensile stress.) As these stresses occur cyclically, the crown will eventually fracture. (B) The usual site of fracture is on the palatal aspect of the crown.

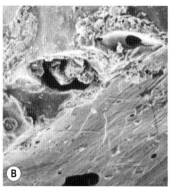
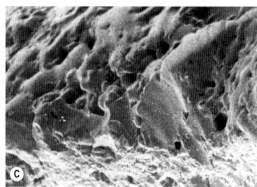

Fig. 22.13 (A) The internal fit surface and margin of an air-fired all-ceramic crown. Note the extensive air voids – seen as black dots – spread across the whole of the fit surface. (B) The margin at a higher magnification. An air void is present with a part-sintered particle included within it. (C) Another part of the margin. The flow of the ceramic has been limited such that there are defects on the crown surface and although the sintering process has occurred, incomplete glazing has resulted.

and form sites of crack initiation. This is a particular problem with crowns manufactured without vaccum firing (Figure 22.13).

As the crown cools down after firing, the outer surface of the crown is likely to cool more quickly than the inner (fit) surface. This means that there is a outer compression stress while the inner surface of the crown is set under tension. If this is followed by cementation and there are any small areas where the crown–cement–tooth interfaces are incomplete or defective, there will be a risk of fracture as the ceramic is unsupported. Additionally, residual voids within the ceramic as a result of the firing process are also areas of weakness which will aid in crack propagation across the restoration surface. Glazing can reduce surface microcracks, but this cannot be done on the fit surface. Such problems have led to the development of alternative ways of preventing crack propagation in the production of modern dental ceramic crowns.

METHODS OF REINFORCING DENTAL CERAMICS

There are several ways of reinforcing dental ceramics:

- Producing a **coping** over the preparation which is resistant to fracture and covering this with conventional ceramic
- **Casting** or **pressing** a block of ceramic
- **Milling** a laboratory-prepared block of ceramic.

Producing a coping in a stronger material

A coping is built in a **metal alloy** to produce a metal-ceramic crown or a stronger polycrystalline ceramic (glass-free) material such as **alumina**, **spinel** or **zirconia** can be used as the core to create an all-ceramic restoration. The conventional felspathic ceramic is then fired onto the coping as a veneer. All of these systems prevent crack propagation from the outer surface of the ceramic through to the tooth surface. They also eliminate the microcracks which form on the fitting surface and which cannot be glazed as previously described. Furthermore, the design of the coping will support the more fragile ceramic. The structure is therefore much stronger. This process must take account of the variation in properties between the two layers, otherwise delamination will occur.

Metal alloy

The first coping material to be used was a metal alloy. Metal alloys are strong and also have the effect of holding the underlying tooth together by bracing. This is advantageous as heavily restored (weak) teeth are commonly crowned to prevent them from breaking. The metal alloy and the ceramic used are optimized to achieve a strong bond to each other both chemically and with respect to their physical properties.

Methods of ceramic retention on the metal coping

The ceramic is retained onto the metal coping by three mechanisms:

- **Compression fit**. This is achieved during the firing process as the ceramic powder slurry will shrink and adapt to the irregularities on the alloy surface. Additionally, the metal underlying the ceramic has a slightly higher coefficient of thermal expansion than the ceramic. This means that on cooling the metal shrinks slightly more and the ceramic has slight residual compression stresses. Ceramic is strong in compression and so can withstand the stresses. However, this stressing must be controlled because if the metal shrinks too much then the ceramic will be overstressed, resulting in the ceramic cracking and crazing. Failure will therefore occur at the metal–ceramic interface. If the coefficient of thermal expansion is higher for the ceramic than the alloy, it will contract more but this contraction is limited by the metal. The ceramic is then under tension and when it cools surface cracks and crazes will form. If the coefficients of thermal expansion are the same for both the ceramic and alloy then no stresses are generated and delamination is unlikely to occur.
- **Micromechanical retention**. During the firing process, as the ceramic powder heats it flows into the surface irregularities of the metal coping. Sometimes the metal surface is roughened by sandblasting with 25–50 μm alumina to increase surface area for bonding. To achieve an effective union between the two materials the ceramic must wet the surface of the metal well.
- **Chemical union**. The chemical union of the alloy and the ceramic is achieved via oxides. These form on the surface of the metal and are formed in the ceramic when it is fired. The oxides then bond so a chemical union is created. The alloy and the ceramic must be compatible for this to occur. A range of alloys may be used; the most important factor influencing the choice is that the melting point of the alloy must be in excess of the fusing temperature of the ceramic powders used. If this is not the case the alloy will melt during the firing process. Similarly, the alloy must be stable at the firing temperature and not distort and flex. Finally, the alloy composition must not affect or influence the aesthetics of the final restoration. For specific information relating to the bonding alloys used, see Chapter 21.

To achieve the best chemical union between the alloy and the ceramic a number of procedures must be carried out. After the coping has been cast, it is cleaned and the surface ground to remove any porosities, fine projections and any residual investment material. The surface micro-roughness aids mechanical retention of the ceramic. This may also be achieved by sandblasting. The casting is then treated with an organic solvent such as carbon tetrachloride to remove any debris and grease deposited during the roughening process, and is usually done by immersion in an ultrasonic bath.

In the case of a noble metal alloy, the casting is returned to the furnace. There it is held under a partial vacuum to allow elements such as gallium, indium, zinc and tin within the alloy to migrate to the surface to form an oxide layer. The temperature at which this process is carried out is just below the firing temperature of the ceramic. Each alloy will have a clearly defined heating cycle and this must be adhered to otherwise the oxide layer formation will be impared. When base metal alloys are used, the formation of an oxide layer is much easier and care must be taken not to produce too thick a layer. Cohesive failure may occur within this thick layer. Heating under vacuum additionally helps to **de-gas** the alloy, which aids even oxide layer deposition.

After the oxide layer has been formed, the casting can be immersed in an acid which is generally 30% hydrochloric acid. This process is called **pickling**. It is designed to increase the concentration of tin oxide at the surface at the expense of the other oxides which have been formed. The casting at this point has a light grey appearance. This process is now infrequently used as it requires considerable care and is not risk free.

The noble metal alloy casting may then be reheated in air to increase the oxide layer thickness. If this is done then care must be taken to ensure that the oxide layer is not too thick. Equally the oxide layer should not be lost by this process. The surface should at this point have a grey-white, matt appearance (Figure 22.14). The ceramic may now be applied.

As bonding alloys have been specially formulated to work well with ceramics, similarly bonding ceramics have been created so that they may react chemically with the alloy (Table 22.4). These ceramics

Table 22.4 Composition of three ceramic powders suitable for use with alloys

Compound	Ceramic powder A	Ceramic powder B	Ceramic powder C
Silicon dioxide	52	52	62
Aluminium oxide	14	15	13
Calcium oxide	Not present	Not present	1
Potassium oxide	11	10	11
Sodium oxide	5	7	5
Titanium dioxide	3	3	Not present
Zirconium dioxide	3	5	>0.3
Tin dioxide	6	5	>0.5
Barium oxide	1	Not present	>0.06
Zinc oxide	Not present	Not present	Not present
Rubidium oxide	>0.01	>0.01	Not present
Boron trioxide carbon dioxide and water	4	3	6

This table show the common additives in contrast to the felspathic ceramics.

that of the alloy. Leucite formation occurs by holding the ceramic at a specific temperature for a period of time and its presence strengthens the ceramic. If the metal coping is titanium then specific ceramics must be used in combination.

The three methods of metal-ceramic bonding are summarized in Figure 22.15.

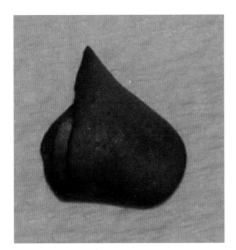

Fig. 22.14 The appearance of the surface of the metal substructure immediately prior to the application of the ceramic.

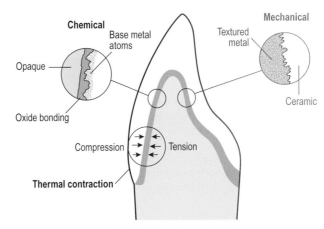

Fig. 22.15 The three modes of retention of the ceramic veneer onto a metal coping.

are feldspathic but which have significant amounts of leucite either added or as part of the felspar derivative used. The leucite lowers the coefficient of thermal expansion of the ceramic to bring it closer to

Problems to overcome with the metal-ceramic system

Unfortunately there are several disadvantages of using a metal alloy coping.

- To accomodate the minimum thickness of metal and ceramic required for strength and satisfactory aesthetics, more tooth needs to be removed so the preparation is less conservative. This inevitably leads to compromise. The minimum bulk of a gold alloy and ceramic is generally considered to be 1.7 mm although most technicians would prefer 2.0 mm. This allows 0.9–1.1 mm of ceramic facing and 0.6–0.8 mm of gold alloy. Most dentists wish to conserve tooth tissue and this in some cases means that tooth reduction is less than ideal. Teeth particularly prone to this are lower incisors, upper laterals and premolars, where there is a risk of encroaching on the dental pulp if a full 2 mm is removed from the preparation (Figure 22.16).

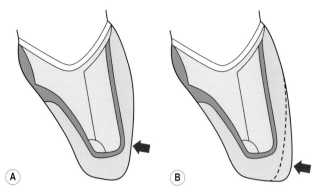

Fig. 22.17 The consequences of inadequate tooth preparation on the (A) shape and (B) amount of ceramic required.

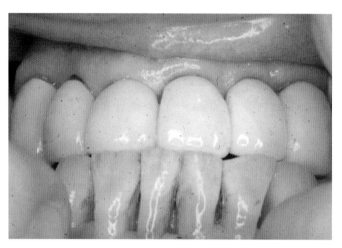

Fig. 22.16 Overbuilt metal-ceramic crowns on the upper incisors due to inadequate reduction during preparation. The result is crowns which have a poor emergence profile, which may compromise periodontal health in the long term. The aesthetics are also suboptimal.

- Figure 22.17 shows the compromises which may be made with inadequate tooth reduction:
  - In Figure 22.17A, the dentist has inadequately reduced the incisal tip, which means that the technician can achieve the correct crown shape only by reducing the amount of ceramic near the incisal tip. This has two consequences: (i) the underlying opaquing agent will show through and the crown will have a white opaque blob near the incisal tip and (ii) the ceramic will be much thinner and is more prone to fracture if loaded.
  - In Figure 22.17B, the technician has done their best to create an aesthetic result by increasing the bulk of ceramic at the incisal tip. Unfortunately the resulting crown has an incisal tip thickness which is nearly double that of the normal tooth. This impedes normal function as well as having an inferior appearance.

- The strength of the metal coping may result in fracture of the underlying core if this is thin and therefore weak. In this case the core will fracture within the crown.
- The metal coping must be disguised otherwise the metal will shine through, resulting in an unaesthetic restoration. This presents difficulties for the clinican and the technician in obtaining a succesful aesthetic result that is anatomically ideal. The aesthetics of the metal-ceramic crown are compromised when compared with an all-ceramic crown as the dark alloy coping must be masked. Figure 22.18 shows the effects of light behaviour in relation to a metal-ceramic crown.

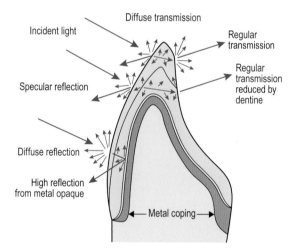

Fig. 22.18 Diagrammatic illustration, of the behaviour of light in a metal-reinforced ceramic crown. The incisal tip, where no core metal is present, allows transmission. However, near the midline of the tooth the underlying opaquing agent reflects the light back. A similar effect is produced in the approximal areas. Light also reflects, refracts and is transmitted through the ceramic.

It is essential that good communication is established between the dental technician and dentist so that problems such as inadequate tooth reduction can be discussed and the best compromise achieved.

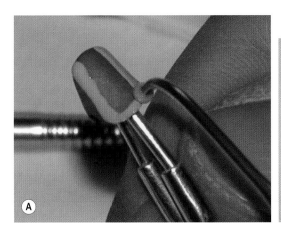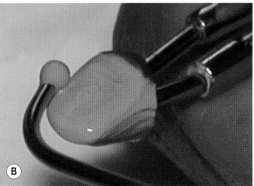

Fig. 22.19A,B Application of an opaque layer of ceramic to the surface of the metal coping.

- It is extremely challenging for the dental technician to construct an aesthetic metal-ceramic crown. They must apply an opaque layer of ceramic to prevent the grey metal substructure showing through (Figure 22.19). The colour of the opaquing agent is determined by the shade of the subsequently applied ceramic which has been selected by the dentist. This layer is a masking material and has no light reflective properties. The dental technician must then use shading and tinting of the ceramic to achieve the right level of reflection and translucency in the ceramic. However, even well-constructed metal-ceramic restorations are less life-like or less natural than than a commensurate all-ceramic one (Figure 22.20).

Alumina

The aesthetic disadvantages of using a metal coping may be circumvented by using a non-metallic material. A tougher crystalline material such as alumina can produce a strengthened coping. The alumina particles prevent the peneration of a crack which has developed in the weaker superficial phase of the material from passing further. This principle was discovered in the early 1960s when alumina was added to the normal feldspathic ceramics and is often referred to as **dispersion of a crystalline phase**. The alumina crystals are much less likely to crack than the surrounding glass and stop the crack propagating. This is also known as a **crack stopping**. The limitations of the original aluminous porcelains was that the core material laid down first on the model was primarily the alumina. There was a limit as to how much alumina could be included before the opacity of the core affected the aesthetics of the crown. The maximum included in the core materials was 45–50% alumina. This addition did, however, make a substantial improvement in the flexural strength of all-ceramic crowns. An aluminous ceramic crown has a flexural strength of about 120–140 MPa.

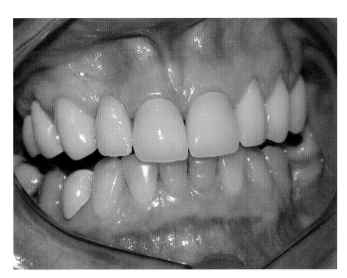

Fig. 22.20 A case restored with metal-ceramic units; bonded crowns 15, 14, 11, 21, 22, 23, 24 and 44 and a cantilever bonded bridge 13/12. While the aesthetics are more than acceptable, metal-ceramic restorations are less life-like than their all-ceramic equivalents.

Glass-infiltrated alumina

More recently the core structure has been modified and the aesthetics enhanced. Vitafabriken has developed a system whereby the core structure is prepared by a **slip casting process**. A duplicate of the preparation die is prepared in a proprietary refractory material and then a fine slurry of alumina powder (**slip**) is laid down on the surface to form the cast. Once the water from the slurry has evaporated, the die and coping are heated to a temperature in excess of 1100°C for a period of 10 hours – the first stage of the sintering process. This is sufficient to allow the alumina particles to be 'tacked' together but is insufficient for them to fuse completely by sintering. After the heating cycle, the die is allowed to cool. The coping produced in this fashion is friable with very low strength, and it is porous (Figure 22.21).

The porous structure is carefully coated with a slurry of glass, usually containing **lanthanum**. This has a low viscosity and on heating will flow through the porous alumina core filling the voids and producing a glass-infiltrated ceramic (Figure 22.22), that is the resultant crown consists of about 85% alumina. Advantages of this method are that the material is much stronger than the conventional core material and the presence of the glass makes the material more translucent and reduces the problem of having an opaque core. The resulting restoration exhibits good aesthetics (see Figure 22.23). The aesthetics achieved using a alumina core are better than when the glass infiltrates the alumina as there is some transmission of light through the core.

Laboratory fabrication stages

Box 22.1 shows the laboratory sequence for the construction of an Inceram Alumina (Vita) crown. This restoration has an alumina core with conventional feldspathic ceramic applied to the coping to create the final restoration.

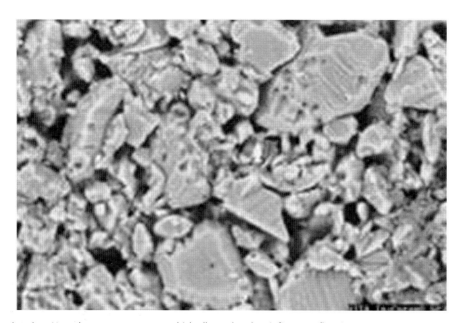

Fig. 22.21 Alumina after sintering. Note the porous structure, which allows the glass infitrate to flow in.

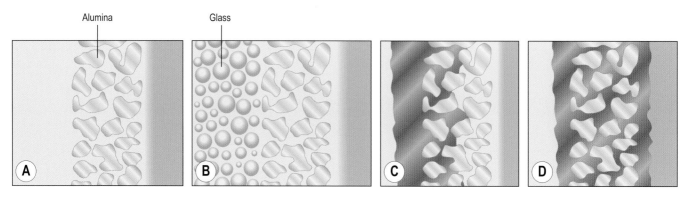

Fig. 22.22A–D Glass infusion of the sintered alumina. As the material heats, it melts and flows by capillary action to form a non-porous mass. (A) The sintered alumina. (B) Glass slurry painted on the outer surface of the alumina. (C) Glass flowing into the spaces in the sintered alumina by capillary action as heat is applied. (D) The glass has fully infiltrated the alumina and the material produced is a solid glass alumina construct.

Box 22.1 Sequence of glass infiltration of slip. *Images courtesy of Vita Fabric*

Step 1	Step 2	Step 3	Step 4	Step 5	Step 6
The prepared working model	The model is duplicated using a silicone impression rubber material	A second die is prepared using refractory material	The ceramic material used to construct the slip is mixed according to manufacturer's instructions to slurry	The slip material is applied to the die to build up the coping using a paint brush	The slip is then sintered in a furnace at low temperature to give a friable coping

Step 7	Step 8	Step 9	Step 10	Step 11	Step 12
Careful adjustments are made to the coping to provide correct contour	The glass powder in the form of a slurry is applied to the coping using a paintbrush	The glass coated coping is then placed on a platinum foil sheet for firing	The copings after firing, during which time the glass infiltrates the porous coping	The coping is then trimmed and the finished coping has a slightly golden colouration	The glass infiltrated coping on the original model ready for the build up of the crown in ceramic

Another well-known proprietary alumina-reinforced crown is the Procera AllCeram (Nobel Biocare) (Figure 22.23). This system is slightly different to the one illustrated above as the morphology of the die is digitized and sent electonically to a dental laboratory in Stockholm, Sweden. The alumina coping is produced by the Nobel Biocare laboratory. It is then returned to the dental laboratory in the country of origin where the veneering ceramic is applied to the alumina coping to complete the restoration.

Techceram is a similar system in that it is based on an alumina core. In this case, a special die is produced and alumina is sprayed onto the die using a thermal gun spray to construct the core. It is sintered at 1170 °C and has a density of 80–90%. As with Procera AllCeram, conventional feldspathic glass is then added to the coping.

Spinel

Another non metallic material that is used as a coping is **spinel** (chemically **magnesium aluminium oxide**). This material has the advantage that is it more aesthetic than alumina but has a slightly lower strength. It is also a polycrystalline (glass-free) ceramic.

Zirconia

The last and increasingly popular non-metallic coping material is **zirconium dioxide**, also known as **zirconia**. It is found as a naturally occuring mineral in igneous rock (Figure 22.24) and also in sand.

Zirconia exists in different forms which change with temperature. The most dramatic structural change occurs at relatively high temperature and leads to a large volumetric expansion. This can lead to cracking as the zirconia cools. For its use in dental applications zirconia has to be stabilized and this is usually achieved by adding a doping agent such as **yttria** (yttrium oxide). This combination when heated forms a mixture of structural phases that above 1000 °C are tetragonal zirconia polycrystals. For the dental application, a trace of alumina is present to prevent leaching of the yttirum oxide.

> **Doping agent:** an impure material added to the pure material to enhance one or more of its properties.

The resulting material has a high flexural strength of 650 MPa and it is resistant to degradation. It also has high fracture toughness and low thermal conductivity. The material is more opaque than the previously described polycrystalline (glass-free) core materials such as spinel. It is homogeneous when fully sintered, with minimal risk of microfractures. It is inert and therefore biocompatible.

The materials produced for dentistry have variying properties depending on the manufacturer – this relates to particle size and distribution and additives included. The majority of the systems rely on the coping being prepared using some form of CAD-CAM system. However, Vita produce a Inceram Zirconia core powder that may be use to produce a slip casting, which may be glass infiltrated as described above. This material is a zirconia/alumina mixture.

Those companies producing blocks for milling will either provide a pre-sintered block, which is milled in the softened or green state, or a block that has been processed to form the dense ceramic. This is often referred to as **HIP (hot isostatic pressing) zirconia** and is much harder to mill. The perceived advantage of the milled approach is that the block of ceramic is prepared in the manufacturer's laboratory and is less variable in its structure as it will be free of large air voids.

As zirconia is chemically inert, and, unlike other ceramic materials, it cannot be etched or silanated without being treated. However, if the

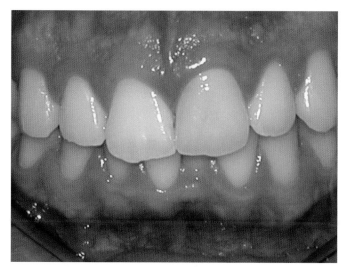

Fig. 22.23 Tooth 21 restored with a Procera AllCeram (Nobel Biocare) crown. Note the excellent biocompatility of the ceramic with the gingival tissues and the aesthetics.

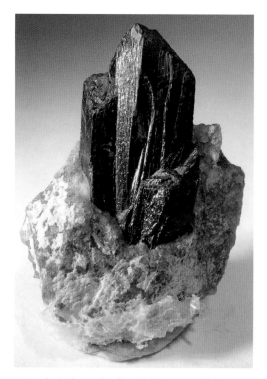

Fig. 22.24 A geological sample of baddeleyite, one of the sources of zirconia.
(Rob Lavinsky, "http://www.irocks.com/" iRocks.com – CC-BY-SA-3.)

surface of zirconia is sandblasted with aluminium oxide (for example by using Rocatec, 3M ESPE), small particles of the oxide will coat the zirconia surface by a tribochemical reaction (see Chapter 19), permitting bonding to a silanating agent and thereby a chemical bond to resin adhesive. This would then allow the restoration to be bonded onto the tooth tissue; whereas without this surface treatment, the restoration may only be luted onto the preparation (see Chapter 11).

Figure 22.25 shows a zirconia coping and a completed zirconia-based crown. Once the coping has been constructed, the remaining crown form is built up using conventional feldspathic ceramics such as IPS e.max Ceram (Ivoclar Vivadent) layering ceramics. These have been formulated to match the thermal properties of the core material. There are other methods of producing zirconia- based ceramic restorations, such as IPS e.max ZirPress (Ivoclar Vivadent), which is pressed onto the zirconia coping. This latter ceramic contains fluorapatite and masks the zirconia core. These are discussed later in the chapter.

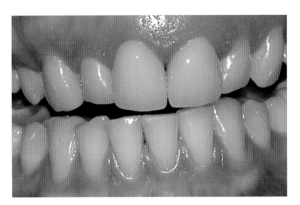

Fig. 22.26 Zirconia based all-ceramic crowns on 11 and 21. Note the excellent aesthetics and biocompatibility with the gingival soft tissues.

Commercially available products

Table 22.5 lists examples of commercially available sintered ceramics.

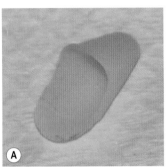 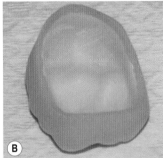

Fig. 22.25 (A) A zirconia coping for an incisor tooth and (B) a completed zirconia-reinforced crown for a molar. Note the relatively opaque zirconia coping with a conventional feldspathic ceramic laid down on it to complete the restoration.

Restorations based on zirconia are showing great promise due to their strength and excellent aesthetics (Figure 22.26). Long-span (posterior) bridges are possible using zirconia substructures and early results of studies suggest that it may offer an alternative to metal-ceramic restorations in some cases.

As with metal alloys, it is the responsibility of the dentist to prescribe a specific ceramic for the intended restoration in detail on the laboratory prescription.

Casting and pressing ceramics

Casting a wax pattern of the proposed restoration is a common technique in the production of gold restorations (Chapters 20 and 21). The lost wax technique also has the advantage that the occlusal

Table 22.5 Some sintered ceramic products currently available on the market

Product	Manufacturer	Type of ceramic	Clinical application
Cerabien	Noritake	Alumina	Frameworks for all-ceramic crowns and bridges
DC-Crystall	DCS Dental	Alumina based	Translucent frameworks
Finesse All Ceramic	Ceramco	Low fusing	Inlays/onlays, anterior and premolar crowns, veneers
Fortress	Mirage	Leucite reinforced	Veneers
In-Ceram Alumina	Vita	Alumina	Crowns
In Ceram Spinell	Vita	Spinel	Crowns
In Ceram Zirconia	Vita	Zirconia	Veneers, crowns and anterior bridges
IPS d.SIGN	Ivoclar Vivadent	Fluorapatite leucite glass ceramic	Metal bonding ceramic
IPS e.max Ceram	Ivoclar Vivadent	Nano-fluorapatite layering glass ceramic	Veneers, veneering of other copings/suprastructures
Lumineers	Cerinate	Leucite-reinforced ceramic	Very thin veneers
Noritake Super Porcelain EX-3	Noritake	Pressable ceramic	Veneers, crowns
Noritake Super Porcelain TI-22	Noritake		For bonding to pure titanium
Optec-HSP	Jeneric/Pentro	Leucite reinforced	veneers
Procera AllCeram	Nobel Biocare	Die scanned, sent to Sweden and alumina coping made	crowns
TechCeram	TechCeram	Sprayed	Inlays/onlays, crowns, veneers

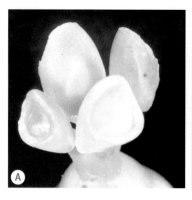

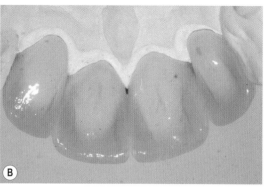

Fig. 22.27 Four crowns manufactured using a cast ceramic (Dicor). (A) The restorations after casting but before the sprues have been removed. (B) The same crowns on the model after characterization has been placed. Note their extreme translucency.

morphology of the restoration may be verified when the models are mounted on an articulator. This has encouraged manufacturers to consider attempting to use this technique in the production of ceramic crowns. These materials are known as **casting**, **pressing** or **injection moulded ceramics**.

Casting ceramics

The first attempt was the casting of glass ceramic. A glass ceramic is a material that is produced in the required shape and then subjected to heat treatment to produce partial **devitrifiction** (partial crystallization of the glass). This 'ceraming' process produces crystalline needle and plates which act as crack stoppers. The first commercial process in dentistry was by Corning Glass and was marketed as Dicor.

In this process, the restoration is waxed up on a conventional laboratory model (made of epoxy resin), invested in a proprietary investment developed specifically for this purpose and cast in a similar way to a gold restoration. The glass casting is devested and sandblasted to remove the investment and clean the surface (Figure 22.27). The sprues are then removed and the casting covered by an **embedding material** to protect it. This also helps to produce uniform heating as the casting is then subjected to a carefully controlled heat process over a period of hours. During this process microscopic plate-like crystals are formed, called **mica**. Once this process is complete the restoration is ground as necessary and a thin veneer of conventional

felspathic ceramic placed over the surface to complete the restoration in form and aesthetics.

The glass ceramic approach has become less popular in the past 10 years for two reasons:

- The strength of the final restoration was not as good as was expected
- The translucency of the restorations was too high. To attempt to overcome this, the dentist had to carefully vary the shade of the cement in order to achieve a satisfactory shade match. There is also a tendency for the incisal tips and sides of the crown to appear grey. For these reasons, Dicor is no longer available.

Pressing ceramics

More recently, the lost wax approach has been pursued by those manufacturers who have adopted the process of hot pressing. An ingot of the ceramic, usually a leucite or zirconia-reinforced feldspar, is used in the manufacturing process. The intended restoration is waxed up and invested in a refractory investment. The wax is then burnt out and the mould placed in a specially designed pressing device, which heats the ingot to 1180 °C. The material softens, and the softened mass is driven into the mould space by an alumina plunger. The resulting restoration is then removed from the investment and coloured using veneering ceramics to achieve the required shade (Figure 22.28).

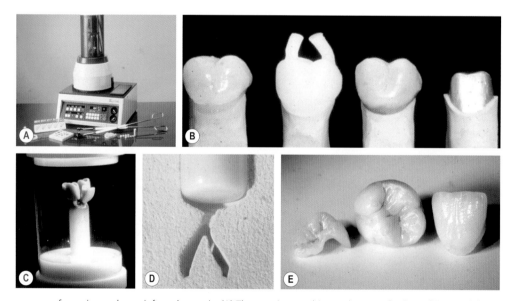

Fig. 22.28A–E The sequence of pressing a glass-reinforced ceramic. (A) The pressing machine and range of coloured ingots. (B) Sequence of the process from the die, waxing and casting to finished restoration. (C) The casting ring with three crowns and sprues. (D) Cross-section of the casting ring showing the alumina piston in position after pressing. (E) The finished restorations with surface characterisation.
Courtesy of Ivoclar Vivadent.

Table 22.6 Some hot pressing and injection moulding ceramic products currently available on the market

Product	Manufacturer	Type of ceramic	Clinical application
IPS e.max Press	Ivoclar Vivadent	Lithium disilicate glass ceramic	Thin veneers, veneers, inlays, onlays, crowns and anterior bridges (maximum three units)
IPS e.max ZirPress	Ivoclar Vivadent	Nano-fluorapatite glass ceramic	Veneers, crowns, anterior and posterior bridges
IPS Empress	Ivoclar Vivadent	Leucite reinforced glass ceramic	Anterior onlays and crowns
IPS Empress 2	Ivoclar Vivadent	Lithium disilicate glass ceramic	Onlays and crowns
IPS Empress Esthetic	Ivoclar Vivadent	Leucite reinforced glass ceramic	Veneers, inlays, onlays and crowns

Unlike the Dicor system, the pressed ceramic is not so translucent and a range of different shades allows the body colour of the tooth to be achieved with some level of accuracy. However, to achieve the ideal aesthetic result, the buccal surface of the crown should be cut back by about a third and a conventional feldspathic ceramic used to build up the requisite form and shade.

However, the pressing process is not without problems as positioning the dies in the investment ring is critical. If they are too close to the piston, once the pressing process commences the piston travels a fixed distance and can encroach on the mould space, causing a miscast. It is also very easy to see how the bulk of the characterization of the crown is achieved by surface veneering. This has the disadvantage that with time, even ceramics will wear, and this will result in slow loss of surface stain.

Commercially available products

Ivoclar Vivadent's IPS e.max Press (Table 22.6) is available in four levels of translucency (HO (highly translucent), LT (low translucency), MO (medium opacity) and HO (high opacity)). It may be used in a number of ways by the dental technician, namely **cast and stain**, **cast and cut-back** and **veneer with layering ceramic**. An opalescent ceramic such as IPS Empress Esthetic Veneer (Ivoclar Vivadent) may be used for this purpose while IPS Empress Universal Shade/Stains, also by Ivoclar Vivadent may be used to inculcate individual surface characterization. This latter material is presented in paste form and is only used with Empress products. The choice of technique will depend on the demands of the case. Low translucency is used for crowns usually in combination with the cut-back technique, medium opacity is used with a layering material (this is available in five shades MO 0 to MO 4) whereas high opacity is used for cases with a very discoloured core and comes in three shades (HO 0 to HO 2). Staining materials are also available (shades/essence): 16 Vita A–D shades and four bleach shades in total. Two sizes of ceramic ingot are produced, the choice of which depends on the size of the restoration to be constructed.

An alternative method utilizes a **press-on technique** where a fluorapatite glass ceramic is pressed onto a zirconia framework. Here the prepared coping is placed on the die and the wax-up and pressing are carried out as described above. This technique may be used to construct crowns, multiunit bridges and suprastructures. One such product is IPS e.max ZirPress (Ivoclar Vivadent), available in three different levels of opacity in A–D shades and four bleach shades. Two gingival shades are also available. Unlike the IPS e.max Press, the ingots are supplied in one size as several ingots may be pressed at the same time. Three translucencies are available: highly translucent (HT) is used with the fully anatomical technique and then stained whereas the low translucency (LT) is used with the cut-back technique. Medium opaque (MO) is also available.

CAD-CAM

More recently, developments in digital technology have led to the introduction of computerized design and manufacture of ceramic restorations. This is described by the acronym **CAD-CAM**. There are broadly two methods to produce the restoration (Figure 22.29):

- The first method involves recording a conventional elastomeric impression and constructing a working model cast from it. This model is then scanned.
- In the second method, a digital impression of the preparation and surrounding teeth is captured using an intraoral scanning device. The clinician can, at this stage, design and customize the restoration on-screen using a **virtual wax knife** and the computer's large database of tooth morphology designs to incorporate the most appropriate forms into the restoration. This digitized information is then transferred to the three-dimensional (3D) milling machine, where the restoration is milled using diamond cutters from a block which has been optimized to enhance the physical properties of the ceramic.

The restoration may then be finished by the technician. With the CAD-CAM scanning and milling technique, the patient can receive their restoration the same day without having to return to the clinic for a second fit appointment. This also obviates the need for a second local anaesthetic injection. The milling of the restoration takes a matter of minutes so the patient can wait for this to be done. Some dental practices site the milling machine in the waiting room so that the patient can watch their restoration being 'magically' created from the ceramic block. Using this technique means that there is no laboratory fee for the dentist, which helps to offset the large start-up costs. Some systems allow the milled restoration to then be characterized and finally fired. Depending on the restoration, the ceramic may then be etched and silanated prior to cementation.

CAD-CAM scanner systems

As with conventional impression taking, the preparation and adjacent and opposing teeth need to be recorded. This may be done digitally, and a number of methods of digital impression recording have been used. The first method was a tactile method where fine, hair-like projections touched the preparation and a digital image was produced. This method has been superseded by **optical** image capture. Some of the systems on the market take still images like a normal camera while others use video capture. The latter method is reputed to be most accurate and is used in some of the most popular systems. In order for the scanner to 'see' the preparation and other teeth, a

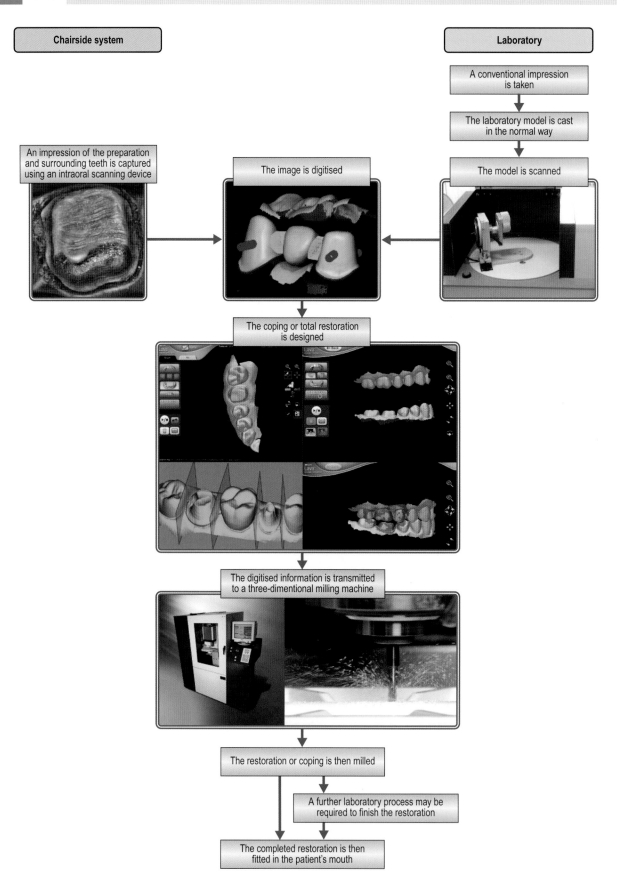

Fig. 22.29 Flow diagram showing the different ways in which CAD-CAM has developed. The left side shows how the whole process may be completed at the chairside with the impression taken by optical means and the restoration milled out of a processed ceramic block. The right side shows a system relying on conventional clinical procedures, but with sensitive processes mechanized in the laboratory.

fine powder must be applied. This is usually a pigment suspended in ethanol (such as Ivoclar Vivadent's IPS Contrast Spray Chairside) and appears as an opaque white or grey powder. However the layer needs to be as thin as possible and also uniform in thickness which can be problematic in the mouth.

Commercially available products

Some of the currently available CAD CAM systems are shown in Table 22.7 and Figure 22.30.

Table 22.7 Some CAD-CAM scanner products currently available on the market

Product	Manufacturer	Comments
Cadent iTero	Cadent	Confocal oral scanning device for passing to recommended laboratory for milling
Cerec 3D	Sirona	Oral scanner: impression and either chairside or laboratory based production of restoration
etkon-CADCAM	Straumann	Confocal oral scanner digitized image to laboratory for processing
Everest	KaVo	Laboratory-based systems for scanning models and then milling
inLab	Sirona	Laboratory-based systems for scanning models and then milling
inVizion	3D Systems	Laboratory-based systems for scanning models and then milling
Lava C.O.S.	3M ESPE	Intraoral scanner and full laboratory system
Scan 2000 Mill200 (CNC tool machine)	Bien-Air Dental S.A.	Laboratory-based systems for scanning models and then milling

Laboratory scanning devices

Laboratory scanning devices usually consist of a laser scanner that performs a number of traverses over the conventional model. Algorithms in the computer program look for a best 'fit' of these scans, determined by the preparation shape. An older but very successful design uses a moving head which migrates over the model to produce another model. Figure 22.31 shows the two types of scanner. The scanning devices are considered to be very accurate and cement lutes of the final restoration are now in the region of 25–50 μm.

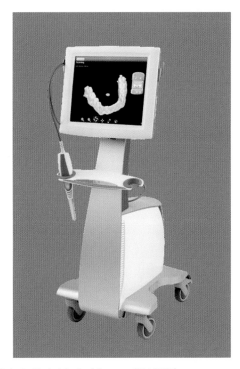

Fig. 22.30 Lava Chairside Oral Scanner (3M ESPE).

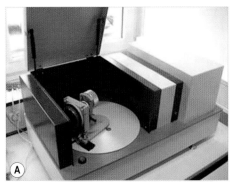

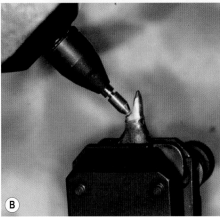

Fig. 22.31A,B Optical laser scanner (3M ESPE) and contact scanner (Nobel Biocare).

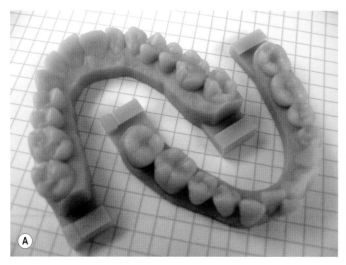
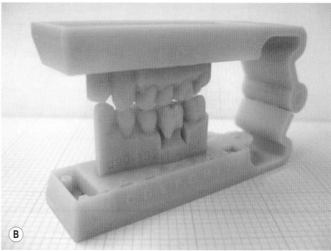

Fig. 22.32A,B Models milled from polyurethane for constructing a crown for tooth 36 using Lava (3M ESPE).

Materials used in CAD-CAM systems

In the systems that require the construction of a model, polyurethane is used and the models are milled out of this material. Furthermore the occlusal relationship must also be transferred to an articulator by the intraoral scanning (Figure 22.32).

The restoration frameworks and copings are now more frequently constructed of zirconia. This may be in one of two forms:

- The first is in its **presintered state**.
  - Advantages: Phase change during later heating stops crack propagation and the material is much easier to mill in this state as it is softer. It is less demanding and wearing on the cutting tools used.
  - Disadvantages: The milled coping or framework must be made much larger than the final restoration as it shrinks significantly during firing which may compromise its subsequent fit.
- The other form is the **hard state HIP zirconia**, which may also be milled to overcome the disadvantages. However, the cutting tools used to mill it must be very durable.

Both the Lava (3M ESPE) and the IPS e.max ZirCAD (Ivoclar Vivadent) systems use zirconia in the partially sintered 'chalk-like' state. When the ingot is machined, it is 20% larger than its final size as when it is sintered, the milled restoration shrinks. In the case of Lava, this is done at a **milling centre**, which is an 3M ESPE accredited dental laboratory. The framework may then stained by the application of a colouring which is available in seven shades. The coping or framework produced by both of these systems is then either conventionally veneered or in the case of the Ivoclar Vivadent product may have ZirPress pressed onto it. A zirconia liner may be used to create a sound bond between the two materials.

The IPS e.max ZirCAD product is available is seven block sizes and in three shades. The smaller blocks are used for single units and the larger ones for longer span bridge frameworks. Another Ivoclar Vivadent product is IPS e.max CAD, and this is also milled in soft state and then crystallised at 850 °C. In the soft state it is blue/mauve in colour and comes in three levels of translucency and in two sizes. It is available in 16 Vita shades (A–D) and four bleach shades (BL). Finally a glaze is available for glazing uncrystallized full contour IPS e.max CAD restorations. IPS e.max Ceram Glaze Spray (Ivoclar Vivadent) is applied in a thin layer.

Commercially available products

Some of the commonly use machinable ceramics currently available are shown in Table 22.8.

RESIN-BONDED CERAMICS

Some ceramics may be bonded onto tooth tissue by the use of a resin-based composite adhesive if they are firstly chemically treated. The restoration derives its strength from the bond which forms between the ceramic and the underlying tooth tissue. It is important therefore not to load these restorations until they have been bonded into place and the bond has been fully formed otherwise the unsupported ceramic will fracture. The types of ceramic used for this purpose include feldspathic ceramic, leucite containing feldspathic glass, glass ceramic, hot pressed ceramic and block forms of these ceramics for use in milling machines using the CAD-CAM technique. A refractory die is made and the ceramic is built up and then sintering onto it. The fitting surface is then etched with hydrofluoric acid and silanated prior to being sent to the clinic for fitting. Alternatively, the ceramic block is milled before etching.

Table 22.8 Some machined ceramic products currently available on the market

Product	Manufacturer	Type of ceramic	Clinical application
Celay	Vident	Pre sintered Spinel, Zirconia, Alumina	High translucency all-ceramic crown framework
Cercon	DeguDent (part of Dentsply)	Cercon zirconia – cerconoxide	Crowns; anterior bridges (up to 47 mm), anterior resin retained bridges (0.5 mm thickness), splinted crowns, posterior bridges up to 47 mm
Cerec 3D	Sirona	Feldspar ceramic	Inlays, onlays crowns, veneers
Everest G Blank	KaVo	Leucite reinforced glass ceramic	Inlays, onlays, veneers and crowns
Everest T Blank	KaVo	Bio-titanium	Copings, abutments and crowns
Everest ZH Blank	KaVo	Yttrium-stabilized hard zirconium dioxide	Larger bridge substructures
Everest ZS Blank	KaVo	Yttrium-stabilized soft zirconium dioxide	Coping and abutments
In Ceram Alumina	Vita	Alumina	Crowns
In Ceram Spinell	Vita	Spinel	Crowns
In Ceram Zirconia	Vita	Zirconia	Crowns, bridges
InVizion YZ Cubes	Vita	Yttrium-stabilized zirconia	Substructure for crowns
IPS e.max CAD	Ivoclar Vivadent	Lithium disilicate glass ceramic	Veneers, inlays and crowns, aesthetic copings and abutments (three-unit anterior bridges), implant suprastructures
IPS e.max ZirCAD	Ivoclar Vivadent	Zirconium oxide	Crowns, anterior and posterior bridges, telescopes and implant suprastructures
IPS Empress CAD	Ivoclar Vivadent	Leucite reinforced glass ceramic	Veneers, inlays, onlays and crowns
KaVo Everest CAD/CAM system	KaVo	Yttrium-stabilized zirconium dioxide (feldspar type)	NB: these are Vitablocs made for the milling machine in a variety of ceramics
Lava	3M ESPE	Partially stabilized zirconia	Crowns; veneers, anterior resin-retained bridges, anterior bridges (up to 41 mm), splinted crowns, posterior bridges (up to 41 mm), implant retained crowns and bridges cemented onto a titanium base, implant abutments
Opalite	DTS	All zirconia, just add stain	Crowns
Procera	Nobel Biocare	Partially stabilized zirconia	Implant abutments
Procera	Nobel Biocare	Alumina	
Vita TriLuxe Bloc	Vita	Fine structure feldspar block with three gradations of colour	Anterior crowns, veneers
VitaBlocs Mark II	Vita	Flespathic ceramic made for Cerec/inLAB	Crowns, veneers
Zerion	Straumann	Zirconium dioxide	Substructure for bridges

The restorations most commonly constructed from this ceramic and best suited to this technique are veneers (Figure 22.33), resin-bonded crowns, inlays and onlays. Excellent aesthetics are produced by these ceramics as they have a high translucency, fluorescence and opalesecence.

There have been attempts to produce a core material for bonding, based on a lithium disilicate glass. The presence of silica means that

Resin-bonded crown: a minimally invasive restoration made of feldspathic or leucite ceramic. It is bonded onto the tooth using a resin-based composite adhesive after silanation. It can be considered as a veneer that extends to cover the entire crown of the tooth.

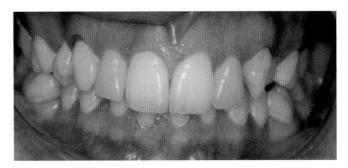

Fig. 22.33 Ceramic labial veneers used to restore congenitally peg shaped 12 and 22.

it may be etched to aid bonding to tooth tissue. Aesthetically it is not suitable for full crown construction and it is currently used as a core material that is overlaid with conventional feldspathic ceramic. The material has a crystalline structure that is different from most of the other glasses as up to 70% is in the form of needle-shaped crystals which are randomly orientated. This is very effective at preventing crack propagation. This material is about three times stronger than a conventional feldspathic ceramic.

INDICATIONS AND CONTRAINDICATIONS OF CERAMIC RESTORATIONS

Ceramic restorations are indicated for most dental applications. These include veneers, inlays, onlays, crowns, bridges, implant supra- and sub-structures and denture teeth (Chapter 23). Different systems (ceramic and the core material) have different indications and contraindications and it is important that the dentist prescribes restorations which will work in the situation in which they are placed. This information may be found in the directions for use and promotional literature provided by the manufacturer. Common contraindications include:

- Parafunction
- Short clinical crowns
- Immature teeth
- Unfavourable occlusion
- Subgingival preparations (mainly for adhesive cementation).

TOOTH PREPARATION

The dentist should consult the manufacturers' literature for the recommended tooth preparation so that the intended material will perform adequately in the mouth. However, there are some general principles for preparation design when working with dental ceramics:

- There should be rounded internal line angles and edges, otherwise stress concentrations form.
- There should be sufficient reduction to allow for strength of material, usually 1.5–2 mm occlusally.
- Feather edges should be avoided as this insufficient reduction will prevent proper ceramic build-up and there is potential for fracture as insufficient bulk of material will lack strength.

If a tooth is being prepared to receive a zirconia-based restoration, the margins are finished to a **chamfer**. This preparation is more conservative as a shoulder is not required for support and sufficient thickness of material unlike conventional ceramics.

BISCUIT TRY-IN

The use of ceramic on an occluding surface of a restoration presents problems:

- More tooth tissue needs to be removed to accommodate a thicker layer of material for strength (see above)
- There is a large volumetric shrinkage
- It is abrasive in the unglazed state.

The large volumetric shrinkage which is seen when ceramic is fired makes the creation of exact and accurate occlusal contacts very difficult, if not impossible. The biscuit try-in appointment allows the dentist to verify and make adjustments to the ceramic to get the occlusion correct. Any adjustment to the glazed surface will expose the underlying surface, which is very abrasive and may cause significant wear to the opposing dentition. In severe cases, substantial tooth tissue loss may result. Furthermore, stress concentrations may occur on this abraded surface which may subsequently manifest in fracture of the ceramic. As has been described previously, ceramic is porous and glazing will seal the surface to prevent ingress of oral fluids, which may also have a detrimental effect on the ceramic, leading to failure.

In order to overcome the latter two problems, many dentists recommend a try-in appointment in the biscuit or unglazed state. This stage is called a **biscuit try-in**. Any necessary adjustments may then be made and the restoration returned to the dental laboratory for final glaze application prior to cementation at a subsequent appointment. This will ensure a smooth, sealed surface that will not cause any differential wear on any opposing surfaces. However, if only a small amount of ceramic has been adjusted or if the restoration cannot be returned as it has had to be fitted prior to occlusal verification (such as a veneer or inlay), the adjusted roughened ceramic surface should be polished with diamond impregnated burs and rubber wheels and a ceramic polishing material (Figure 22.34). This step has only recently become possible as products for polishing have become available. Even with these new polishing aids, the ideal and best solution is a glazed surface that will yield the most desirable finish.

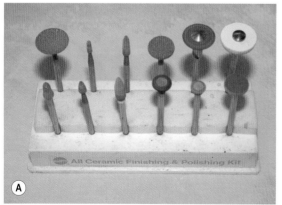
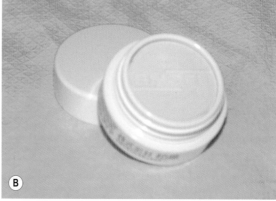

Fig. 22.34A,B A bespoke ceramic polishing kit and Dura-Polish (Shofu), a ceramic polishing paste specially designed for polishing the rough ceramic surface after adjustment to create a sealed surface as an alternative to reglazing.

Table 22.9 compares the advantages of reglazing and polishing ceramic surfaces.

Table 22.9 Reglazing versus polishing ceramic surfaces

Reglazing	Polishing
Better result achieved	Can be done intraorally
Surface resealed	No need for a further appointment

The dentist should ensure that the patient does not occlude on unsupported ceramic otherwise the ceramic will fracture. This is especially true with thin edges of veneers, inlays and onlays. The restoration should therefore be bonded in situ and then the occlusion verified. Any adjustment may then be made and the adjusted surface polished intraorally.

A general rule and good advice is to have like surfaces opposing each other so that no differential wear will occur.

CEMENTATION

As discussed in the Chapter 11 on bonding, indirect restorations may either be luted or bonded onto the prepared tooth. Generally, most metal-ceramic and reinforced-ceramic indirect restorations are luted but some ceramics can be bonded, such as the resin-bonded ceramics. The fitting surface is usually treated with hydrofluoric acid and then silanated. This silanated surface will then bond with the resin-based composite adhesive, facilitating bonding to tooth tissue. The fitting surface of a zirconia restoration is micromechanically rough and micromechanical retention will be achieved with the luting cement. For detailed information on cement selection, which technique to use and how, see Chapter 11.

SUMMARY

- Ceramics are widely used in dentistry for a range of applications such as veneers, inlays, onlays, crowns and bridges.
- They have excellent aesthetics but are brittle, which may cause them to fracture during use.
- Reinforced cores may be used to strengthen the overlying ceramic. Materials used as core materials include metal alloys, alumina, spinel and zirconia.

- Zirconia has shown great promise and may now be used in very challenging situations (for example long-span bridges) and even replace the metal-ceramic restoration in the longer term.
- Development in the field of information technology has enabled CAD-CAM systems to become commercially available; the dentist can take optical impressions and construct a ceramic restoration on a model or mill it from a block of optimized ceramic.
- It is important that if ceramic is adjusted, it is either reglazed or polished to re-create the seal on the surface which may otherwise cause wear on opposing teeth and stress concentrations within the ceramic and catastrophic failure.

FURTHER READING

McCabe, J.F., Walls, A.W.G., 2008. Applied Dental Materials, ninth ed. Blackwell Munksgaard, Oxford (See Chapter 11).

Powers, J.M., Sakaguchi, R.L. (Eds.), 2006. Craig's Restorative Dental Materials, twelfth ed. Mosby Elsevier, St Louis (See Chapter 18).

van Noort, R., 2007. Introduction to Dental Materials, third ed. Mosby Elsevier, Edinburgh (See Chapters 3.4, 3.5, 3.6 and 3.7).

SELF-ASSESSMENT QUESTIONS

1. Why are modern all-ceramic crowns generally prepared with a subframe of alumina or zirconia?
2. What is the difference between decorative porcelains and dental ceramics?
3. What is the advantage of hand constructing a ceramic crown over use of the modern hot pressing techniques?
4. What advantages does the CAD-CAM system have over conventional ceramic crown manufacture?
5. Why is it essential that any areas of unglazed ceramic are re-polished prior to cementation?
6. What are the disadvantages of using zirconia or alumina cores, particularly for anterior all-ceramic crowns? What problems can occur when covering a coping with feldspathic ceramics?

Polymers in prosthodontics

INTRODUCTION

A **denture** is a removable dental prosthesis. It can be a **full** (sometimes also referred to as **complete**) denture, where it replaces all the teeth in an arch. It can also be a **partial** denture, replacing one or more teeth with some natural teeth remaining in the arch. This chapter discusses the resin polymers used in the construction of both types of denture and other associated materials.

DENTURE BASE RESINS

The **denture base** is the part of the denture which is in contact with the oral tissues and supports the teeth (Figure 23.1). The denture base may be constructed of a **metal alloy** (discussed in Chapter 21) or a 'plastic' such as an **acrylic**.

What is required of a denture base resin?

The material of which the denture base is constructed must have certain requirements to perform satisfactorily (Box 23.1). While

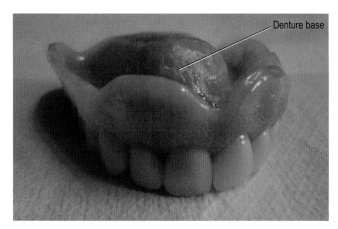

Fig. 23.1 A complete upper acrylic denture.

Box 23.1 Requirements of a denture base resin

From the perspective of both the dentist and technician, the material should:
- Be of adequate strength to withstand occlusal loading
- Be easy to manipulate and process
- Not produce toxic fumes or dust during processing
- Remain unstained and unaffected by fluids and temperature changes in the oral cavity
- Be simple to repair when necessary
- Maintain its shape, form and aesthetics in normal function
- Be biocompatible
- Be radiopaque.

From the patient's view point the denture should:
- Fit well and be comfortable in use
- Not traumatize the tissues
- Be easy to clean
- Be aesthetically pleasing both immediately on placement and in the longer term
- Allow good heat diffusion to retain normal perception of thermal stimuli
- Permit food to be tasted normally so that food can remain appealing.

many materials can achieve some of these requirements, no material currently available achieves all of them. The materials which fulfil most of these criteria are the resin polymers and more specifically **polymethylmethacrylate (PMMA)**.

Constituents

PMMA is a polymer formed from the addition reaction of the monomer **methylmethacrylate (MMA)**. Although PMMA is available as gel, sheet or blank, the powder/liquid presentation is most widely used. The powder is **PMMA polymer** and the liquid is **MMA monomer**.

Polymer

The PMMA polymer powder is composed of small spheres called **beads** or **pearls**. It may also be in a fine **granular form** in some products. This enables the polymer to dissolve more readily in the monomer as its surface area to volume ratio is higher. The size of these particles is approximately 150 μm in those resins which are processed by heat, the most commonly used method. Other chemicals are added to the PMMA polymer to modify the final product (Table 23.1). For example, PMMA is inherently translucent and so pigments and opacifiers must be added to change its appearance unless a clear acrylic is desired.

Table 23.1 Typical chemical constituents of the powder component of a heat-cured resin

Constituent	Percentage (%)	Reason for inclusion
Polymethylmethacrylate	95–98%	Principal component
Benzoyl peroxide	1	Initiator
Titanium dioxide Zinc oxide	Small amount	Increases opacity to match the translucency of the oral soft tissues
Inorganic pigments	1	Varies colour, respectively:
Mercuric sulphide		Red
Cadmium sulphide		Yellow
Ferric oxide		Brown
Dibutyl phthalate	Small amount*	Plasticizer
Dyed synthetic fibres – nylon or acrylic	Small amount	Simulate anatomical structures such as capillaries within the denture base material

*Phthalates are now regarded as hazardous materials, which, when used in excessive concentrations, are potential carcinogens. Manufacturers are looking at alternatives to these chemicals, such as citrates and benzoate esters.

Benzoyl peroxide coats the surface of the polymer beads. It is important that these beads are not contaminated as only a very small amount of polymer is required to start the reaction. Contamination can potentially initiate a premature polymerization reaction. If kept in good condition, the powder is very stable and as such has a very long shelf-life.

Monomer

The liquid monomer is mainly MMA. This is a volatile liquid whose boiling point is 100.3 °C. It is toxic if inhaled for a prolonged period

and it is also highly flammable. It should therefore be handled in a well-ventilated room or preferably a fume cupboard. As with the powder, additional chemicals are added to the liquid to modify the final product (Table 23.2). In some products higher methacrylate monomers such as ethyl and butyl are substituted for the methylmethacrylate because they are less irritant.

Table 23.2 Chemical constituents of the liquid component of a denture base resin

Constituent	Percentage (%)	Reason for inclusion
Methylmethacrylate	97	Monomer
Hydroquinone	0.003–0.1	Inhibitor – prevents monomer polymerizing during storage
Ethylene glycol dimethacrylate (substituted for the main monomeric component)	2–14	Cross-linking agent
Dibutyl phthalate, butyl and octyl methacrylate	Small amount	Plasticizer
For chemical activation the following is added:		
Organic amine: N,N-dimethyl p-toluidine or N,N-dihydroxyethyl-p-toluidine	0.8	Accelerator*

*An organic amine such as N,N dimethyl p-toluidine or N,N dihydroxyethyl-p-toluidine may be added to those materials which undergo chemically 'cold curing' polymerization.

Cold, chemical or **self-cure acrylics:** synonymous terms applied to this group of materials where the accelerator of the polymerization reaction is a chemical rather than heat. This is usually a tertiary amine or sulphinic acid such as N,N dimethyl p-toluidine or N,N dihydroxyethyl-p-toluidine.

The polymerization reaction may be initiated prematurely either by ultraviolet light or by free radicals forming spontaneously within the liquid. In order to prevent this occurring, the monomer is supplied in a dark bottle and **hydroquinone** is added to the monomer to preferentially react with any random free radicals which may be produced. The action of the hydroquinone produces stabilized free radicals which are not able to initiate the polymerization process. In this respect the hydroquinone acts rather like a sponge, mopping up free radicals until it is saturated. During the polymerization process all the hydroquinone must be used up before the polymerization reaction may take place.

It is advantageous that the mechanical properties of the acrylic are improved to increase the wear and fracture resistance of the material and also its resistance to the action of organic solvents which may cause surface cracking or crazing. This is achieved by adding **cross-linking polymers** such as **diethylene glycol dimethacrylate**. These different monomer units (**co-polymers**) can react with another growing chain at each end of the molecule when the polymer chains are growing so linking the chains. They are present in relatively small amounts and they have little effect on the transverse strength or hardness of the denture base material.

Craze: a very small surface defect in the resin. Crazing appears as areas of cloudiness on the denture surface.

Plasticizers are often added to acrylics to vary their mechanical properties. Chemicals such as **dibutyl phthalate** do not take part in the polymerization reaction but are distributed throughout the polymerizing mass. They prevent the interaction between polymer molecules. Since they are not part of the structure, the plasticizer leaches out slowly as the denture becomes saturated with water. This presents two problems:

- The denture becomes harder with the loss of the plasticizer
- The plasticizer will migrate out into the oral fluid.

Concerns have been voiced with respect to the biological effects of the phthalates and manufacturers are looking at alternative plasticizers for use in denture base resins. Other chemicals such as the esters **octyl** or **butyl methacrylate** can also be used for materials which are made intentionally softer such as soft denture linings. Since these methacrylates will polymerize as part of the overall polymerization process, they are much less likely to leach out with time. Failure to initiate polymerization of these materials will, however, lead to leaching of the monomer and subsequent hardening of the denture base over time.

Alternative presentations

A few manufacturers supply the denture base material in a gel form. Here all the components are mixed together and formed in a thick sheet. The nature of the material precludes the use of chemical initiators and storage of the unprocessed material is important. It is generally recommended that the sheets are stored in the refrigerator in the dark before heat processing in the normal way.

Setting reaction

The reaction is initiated by an organic peroxide such as **benzoyl peroxide**, which produces **free radicals** either by heating (**heat-cured acrylics**) or reacting with a chemical accelerator such as an organic amine.

The reaction is highly exothermic and this temperature must be carefully controlled as the volatile monomer, whose boiling point is 101°C, may vaporize during processing. Since the processing is carried out in a plaster mould, this heat is slow to dissipate and there is a risk of gas bubbles being produced. These bubbles of gas can become entrapped in the denture base resin, leading to **gaseous porosity** (Figure 23.2).

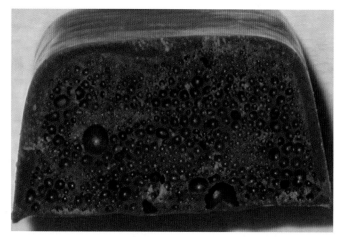

Fig. 23.2 An aerated chocolate bar to illustrate gaseous porosity in acrylic.

Fortunately, a large proportion of the reacting chemicals is polymer (75%) so the amount of heat produced as a result of the chemical reaction is reduced. Various processing regimes have been established to reduce the heat production.

As the setting reaction is a **polymerization** reaction, shrinkage of the material occurs. This dimensional change must be compensated for during the manufacturing process otherwise the final denture or appliance will not fit. This shrinkage is of the order of 6% for the recommended 3:1 polymer:monomer mix. As a result of shrinkage, internal strains are set up within the material. Some of these strains will be relieved as the curing cycle is taken above the glass transition temperature of the denture base material allowing flow to occur.

Structure

During the processing of the denture base material, the addition of the monomer to the polymer powder leads first to the softening of the outer surface of the polymer beads and part dissolution of the outer structure. Since the monomer is primarily the same as the polymerized beads, the material becomes a coherent mass which will then set. It is often difficult to observe any difference between the original beads and the repolymerized PMMA under the microscope, although there may be some differentiation particularly where cross-linking agents are used to any extent. Cross-linking agents help to ensure that there is a network of molecules rather than long chains or branched chains that reduce the strength of the final material.

Properties

Mechanical properties

PMMA has low tensile strength and a low elastic modulus. This means that it will flex in use. This flexure due to cyclical loading will, over time, result in fracture of the denture base. This is known as **fatigue fracture**. The process takes some time and is the least likely reason for fracture to occur. It also depends on the degree of flexure and the load applied. For example, an upper denture will flex about the midline of the palate, particularly if there is a bony ridge in this region. The degree of loading is determined by the chewing force applied during mastication.

Fracture of the denture base (particularly impact fracture) is not an uncommon occurrence. Many patients attempt their own repair by using a cyanoacrylate adhesive such as Super Glue® (Loctite). This should be strongly discouraged as the cyanoacrylate cement can react with the PMMA, damaging the denture surface. The repair will also fail quite quickly as the cyanoacrylate will hydrolyse and breakdown. At this point it is very difficult to accurately position the fragments for further repair. If the PMMA has been contaminated, the acrylic must be cut back to remove all traces of the cement and then the denture repaired using cold-cure acrylic.

Its **fracture toughness** is also low and as it behaves as a brittle material on impact, a denture will frequently fracture if dropped onto a hard surface. To avoid this, patients should be advised to clean their denture over a bowl of water rather than directly over an empty

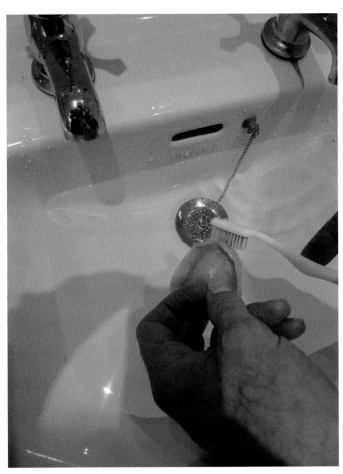

Fig. 23.3 An acrylic denture being cleaning over a sink filled with water to prevent its fracture should it be inadvertently dropped during the cleaning process.

hard ceramic bathroom basin (Figure 23.3). Dentures dropped on this type of surface will break very readily.

Thermal properties

As would be expected from a resin, PMMA has a high coefficient of thermal expansion. It also has a relatively low glass transitional temperature. This does not present too much of a problem during normal function, as the variation of the temperature in the mouth is relatively low with a range of less than 50°C. However there can be problems where a polymeric denture base is used to support ceramic teeth. Due to the difference in coefficients of thermal expansion of these materials, the ceramic teeth may be lost due to variations in the contraction and expansion characteristics of the two materials during thermal cycling. PMMA has low thermal conductivity and diffusivity. This is problematic for two reasons:

- During processing, the heat produced as a product of the exothermic reaction cannot escape; this may cause gaseous porosity of the denture base
- The low diffusivity means that the transfer of heat from one side of the denture to the other is slow, that is, it takes time for heat to permeate the denture base and reach the underlying soft tissues. This has two consequences:
  - The patient's sensation of hot food is often reduced

- The oral mucosa may become less keratinized. If the patient subsequently loses the denture or has it replaced by a fixed restoration, this oral mucosa is not protected. Mucosal burns may result if ingested foods are too hot. These patients should always be warned to exercise caution when drinking hot drinks for a few days after placement of the new restoration.

The softening temperature of PMMA ranges from 75 to 95°C and within this range the denture may distort. Thus patients should be warned against cleaning their acrylic dentures in very hot water or placing them in very hot water. Failure to do so will result in distortion of the denture base which will then no longer fit snugly.

Dimensional stability

During use, PMMA absorbs fluid. This water sorption causes the denture base to expand by about 2%, which is considered to be high. The polymer is sufficiently accurate for the proposed applications, in other words it achieves a close fit to the denture-bearing tissues despite the various inaccuracies encountered during the processing procedures.

The polymerization shrinkage which occurs during curing partly compensates for this expansion improving the fit of the denture. For this reason, it is essential to keep the denture wet as drying out of the PMMA denture base will cause shrinkage and crazing. Long-term water sorption often causes the polymer to discolour and stain. This is particularly the case if the patient drinks a lot of tea, coffee or red wine. However, generally its colour stability is good.

The dental technician must be careful to use the correct proportions of the monomer and polymer. It is generally accepted that for a heat-cured prosthesis, the powder:monomer ratio should be in the region of 3:1. Failure to follow these proportions can result in the formed prosthesis having inferior properties. If the ratio of polymer powder to monomer is too high, there will be insufficient monomer to wet the polymer and a granular resin structure will be produced. Excess monomer leads to increased shrinkage. The pure monomer shrinks by 21% but with correct proportioning, a 7% shrinkage may be achieved, which correlates to a 2% linear shrinkage. If a good technique is used during processing, this may be reduced to 0.5%, although stresses will be incorporated within the material, which will need to be relieved during the curing process. Manufacturers provide vials to ensure that the correct proportions should be used. The optimum ratio is usually 3 or 3.5:1 by volume or 2.5:1 by weight.

PMMA, even when it has been properly processed, retains some residual monomer in the order of 0.2–0.5%. The presence of free monomer leads to two problems:

- It (or the benzoic acid which can also leach out) is an irritant to oral soft tissues. Improper processing will compound this problem. Concern has been expressed that it may cause an allergic reaction but has largely been dismissed as the reaction of the oral soft tissues is irritancy to the monomer and not a true allergy
- It acts as a plasticizer so softening the polymer, making the denture base weaker and increasing its flexibility. Fracture may also result.

The polymer may creep under load over the long term and deform the denture base. This phenomenon is more marked with cold-cure acrylics and can create greater problems. The addition of cross-linking agents is an attempt to minimize this effect.

Loss of material due to water solubility is low. However, the presence of organic solvents such as alcohols and chloroform has an adverse effect on methacrylates.

Prior to mixing the polymer and monomer, the containers should be thoroughly shaken to ensure an even distribution of the powder ingredients as some additives which are required to participate in the curing process may settle at the bottom of the container. This will also ensure that any pigments which are mixed with powder are evenly distributed.

Crazing

As mentioned earlier, crazing is the presence of fine cracks on the surface of the acrylic. They represent localized areas of plastic deformation of the polymer caused by stress relief of internal strain. Tensile stresses will also cause rupture of the polymer chains leading to a weakened denture. These areas may be filled with microscopic voids and a crack may result if the crazed area can no longer support stress.

A crack is formed as a result of brittle fracture, as the walls of voids in the region are thin in the region of the fracture. The crack grows under externally applied load such as a patient biting, eventually leading to a continuous crack. This can cause fracture of the denture base. Crazes may be caused by heat, the action of organic solvents (for example alcohol or if the monomer comes into contact with resin during a denture repair) or differences in coefficients of thermal expansion around (dissimilar) inclusions that form stress concentrations. The most obvious example of this is ceramic denture teeth on a PMMA denture base or the inclusion of stainless steel clasps. The adhesion of PMMA to metal components and ceramic teeth is primarily by mechanical retention.

Crazing may also be seen if the denture is not kept moist at all times during its life. This is due to mechanical stresses set up within the denture base as it contracts and expands during the drying and wetting cycle. The cross-linked resins are less likely to craze as they contain fewer lines of weakness (Figure 23.4).

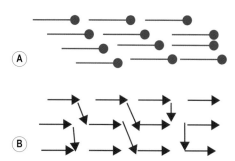

Fig. 23.4A,B (A) Polymer with no cross-linking; and (B) a cross-linked polymer.

In order to prevent crazing, the polymer should not be allowed to dry out and so the finished denture should always be supplied to the dentist in water (Figure 23.5). The patient should then be advised to store the prosthesis in water when it is not in use. Wrapping in gauze or cotton wool is inadequate as the resin does not remain saturated.

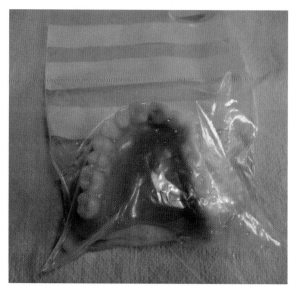

Fig. 23.5 A complete upper acrylic denture being stored in a sealed polythene bag containing water to prevent the acrylic drying out.

Shade of denture base acrylics

Denture base acrylics are available in different shades to match the patient's natural gingival tissues. This is more significant in patients whose mucosa is more pigmented. Some acrylics are available with small fibres of red acrylic in them which mimic small blood vessels and these are called **veined** materials (Figure 23.6). These fibre inclusions are frequently coated with a coupling agent, commonly triethoxysilane, to improve their wettability.

Fig. 23.6 Acrylic fibres used to vein denture base acrylic.

Radiodensity

PMMA denture base resins are radiolucent. In case of accidental ingestion or inhalation of the denture or parts of it, it would be desirable if all components were radiopaque to facilitate identification by medical radiographic investigation. Radiopacity can be achieved by the addition of chemicals such as 10–15% **bismuth** or **uranyl salts**. Unfortunately their addition adversely affects the properties of the denture base material, increasing transverse deflection and water sorption, so making handling of the unset polymer more difficult.

Other properties

PMMA has a low density so it is relatively light in weight, making the denture easier to wear. It does not taste or smell. It is relatively cheap and easy to process, hence its widespread use both historically and in modern practice.

TYPES OF ACRYLIC

Acrylics can be categorized based on their means of curing or their properties:

- Heat-cured
- Cold-cured
- Light-cured
- Injection technique
- High-impact acrylics.

Heat-cured acrylic

The term used to describe the use of a heat-cured acrylic to process a denture is **dough moulding**. The process is described below.

When the polymer and monomer are mixed they initially form a sand-like mixture. This changes to a tacky mass as the surface of the polymer beads start to dissolve in the monomer. Under normal conditions once the polymer and monomer have been mixed then the mixture is left undisturbed in the mixing container until the dough stage is reached (Figure 23.7).

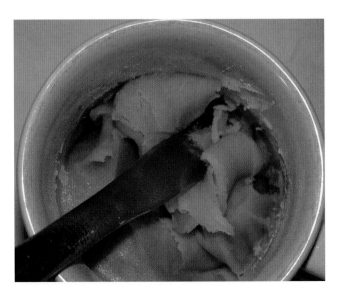

Fig. 23.7 Acrylic left undisturbed after mixing.

The next stage is described as the **dough stage**. As the name implies, the mixture at this point is similar in appearance to the dough used in bread making. The mixture does not stick to the container walls and 'snaps' when pulled apart (Figure 23.8). Failure to pack the mixture into the mould at the dough stage will result in the material becoming too rubbery and stiff. It cannot then be moulded properly.

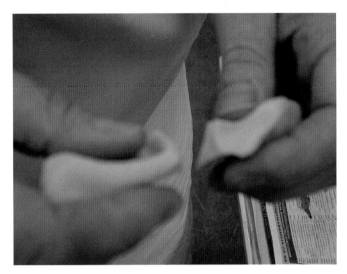

Fig. 23.8 Acrylic dough at the snap stage. Note the clean separation of the material when pulled apart.

The time it takes to achieve the desired consistency 'dough time' depends on a number of factors:

- The **particle size of the polymer**. The smaller the bead diameter, the more rapidly the dissolution of the bead in the monomer. The reaction therefore proceeds more quickly.
- The **molecular weight of the polymer**. The lower the molecular weight, the faster the reaction will proceed.
- A higher **temperature** will produce a quicker reaction.
- The **presence of a plasticizer**. This will reduce the dough time.
- Polymer/monomer ratio. The higher the ratio the shorter the dough time.
- The **type of polymer**. If the polymer is granular, the permeation of the monomer is greater. This means they will dissolve more readily and the reaction time will be quicker (see Chapter 1).

Colouring of the acrylic

PMMA is naturally transparent and so colouring agents must be added, for example, to mimic gingival tissue. These pigments may be incorporated within the polymer beads or mixed in with the powder. Their inclusion in the polymer beads imparts an overall colour whereas their inclusion with the powder can give a slightly variable colour, which is more akin to the oral mucosa. The colouring agents have very intense colours and very little of the agent is needed to produce the coral pink shade needed for most denture base resins. If the colouring agents are on the surface of the bead then the polymer should be added slowly to the monomer as the pigment may be washed off if it contacts the monomer too rapidly. This can lead to streaking of the colouring agent. If only a little powder is used then a lighter shade may result as there is less pigment in the mix.

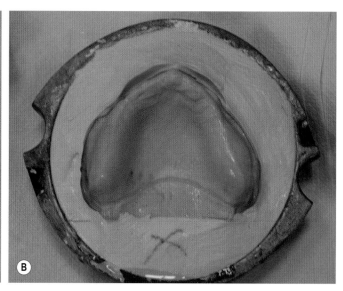

Fig. 23.9 The flask has been opened and the wax boiled out, leaving (A) the denture teeth and (B) the working cast encased in plaster of Paris.

Process

The waxed up denture is sealed onto the master model and invested in plaster of Paris in a **split metal flask**. After the plaster has set the flask is opened and boiling water is used to remove the wax (Figure 23.9). This must be done very thoroughly to remove all traces of wax. Care must be taken not to disturb any teeth or clasps, which at this point are held in the mould solely by mechanical interlocking of any undercuts with the plaster.

It is imperative that all traces of wax are thoroughly removed from the flask prior to packing the acrylic otherwise the wax will prevent bonding between the denture teeth and the denture base polymer.

The surface of the plaster is then cleaned and a separator is applied to prevent the resin dough impregnating the gypsum, which would produce a rough surface. It also reduces water ingress into the acrylic. This separator is usually **sodium alginate solution** (Figure 23.10) but

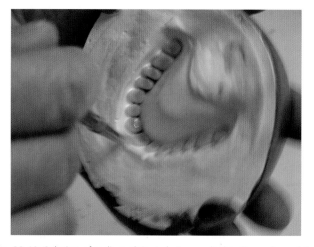

Fig. 23.10 Solution of sodium alginate being applied to the surface of the gypsum.

sometimes **potassium** or **ammonium alginate solutions** may be used. These solutions form an insoluble calcium alginate coating on the surface of the plaster that is largely effective at eliminating water ingress into the body of the denture. Any slight percolation can lead to crazing.

An excess of the acrylic dough is then placed into the part of the flask containing the teeth and a thin polythene sheet placed on it. If an excess is not used then **shrinkage porosity** will result. The flask is closed and placed into a press, and pressure applied so that the dough is forced into all parts of the mould and the excess is expressed out of the press (Figure 23.11).

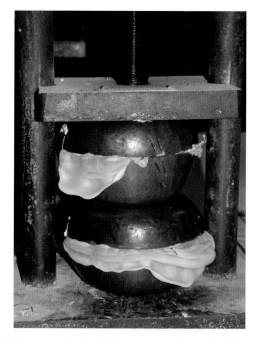

Fig. 23.11 Excess acrylic dough being expressed from the flask.

The flask is then opened and the excess is removed. This is called **trial packing** and may be repeated several times until no excess is expressed. At the last closure the polythene sheet is removed with any residual excess. The flask is finally closed and placed under pressure in a water

During the packing of the resin at the dough stage, it is essential that sufficient material is tamped into place so that the material remains under pressure during the processing. Failure to do this will mean that any air voids incorporated during the packing will not collapse. They will then become a source of porosity and weakness.

bath most commonly 73°C for 8 hours or longer. For convenience, this is normally carried out in the laboratory overnight. During the process, the temperature of the water bath is slowly raised to reduce the risk of the monomer vaporizing and gaseous porosity occurring in the final product. Nearly complete conversion of the monomer results in a minimum amount of unreacted monomer remaining.

On completion of the polymerization cycle, the flask is removed from the water bath and allowed to cool slowly at room temperature before it is opened. Slow cooling prevents stresses forming by plastic deformation within the polymer as there is a difference of contraction between the gypsum and acrylic. It also allows some stress-relieving flow of the material. The higher the temperature the acrylic is cured at the more likely it is to distort as it will have more residual stress.

Finally, the denture is carefully removed from the gypsum model avoiding flexure and breakage (Figure 23.12). The acrylic **flash** is removed and the non-tissue-bearing surfaces are **polished** (Chapter 19).

The processing temperature is dependent on the exact composition of the polymer/monomer mix being used. There is a risk that the monomer may be heated too much, causing it to vaporize. Since the polymerization reaction is exothermic, the temperature of the water bath does not represent the temperature within the flask while the polymerization reaction occurs. Slow processing and slow heating means that the heat of reaction may be dissipated more readily and the gypsum will slowly absorb the heat which is generated. Manufacturers' processing instructions should be followed exactly to ensure that processing faults are minimized.

Cold-cured acrylic

Constituents

Cold-cured acrylic resins do not rely on heat to initiate their cure. Instead they contain a **tertiary amine** which acts as an initiator. **N,N dimethyl-*p*-toluidine** or **sulphinic acid** are commonly used. The chemical composition is otherwise the same as the heat-cured acrylics. They are also called **self-cured**, **chemically cured** or **autopolymerized** resins or **pour acrylics**. They are available as two types (Table 23.3).

As Type 2 cold-cured resin does not contain MMA, it is used for patients who are sensitive to MMA. Type 2 is also less irritant to the soft tissues but the softening temperature is lower (for MMA it is 90°C and for ethyl methacrylate it is 67°C). This means that the risk of distortion in use or on cleaning is greater. The type 2 materials are similar to those used to construct temporary crowns and bridges (Chapter 14); an example of such a material is Trim II (Bosworth).

Table 23.3 Two types of cold-cure acrylic resin available on the market

	Type 1	Type 2
Powder	Polymethylmethacrylate	Polyethyl methacrylate
	Benzoyl peroxide	Benzoyl peroxide
	Pigments	Pigments
Liquid	Methylmethacrylate	Butyl methacrylate
	Di-n-butylphthalate	Amine
	Amine	

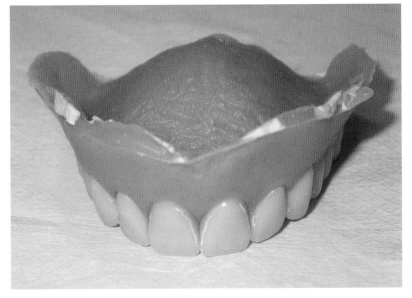
Fig. 23.12 An upper complete acrylic denture immediately on removal from the flask after processing. The flash is now removed and the polished surfaces polished.

Properties

Polymerization efficiency

As the polymerization process is less efficient than the heat-cured method, a higher percentage of residual monomer remains, in the order of 3–5%. It is believed to be due to the lower molecular weight of the formed polymer chains and also due to the lack of propagation of the chain during the polymerization process. Residual monomer functions as a plasticizer which softens the material, so lowering its mechanical properties. Over time and during use, however, the monomer will leach out of the material with the result that its properties improve and will eventually approach those of heat-cured acrylics. However, leaching of the monomer on the oral mucosa is a potential cause of irritation in some patients.

The average size of polymer beads in these materials is smaller than in heat-cured varieties to facilitate the monomer dissolving the polymer.

Porosity

Porosity is more of a problem than with the heat-cured acrylics. This is due to air dissolved in the monomer which is not soluble in the polymer at room temperature. Porosity can be reduced by polymerizing the material under pressure. Again, excess material within the mould will ensure that the prosthesis will remain under pressure during the curing process and ensure that porosity is minimized.

Mechanical properties

Acrylics which have been cold cured are not as strong as those that are heat cured, achieving approximately up to 80% the strength of heat-cured polymers. This in part is due to the lower molecular weight of the formed polymer. There is less conversion of the monomer to polymer. As a result they show more initial deformation, creep and slower recovery than their heat-cured counterparts. However, they also show less build up of internal strain as no external heat source is used and so the degree of shrinkage is also less.

Stability

- As with other dental materials containing a tertiary amine, cold-cured acrylics tend to have poorer long-term colour stability with the material yellowing with time.
- Cold-cured acrylics are reputed to show less dimensional change on setting with only a 0.1% dimensional change seen on polymerization. This is due to the reduced level of conversion of the monomer.
- Cold-cured acrylics have a greater exothermic reaction than heat-cured materials because they contain an excess of initiator. It is this initiator which contributes most significantly to the exothermic reaction.

Indications

These products are used either in the dental laboratory or at the chairside for minor denture repairs, in the manufacture of removable orthodontic appliances and for chairside denture relines. Chairside relines are notoriously difficult to carry out as it is difficult to control over the amount of denture material that is removed and the subsequent thickness of the denture base after relining. This usually results in a thicker base and affects the vertical dimensions of the denture. Additionally, the patient may complain about the unpleasant taste, which is the result of leaching of the various components from the denture base.

The procedure of a cold-cure repair

The steps for repairing a fractured denture using cold-cured acrylic are as follows:

1. The parts of the fractured denture are secured together with wire and sticky wax splinting (assuming they can be localized exactly, otherwise an impression will have to be taken to localize them).
2. A plaster model is made by pouring plaster into the fit surface of the splinted denture and allowed to set.
3. The denture segments are removed from the plaster cast and the surfaces adjacent to the fracture cut back to achieve a 5 mm separation, avoiding 'V' shaped edges to reduce the risk of stress concentrations.
4. All the wax is thoroughly removed from the denture by immersing it in hot water but at a temperature of less than 70°C. The use of sticky wax with a melting point of less than 50°C ensures that the wax can be removed without damage to the denture fragments.
5. An alginate separating medium is applied to the gypsum and denture fragments are replaced on it.
6. The cold-cured material is mixed and applied into defect. In some cases the cut-back surface is painted lightly with monomer. Monomer/polymer layers are then built up using a brush or the cold-cured dough is packed into the defect.
7. The model and resin repair is then placed in a vacuum flask to polymerize under a pressure of 250 kN/m² at 40–45°C for 30 minutes.
8. The repaired denture is then removed from the model, any flash removed and the acrylic polished.

Light-cured acrylics

Some acrylics are cured by the application of visible light energy in a similar manner as resin-based composite setting by free radical addition polymerization. These materials are presented as a prefabricated sheet of material which can be adapted to the surface of a model. The chemical constituents are therefore similar to resin-based composite materials (Chapter 7). **Urethane dimethylacrylate** and high molecular weight acrylic resin monomers are blended with an organic filler of acrylic beads, and **microfine silica** is added to optimize handling. This mixture when cured becomes part of an interpenetrating polymer network.

A blue light absorber (**camphorquinone**), accelerator (**amines**) and pigments are also required and are supplied fully compounded in a light tight package. The dental technician lays down the material on the model or denture being constructed or modified, moulding it into the desired shape. It is then placed into a light box and cured for 5–10 minutes, depending on the recommendations of the manufacturer. Since the polymerization process is carried out in air, the surface of the material is treated with a barrier chemical such as **carboxymethylcellulose**. This prevents oxygen inhibition of the polymerization reaction.

This type of acrylic is usually used in following applications:

- To form the baseplate of the denture on which a conventional PMMA suprastructure is added
- Construction of orthodontic appliances
- Construction of the gum work portion of metal-based partial dentures
- Repair of fractured acrylic dentures
- Hard relines
- Construction of special (impression) trays.

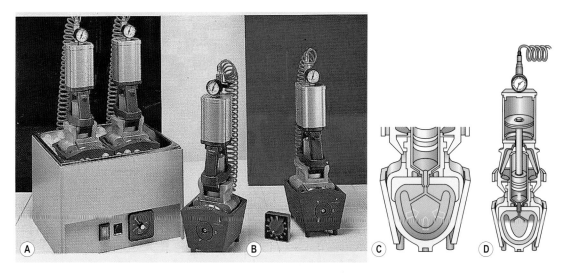

Fig. 23.13 Injection moulding system (Ivoclar Vivadent) in (A) the water bath and (B) before placement. (C, D) The injection moulding device and close up showing the ducts leading from the injection chamber to the denture mould.

Injection technique

In an attempt to overcome the large volumetric shrinkage of PMMA, some systems are designed to maintain pressure on the acrylic as it cures. The denture is flasked and the wax boiled out together with a wax sprue which is added to the denture. A high pressure injection cylinder is then connected to the flask. The acrylic is mixed and placed into the cylinder. When the material has reached the desired consistency it is injected into the mould under pressure. This high pressure is maintained during the polymerization reaction so more material is pushed into the flask to compensate for the polymerization shrinkage (Figure 23.13).

High-impact acrylics

One of the inherent problems with acrylics is their brittleness. If a denture is inadvertently dropped, it may fracture. High-impact acrylics are those in which a reinforcing agent (such as **butadiene-styrene rubber**) is added to confer some resistance to fracture. These rubber particles are grafted onto the MMA to become incorporated into the acrylic matrix. They are presented as a powder/liquid and processed in the same manner as conventional heat-cured resins.

These acrylics are mainly used to make more high-quality prostheses as they are more expensive. If the patient is investing in a more expensive prosthesis, it is cost-effective to invest in a better quality acrylic to maximize its lifespan and performance.

Other dental appliances constructed with acrylic

As well as full and partial dentures, acrylics are used to construct other dental appliances. **Occlusal splints** such as **Michigan splints** (Figure 23.14) are constructed usually in the clear variety which is chemically similar to the acrylic used as a denture base material, except with the omission of any pigments. This type of splint is constructed in the same manner as a denture, i.e. by the lost wax process followed by flasking and packing.

Clear acrylic is also used when a **clear palate** has been requested by either the patient or the dentist (Figure 23.15). The purpose of this is an 'improved' appearance for the more discerning patient. The processing is of necessity in two stages and this adds to the cost. Whether this is justifiable is debatable.

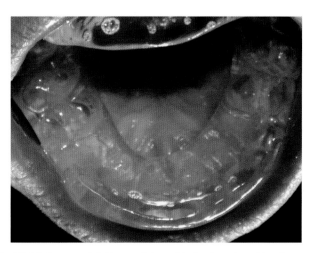

Fig. 23.14 An upper Michigan splint used to treat nocturnal bruxism.

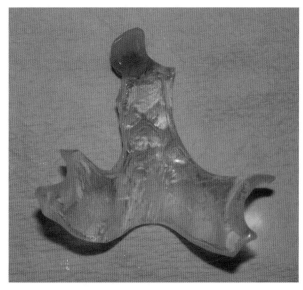

Fig. 23.15 A partial upper denture with a clear acrylic palate.

Special (impression) trays may also be constructed using acrylic (Figure 23.16). Special trays are used to construct the master model when an even amount of impression material is used over the full extension of the denture base. This is to minimize any distortion within the impression material and to therefore produce a working cast as accurately as possible. The acrylic tray also confers rigidity, such that the tray will not distort and the cast model will be accurate (also see Chapter 15).

After a period of time, the retention and stability of a denture can decrease due to the alveolar resorption that continues to occur after the loss of teeth. Instead of constructing a new denture, the existing denture may be **rebased** or **relined**. A **rebase** procedure involves replacing the denture base in contact with the tissues while a **reline** provides a new fitting surface, usually inside the existing denture base. These procedures improve the quality and accuracy of the fit of the denture while preventing its flexure on the denture-bearing tissues, a phenomenon which is likely to lead to denture fracture, particularly around the midline. The materials used for these can either be **rigid** or **soft**. Rigid materials have previously been discussed in this chapter and soft lining materials are discussed later.

Flexible dentures

More recently, dentures have been manufactured using a biocompatible nylon thermoplastic. There is little information available about these materials but they are claimed to be flexible and unbreakable. Two examples of such products are Sunflex Partials and Valplast Flexible Partials (Figure 23.17). The nature of the material means that it might be unnecessary to fit conventional clasps to partial dentures as the denture will be retained without them.

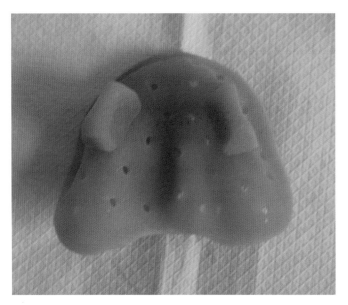

Fig. 23.16 An upper acrylic special tray used in the construction of a full upper denture.

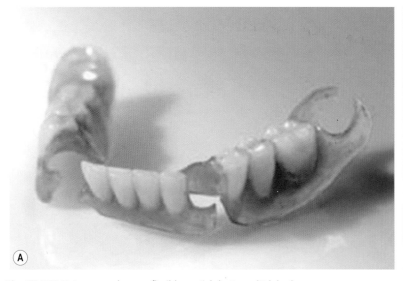
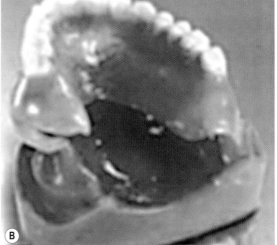

Fig. 23.17A,B Lower and upper flexible partial dentures (Valplast).

The material can be used to construct both the denture base and the clasps. Clasps may be made tooth coloured, which camouflages them when in situ against a natural tooth. It is claimed that the material is more stain resistance than a conventional PMMA-based acrylic as it will not warp or become brittle. As there is no monomer in the material, it could be considered for those patients allergic to MMA.

To fit the denture initially or if clasp adjustments are required, the denture is placed in very hot water for a minute prior to placement into the mouth of the patient. As the material is thermoplastic, it will soften and on cooling gain its new shape.

As the nylon material is microscopically porous, the dentures look unaesthetic in use as the denture base is more difficult to adjust and polish. This is done with soft brown rubber points, which need to be kept moving during the procedure as localized heat may burn and distort the prosthesis. Some fibres may approach the surface during adjustment and these can be removed using a sharp scalpel blade, suggesting that the claims for stain resistance may not be borne out in practice.

Commercially available products

Denture base acrylic materials are used almost exclusively in the dental laboratory although some cold-cured products may be used in the dental surgery. See Table 23.4.

Table 23.4 Some denture base acrylics currently available on the market

Product	Manufacturer	Description of product	Comments
Coe Kooliner	GC	Hard reline	
Delphic	Schottlander	Hot and cold cure	Acrylic tooth repair
Duraliner II Denture Rebase	Reliance	Chairside hard reline material	
Enigma High Base	Schottlander	Heat cure	High-impact denture base acrylic
Formatray	Kerr Hawe	Cold cure	Special trays, denture base plates
GC Reline	GC	Cold cure	Chairside relining material
GC Unifast III	GC	Cold cure	Denture repair
GC Unifast TRAD	GC	Cold cure	Repair of partial dentures
Hyflo	Hygenic	Fast temporary or duplicate dentures	
Hygenic Cold Cure Resin	Hygenic	Cold cure	Repairs
Hygenic Perm	Hygenic	Repairs and relines	
Hygon Tray Material	Hygenic	Cold cure	Special trays, denture base plates
Hypar	Hygenic	Heat cure	Cross-linked, cheap
Hy-Pro Lucitone	Dentsply	Denture base resin	
Individo Lux	Voco	Light cure	Special trays
Lucitone 199	Dentsply	High impact acrylic	Denture repair and denture base construction
Lucitone Fas-Por	Dentsply	Cold cure	Repairs
Microlon	Hygenic	Heat cure	Cross-linked
MultiTray	3M ESPE	Light cure	Special trays
Onepart Versyo	Heraeus	Injectable, light cure	Denture base
Optilon High Impact	Hygenic	High impact acrylic	Denture base
Orthodontic Resin	Hygenic	Cold cure	Orthodontic appliances
Orthoresin	Dentsply	Cold cure	Orthodontic appliances
Paladon 65	Heraeus	Heat cure	Denture base
Palaimpact	Heraeus	High impact acrylic	Denture base
Palapress	Heraeus	Cold cure	Metal partial denture saddles, repairs and relines
Palapress Vario	Heraeus	Cold cure	
Palatray XL	Heraeus	Light cure	Special trays
Palavit L	Heraeus	Cold cure	Special trays
PalaXpress	Heraeus	Injection, cold cure	Denture base material

(Continued)

Table 23.4 (Continued)

Product	Manufacturer	Description of product	Comments
Pegasus denture base	Schottlander	heat cure	Denture base
Pegasus pourable cold cure	Schottlander	Cold cure	Denture base
Pegsus Plus repair	Schottlander	Cold cure	Denture repair
Profibase	Voco	Light cure	Special trays
Repair-Synthetic	Hygenic	Cold cure	Denture repairs, partials, splints and flasked relines
RR	Dentsply	Cold cure	Rapid repairs
Selectaplus	Dentsply	Cold cure	Metal partial denture saddles and relines
Special Tray	Dentsply	Cold cure	Special trays
SR Ivolen Cold Cure Polymer	Ivoclar Vivadent	Cold cure	Special trays
Stellon QC 20	Dentsply	Heat cure	Full or partial denture base material
Trevalon	Dentsply	Heat cure	Full or partial denture base material
Triad Dualine	Dentsply	Dual cure	Relining
Triad VLC	Dentsply	Light cure	Orthodontic appliances
Ufi-Gel Hard C	Voco	Methylmethacrylate free, cold cure	Chairside hard relining material
Versyo Direct	Heraeus	Injectable, light cure	High viscosity

DENTURE TEETH

Denture teeth may be constructed from:

- PMMA
- Bis-GMA
- Ceramic.

PMMA denture teeth

PMMA teeth are the most commonly used denture teeth. They tend to be more **highly cross-linked resins** with improved mechanical properties, in particular hardness and wear resistance. This resists crazing and the increased abrasion resistance maintains occlusal vertical height over the longer term.

The aesthetics of the best quality denture teeth are excellent and it can be impossible to detect that they are artificial while in use even to the trained eye. Artificial teeth must also be **translucent** and opalescent, and be available in all shapes and sizes (**moulds**) and shades. Various pigments may be used to provide the different shades required. As natural teeth fluoresce, it is desirable that denture teeth have the same fluorescence as natural teeth so that under ultraviolet light any differences are imperceptible.

PMMA denture teeth are constructed by one of two methods:

- *Injected into a mould.* This method can be further divided into dough moulded or injection moulded processes, where the acrylic powder is softened by heating and forced into the mould under pressure.
- *Built up in layers.* This method provides the best aesthetics as it more closely copies natural teeth.

Occlusal vertical height: distance between two fixed points which determines the vertical height of the lower one-third of the face. This is a physiological point at which with the musculature at rest there is normally 2 mm between the incisal tips of the upper and lower incisors.

Choice of teeth

There are specific clinical indications that determine the choice of denture teeth. Ceramic teeth were very popular but have now been replaced by acrylic teeth as the first choice. Ceramic teeth are durable but noisy as they make a clicking noise during the mastication. Furthermore, they are unsuitable for use in cases where there is reduced ridge support or little interocclusal clearance. This is because they have been shown to transmit more force to the ridge. These teeth also have to have sufficient bulk or they can fracture as they are brittle.

Many clinicians will base their choice of denture teeth on cost which is driven by the expectation and preferences of the patient. The better quality, more highly cross-linked, layered and aesthetic teeth are more expensive. Not only do they look better but as their wear resistance is better their life expectancy is also greater. The more cost-effective teeth, while perfectly functional, will tend to wear more quickly and are not as aesthetic (Figure 23.18).

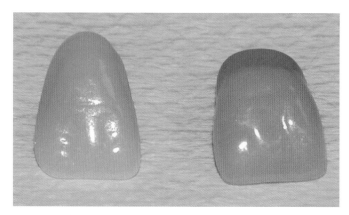

Fig. 23.18 A basic denture tooth (left) and a top-of-range one (right). Note the improved aesthetics of the tooth on the right; it is composed of layers of acrylic to copy the natural situation.

Bonding the denture teeth to the denture base

It is obvious that the denture teeth need to bond effectively to the denture base for the denture to function. Failure to achieve adequate bonding will lead to stress concentrations and debonding of the tooth from the denture base. In fact, this is a common reason for denture repair. A chemical union is desirable but can be difficult to achieve. The highly cross-linked resins of which the tooth is formed have a decreased ability to bond. Uncross-linked or lightly cross-linked resins bond best and commonly teeth are constructed with a base layer formed of less cross-linked resin. Additionally, the resin at the base of teeth may be softened with monomer to enhance chemical adhesion; micromechanical retention of the base can also be achieved by roughening.

Both the chemicals used to construct the denture teeth and denture base need to be chemically compatible. Heat curing achieves a better union between a tooth and the denture base than the cold-curing method. Some highly cross-linked acrylic teeth are treated with 4 META (4-methacryloxyethyl trimellitic anhydride) to enhance the bond strength.

As well as chemical compatibility, it is important that the properties of the denture teeth (modulus of elasticity and coefficient of thermal expansion) are similar to that of the denture base material. This will prevent crazing and cracking around the base of the teeth and potentially loss of the teeth.

Commercially available products

See Table 23.5. Modern resin teeth are often made of a cocktail of resins including a range of dimethacrylates such as bis-GMA and urethane dimethacrylates. These improve the wear characteristics and also the cross-linking.

Table 23.5 Some acrylic denture teeth currently available on the market

Product	Manufacturer	Anterior/posterior	Comments
Acrotone	Wrights	Both	A more cost-effective tooth
Basic 6	Heraeus	Anterior	
Basic 8	Heraeus	Posterior	
Cosmo HXL	Dentsply		
Delphic	Schottlander	Both	A more cost-effective tooth
Dentacryl HXL	Dentsply		
Duratomic	Myerson	Posterior	
Enigma	Schottlander	Both	
Gnathostar	Ivoclar Vivadent	Posterior	Mid-range tooth
Monarch	Wrights	Both	
Natura	Schottlander	Both	Mid-range tooth
Optognath	Heraeus	Posterior	
Optostar	Heraeus	Anterior	
Premium 6	Heraeus	Anterior	
Premium 8	Heraeus	Posterior	
Senator	Wrights	Both	Mid-range tooth
Special	Myerson	Both	
SR Antaris	Ivoclar Vivadent	Anterior	
SR Ivostar	Ivoclar Vivadent	Anterior	Mid-range tooth
SR Ortholingual DCL	Ivoclar Vivadent	Posterior	Lingualized
SR Orthoplane DCL	Ivoclar Vivadent	Posterior	Simple occlusal anatomy
SR Orthosit PE	Ivoclar Vivadent	Posterior	Semi-anatomical
SR Orthotyp DCL	Ivoclar Vivadent	Posterior	Semi-anatomical
SR Postaris	Ivoclar Vivadent	Posterior	
SR Postaris DCL	Ivoclar Vivadent	Posterior	Double cross-linked, increased wear resistance, especially for partial dentures
SR Vivodent DCL	Ivoclar Vivadent	Anterior	Double cross-linked, increased wear resistance, especially for partial dentures
SR Vivodent PE	Ivoclar Vivadent	Anterior	Pearl effect, especially used for complete dentures
Vitapan	Vita	Both	

Ceramic denture teeth

Denture teeth made of ceramic have been available for many years. The aesthetics of these teeth are excellent as is their wear resistance. However, they have a number of disadvantages:

- The primary form of retention to the denture base is mechanical, and ceramic teeth have a retention hole cut into their undersurface into which the PMMA is forced. This is termed a **diatoric hole**. The absence of a chemical bond between the teeth and the denture base resin may cause the teeth to become detached during the lifetime of the denture. Attempts to provide some chemical union rely on silane coating of the ceramic teeth (see Chapter 7) but silane bonding is relatively unreliable.
- They are very hard and so cannot easily be adjusted. If adjustments are made, the surface glaze is removed. This may only partly be recovered by polishing.
- They make a different noise to natural teeth when they contact each other during function. This chattering, clicking sound is more unnatural.
- They are brittle and so are more likely to chip and fracture.

Although ceramic teeth are still used, they have been largely superseded by acrylic teeth whose appearance, mechanical properties and versatility are much better.

SOFT LINING MATERIALS

Unfortunately some patients find wearing dentures uncomfortable. This may be due to anatomical problems or excessive forces being transmitted to the underlying tissues. The use of a material whose glass transition temperature is in the region of the temperature of the oral cavity will absorb some of the energy of mastication and decrease impact forces on the denture-bearing tissues compared with a hard material. These materials are referred to as **soft lining materials**. They flow under static load but are elastic under the intermittent loads produced during mastication. Soft lining materials are of two types:

- Plasticized acrylic resins
- Silicones.

Plasticized acrylic resins

One of the common soft lining materials are the plasticized acrylic resins. These can be both heat and chemically cured. The polymer in these cases is either methyl or ethyl methacrylate. They are presented as a powder and a liquid. The primary difference between a conventional PMMA and these materials is that the liquid contains a large amount of plasticizer. This plasticizer limits the degree of tangling of the polymer chains. The soft liner can change shape quickly as there is little cross-linking of the polymer chains.

As might be expected, the heat-cured varieties are more durable. There are some problems with this type of material:

- The tendency for the plasticizer to slowly leach out means that over time the lining becomes harder
- There is also the potential for tissue reaction to the soft liner.
- In general these soft liners have a finite life (see below).

Higher acrylic esters such as **octyl methacrylate** are used as plasticizers. The resulting material is a copolymer. Other compounds such as oily organic esters without reactive groups (such as **dibutyl phthalate**), rubbers and inorganic fillers which do not polymerize may also be added. If present in sufficient amounts the polymer becomes rubbery as the oils plasticize (soften) the polymer. The use of dibutyl phthalates is now regarded as unsatisfactory and citrates are now being considered as alternatives. These materials should therefore be regarded as semi-permanent and have a lifespan of about 6 months.

One of the advantages of using a higher methacrylate such as butyl methacrylate is that the glass transitional temperature decreases to below oral temperature. This means that the material is softer and little or no plasticizer is required. These soft liners are unlikely to support fungal growth and may be polished.

Silicone

One of the more successful soft lining materials is **silicone rubber**. The nature of the material means that there is no need for the addition of plasticizing agents and the material retains its rubbery consistence for long periods of time. The disadvantages are:

- They generally do not bond to the denture base and require some form of adhesive to achieve success. This means that they are likely to debond with time.
- The material is also unsuitable for polishing and has to be left in the finished state. Thus, they are prone to bacterial contamination and growth of *Candida albicans*.
- They occupy space and as their thickness increases, the thickness of the denture itself is reduced. This will affect the strength of the denture base.
- Due to the material being soft, finishing by polishing is difficult. Certain products are available, such as GC Reline Modifier, which remove surface roughness and manufacturing defects when added.

> ***Candida albicans:*** a white fungus that grows both as yeast and filamentous cells that cause oral infections in humans particularly on the palate under dentures.

The silicones can be either chemically or heat activated, the chemically cured material being provided as two components and setting by a condensation reaction similar to a condensation silicone impression material. The delivery of this is simple. The denture is relieved to permit sufficient soft liner to be placed. Adhesive is applied to the denture surface and the silicone is placed using a compression moulding technique. The heat-cured varieties are one-component pastes, which are again applied using compression moulding techniques.

Silicone relining materials are indicated for patients who present with pain under their denture. This is due to the thin mucosa being 'nipped' between the underlying bone and the hard denture base material. Chronic soreness may also be due to bruxism and the elastic properties of the material decreases the trauma on the denture-bearing tissues. Two grades of softness are available to the dentist and the one selected will depend on the diagnosis.

Soft liners

The soft liners are used over sharp (knife edge) bony alveolar ridges, sensitive mucosa or pressure points where localized high pressure may be uncomfortable for the denture wearer. They provide a cushion between the denture and the denture-bearing tissues to decrease masticatory pressure.

They may be used after oral surgery where a denture is required to be worn, especially after dental implants have been placed, as an aid to wound healing. The flow properties of the soft liners offer the possibility that as the tissues heal, the liner will flow and follows the contours of the tissues.

They are useful where severe undercuts are present as their resilience allows them to enter these regions. Equally they may be able to utilize undercuts to increase retention and for this reason are often used as the material of choice for the fitting surfaces of obturators and other devices such as facial prostheses to restore congenital or acquired defects.

Soft liners tend to be used in the medium term, ranging from weeks through months to years.

> **Obturator:** a prosthetic device used to restore congenital or acquired defects of the hard palate and nasal cavity. The device forms a physical barrier between the mouth and nose, allowing the patient to eat and swallow normally without displacement of food into the nasal cavity.

Extra soft liners

These products are used for patients who have severe ridge resorption or whose dentures are causing pressure points. These products will allow the inflamed tissues to resolve before a new denture is made or a relining or rebasing procedure is done. They are usually used for only for a few days or weeks.

In general, the use of soft liners is contraindicated in patients who produce little saliva. Without the saliva lubricating the interface between the denture and the mucosa, the mucosa may be traumatized, particularly where silicone materials have been used.

>
> Usage of soft liners is not a panacea. It is not a good idea for patients to get used to soft-lined dentures in the long term as the chewing ability is reduced.

Care and cleaning

Cleaning can be a problem with soft lining materials, as due to their softness food can get embedded into the rough surface. Removing this food and plaque is difficult as cleaning can damage the surface due to the poor abrasion resistance and low hardness of the material. Cleaning should therefore be done with care. Bleaching products and high temperatures should be avoided, otherwise the material may become white and hard.

Commercially available products

Some of the currently available soft liners are shown in Table 23.6.

TISSUE CONDITIONERS

Tissues conditioners are soft elastomers that are applied to the fitting surface of the denture to allow more even distribution of load as a temporary measure. This may be to promote healing of inflamed tissues by cushioning the forces of mastication or allowing healing after a period of wearing an ill-fitting denture or following oral surgery.

They are materials contain **polyethylmethacrylate**, **ethyl alcohol** and an aromatic ester such as **butyl phthalylbutylglycolate**. Both the alcohol and ester are plasticizers which soften the polymer. When mixed, the material is gel like in nature with its consistency and viscoelasticity being dependent on the powder:liquid ratio, the relative amounts of the constituents and the molecular weight of the powder.

> **Viscoelastic behaviour:** a viscoelastic material is one which behaves both as an elastic solid and a viscous liquid. Under prolonged load the properties of a viscous fluid come into play and this leads to slow displacement. Rapid movement has less effect and the material acts as an elastic solid.

No chemical reaction occurs and the process is purely a partial solution of the polymer. The liquid solvent readily permeates the polymer allowing the plasticizer to rapidly enter it. The small beads of powder dissolve while the larger ones swell as the solvent is taken up by them. The product of this process is a very soft material, which is a gel.

Unfortunately the alcohol and the plasticizer both leach out very quickly. Thus the material becomes stiffer and material requires replacing every few days. This process can continue for a few weeks but requires monitoring.

Table 23.6 Some soft lining materials currently available on the market

Product	Manufacturer	Type of material	Notes
Coe Soft Self-Cure	GC		Chairside tissue conditioner with no chemical reaction using a solvent base
Elite Relining	Zhermack	Silicone	Chairside or laboratory reline
Eversoft	Dentsply	Plasticized methacrylate	Laboratory reline
GC Reline Extra Soft	GC	Silicone	Chairside reline
GC Reline Soft	GC	Silicone	Chairside reline
Luci-Sof	Dentsply	Silicone	Laboratory reline
Molloplast B	Myerson	Silicone, heat cure	Laboratory reline
Ufi Gel SC Soft	Voco	Silicone	Chairside or laboratory reline

Properties

The material is soft and elastic in nature and able to undergo plastic flow for 24–36 hours after placement in order to decrease trauma to the tissues and record the shape of the denture-bearing tissues.

Biocompatibility

These materials are biocompatible. They are non-irritant as they contain no acrylic monomer. Some products may inhibit the colonization of oral microorganisms while others allow microorganisms to colonize the surface of the material readily. However, in practice this should not pose too much of a problem as the material is not used for very long (a few days) before being replaced.

Care and cleaning regimen

Although cleaning the material with sodium hypochlorite solution is effective, unfortunately, it is damaged by the chemical. Patients should therefore be advised to clean the product with soap and water only.

FUNCTIONAL IMPRESSION MATERIALS

In common with tissue conditioners, these viscoelastic materials are applied to the fitting surface of the denture with the intention of recording the denture-bearing tissues under functional stresses.

The material is mixed at the chairside and applied to the fitting surface of the denture when the material has reached the correct consistency. The denture is inserted into the mouth and the prescribed time must elapse before the material reaches a sufficiently 'set' stage to allow the patient to be dismissed. The patient is encouraged to wear the denture and use it in normal functions for 24–48 hours. The soft nature of the material will deform plastically to record the denture-bearing tissues, so producing the functional impression. This can then be sent to the dental laboratory to be converted into a hard or soft permanent lining, which is fitted at the next appointment.

Commercially available products

Some of the currently available tissue conditioners and functional impression materials are shown in table 23.7 and fig 23.19.

Table 23.7 Some tissue conditioners and functional impression materials currently available on the market

Product	Manufacturer	Notes
Coe Comfort	GC	
Functional Impression Tissue Toner (F.I.T.T.)	Kerr Hawe	Functional impression material
GC Tissue Conditioner	GC	Also used for soft relining and functional impressions
Visco-gel	Dentsply	Also a temporary soft denture liner

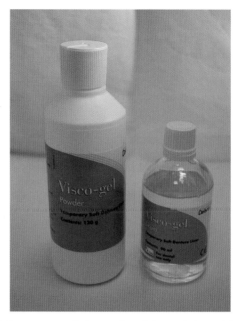

Fig. 23.19 A temporary soft denture liner (Visco-gel, Dentsply).

MOUTHGUARDS

Mouthguards, also referred to as **gum shields**, are worn to protect the oral structures during contact sports activities. They usually cover the teeth and gingivae in the maxillary arch up into the sulcus and work by dissipating forces to a wider area thus reducing their harmful localized impact. They are made in various thicknesses depending on the forces they are likely to meet. For example, sports which involve high velocity objects (hard balls, sticks or boxing gloves) will require a heavier gauge mouthguard than other sports where players will not encounter a hard object or ball. The gauge ranges from **light** to **extra heavy**.

They are made of **polyvinyl acetate-polyethylene**, a copolymer, also called **ethylene vinyl acetate** (**EVA**). Other materials such as **polyurethane**, **rubber latex**, **polyvinyl chloride** and **vinyl plastisol** are also used. These are thermoplastic polymers and are supplied in 14 cm square blanks 1.6–3 mm in thickness.

Properties

Clearly the main property of any material used in the construction of a mouthguard is its ability to absorb impact energy. Equally, however, to ensure that the appliance is worn it must be comfortable, fit well and not have a taste. Polyvinyl acetate-polyethylene fits these criteria and it also has the advantage of being the easiest to fabricate of all the available mouthguard materials. The thicker the material, the more impact energy it can absorb to dissipate the force, so decreasing transmitted force to the teeth and surrounding structures. However, there is a balance to be struck as the mouthguard should be thick enough to absorb an adequate amount of impact while not being too thick, so that the wearer finds the appliance bulky, uncomfortable and difficult to wear. A reasonable minimum thickness is therefore about 4 mm.

Dimensional change

The material will shrink when it is made into the mouthguard. Shrinkage of 30% has been reported with single sheets. To

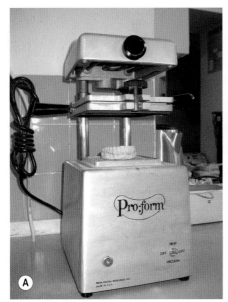 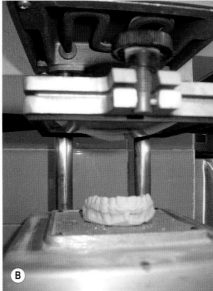 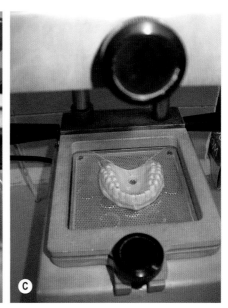

Fig. 23.20A–C The stages in the process of fabrication of a vacuum-formed mouthguard. (A) The machine used to construct blow-down devices. The sheet of vinyl is placed in the tray area and the heating element is switched on. (B) After a few minutes the vinyl heats and sags. (C) At this point the tray is pushed down over the model with the suction motor on. The thermoplastic vinyl is then pulled tightly over the model by the vacuum, so forming the device. The device is then removed from the model, and trimmed and finished.

compensate for this shrinkage many mouthguards are laminated by being constructed from two sheets. To achieve a final thickness of 4 mm, two 3 mm sheet are used. In the same way, some technicians bond a harder material to the softer polyvinyl acetate-polyethylene to increase protection.

After wearing the appliance for some time, the properties of polyvinyl acetate-polyethylene change. The material's flexibility increases and it is more able to absorb impact energy; however, a decrease in tensile strength is seen. Wear will occur during use as a result of biting or chewing the mouthguard. If a harder material is used in the construction of the appliance this phenomenon is less of an issue. Tears can also occur with the softer materials and staining is also common with time.

When compared with polyvinyl acetate-polyethylene, polyurethane is stronger, harder and be able to absorb energy. Unfortunately it absorbs more water and higher processing temperatures are required for its manufacture. Latexes and vinyl plastisols are only slightly less strong, hard and absorb less energy than polyvinyl acetate-polyethylene but are difficult to process. It is very difficult to trim and polish this material well.

Fabrication

Three types of mouthguard are available:

- Custom-made
- Mouth-formed
- Stock.

Custom-made appliances

These are constructed by taking an upper full sulcus impression (usually alginate) and pouring a stone (usually Kaffir D) model. The vinyl blank is then heated and then when it reaches the correct temperature it is blown down by suction over the model on a **vacuum-forming machine**. The dental technician can then trim it up to the desired sulcular extension (Figure 23.20). Soft bite splints are fabricated in the same way, usually from a blank 2 mm in thickness.

This type of mouthguard is regarded as being the best type with respect to its fit, durability, and comfort. The only disadvantage is that it is more expensive, due to the more involved manufacturing process.

 It is advisable to take both upper and lower impression when constructing a mouthguard. This allows the dental technician to indent the lower teeth into the thermoplastic vinyl which will afford them some protection during use.

The blanks come in a range of colours, stripes and patterns. Other patterns may be made in the mouthguard such as flags by using transfers (Figure 23.21).

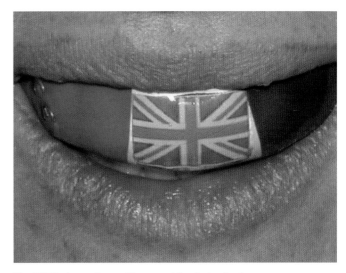

Fig. 23.21 A mouthguard for use while playing hockey.

Some dental technicians incorporate name tags so that the appliance can be more readily identified if lost. Metallic strips are also inserted into the body of the mouthguard to provide radiopacity for the appliance. This will aid identification and localization prior to medical retrieval in case of ingestion or inhalation during use.

The custom-made mouthguard should be rinsed in cold water after use and stored on the model it was constructed on and kept in a hard box to prevent permanent deformation.

Mouth-formed appliances

Other products are available in pharmacies; the user places the blank in very hot water and then inserts it into the mouth to mould it to the desired shape. These are less desirable than the professionally constructed type as they are tolerated less well, are more liable to be dislodged during wear and may lack the appropriate thickness for adequate protection. Their comfort and durability may also be poor, but they are less expensive than custom-made devices.

Stock mouthguards

These are also available over the counter and require no moulding. They are most commonly made of polyvinyl chloride although some are made of polyvinyl acetate-polyethylene or polyurethane. They are the least satisfactory of the three types described; however, a badly fitting mouthguard is still better than no mouthguard at all. Use of any mouthguard decreases the damage to the dentition and surrounding structures, and all contact sports participants should be strongly encouraged to wear one.

DENTAL APPLIANCE CLEANING AND CARE

Good denture hygiene is as important as good oral hygiene. It is important that the dental team gives instructions to patients on the care and cleaning regimen of any removal dental appliance. Good denture hygiene will help to prevent the growth of bacteria and fungi such as *Candida albicans* on the denture.

Any food debris and plaque should be removed by gentle brushing with a soft brush. This should be done under a running cold tap, as the use of hot water may release processing stresses leading to permanent deformation and distortion of the appliance. Ordinary toilet soap should be used to clean the denture. Abrasive dentifrices should not be used as these may scratch the acrylic surface, leading to plaque retention and poorer denture hygiene.

After the denture has been manually brushed, it should be steeped in Milton's solution in a concentration of one teaspoon to a tumbler full of cold water for 30 minutes. There is a potential risk that if the denture is left in the bleach for any longer than this, the pink pigments

may be bleached out of the acrylic used in the construction of the gingivae and denture base. After this time the denture should be removed, rinsed and placed in water until it is to be worn again. This is because the acrylic absorbs water and this maintains the water contact in the material. Failure to do this will cause the acrylic to dry out, causing crazing and permanent damage.

SUMMARY

- Denture base materials are acrylic resin-based materials and are processed either by heat or cold curing.
- The processing in the laboratory is designed to reduce the risk of porosity and produce a highly polished appliance.
- The properties of the resin mean that care must be taken to limit the processing shrinkage.
- The properties of most denture materials mean that they are at risk of fracture if dropped.
- Bonding of denture teeth to the denture requires either mechanical or chemical reaction between the two components. Ceramic teeth will only be retained mechanically.
- Soft liners may be applied to the denture base to improve comfort, but they are a short term option, particularly when they contain plasticizers.

FURTHER READING

McCabe, J.F., Walls, A.W.G., 2008. Applied Dental Materials, ninth ed. Blackwell Munksgaard, Oxford (See Chapters 12–15).

Powers, J.M., Sakaguchi, R.L. (Eds.), 2006. Craig's Restorative Dental Materials, twelfth ed. Mosby Elsevier, St Louis (See Chapter 21).

van Noort, R., 2007. Introduction to Dental Materials, third ed. Mosby Elsevier, Edinburgh (See Chapter 3.2).

SELF-ASSESSMENT QUESTIONS

1. What are the advantages of using heat-cured acrylic resin rather than chemically cured resin in the construction of a denture?
2. What are the disadvantages of using plasticizers in acrylic resin?
3. Methylmethacrylate is a poor thermal conductor. Why can this be a problem if it is used as a denture base material?
4. What precautions should be taken when cleaning a plastic denture?
5. What problems can occur during the curing cycle of a heat-cured methylmethacrylate-based denture?

Index

Note: Page numbers followed by "*f*", "*t*" and "*b*" refers to figures, tables and Boxes respectively.

Index

Index

Index

Index

Index

11-12-14